Routine Radiologic Examination Series

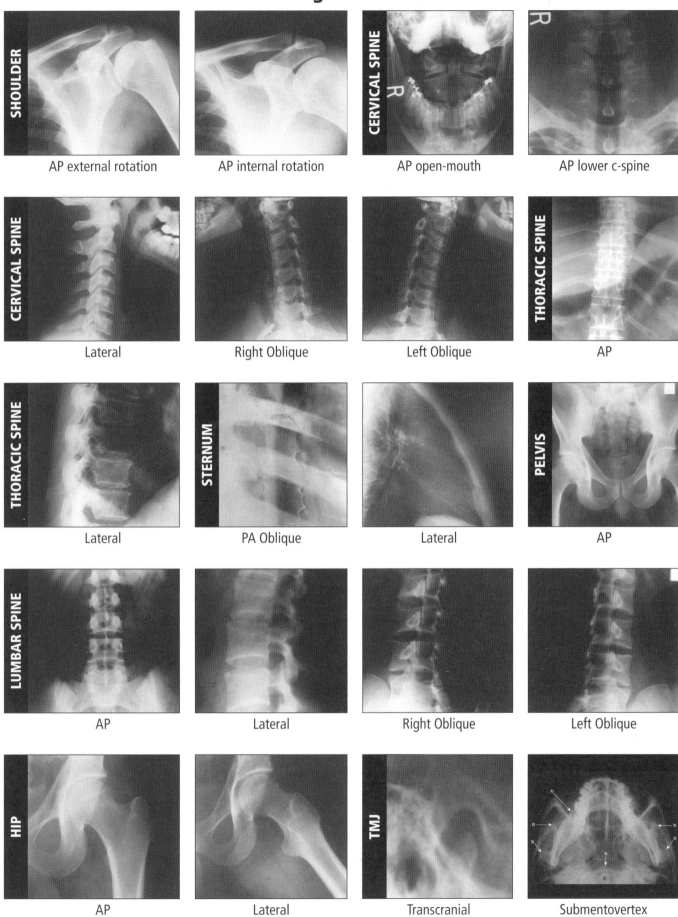

SHOULDER — AP external rotation	AP internal rotation	**CERVICAL SPINE** — AP open-mouth	AP lower c-spine
CERVICAL SPINE — Lateral	Right Oblique	Left Oblique	**THORACIC SPINE** — AP
THORACIC SPINE — Lateral	**STERNUM** — PA Oblique	Lateral	**PELVIS** — AP
LUMBAR SPINE — AP	Lateral	Right Oblique	Left Oblique
HIP — AP	Lateral	**TMJ** — Transcranial	Submentovertex

FUNDAMENTALS OF MUSCULOSKELETAL IMAGING

THIRD EDITION

Contemporary Perspectives in Rehabilitation

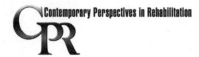

Steven L. Wolf, PT, PhD, FAPTA, Editor-in-Chief

Spinal Cord Injury Rehabilitation (New!)
Edelle Field-Fote, PT, PhD

Vestibular Rehabilitation, 3rd Edition
Susan J. Herdman, PT, PhD, FAPTA

Pharmacology in Rehabilitation, 4th Edition
Charles D. Ciccone, PT, PhD

Modalities for Therapeutic Intervention, 4th Edition
Susan L. Michlovitz, PT, PhD, CHT, and Thomas P. Nolan, Jr., PT, MS, OCS

Wound Healing: Alternatives in Management, 3rd Edition
Luther C. Kloth, PT, MS, CWS, FAPTA, and Joseph M. McCulloch, PT, PhD, CWS, FAPTA

Evaluation and Treatment of the Shoulder: An Integration of the Guide to Physical Therapist Practice
Brian J. Tovin, PT, MMSc, SCS, ATC, FAAOMPT, and Bruce H. Greenfield, PT, MMSc, OCS

Cardiopulmonary Rehabilitation: Basic Theory and Application, 3rd Edition
Frances J. Brannon, PhD, Margaret W. Foley, RN, MN, Julie Ann Starr, PT, MS, CCS, and
Lauren M. Saul, MSN, CCRN

For more information on each title in the *Contemporary Perspectives in Rehabilitation* series, go to
www.fadavis.com.

FUNDAMENTALS OF MUSCULOSKELETAL IMAGING

THIRD EDITION

Lynn N. McKinnis, PT, OCS
Butler, Pennsylvania

Concordia Visiting Nurses
Staff Physical Therapist
Cabot, Pennsylvania

St. Francis University
Adjunct Instructor
Department of Physical Therapy
Loretto, Pennsylvania

University of Montana
Faculty Affiliate
School of Physical Therapy & Rehabilitation Science
Missoula, Montana

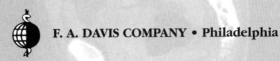

F. A. DAVIS COMPANY • Philadelphia

F. A. Davis Company
1915 Arch Street
Philadelphia, PA 19103
www.fadavis.com

Printed in the United States of America

Last digit indicates print number: 10 9 8 7 6 5 4

Publisher: Margaret Bublis
Acquisitions Editor: Melissa A. Duffield
Manager of Content Development: George W. Lang
Senior Developmental Editor: Jennifer Pine
Art and Design Manager: Carolyn O'Brien

As new scientific information becomes available through basic and clinical research, recommended treatments and drug therapies undergo changes. The author(s) and publisher have done everything possible to make this book accurate, up to date, and in accord with accepted standards at the time of publication. The author(s), editors, and publisher are not responsible for errors or omissions or for consequences from application of the book, and make no warranty, expressed or implied, in regard to the contents of the book. Any practice described in this book should be applied by the reader in accordance with professional standards of care used in regard to the unique circumstances that may apply in each situation. The reader is advised always to check product information (package inserts) for changes and new information regarding dose and contraindications before administering any drug. Caution is especially urged when using new or infrequently ordered drugs.

Library of Congress Cataloging-in-Publication Data

McKinnis, Lynn N., 1959–
    Fundamentals of musculoskeletal imaging / Lynn N. McKinnis. — 3rd ed.
        p. ; cm.
    Includes bibliographical references and index.
    ISBN 978-0-8036-1946-3
1. Musculoskeletal system—Imaging. 2. Musculoskeletal system—Diseases—Diagnosis. 3. Radiography in orthopedics.
I. Title.
    [DNLM: 1. Diagnostic Imaging—methods. 2. Musculoskeletal Diseases—diagnosis. 3. Musculoskeletal System—injuries.
    4. Physical Therapy Modalities.   WE 141 M4785f 2010]
    RC925.7.M356 2005
    616.7'07548—dc22   2009043023

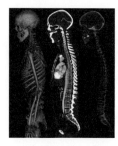

Contrast-enhanced CT study of the body, made possible by volumetric imaging capabilities and advance software applications. On the left is a three-dimensionally reformatted image display, showing the skeleton and organs. In the middle is a two-dimensional, sagittally reformatted image, displayed in a *mediastinal window,* meaning both contrast-enhanced soft tissues and bone are displayed. On the right is a "scout" image used in planning the exam and to establish where the target organs are located. This image appears similar to a radiograph. The data for these images were obtained in one exam in less than 17 seconds. The scanner used was *Aquilion 64,* the first true volumetric 64-slice CT scanner, able to acquire 64 simultaneous slices of 0.5-mm thickness with each 350-millisecond gantry revolution. *(Courtesy of Toshiba Medical Systems, Europe.)*

This book is dedicated with love
to my Mom, who finds joy in her work
to my Dad, who takes pride in his work
to my husband, Dave, who lives his work
and to our children, Jesse and Ann,
for whom I wish all these things.

FOREWORD

In my capacity as an educator, my knowledge of radiographic anatomy has been learned through the evolution of information resources over the 35 years of teaching Human Anatomy to medical and physical therapy students, and reviewing anatomy with residents specializing primarily in physical medicine and rehabilitation. Although I teach throughout the total curriculum in the medical student anatomy course, my primary responsibilities are contained in modules that emphasize the back and limbs. As a clinician and researcher, my primary focus has been on neurorehabilitation, particularly as it pertains to patients with stroke. As such, the "true value" of applying fundamentals of musculoskeletal imaging became somewhat rote and less than optimally relevant. That perspective changed radically 10 months ago.

Although my wife spent the first 6 years of her career as a physical therapist practicing primarily with neurological patients, most of her subsequent career focused on orthopedics. While we often discussed difficult cases, I never truly appreciated the importance of maximizing information until she sustained a total tear of her anterior cruciate ligament. Her efforts to strengthen her knee were well intended and persisted for over 9 months, but the instability she encountered during efforts at lateral and rotational movements led to the inevitable surgery resulting in an allograft taken from a cadaver tibialis anterior tendon. This history brings me full circle to Lynn McKinnis and the third edition of *Fundamentals of Musculoskeletal Imaging*.

When reviewing my wife's rehabilitation plan with physical therapists following her case, I was pleased to learn how much they had depended on the second edition of *Fundamentals* to reinforce their visualization of knee anatomy. While each had undoubtedly been well trained in the best procedures to undertake in her treatment, the reference to this text was highlighted with considerable comfort since they had been exposed to very little formal radiographic anatomy during their training. The ability to see what they were doing was much appreciated. The only "missing" piece was the presentation of data that imaged the torn and subsequently repaired ligament in question with greater detail. In fact, one therapist lamented the fact that there was little taught in the classroom and amplified during clinical rotations about the application of computerized tomography (CT) and magnetic resonance imaging (MRI). Often the "learning" that ensued was driven by dialogue with orthopedic surgeons willing to take time away from busy schedules to orient the therapists to musculoskeletal pathologies rendered remarkably clear through contemporary imaging techniques. Obviously a knowledge gap existed.

This "void," both in their education and in the first two editions of this text, has now been filled. In fact, the third edition of *Fundamentals* mimics McKinnis's own maturation in the presentation of materials. This text has always been intended to educate physical therapy and other health sciences students as well as clinicians to better understand imaging so that more comprehensive patient evaluations could be effected and interprofessional communications enhanced, ultimately benefiting the patients we serve. With the addition of over 100 CT and MRI images of normal and pathological anatomy liberally distributed over all the anatomically specific chapters, the reader is now far better positioned to visualize anatomy. Moreover, information about how these forms of imaging are generated and interpreted has been distributed into separate chapters on Computerized Tomography, Magnetic Resonance Imaging, and Diagnostic Ultrasound (Chapters 4–6) presented with extraordinary clarity by Hilmir Agustsson. All the images in these chapters as well as throughout the text have been labeled with sufficient (but not overwhelming) detail to facilitate understanding. Throughout the text, over 90 previous radiographs have been replaced with digital radiographic images.

An entire chapter of chest (thoracic) radiography has been added to the third edition (Chapter 10). This comprehensive information is invaluable for any clinician since enhanced knowledge about normal and pathological images of the heart and lungs may be relevant to pacing treatment of musculoskeletal pathologies among those patients with concomitant cardiopulmonary problems. Alternatively, the chapter can serve as a "stand alone" for those students or clinicians wishing to visualize anatomy within the context of treatment of patients with respiratory or cardiac diagnoses. Like all other chapters, this addition not only offers typical radiographic images, but also provides nuclear medicine studies, CT angiograms, MR angiograms, and echocardiograms.

The third edition of *Fundamentals* includes updated American College of Radiology Appropriateness Criteria for 160 musculoskeletal conditions, provided in detail with the accompanying CD-ROM. This information is intended to foster a better understanding of the relevance of a specific image to the conditions being studied and treated, and better positions therapists to make recommendations to physicians about alternative images that might either clarify a pathological concern or dictate a decision on optimization of a treatment plan.

Last, McKinnis and contributors have done a remarkable job of not only updating references for each chapter but often they have clustered these references to the subject matter categories. The self-test quizzes remain a stalwart of this book as to the summary points at the end of each chapter. But perhaps the most relevant feature may not be the content itself but what the process in composing this book represents to present and future clinicians. A very genuine and comprehensive effort has been set forth to marry an information base with justification of treatment decisions. This information is derived from past and emerging technologies, which all clinicians must embrace to be contemporary while optimizing communication and decision making with referral sources. This bridge between technology, represented here through new forms of imaging that enhance resolution of normal and pathological musculoskeletal states, and treatment is becoming commonplace throughout the medicine–rehabilitation interface and has become the cornerstone for successful communication. Witness such linkages in brain-computer interfaces or robotics, for example, *Fundamentals*, is a showcase representation of this interface. The evolution of this book over three editions spanning 13 years captures Lynn McKinnis's journey to becoming a better clinician while absorbing the impact of the rapidly changing world of radiographic imaging. I think we can all improve our commitment to our patients by joining her.

Steven L. Wolf, PhD, PT, FAPTA, FAHA
Series Editor, Contemporary Perspectives in Rehabilitation

PREFACE

To the Reader, a Non-Radiologist

In 1997, the first edition of this book posed the question: *What is to be gained in patient care if rehabilitation clinicians have an understanding of radiology?* In 2005, the second edition drew on the experiences of educators, students, and clinicians to provide concrete examples of the answer: *The correlation of imaging findings to clinical findings can result in more comprehensive patient evaluations, more specific treatment plans, and better patient outcomes.*

In 2010, the third edition of this book remains rooted in the fundamentals of imaging while acknowledging that today it is almost as commonplace for a patient to bring their MRIs to the physical therapist (on disc!) as it was for them to bring their x-rays to them (on film!) 10 years ago. The goal of this third edition is to continue to be an excellent primer—the place to gain an overview of musculoskeletal imaging and a foundation to build clinical work upon. Its *tangent* goal is to recognize that advanced imaging must now be fully incorporated into the fundamentals. This is not discordant at all. In fact, the juxtaposition of radiographs to MRIs and CTs wonderfully illustrates the point that two-dimensional radiographs are not only the starting point in the diagnostic investigation but also serve as road maps for understanding multiplanar advanced images.

This edition preserves the vision of the original edition: *to provide an organized introduction to the fundamentals of musculoskeletal imaging.* This includes presenting (1) an awareness of the capabilities and limitations of the different imaging modalities, (2) an understanding of the information given on the radiologist's report, and (3) the ability to view images independently. Viewing the image independently is a critical skill, especially if the rehabilitation clinician is seeking information not provided on the radiologist's report, which is written from and to a medical physician's perspective. The information the rehabilitation clinician seeks can be of a different nature.

Changes in the third edition begin with the addition of three new chapters by Hilmir Agustsson. The greater emphasis on advanced imaging required an expansion of one prior chapter into three separate new chapters: Chapter 4, *Computed Tomography*; Chapter 5, *Magnetic Resonance Imaging*; and Chapter 6, *Diagnostic Ultrasound*. Each chapter provides a concise explanation of the technology, how to view the images, and the clinical applications of each. Of note in Chapter 4 is the addition of 16 brain scans. Although neurological imaging is outside the scope of this text, an overview of normal brain tissue in common scanning planes and examples of pathologies serves to provide the reader with a foundation for looking at other neurological texts.

A most surprising new chapter is Chapter 10, *The Chest Radiograph and Cardiopulmonary Imaging*. This addition evolved from educators who requested information on cardiopulmonary imaging—certainly outside the scope of a musculoskeletal text! Yet, the biggest surprise to this author was how well it worked out. First, it is important to recognize that the chest radiograph is the most commonly made radiograph on any given day in any country in the world. It is undeniably a standard tool of basic health care. In that respect, it is easily covered with the other radiologic fundamentals of this book, especially following the related anatomy of Chapter 9, *Radiologic Evaluation of the Thoracic Spine, Sternum, and Ribs*. In another respect, the results of the chest radiograph will determine what *treatment* we can do safely with our patients—whether it is of a musculoskeletal or cardiopulmonary nature. The final consensus is that it is very fitting for physical therapy students and clinicians to understand the fundamentals of the chest radiograph.

The enclosed CD-ROM is most valuable for providing two excellent teaching devices:

- *Interactive CD-ROM exercises* designed to teach the reader to identify *normal anatomy* on every radiograph in the routine radiographic examination of each body region. Exercises in the interpretation of images and identification of *pathology* is also presented.
- The entire current *American College of Radiology (ACR) Musculoskeletal Appropriateness Criteria* for 160 musculoskeletal conditions. These criteria have been developed to guide clinicians in choosing the best diagnostic imaging test for defining a specific musculoskeletal condition. The imaging modalities are ranked, according to the literature, for their efficacy in defining a proposed diagnosis with respect to specificity, time, cost, radiation risk, and invasiveness. Not every physician can be aware of what imaging modality is best in every situation. And because physical therapists are often in a position to make imaging recommendations, they must be aware of and have ready access to this resource!

The Davis*Plus* website (http://davisplus.fadavis.com) now provides student support with an easily accessible active search glossary, additional Focus On articles, and instructor accessible *case studies* that demonstrate the integration of imaging information to physical therapy intervention.

For the reader who has never viewed medical images before, this text still strives to be a primer and teach imaging in logical steps. It hopefully reads like learning to swim in the shallow end of the pool instead of being thrown into the deep end! So, it is desirable to wade through these chapters in the order intended. Read the first three chapters to gain a foundation in radiologic science, search patterns, and common pathological and fracture characteristics on radiograph.

Read the next three chapters to understand advanced imaging modalities. After that, you can paddle around the next 11 anatomy chapters at your leisure.

Each anatomy chapter has a similar organization. The *complete routine radiologic evaluation series* is the heart of each chapter. Radiologic observations are taught for each projection with illustrations to point out anatomic relationships. The tracings of the radiographs are most valuable for teaching the reader to "see" radiographic anatomy. Ideally, the reader will make their own tracings of the radiograph with a transparency sheet and marker, and then compare their results to the printed tracing. Drawing is an invaluable intellectual exercise for teaching anatomy and will enhance the reader's perception of radiographic anatomy in a dimension not afforded by point-and-click exercises. And new to this edition, advanced imaging also accompanies the routine radiographs. The remainder of each chapter discusses and provides imaging examples for trauma and pathologies commonly seen at that body region. Self-tests using unknown radiographs are presented at the end of every chapter to challenge the reader's visual interpretation skills.

It is the wish of this author that the reader finds satisfaction in gaining a new vision with which to see anatomy and the potential to develop the skill of correlating imaging findings with clinical findings. It is hoped that this skill will become a valuable tool that contributes to the rehabilitation of patients and furthers individual professional growth.

Lynn N. McKinnis, PT, OCS
119 Kemar Drive
Butler, Pennsylvania 16002

CONTRIBUTORS

Hilmir Agustsson, MHSc, PT, MTC, CFC
Professor
School of Health Related Professions
University of St. Augustine
St. Augustine, FL

J. Bradley Barr, PT, DPT, OCS
Professor
Physical Therapy Department
Creighton University
Omaha, NE

Ellen J. Pong, DPT, MOT, OTR/L
Physical and Occupational Therapist
Sacred Heart Health System
Pace Rehabilitation
Pace, FL

Adjunct Instructor
University of St. Augustine for Health Sciences
St. Augustine, FL

Corlia van Rooyen, MPT, RHT
Rototuna Physiotherapy
Hamilton, New Zealand

REVIEWERS

Lawrence P. Cahalin, PT, MA, PhD
Clinical Professor
Northeastern University
Department of Physical Therapy
Boston, MA

Nancy Ciesla, PT, DPT, MS
Physical Therapy Clinical Specialist
Johns Hopkins Hospital
Baltimore, MD

Francis Golier, MD
Tarrytown Cardiology
Tarrytown, NY

Steven H. Tepper, PT, PhD
President, Rehab Essentials, Inc.
Coordinator, tDPT Program
University of Montana
Missoula, MT

ACKNOWLEDGMENTS

This third edition is enhanced by new images that were discovered and made accessible via the digital wonders of the world wide web and e-mail. Many individuals took the time to send images, patiently answer questions, and share teaching files of archived cases. I am especially grateful to the generosity of Nick Oldnall at http://www.xray2000.co.uk; John C. Hunter, MD, at the University of California, Davis School of Medicine; Laughlin Dawes, MD, of Perth, Australia, and his images at http://www.radpod.org; and Morten Weibye at http://www.medcyclo.com by GE Healthcare.

This third edition stands on the shoulders of the earlier editions and is indebted to the kindness of many exceptional professionals. For providing the core radiographs that made this book possible and for generously sharing their time, knowledge, and materials during the development of the first edition, much appreciation is extended to the following radiologists and hospital radiology staffs: Arthur Nussbaum, MD, and Peter Fedyshin, MD, at the University of Pittsburgh Medical Center (UPMC) Passavant; Jeffrey Towers, MD, at UPMC Montefiore; Lance Cohen, MD, formerly of Children's Hospital in Pittsburgh; Margie Brindl, retired Administrator of Undergraduate Medical Education in Radiology at the University of Pittsburgh; Linda Barto, RTR, formerly of Butler Memorial Hospital, Butler, PA; Sarah Hample, RTR, private practice; and to my first boss and lasting mentor, Charles W. Etter, PT, who teaches by example what it is to be your best.

Grateful appreciation is extended to my colleague Hilmir Agustsson, MHSc, DPT, MTC, CFC, for sharing his ideas, enthusiasm, and labor of love for teaching imaging. Research assistant Ellen J. Pong, DPT, MOT, always produced more than expected and became invaluable for her glossary compilations as well as her friendship and moral support. Special thanks to J. B. Barr, PT, DPT, OCS, for providing new insights to the integration of imaging in daily practice, and to his students in Creighton University's Transitional DPT program, 2000–2004, whose course work generated case studies. Many thanks to Corlia van Rooyen, MPT, RHT, who advanced the clinical aspect of the hand and wrist information. And a sincere thank you to Michael Mulligan, MD, for being a ready source of radiologic expertise, sage counsel, and friendly advice.

Thank you to the dedicated staff at F. A. Davis, and especially to Margaret Biblis, Publisher, Jennifer Pine, Developmental Editor, and Melissa Duffield, Acquisitions Editor, for their devotion, expertise, diplomacy, and sense of humor during the long journey of three editions. They were the best of traveling companions.

Heartfelt thanks to my family. To my parents, Francis and Berniece Nowicki, for a lifetime of love and support in all endeavors, and for pointing me toward physical therapy in the beginning. And to Jesse and Ann, for their happy spirits, love, patience, and unflagging belief that Mom's book is pretty neat. New to this edition is the contribution of Jesse's pencil drawings that appear on each chapter's title page. These drawings depict people engaged in everyday activities and exude a warmth that reminds us that imaging begins and ends with the patient.

And thanks to my best friend and husband, David Lindsey McKinnis, MEd, PT, who taught me how to teach, how to write, and how to achieve. His most tangible contribution to the book was drawing the original line art. These drawings simplified difficult material and greatly enhanced the practical use of the text. His most intangible contribution was in giving me the belief in myself that I could write it.

CONTENTS IN BRIEF

TABLE OF CONTENTS

Chapter 6   **Diagnostic Ultrasound ... 147**
Hilmir Agustsson, MHSc, DPT, MTC, CFC

Chapter 7   **Radiologic Evaluation of
the Cervical Spine ... 159**

GENERAL PRINCIPLES OF MUSCULOSKELETAL IMAGING

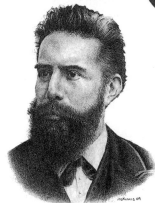

RÖNTGEN

Why Study Imaging?

Traditionally the field of imaging has been the domain of the physician. Rehabilitation clinicians have generally excluded themselves from interaction with imaging. This self-built professional boundary evolved from a misconception that information gained from viewing images was pertinent only to the medical diagnosis and therefore pertinent only to the physician. Studying the patient's diagnostic images was rarely considered, and simply reading the radiologist's "x-ray report" was accepted as sufficient. It was a long-held erroneous belief of clinicians that, even if images contained a

wealth of information to enhance patient treatment, clinicians were incapable of finding it on their own.

Traditions change. Rehabilitation clinicians have discovered that their knowledge of functional anatomy is an excellent foundation for visually comprehending diagnostic images as well as correlating clinical findings with imaging findings. The inclusion of diagnostic imaging courses in educational and professional settings is giving clinicians the confidence to dialogue with radiologists, gain relevant information from the radiologist's report, and most significantly, *view diagnostic images with their own eyes.*

Traditions change slowly. Although it is accepted as logical that rehabilitation clinicians need to be aware of the patient's medical diagnosis, it is considered novel by some that these clinicians view diagnostic images themselves. For others the idea is more than novel—it can appear threatening if it is mistakenly perceived by physicians as a move toward diagnosis or second-guessing the diagnosis or if it is mistakenly perceived by clinicians as either an opportunity or a responsibility to do just that. *Professional collaboration to enhance the quality of patient care is the single most important goal.*

Traditions change for good reasons. Why do clinicians need to view diagnostic images?

1. *A more comprehensive evaluation is obtained.* The success of rehabilitation depends on the effectiveness of the clinician's evaluation. The more thorough the evaluation, the more substance the clinician has on which to build the rehabilitation program. Many of the clinician's evaluation tools—observation, palpation, goniometry, manual muscle testing, ligamentous stress testing, joint-end feels, joint mobility testing—are dependent on the clinician's own perceptive skills and have an inherent degree of subjectivity and limitation. Imaging can provide an objective, visual aspect to the evaluation that makes the expertise of the clinician more comprehensive. Supplementing the initial evaluation and re-evaluations with musculoskeletal images increases the clinician's awareness of the patient in an added dimension. The clinician's knowledge of functional anatomy becomes more dynamically effective by allowing direct visualization of the processes of growth, development, healing, disease, and dysfunction.

2. *The information the clinician seeks is often of a different nature than the information the physician seeks and of a different nature than may be described in the radiologist's report.* For example, a physician needs to know whether a fracture of the distal radius that has united with a malunion deformity is clinically stable; if so, the cast can be removed and the patient can be sent for rehabilitation. The rehabilitation clinician, however, also needs to know the severity and configuration of the malunion deformity. By viewing the patient's radiographs, the clinician becomes aware of how the adjacent joints of the hand, wrist, forearm, and elbow have the potential to be affected by the deformity. The clinician's treatment goals may thus be modified from obtaining full premorbid range of motion to obtaining a lesser degree of motion, adequate for function but minimizing the abnormal joint arthrokinematics that may accelerate degenerative changes in the joints.

These are the starting points for the relatively new idea of a frequent intersection between the fields of rehabilitation and imaging. The future holds potential for other synergies that can advance the scopes of both fields. For example, the goal of accurately correlating and quantifying palpable joint motion findings with radiologic evidence would require the collaborative expertise of both orthopedic physical therapists and musculoskeletal radiologists. *Collaborations require an understanding of what each party has to offer.* The goal of this text is to provide an understanding of imaging fundamentals so that the content, possibilities, and limitations of diagnostic images can be appreciated.

What Is Radiology?

Radiology is the branch of medicine concerned with radiant energy and radioactive substances including x-rays, radioactive isotopes, ionizing radiation, and the application of this information to prevention, diagnosis, and treatment of disease.[1] Physicians specializing in radiology are called *radiologists*. Professional technicians that produce the images are *radiographers*.

Many subspecialties exist within radiology. Although most imaging studies are produced by ionizing radiation, *nonionizing* studies, such as diagnostic ultrasound and magnetic resonance imaging (MRI), are used extensively. Additionally, the ability to image areas of the body that had previously been inaccessible to nonsurgical evaluation has made *interventional* and biopsy procedures possible using diagnostic imaging for guidance. Virtually all systems of the body can be evaluated by the tools of radiology. This expanded scope of practice has required new titles to encompass the growth of the field, and descriptors such as *diagnostic imaging* or *medical imaging* are common and used interchangeably at times with *radiology.*

What Is Musculoskeletal Imaging?

Musculoskeletal imaging is the subspecialty of radiology concerned with the diagnostic evaluation of the musculoskeletal system. Musculoskeletal imaging is the latest term for what was previously called *musculoskeletal radiology* and *orthopedic radiology*. These changes in terminology reflect advancements in technology, the variety of imaging modalities available, and the ability to image not only bone but all tissues of the musculoskeletal system.

The fundamental tool of the musculoskeletal radiologist is *conventional radiography*. Although many advanced imaging modalities are now commonly used in musculoskeletal imaging, conventional radiography remains the most effective means of demonstrating a bone or joint abnormality.[2] Conventional radiography screens for a significant portion of pathologies, with little risk to the patient and with extreme time- and cost-effectiveness. Thus, *conventional radiography is the first-order diagnostic study, or the first imaging procedure to be done following the clinical examination.* Conventional radiographs were a staple of medical management in the 20th century and are continuing that role into the 21st century.

Historical Perspective[3–16]

The discovery of x-rays by Wilhelm Conrad Röntgen in 1895 and the subsequent discovery of radioactive elements by Marie Curie in 1898 mark the beginning of the transition from classical physics to quantum theory. These events can be seen as the foundation for the following century's advancements in radiology and other fields of science.

Turn-of-the-Century Sensationalism

In the year following his discovery, Röntgen, a meticulous researcher, explored almost every possible application of x-rays to medicine. The sensationalism of x-rays also had immediate effects outside the world of medicine. X-rays aided in the detection of art forgeries, jewel smuggling, and counterfeited rare stamps and also assisted in forensics and archaeology. Popular interest was pandemic. Turn-of-the-century lingerie advertisements promised "x-ray proof" underwear to protect feminine modesty from the gaze of lecherous scientists. A politician, capitalizing on the public's irrational fears, submitted a bill to ban x-rays in opera glasses. X-rays also provided entertainment value to a curious public. Photographers hawked "x-ray portraits" to their customers (Fig. 1-1). Fluoroscopes were popular attractions at carnivals. Shoe store patrons could view their foot bones inside new shoes. Comic book superheroes were given "x-ray vision."

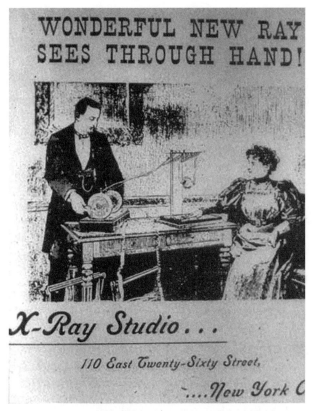

Figure 1-1 Historical newspaper ad illustrating the public's fascination with the possibilities presented by the "new rays." X-ray studios, like this one in New York, opened in cities and towns across the country to take "bone portraits" of subjects who often had no physical complaints.

The 1910s and 1920s

Military use of x-rays began the year after their discovery. Later, during World War I, thousands of recruits in Europe and America were screened for tuberculosis via chest films. In war conditions the effectiveness of clinical radiology was well established. Hand-held fluoroscopic equipment allowed immediate visualization of the location of bullets, extent of fractures, and need for emergency surgery. Marie Curie, with her 17-year-old daughter Irène, established over 200 radiologic posts throughout France and Belgium and drove one of her fleet of hand-cranked Renault trucks, which housed portable x-ray units. It is estimated that Curie's outfits made over a million radiographs during the first winter of the war.

Sonar technology was developed at this time to track submarines and locate icebergs. Spin-offs of sonar technology later evolved into *diagnostic ultrasound*.

These decades also saw the development of nuclear physics with the significant contributions of Max Planck's theory of quantized energy, Albert Einstein's theories of relativity and the photoelectric effect, Arthur Compton's theory of the particle nature of light, Ernest Rutherford's identification of the components of radiation, and Neils Bohr's model of the atom.

The 1930s and 1940s

In the 1930s, *nuclear medicine* was pioneered with the development of the cyclotron by Ernest Lawence. The cyclotron, a form of particle accelerator, became the leading instrument for studying nuclear physics and was the primary source for the creation of radioactive substances used in medical imaging and the treatment of cancer. Radioactive iodine treatments were first used to stop the spread of thyroid cancer in patients.

Irène Joliot-Curie, with her husband Frédéric, won the Nobel Prize in chemistry in 1935 for their synthesis of artificial radioactivity. Enrico Fermi expanded on this work, demonstrating that single neutrons were more effective than alpha particles at creating radioactivity. His research eventually led to the achievement of fission—the splitting of atoms.

In the fields of diagnostic radiology, radiation therapy, and research, little consideration was given to the adverse affects of radiation exposure. Radiation burns, leading to cancerous lesions and aplastic anemia, shortened the life spans of many workers, physicians, and researchers. The average age of death of a radiologist in the 1930s was 56. Marie Curie died in 1934, at age 67, from radiation-induced leukemia. Her notebooks are still radioactive today. Irène and Frédéric Joliot-Curie died at the ages of 59 and 58, respectively, in the 1950s, of radiation-induced illnesses.

Sadly, it was the cataclysmic destruction of life by the detonations of atomic bombs in 1945 that initiated a conscious worldwide effort to reduce radiation exposure in medicine. Lead-lined gloves and aprons, however, would not become accepted standards of protection for all workers until a decade later.

The 1950s and 1960s

In the 1950s, radiation protection was advanced by a change in philosophy of governmental regulatory agencies, based on recommendations by scientific advisory groups. The original idea of setting a *maximal permissible dose* of radiation exposure was replaced by *effective dose limits.* This philosophy recognized that no dose exists below which the risk of damage does not exist and, thus, no dose is "permissible." However, the benefit of performing radiographic procedures when needed usually far outweighed the risk of possible biological damage. Thus the principle that an individual's dose should be kept *as low as reasonably achievable (ALARA)* remains the foundation for the recommendation of effective dose limits for occupational, diagnostic, and therapeutic exposure.

These decades saw the early development of most of the advanced imaging modalities in use today. However, clinical application was not possible because of the extreme costs of new technology and the limited capabilities of computers at that time. Indeed, conventional radiography only received its first image intensifier and television viewing system in 1955. The first automatic x-ray film-processing system was marketed by Kodak in 1956.

The 1970s and 1980s

In the 1970s *computed tomography (CT)* merged x-ray technology to the computer. Cross-sectional images were now possible, allowing visualization of anatomy that previously had only been possible to see via surgery. Intel developed the first microprocessor at this time. Both fields were relatively primitive—a single anatomic slice required 4.5 minutes of scanning and 1.5 minutes of computer reconstruction to generate one image. In comparison, today one slice is imaged in less than a second.

The first analog waveform image was converted to a digital image in 1978, creating the new era of *digital radiography.* *Digital subtraction angiography* and other digital enhancements to imaging modalities accelerated the subspecialty of *interventional* and *invasive radiology.* Many pathological conditions, previously treated surgically, could now be treated percutaneously under image guidance, with minimized risk to the patient.

Magnetic resonance imagining (MRI), approved for clinical use in 1984, revolutionized imaging of the central nervous system and musculoskeletal system by providing information on all tissues of the body in multiple planes. A decade later, a variation of this imaging modality, *functional MRI (fMRI),* would demonstrate how the brain works by visualizing changes in the chemical composition of various regions of the brain during thought or movement.

The 1990s to the Present

True digital imaging in conventional radiology became possible in the 1990s with the use of *charge-coupled devices (CCDs).* A CCD, the same device as in any digital point-and-shoot camera, translates light photons into a computer reconstructed image. Over the past 20 years, the conversion of most radiology departments from film-based imaging to digital imaging has heralded not only changes in technology but in the practice of radiologic medicine itself.

The backbone of a modern radiology department is a *Picture Archiving and Communication Systems (PACS).* PACS are computer programs developed to view, file, store, and transmit images. Viewing software can also analyze or reformat data to assist in diagnosis. *Computer-assisted diagnostics,* first put to use in identifying subtle microcalcifications in mammography, utilizes the mathematical analysis of pixels to help identify density or chemical variants in many imaging modality studies. As for this *pattern recognition* of abnormalities, computers have been shown to be competent on *sensitivity*—that is, being able to identify what is not normal. At present, humans are still the best interpreters of *specificity*—that is, being able to identify what a pathology actually is.

Interdisciplinary collaboration between radiologists, surgeons, and engineers has enabled the acceleration of three dimensional *image-guided surgery, computer-assisted surgery,* and *surgical robotics,* which have enhanced or even replaced existing invasive procedures. Also a convergence of diagnostic radiology and radiation therapy has advanced the treatment of many cancers by allowing image-guided delivery of site-specific chemotherapy or radiofrequency ablation of tumors. Another vanguard of the millennium is *molecular imaging,* which combines advances in imaging with cellular biology to improve our understanding of normal and disease processes.

Radiology has been described for over a century as both an art and a science. Traditionally, one has enhanced the other. Neither art nor science could exclude each other. The rapid advancement of technology threatens to give science the upper hand, but such advanced knowledge in the hands of a health professional will always underscore the human role in healing other humans. Science is a tool for humanity, especially in the health professions.

Essential Science[7,8,15]

What Is a Radiograph?

A *radiograph* has been defined for over a century as an x-ray film containing an image of an anatomic part of a patient (Fig. 1-2). Production of a radiograph requires three things: (1) the x-ray beam source, (2) the patient, and (3) the x-ray film or other image receptor. The term *image receptor* encompasses both film and digital technologies.

Over the years many terms have been used for a radiograph. The medical community established the term *roentgenograph* to honor its discoverer, Wilhelm Röntgen. During World War I, however, American radiology societies excluded the "German-sounding" term and substituted *radiograph.* Later advancements in radiography necessitated a designation between the simple radiograph and more complex radiographic studies. The phrases "plain-film radiograph," "standard radiograph," and "conventional radiograph" have all been used to define a simple radiograph—one made without modification to

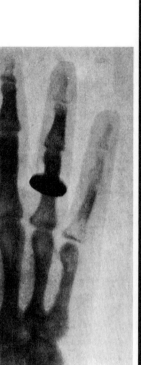
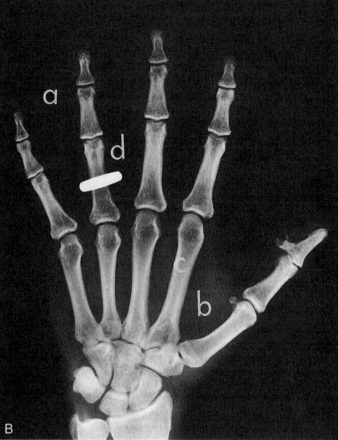

Figure 1-2 (A) This image (produced January 17, 1896, at the Physical State Laboratory in Hamburg, Germany) is similar to what Wilhelm Röntgen first saw of his hand during his historic experiments with a primitive x-ray tube and fluorescing cardboard in his laboratory in 1895. Radiographs of the hand were commonly made in the months following his discovery, as demonstrations at scientific meetings, and to "test" equipment before use. **(B)** Modern radiograph of a hand: *a*, blackened area of the film representing that area where only air is interposed between the beam source and the film; *b*, gray shadow where soft tissues absorb part of the beam before it reaches the film; *c*, mostly white area where calcium salts in bone absorb more x-rays than soft tissues do and the film is exposed only lightly; *d*, solid white area where the dense metal of the wedding ring absorbs all of the x-rays and so no area of the film is exposed underneath it. Note that in contrast to the historic x-ray image in part A, this is a doubly reversed print. This is what the clinician sees when he or she views radiographs on film or when radiographs are printed for publication. *(From Squire and Novelline,[12] pp. 2–3, with permission.)*

the equipment (as in fluoroscopy) or addition of contrast media (as in arthrography).

Today, common verbal usage for a conventional radiograph includes referencing the patient's "plain films," "films," or "x-rays." This casual usage presents some problems. For one, x-rays are invisible to the human eye, so it is not possible to actually "look at x-rays"! Also, film may not be the actual recording medium. Although the use of casual terms may be insignificant in some exchanges, it is significant in communicating with the interdisciplinary team. It is correct to refer to the patient's "conventional radiographs." This language has also become the standard in medical publications.

The advent of computer technology in radiography has added new vernacular to imaging vocabulary. "Hard copy" refers to a radiograph viewed on traditional film. "Soft copy" refers to a radiograph viewed on a monitor. Some x-ray imaging systems produce the soft copy for immediate viewing and a hard copy for the archives.

What Is Radiation?

Radiation is energy that is transmitted through space or matter. The different forms of energy used in medicine include mechanical, electrical, thermal, nuclear, and electromagnetic energy. All these energy forms can be transmitted as radiation, such as mechanical energy in the form of ultrasound waves, heat from an infrared lamp, nuclear energy in the form of gamma rays or alpha particles, and electromagnetic energy in the form of visible light or x-rays. The higher-energy forms of radiation, such as x-rays and gamma rays, have the ability to *ionize* atoms in matter. Ionization is the process by which a neutral atom gains or loses an electron, thus acquiring a net charge. Ionization has the ability to disrupt the composition of matter and, as a result, disrupt life processes. Protection against excessive exposure to ionizing radiation is of significant importance in radiology. Recommendations for *effective dose* (the average of all tissue and organ absorption) *limits* is listed in

TABLE 1-1 ● *Effective Dose Limit Recommendations*

Population and Area of Body Affected	Dose Limits	
	Traditional Unit	*SI Unit*
Occupational Exposures		
Effective dose limits		
Annual	5 rem	50 mSv
Cumulative	1 rem × age	10 mSv × age
Public Exposures (Annual)		
Effective dose limit		
Continuous or frequent exposure	0.1 rem	1 mSv
Infrequent exposure	0.5 rem 1.5 rem	5 mSv
Equivalent dose limit for tissues and organs		
Lens of eye	5 rem	15 mSv
Skin, hands, and feet		50 mSv
Embryo–Fetus Exposures (Monthly)		
Equivalent dose limit	0. 05 rem	0.5 mSv
Annual average effective dose from naturally occuring radioactive materials and cosmic radiation for a person in the United States		3 mSv
Average Effective Dose For Common Imaging Modalities		
Whole body CT scan		10 mSv
Mammogram		0.7 mSv
Chest radiograph		0.1 mSv
Bone densiometry (DEXA)		0.01 mSv
Modified from NCRP Report No. 116: Limitation of Exposure to Ionizing Radiation. National Council on Radiation Protection and Measurements, Bethesda, MD, 2006 and available at www.radiologyinfo.org, accessed 2009.		

TABLE 1-2 ● *Radiation Units of Measurement*

Quantity of Ionizing Radiation	Traditional Unit	SI Unit	Equivalents
Intensity in air	roentgen (R)	C/kg	$1 R = 2.58 \times 10^{-4}$ C/kg
Radiation absorbed dose	rad	gray (Gy) (J/kg)	100 rads = 1 Gy
Radiation dose equivalent	rem	sievert (Sv) (J/kg)	100 rem = 1 Sv
Radionuclide decay rate	curie (Ci)	becquerel (Bq) (nuclear decay per second)	$1 Ci = 3 \times 10^{10}$ Bq

Table 1-1, as well as a comparison of natural and diagnostic exposures.

Ionizing radiation exists in two forms: *natural* or *background* radiation and artificial radiation. Natural radiation includes cosmic radiation from the sun and other celestial bodies as well as radioactive elements present on Earth that may be absorbed through food, water, or air. Artificial radiation sources include the nuclear industry, the radionuclide products industry, and the medical and dental industry. Medical and dental x-ray exposures constitute the greatest artificial source of radiation exposure.

Units of Measure in Radiologic Science

Four units of measurement are used to express a quantity of ionizing radiation: the roentgen (R), the rad (radiation absorbed dose), the rem (rad equivalent man), and the curie (Ci). The curie measures the number of nuclear decays per second produced by a given sample of a radionuclide and is equal to the radioactivity in 1 gram of radium. These traditional units have been in use since the 1920s and are the most familiar to those who work in radiology. Metric measurements for radiation exist in the Système International d'Unites or SI units, but these have not been fully adopted in the United States. It is not uncommon to see both sets of units in publications. Table 1-2 compares these measurements.

In diagnostic radiology, 1 roentgen is considered equal to 1 rad and to 1 rem. This simplifying assumption is accurate to within 15% and thus is sufficient for nearly all considerations of diagnostic exposure. However, these terms

cannot be used interchangeably, because each unit has a *precise application*. The roentgen measures the x-ray beam's ability to ionize air, the rad measures how much radiation energy the patient absorbs from the beam, and the rem measures the effect of that radiation on a person's body (1 rad of x-rays produces 1 rem of effect on the body, but 1 rad of alpha particles produces 20 rem of effect). Typically the rem is used to measure the scatter radiation that reaches the radiographer, whose cumulative exposure is monitored by a radiation badge device. Furthermore, in diagnostic radiology a roentgen, rad, or rem is a very large quantity. In practice, quantities 1,000 times smaller are used: milliroentgen (mR), millirad (mrad), and millirem (mrem).

What Are X-rays?

X-rays are a form of ionizing electromagnetic radiation, similar to visible light but of shorter wavelength. On Earth, x-rays are almost always of human origin. The various forms of radiant energy are grouped according to their wavelengths in what is called the *electromagnetic spectrum* (Fig. 1-3). The shorter the wavelength in the electromagnetic spectrum, the higher the energy of the radiation and the greater its penetrating power.

X-rays can be produced in a range of wavelengths varying from 10^{-8} to 10^{-11} cm. *Soft x-rays* are the longer-wavelength x-rays, located near the ultraviolet band in the electromagnetic spectrum. In medicine, soft x-rays are used for treatment of superficial malignancies such as those of the eye and skin. *Hard x-rays* are the shorter-wavelength x-rays, located closer to and overlapping the gamma-ray range. Hard x-rays are used in general diagnostic radiography. The highest-energy hard x-rays and soft gamma rays are used in the therapeutic treatment of deep tissue tumors.

How Are X-rays Produced?

The production of x-rays requires three things: a source of electrons, a force to move them rapidly, and something to stop that movement rapidly. These conditions are all met by the x-ray tube and an electrical supply. The x-ray tube consists of a cathode (negative terminal) and an anode (positive terminal) enclosed within a glass envelope, which maintains a vacuum (Fig. 1-4). The source of electrons is a heated thoriated tungsten filament in the cathode assembly.

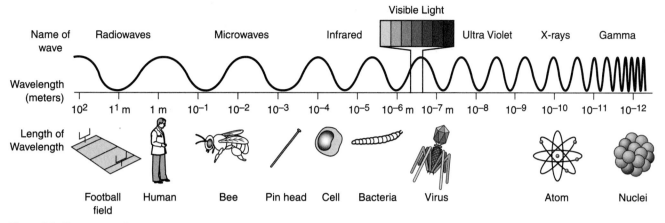

Figure 1-3 Electromagnetic spectrum.

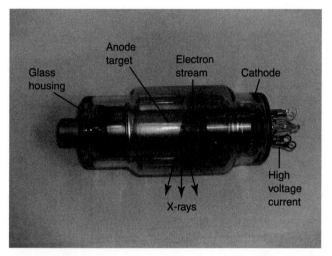

Figure 1-4 X-ray tube used in portable medical radiography. Dimensions are 5.3 inches by 2 inches. *(Courtesy of Superior X-ray Tube Co., Woodstock, Illinois.)*

Production of x-rays begins when kilovoltage (thousands of volts) is applied between the anode and the filament. Electrons emitted from the hot filament are accelerated and strike the anode, where they decelerate and thus create x-rays via an energy conversion.

How Do X-rays Interact With the Patient?

X-rays produced in the tube are beamed through a series of lead shutters and travel out of the tube through a collimator. The collimator controls the size and shape of the x-ray field coming out of the x-ray tube. At this point, the beam of x-ray photons is described as primary radiation. Prior to making the actual exposure, the radiographer uses a light source on the collimator to project a representation of the x-ray field onto the patient. Cross hairs on the light source help define the position of the focal or central ray, the theoretical center of the x-ray beam. The central ray is positioned over the area of anatomic interest. The patient is then exposed to the x-ray beam.

The primary x-ray beam then passes through the patient and undergoes a process of *attenuation*. Attenuation is a reduction in the number of x-ray photons in the beam. Attenuation is the result of x-ray photons interacting with matter and losing energy through either scattering or photoelectric absorption.

How Is the Image Made?

When the the x-ray beam passes through the patient, it is attenuated in different amounts, depending on the density of the tissue it has passed through. The x-ray beam that emerges from the patient is referred to as remnant radiation. This remnant beam contains an aerial image of the patient. The remnant beam is intercepted by an interpretation device called an image receptor. The information gathered at the receptor is, at this point, invisible. It is known as the latent image. The latent image information is processed in a method specific to the type of image receptor used, and a visual image is produced, which is the radiograph.

Basic Requirements for Any X-ray Imaging System

The basic requirements for any x-ray imaging system are the same: to generate x-rays in the x-ray tube, beam the x-rays to the patient, capture the x-rays from the remnant beam exiting the patient, convert them into something measurable that yields a latent image at a receptor, and then convert the latent image into a visible image (Fig. 1-5). There are many technologies available that can do this. Yet how we identify anatomy will remain the same regardless of what technology was used to capture the image. This is because *the shade of gray that represents anatomy is determined by the molecular interaction of x-rays with body tissues, not by the type of image receptor used.*

● Image Receptors: Different Ways to Capture the X-rays[8,9,14–17]

There are three major classifications of diagnostic radiographic imaging based on the type of image receptor used to capture the x-ray image. These are film/screen radiography, fluoroscopic imaging, and computed or digital imaging.

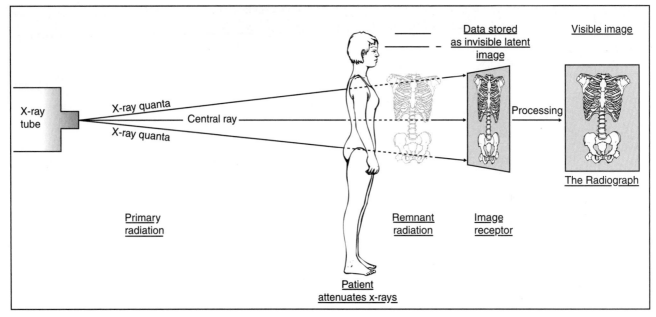

Figure 1-5 Components of a basic x-ray imaging system.

The Gold Standard: Film/Screen Radiography

Film/screen technology has been considered the gold standard against which all new imaging technologies are measured. The greatest challenge for the developers of digital imaging is to match the image quality, cost, reliability, and ease of use of film/screen technology.

The phrase "film/screen" refers to the combination of photographic film with crystal-coated *intensifying screens*. The purpose of the screens is to utilize the luminescence of crystals to decrease the amount of radiation required to make an image.

The film/screen receptor is housed in a *cassette* (Fig. 1-6). Cassettes are lightproof plastic cases that sandwich the x-ray film between intensifying screens and reflective layers. A major goal in the design of cassettes is to reduce patient radiation dose as much as possible. It is estimated that 99% of the photographic effect on a film/screen radiograph is due to

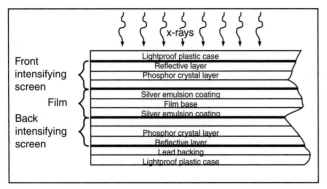

Figure 1-6 Cross section of a modern film/screen cassette image receptor.

screen light, with only 1% due to the direct action of x-ray photons.

The x-ray film itself is a type of modified photographic film that is sensitive to both light and radiation. When the aerial image in the remnant x-ray beam reaches the cassette, it carries an energy representation of the structures through which it has passed. The various intensities of both the reflected light photons and the x-ray photons cause chemical reactions within the silver emulsion coated on the film. These reactions produce various shades of gray when the film is developed. Thus, the *final film image is a representation of the radiodensities of the anatomic structures through which the x-rays have passed.*

Will Film Become Obsolete?

No. After 20 years of progressive replacement by digital technology, film continues to be used for general diagnostic radiology in many areas of the world. This is because film is a simple cost solution. Film is at once the image capture, the display, and the archive media, for a cost of about $3 a study. This is significant in light of the fact that over two thirds of the world's population does not have access to the most basic of diagnostic imaging services. Film will remain a simple, effective, and reliable tool of basic health care. However, in facilities where technological infrastructures exist, digital imaging can offer many advantages over film imaging. See Table 1-3 for a comparison of film and digital imaging systems.

Fluoroscopy

Fluoroscopy is a dynamic or continuous radiographic examination. A useful analogy is that a radiograph is to a photograph as fluoroscopy is to a movie. Fluoroscopy provides real-time imaging of physiological function that

TABLE 1-3 ● *Comparison of Film to Digital Imaging Systems*

Disadvantages of Film-Based Imaging Systems	Advantages of Digital-Based Imaging Systems
1. Potential for higher radiation dose to the patient at initial exam or retake exams 2. Necessity of repeat exposures to improve image quality in the case of chemical development errors 3. Time required for chemical development 4. Inability to alter the image technically to enhance viewing 5. Need for physical transport of the film to the radiologist and for the physical presence of the radiologist 6. The necessity for physical transport of films to other clinicians involved in the patient's care 7. Large physical inventory storage space requirements 8. Potential for films to get lost, borrowed and not returned, or damaged by handling 9. Nonreuseability and cost of film and other consumables	1. Potential for less radiation dose to the patient 2. Better quality control of the image (electronic image processing allows for technical alteration of the image; contrast, density, and magnification can be adjusted without repeat exposures) 3. Better disease detection, related to the technical ability to highlight areas of interest while suppressing irrelevant data 4. Immediate access to the image for the radiologist and others involved in the patient's care as well, via a computer network (none of the consultants need to be at the same location; they only need to have computer access) 5. Storage to a hard drive or disk, eliminating need for physical storage space and inventory costs. 6. Immediate access to past films for comparison with present films 7. Improved patient education via ease of access, as in a monitor at the clinician's office 8. Ease of attachment to a patient's electronic record 9. Ease of attachment to an electronic claims form, facilitating faster reimbursement 10. Less environmental impact on the local community 11. Improved archival quality of the images, due to less degradation over time 12. Possibility of computer-assisted diagnostics

allows for active diagnosis during the examination. For this reason, the radiologist is present and controls the examination during interventional and contrast study procedures.

Some components of fluoroscopy are similar to those of film/screen imaging. However, fluoroscopy is more complex and often involves a combination of imaging processes. Two objectives of the fluoroscopic exam are to view the function or procedure in real time and to archive the images for later review.

The major components of a fluoroscopic imaging system are the x-ray tube and the *image intensifier unit,* which serves as the image receptor. The x-ray tube may be mounted above or below the fluoroscopic table. Mounted opposite is the image intensifier unit. These two, connected together, form the *fluoroscopic carriage.* The fluoroscopic table, with the attached carriage, can be tilted to assist in the flow of contrast media.

The imaging process begins as the radiologist moves the carriage over the patient to the region to be examined. The x-rays are generated, the patient attenuates the x-ray beam, and the image intensifier transforms the remnant x-ray beam into an electronic image displayed on a television monitor.

During the examination, static radiographs, or *spot films,* are made for archival records. This can be accomplished by different methods. A spot film device, mounted on the fluoroscopic tower, uses regular film/screen cassettes to make images. *Roll or cut* radiographic film, exposed by the image intensifier, records one image at a time; after development the images are mounted for viewing. Digital fluoroscopic units permit electronic acquisition of spot radiographs, which can be viewed on a monitor or printed to film.

Dynamic imaging records can also be obtained. *Cinefluororadiography* uses movie film to record dynamic images. Videotaping records the dynamic television image. Digital fluoroscopes permit computer monitor playback of digitally stored data.

Computed Radiography

Computed radiography (CR) was available for commercial use in the early 1980s and is now used to perform every common type of radiographic exam. CR is viewed as a film replacement technology that has served as a gateway into complete digital imaging systems.

CR is the process of producing a digital radiograph by exposing a phosphor screen (instead of film) to x-rays. The x-rays are absorbed on the screen. A laser beam scans the screen. This results in emitted photostimulated light that is converted by a photodetector into an electrical analog signal. The analog signal is converted to a digital image viewed on a monitor. This image is referred to as the *soft copy.* Most CR systems today are still attached to laser printers that produce film as an output. This means that although the image is viewed and technically enhanced on a computer monitor, it is then transferred to radiographic film for hard-copy storage.

The major advantage of CR is that it has extremely wide exposure latitude. This means the same reusable detector can be used under practically any diagnostic exposure conditions. Additionally, the CR cassettes have similar internal physical structure and exposure response to screen/film cassettes and so are compatible with current exposing equipment. Thus, few major changes to the equipment and exposure techniques are necessary to acquire an image. The patient radiation dose required to produce an image is not significantly different between the two systems.

Digital Radiography

Digital radiography (DR) has a shorter history than CR. This film replacement technology has been commercially available since the 1990s. Presently there are two approaches to DR: *direct DR* and *indirect DR.* The distinction between the two is in how the digital detector captures the x-rays from the remnant beam.

Direct DR conversion detectors use an x-ray–sensitive semiconductor material, such as selenium, to convert x-rays directly into an electrical charge. This charge is then measured either electrostatically or with a thin-film transistor array. Indirect conversion detectors use an x-ray–absorbing scintillation material, such as cesium iodide, to convert x-ray photons into light photons. This light is then measured with a charge-coupled device or a thin-film diode array. Either detector yields a latent image, which is converted into an analog electrical signal and then digitized. This digital image can then be manipulated to enhance diagnostic analysis. Other important components in a DR system include control and readout electronics, x-ray machine communications and synchronization, image-processing software, and a host computer interfaced to the various components of the system.

Comparing Computed and Digital Radiography

CR and digital radiography produce similar end results: an image that can be technically altered to enhance diagnostic detail, transmitted electronically, and stored digitally. The radiation exposure dose to the patient is also similar.

The differences in the two systems are in cost, resolution, and speed. CR is significantly cheaper than DR at present. CR processing equipment is compatible with film/screen equipment, whereas DR requires total replacement of existing film/screen imaging equipment. In resolution, CR is higher because the image is recorded at a molecular level as in film. However, CR's resolution can be reduced by the laser size and lack of sharpness in the optical reading system. DR is faster than CR in that there are no intermediate steps to delay the next image acquisition. CR is highly portable, whereas portable DR is not affordable in many settings at present.

Understanding the Image[15,18–22]

The radiographic image is the result of the interaction of x-rays with body tissues. Identification of radiographic anatomy by different shades of gray is dependent upon each tissue's varying attenuation of the x-ray beam. How much a tissue attenuates the beam depends on its *radiodensity*.

What Is Radiodensity?

Radiodensity is the combination of physical qualities of an object that determine how much radiation it absorbs from the x-ray beam. An object's radiodensity is determined by a combination of (1) its composition (in terms of *effective atomic number* and volume density) and (2) its thickness. The effective atomic number is a measure of the number of electrons in a substance with which an x-ray photon may interact. *The greater an object's effective atomic number, volume density, and/or thickness, the greater its radiodensity.*

Radiographic Density

Radiographic density is a technical term that refers to the amount of blackening on the radiograph. An inverse relationship exists between the radiodensity of an object and the radiographic density on the radiograph. That is, the greater the radiodensity, the less radiographic density, resulting in a whiter image. The less the radiodensity, the greater the radiographic density, resulting in a blacker image.

The similarity of these terms can be confusing and awkward in daily use. It is more common and efficient to describe the image with the terms *radiodense, radiopaque,* and *radiolucent*.

Radiopaque and Radiolucent

The terms *radiopaque* and *radiolucent* describe greater and lesser degrees of radiodensity, respectively (Fig. 1-7).

Radiopaque is defined as "not easily penetrated by x-rays"; some sources define it as "impenetrable to x-rays." A radiopaque object has such great radiodensity that it will attenuate almost all the x-rays from the beam. No x-rays reach the image receptor, so the radiographic representation of the object is white. In radiographic description, the term *radiopaque* is usually reserved for objects made of heavy metals, such as lead gonad shields, fillings in teeth, and surgical appliances as well as for contrast media such as barium sulfate. Human tissues do not normally possess enough radiodensity to be described as radiopaque; the term *radiodense* is used instead to describe areas of increased radiodensity. There are instances, however, when the body can produce radiopaque structures; examples of this include calcified gallstones or kidney stones.

Radiolucent is defined as "easily penetrated by x-rays." A radiolucent object attenuates very small amounts of x-rays from the beam. Most of the x-rays reach the image receptor, so the radiographic representation of the object is dark. Air is the best example of a radiolucent substance, as seen normally

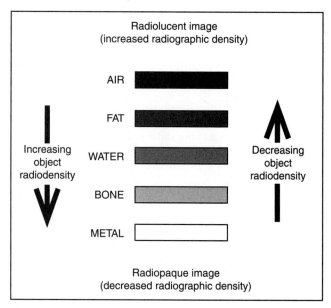

Figure 1-7 Radiographic density (shades of gray) as related to object radiodensity.

on the black background of the radiograph and in air-filled organs of the body. In the radiographic description of bone, the term *radiolucent* is used to identify areas that have decreased radiodensity, usually due to abnormal processes. Examples include osteoporotic bone, osteolytic tumors, and infections.

Radiodensity as a Function of Composition: Anatomy in Four Shades of Gray

The tissues in the human body fall into four major radiodensity categories; thus there are four major shades of gray (radiographic densities) on the radiograph (Fig. 1-8). Identification of tissues is based on the contrast between the radiographic densities of the images. The following paragraphs describe each density's shade of gray, where it normally appears on a radiograph, and where its appearance is an abnormal finding. The list is ordered from least radiodense to most radiodense.

1. *Air (black).* Air is radiolucent. It possesses the least radiodensity of all body structures. Air is seen normally in the trachea, lungs, stomach, and digestive tract. Air is also seen as the black surrounding background of the radiograph, and it can be used in contrast studies as a *negative contrast medium.* An example of an abnormal appearance of air is seen in gas gangrene at a wound site; radiolucent "bubbles" indicate the presence of gas. In the thorax, an abnormal appearance of air is seen in conditions such as pneumothorax (air in the pleural space), esophageal hiatal hernias, and pulmonary abscesses.

2. *Fat (gray–black).* Fat is more radiodense than air. Fat is normally present subcutaneously, along muscle sheaths, and surrounding the viscera. An example of an abnormal appearance of fat is in the visualization of a fat pad displaced from its bony fossa as a result of a joint effusion.

3. *Water (gray).* Water-based tissues are more radiodense than fat. All the soft tissues and fluids of the body—including blood, muscle, cartilage, tendons, ligaments, nerves, and fluid-filled organs—share approximately the same radiodensity as water. This is why conventional radiographs have limited value in assessing the soft tissues: Without the addition of a contrast medium, there is insufficient radiographic contrast to identify tissues. An example of an abnormal appearance of water density is in the distention of a joint capsule as a result of infection, effusion, or hemorrhage.

4. *Bone (white).* Bone is the most radiodense tissue of the body. The teeth image the whitest of all bone because of their high calcium content. A wide range of whitish shades is normal for the skeleton because there are so many thicknesses present. An abnormal appearance of a bone density is seen in conditions such as myositis ossificans or heterotrophic ossification.

Two More Shades of Gray

Two additional substances are often added to this list because of their common usage in medicine (Fig. 1-9).

5. *Contrast media (bright white outline).* Contrast media that are radiopaque are referred to as *positive contrast media.* The most common example is barium sulfate,

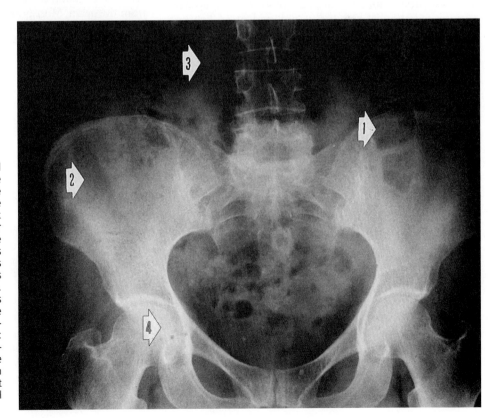

Figure 1-8 The four major physical radiodensities of the human body are demonstrated on this AP view of the pelvis. (1) Air, gas: This is seen in the intestines. (2) Fat: Fat is seen as a dark streak representing the fatty layer next to the peritoneum in the abdominal wall. This stripe, which is the fold of the fat layer as it turns posteriorly toward the patient's back, is known as the flank stripe. (3) Water: Muscles and soft tissues share the same density as water. The psoas muscle extends along the borders of the lumbar spine. (4) Bone: The osseous components of the proximal femur, pelvis, sacrum, and spine are best demonstrated on radiograph because bone possesses the greatest radiodensity of the four natural densities.

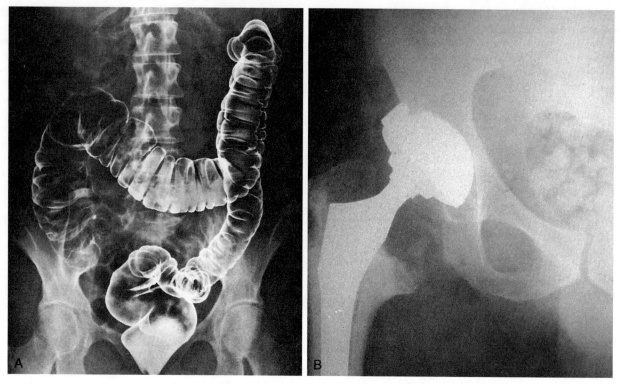

Figure 1-9 (A) Lower gastrointestinal dual-contrast examination. This normal colon is coated inside with barium and distended with air. Contrast media such as barium sulfate are used in gastrointestinal studies to outline the viscera and make them visible. The bright white outline caused by the medium allows detailed visualization of structures not normally visible on plain radiographs. *(From Squire and Novelline,[12] p. 159, with permission.)* **(B)** Total hip arthroplasty. The heavy metals used in the prosthetic components of this joint replacement absorb all the x-rays and cast a solid white image on the radiograph. Any anatomic structures behind the prosthesis are obscured. *(From Richardson and Iglarsh,[16] p. 673, with permission.)*

used in upper and lower gastrointestinal contrast studies. The barium coats the inside of the viscera, allowing visualization of soft tissues not evident on conventional radiographs.

6. *Heavy metals (solid white).* Heavy metals used in tooth fillings, in prosthetic devices such as total joint replacements, in pins and wires used in fracture fixation, or in the lead shields used for gonad protection image as uniformly solid white. An abnormal appearance of a metal density would be seen in unretrieved metal fragments from industrial accidents or weapon discharges.

Listing the effective atomic number and volume density of each of the foregoing substances further illustrates the definition of radiodensity as a function of composition (Table 1-4). Note that whereas air has a higher effective atomic number than fat or water, it has significantly lower tissue density. As a result, air will absorb fewer x-rays than fat and will image blacker.

Radiodensity as a Function of Thickness

The thicker an object is, the more radiodensity it possesses relative to a thinner object made of the same substance. Figure 1-10 illustrates how a stepwise increase in thickness produces progressively lighter shades of gray on the radiograph. So, although an object may be of homogeneous composition, its thicker portions will absorb more x-rays than its thinner portion, and its thicker portions will image lighter.

TABLE 1-4 ● *Radiodensity as Related to Composition of a Substance*

	Substance	Effective Atomic Number	Density (kg/m³)
Increasing Radiodensity	Air	7.78	1.29
	Fat	6.46	916
	Water	7.51	1,000
	Muscle	7.64	1,040
	Bone	12.31	1,650
	Barium	56	3,510
	Lead	82	11,340

The numerous shapes and irregular surfaces of the bones in the skeleton present many different thicknesses for the x-ray beam to pass through. As a result, the radiographic images of bone have variations in the shades of white and are not uniformly white.

How Many Dimensions Can You See?

Understanding how composition and thickness determine an object's radiodensity is part of the foundation for understanding the images of the radiograph. Now consider the contribution of *form* to the radiographic image. The form or shape of an anatomic image will depend on the

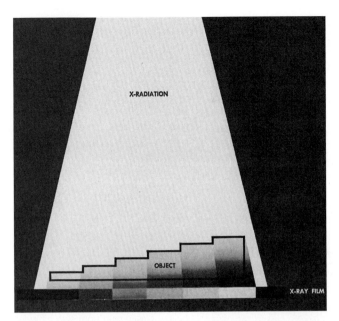

Figure 1-10 Radiographic density as a function of thickness of the object. Here the object filmed is of homogeneous composition and has a stepwise range of thickness. The thicker the object, the greater amount of radiation it absorbs; so the radiographic image is a lighter shade of gray. *(Image courtesy of Eastman Kodak Company. KODAK is a trademark.)*

angle of projection of the x-ray beam. That is, the direction that the x-ray beam passed through the body part will determine its silhouette on film and also alter its radiographic density.

Angles of Projection Over Straight Planes

Look at the three radiographs made of the wedge of wood (Fig. 1-11). The different angles of projection created three very different silhouettes and radiographic densities:

- When the wedge is placed flat on its broad side on the image receptor, the resulting triangular image is of

uniform radiographic density because the x-ray beam traveled through equal thicknesses at all points on the solid wedge.

- When the wedge is placed upright on its base, the resulting rectangular image shows greatest radiodensity present at the center of the image, where the x-ray beam traveled through the greatest thickness from the top of the wedge down to the base.

- When the wedge is placed on its long side, the resulting rectangular image shows a gradual decrease in radiographic density from the thick end to the thin end of the wedge.

If the viewer had no prior knowledge of the form of the object, information regarding the straight planes, dimensions, and whether the object was hollow or solid could easily be deduced by viewing all three images and noting the variations in outline and radiographic density.

Angles of Projection Over Curved Planes

Curved surfaces are slightly more complex than straight planes. Curved surfaces radiograph tangentially as a series of planes. In this instance it is helpful to imagine a curved plane as being at some points either relatively parallel to the image receptor or relatively perpendicular to the image receptor. The portion of the curved plane that is parallel to the image receptor will be relatively thin with little radiographic density. The part of the curve that is perpendicular to the image receptor will absorb more of the beam and image with greater radiographic density.

To illustrate, look at the two radiographs of a hollow plastic pipe (Fig. 1-12).

- The first image is made with the pipe standing on its end on the image receptor. The image is of a circle of equal radiographic density, because the x-ray beam travels down the same length of pipe at all points. The radiographic density of the center matches that of the surrounding air, indicating that the pipe is hollow. The length of the pipe cannot be determined on this one radiograph.

- The second image is made with the pipe lying on its side. The center of the image is the least radiodense area,

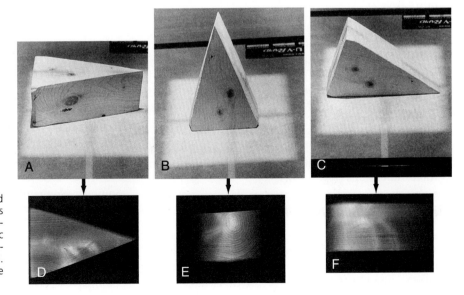

Figure 1-11 (A–F) A wedge of wood radiographed from three different angles produces three distinctly different radiographic images with varying radiographic densities. (Note the whorls representing seasonal growth and the knot in the wood. These present an increased density because of more tightly packed wood cells.)

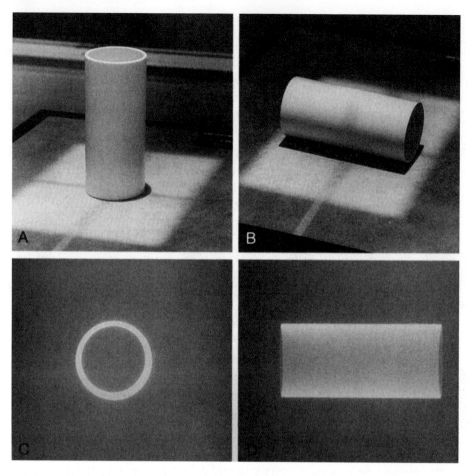

Figure 1-12 (A–D) Radiographs made of a hollow plastic pipe from two different perspectives yield two entirely different images. The first image **(C)** reveals that the pipe is hollow but tells nothing about the length of the pipe. The second image **(D)** reveals the length dimensions of the pipe. Without having seen the first image, it is still possible to deduce that this object is tubular with a less dense center by observing the densities of the margins contrasting with the density of center. *(From Richardson and Iglarsh,[16] with permission.)*

because the x-ray beam traversed only a thickness equal to the sum of two thicknesses of the wall. The image of two very radiodense lines on either margin is a result of the x-ray beam traveling over a greater cumulative distance of the relatively perpendicular curved plane sides of the pipe. This image is consistently found with hollow tubular structures such as the long bones of the skeleton.

One View Is No View

It is plain to see from these examples that more than one projection is required to gain useful information about a structure. A single radiograph provides only two dimensions: length and width. The third dimension, depth, is compensated for by viewing a second radiograph projected at a 90-degree angle to the first image. The adage "one view is no view" is a pertinent reminder that critical diagnostic information is missing if only one radiograph is available for evaluation. At least two images, made as close to 90 degrees to each other as possible, are required to view all three dimensions (Fig. 1-13).

The Perception of a Third Dimension

In evaluating medical radiographs, two projections made at right angles will provide the viewer with the factual dimensions of length, width, and depth. It is up to the viewer's mind's eye, however, to reconstruct form while looking at the

two projections. Knowledge of anatomy in great detail is the heart of the radiologist's science. No matter how advanced the machinery of imaging becomes, the interpretation of the data is still dependent on the viewer's perceptual foundation of anatomy.

The three radiographs of the finger illustrate this concept (Fig. 1-14). The first radiograph is a finger that has been projected in an anteroposterior direction. In the next radiographs, the finger has been coated with barium and radiographed in an anteroposterior and a lateral position. In Figure 1-14A the soft tissues image as a faint gray outline. In Figures 1-14B and 1-14C the barium has collected in the crevices of the skin and the nail, and the illusion of depth is easily perceived by the novice.

The perception of the third dimension in the evaluation of radiographs is critical. The radiologist views most radiographs in this manner, perceiving three dimensions and reconstructing form via a knowledge base of anatomy.

Radiodensity in a Rose

Squire[18] eloquently summarized the fundamentals of radiodensity, form, and perception by describing radiographs not as pictures but as "composite shadowgrams representing the sum of the densities interposed between beam source and film." Squire illustrated her point with this radiograph of three roses (Fig. 1-15). Evaluating a radiograph of something familiar allows the viewer to apply

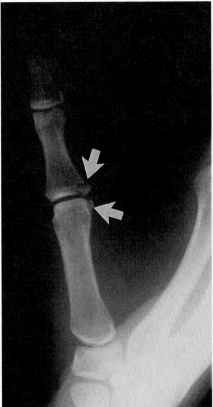
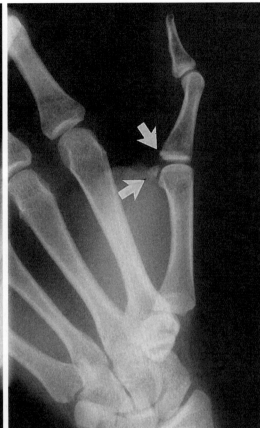

Figure 1-13 These two films of the thumb demonstrate the necessity of viewing two images, as close to 90 degrees to each other as possible, to gather accurate diagnostic information. On the dorsoplanar image on the left, the arrows point to what may be either two bone fragments or two sesamoid bones. On viewing the lateral film, it becomes obvious that the fragment seen at the base of the proximal phalanx was indeed a fracture, whereas the object seen at the head of the metacarpal was a sesamoid bone.

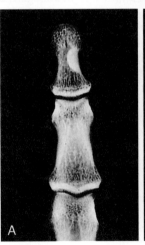
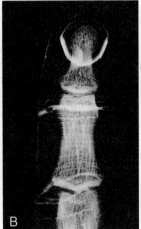
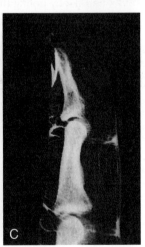

Figure 1-14 (A) Plain film radiograph of a finger. **(B,C)** Plain film radiographs of a finger that has been coated with barium.

confidently the new concepts and terms just presented. Consider the following:

1. Thinking perceptually, the viewer supplies the third dimension by recognizing form and identifying the image as three actual roses, in different stages of bloom.
2. Density and thickness principles are evident in the greater radiographic density of the overlapping petals of the tightly closed bud versus the open petals of the rose that is in full bloom.
3. The single petal is the most radiolucent structure on the image.

4. The leaves are slightly more radiodense than the single petal.
5. The veins of the leaves are denser than the leaves themselves. This is because of the more tightly packed cell structure of the veins, and also because of the added density of the fluid in the veins.
6. The stems are thicker than the other structures, evidenced by their increased radiographic density.
7. The form of the stems can be deduced as tubular by noting the increased density of the margins of the stems versus the less dense centers of the stems. The margins have greater density because they represent curved planes radiographed tangentially.

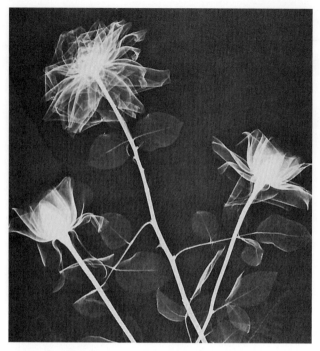

Figure 1-15 Radiograph of three roses. *(From Squire and Novelline,[12] p. 9, with permission.)*

8. As in the veins on the leaves, fluid adds density to the hollow tubular stems.
9. The form of the leaves can be deduced as thin, broad, and flat by noting the dimensions of a leaf flat on the film and another leaf positioned at 90 degrees to the film.
10. The variations in curved plane densities are evident in comparing the radiographic density of the leaf lying flat on the film (parallel to the film) to that of a leaf curling up (relatively perpendicular to the film). The flat leaf is radiolucent. The curled leaf has relatively greater radiographic density.

More to the Radiograph[8,15,18,21]

Understanding how anatomy is repesented as a shade of gray is a good foundation for understanding radiographs. Further comprehension of medical radiographs is gained by understanding radiographic terminology, radiographic identification markers, how to view radiographs, and appreciating the factors that determine *image quality.*

Radiographic Terminology

Position

In radiographic terminology, position is used to discuss the patient's physical position in two ways. First, in reference to general body positions, such as upright, seated, supine, prone, erect, recumbent, or Trendelenburg. Second, in reference to specific radiographic positions that describe which body part is closest to the image receptor or on which surface the body is lying, such as a right anterior oblique (RAO) position.

Decubitus is used specifically in radiology to describe *both* a body positioned on a horizontal surface and the use of a

horizontal x-ray beam. The patient may be lying prone (ventral decubitus), supine (dorsal decubitus), on the right side (right lateral decubitus), or on the left side (left lateral decubitus). Decubitus positions are used to detect air–fluid levels or free air in a body cavity such as the chest or abdomen.

In orthopedic radiology, skeletal radiographs may be made with the patient in the seated, supine, or upright position. *Upright* can denote seated or standing. A distinction between the two may have significance in the evaluation of some joints, especially those of the lower extremities and lumbar spine. In these instances, the positioning words *erect* or *weight-bearing* are used to clearly establish that the joints were under the effects of gravity and weight bearing. Erect or weight-bearing positions are not usually the norm in routine radiographs, so these terms will be marked on the radiograph to inform the reader of the circumstance in which the radiograph was made.

The reference for all positioning terms, directional terms, and planes of the body is the standard *anatomic position.*

Projection

Projection describes the path of the x-ray beam as it travels from the x-ray tube, through the patient, to the image receptor. The most common projection terms are *anteroposterior (AP)*, *posteroanterior (PA)*, and *lateral.* An AP projection, for example, means the x-ray beam entered at the anterior surface of the body, and exited at the posterior surface. See Table 1-5 and Figure 1-16 for a summary of common positions and projections.

Radiologists and radiographers have developed specific patient positions and radiographic projections to comprise the most efficient routine radiographic examinations of the individual bones and joints. Routine radiographic examinations became standardized in the United States in 1989 via a survey of 520 hospitals affiliated with Radiologic Technology Educational Programs. This survey established

TABLE 1-5 ● *Primary Radiographic Projections and Body Positions*		
Projections (Path of the Central Ray)	**Positions**	
	General body positions	**Specific body positions (part named is closest to the image receptor)**
Anteroposterior (AP)	Upright	Right or left lateral
Posteroanterior (PA)	Seated	Right posterior oblique
Lateral	Recumbent	(RPO)
AP or PA oblique	Supine	Left posterior oblique (LPO)
AP or PA axial	Prone	Right anterior oblique (RAO)
Tangential	Trendelenburg	Left anterior oblique (LAO)
Transthoracic		Right lateral decubitus
Inferosuperior		Left lateral decubitus
Superoinferior		Ventral decubitus
Plantodorsal (PD)		Dorsal decubitus
Dorsoplantar (DP)		Lordotic
Lateromedial		
Mediolateral		
Submentovertical (SMV)		
Verticosubmental (VSM)		
Craniocaudal		
Orbitoparietal		
Parieto-orbital		

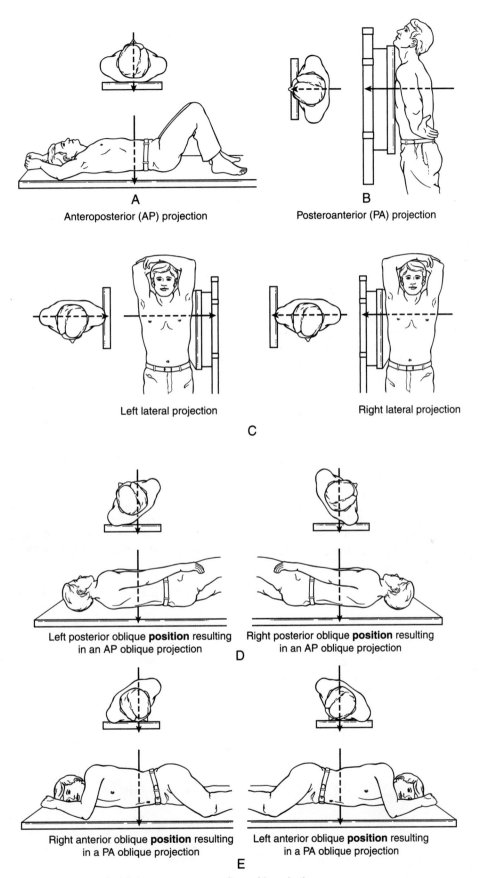

A Anteroposterior (AP) projection

B Posteroanterior (PA) projection

Left lateral projection

Right lateral projection

C

Left posterior oblique **position** resulting in an AP oblique projection

Right posterior oblique **position** resulting in an AP oblique projection

D

Right anterior oblique **position** resulting in a PA oblique projection

Left anterior oblique **position** resulting in a PA oblique projection

E

Figure 1-16 Examples of the most common radiographic projections.

routine projections for all common radiographic procedures and the determination of the most common *optional* or extra projections taken to demonstrate specific anatomic parts or pathological conditions better. The routine and optional projections presented in the anatomy chapters of this text conform to these national norms, as documented by Bontrager.[21]

Anteroposterior, Lateral, and Oblique Projections

The most common projections in routine radiographic examinations of the appendicular skeleton and spine are the *anteroposterior (AP)*, *lateral*, and *oblique projections.*

A general rule in diagnostic radiology is that a minimum of two radiographs made at right angles to each other are necessary to (1) provide information about the dimensions of a structure, (2) locate lesions or foreign bodies, and (3) determine alignment of fractures. Thus the routine radiographic assessment of the long bones of the skeleton requires a minimum of two projections: an AP and a lateral. Oblique projections are additionally included in most routine examinations of the joints for the purpose of greater visualization of the complex anatomic topography of joint surfaces.

An AP projection means the x-ray beam has traveled through the body in an anterior-to-posterior direction. All bones and joints are evaluated by an AP projection with the exception of the hand, which is normally radiographed in a *posteroanterior (PA) projection.* That is, the hand is placed palm down on the image receptor, and the beam is projected through the back of the hand.

A lateral projection means that the x-ray beam has traveled through the body at right angles to the AP or PA projection.

An oblique projection involves rotation of a body part so that the beam traverses the body part at an angle somewhere between the AP and lateral projections. The degree of obliquity varies depending on the anatomic structure being visualized.

The precise positioning of a body part in an AP, lateral, or oblique projection is the responsibility of the radiographer. Accurate positioning guarantees that the body part *will be visualized exactly as planned.* For example, a *true lateral projection* of the cervical spine will directly superimpose the right- and left-side facet joints, allowing clear visualization of the joint surfaces. A correctly positioned *oblique projection* of the cervical spine will permit visualization of the intervertebral foramen of one side of the spine (Fig. 1-17). The opposite is true in the thoracic and lumbar spines, however. In these spinal regions the lateral projection best demonstrates the intervertebral foramina, while the oblique projection best demonstrates the facet joints. See Table 1-6 for a summary of these points.

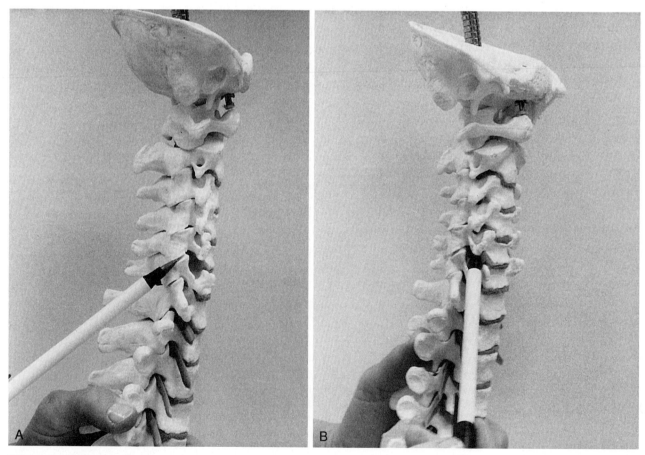

Figure 1-17 (A) The lateral projection of the cervical spine best demonstrates the *facet joints,* indicated by the point of the pen. **(B)** The oblique projection of the cervical spine best demonstrates the intervertebral foramina. The tip of the pen is at the C5–C6 right intervertebral foramen.

TABLE 1-6 ● *Summary of Radiographic Positions That Best Visualize Intervertebral Foramina Versus Zygapophyseal Joints*			
	Cervical Spine	**Thoracic Spine**	**Lumbar Spine**
Intervertebral foramina	Oblique 45°	Lateral	Lateral
Zygapophyseal (facet joints)	Lateral	Oblique 70°	Oblique 45°

Viewing Radiographs

Film or hard-copy radiographs are analyzed on *view boxes,* also called *illuminators.* The radiographs are clipped to the view box surface and illuminated from behind (Fig. 1-18A and B). Additional wattage is used in the form of "hot lights" to focus attention on areas of the image that may not be adequately illuminated on the view box, such as the subacromial region in a routine AP radiograph of the shoulder (Fig. 1-19).

Because film radiographs are transparent, they may be viewed from either side. The custom, however, is to place the radiographs on the view box as if the patient were *facing* the

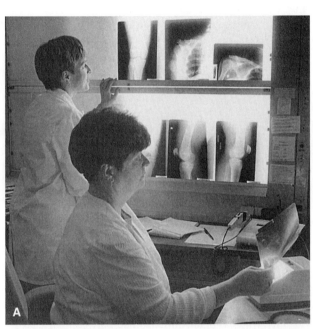
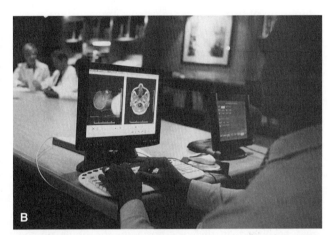

Figure 1-18 **(A)** Radiographs are analyzed on view boxes, also called illuminators. Additional wattage gained from "hot lights" focuses attention on areas that may not be adequately illuminated on the view box. **(B)** Digital image viewed on a LCD monitor.

Figure 1-19 Because of the varying thicknesses and densities of the body, not all areas of anatomy are adequately exposed on one radiograph. Each radiograph is made to expose the area of interest for best visibility. Thus, in the routine anteroposterior projection of the shoulder, the glenohumeral joint is properly exposed, whereas the acromioclavicular joint is overexposed, or too dark. In order to demonstrate the acromioclavicular joint adequately, a separate radiograph must be made.

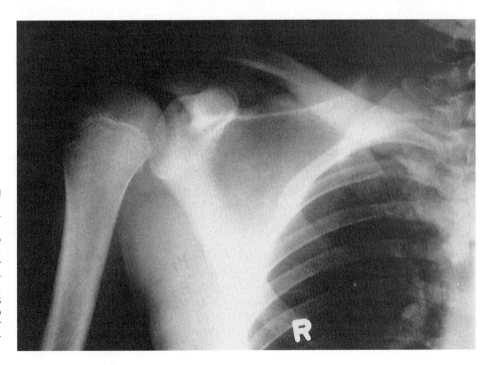

viewer, with the patient in anatomic position; this is true for either AP or PA projections. An exception to the rule is in viewing the distal extremities. Radiographs of the hands and feet are usually viewed with the toes or fingers pointing upward. The limbs are still viewed hanging down, as in the true anatomic position.

Lateral projections are generally placed on the light box so that the viewer is seeing the image from the same perspective as the x-ray tube.

Soft-copy viewing is done on two basic types of monitors: the traditional cathode ray tube (CRT) monitor, and the monitors that can be put in the broad category of "flat-screen" technologies. Flat screen monitors include the older gas plasma displays and the newer active and passive liquid crystal displays. The custom for viewing the patient in anatomic position, facing the viewer, still holds true when radiographs are viewed on a monitor.

Identification Markers

A minimum of two markers are usually imprinted on every radiograph. These are *patient identification* markers and *anatomic side* markers. Markers are placed on the image receptor during the procedure, rather than afterward, to avoid potential mismarkings.

The patient identification information usually includes the patient's name, age, sex, case number, date, and institution.

The anatomic side markers are radiopaque letters that identify the patient's right or left side of the trunk, or right or left limb. These may be either the words *right* or *left* or just the initials *R* or *L*. The letters may sometimes appear backward or upside down on developed films. *Do not* orient the radiograph to obtain a correctly positioned letter. *Always view radiographs as if viewing the patient in anatomic position.* Thus, an AP film of the patient's left lower extremity would be placed on the view box with the fibula on the viewer's right-hand side (Fig. 1-20).

The following are some additional markers that may be used:

Internal (INT) indicates that a limb has been rotated internally.
External (EXT) indicates that a limb has been rotated externally.
Weight-bearing (WTB) or *(ERECT)* indicates that the patient was standing for the examination.
Decubitus (DECUB) indicates that the patient was recumbent.
Inspiration (INSP) and *expiration (EXP)* are used in comparison films of the chest indicating the state of respiration.

The initials of the radiographer are generally placed on the R or L markers to identify the individual responsible for that examination.

Image Quality Factors

The factors by which one evaluates the quality of a radiograph are termed *image quality factors.* The four image quality factors are *density, contrast, detail,* and *distortion.* Density and contrast are *photographic properties* that control

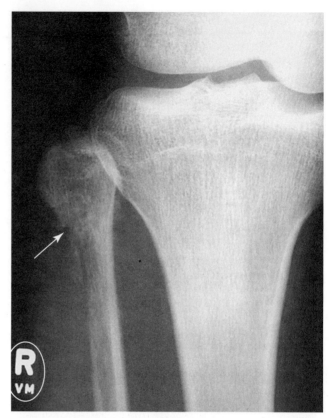

Figure 1-20 Radiographs are viewed as if the patient were standing in front of the viewer in anatomic position. This AP radiograph of the knee is viewed properly. The R marker (circled) tells us this is the patient's right leg, so the film is viewed with the fibula to the viewer's left-hand side. The small letters below the R are the technician's initials. The pathology indicated by the arrow is an osteogenic sarcoma. *(Image courtesy of John C. Hunter, MD, University of California, Davis School of Medicine.)*

visibility, whereas detail and distortion are *geometric properties* that control clarity. Although it is the radiographer who monitors the technical aspect of these factors, the viewer too must have an appreciation of how these factors contribute to or alter the image.

Radiographic Density

Radiographic density is defined as the amount of blackening on the radiograph. The radiographer adjusts radiographic density by varying the current (milliamperage) and the exposure time, which regulate the quantity of x-rays emitted from the x-ray tube during an exposure. The product of current and time is expressed in milliampere seconds (mAs). Additionally, distance affects radiographic density according to the inverse square law. For example, doubling the distance from the beam source will reduce density on the image receptor by a factor of four. Standard distances are usually used in medical radiography, however, so radiographic density is primarily controlled by mAs. The radiographer uses his or her knowledge of human tissue densities, part thickness, and positioning to select an appropriate mAs for each radiograph. An underexposed radiograph has too little radiographic density and appears too white. An overexposed radiograph has too much radiographic density and appears too dark. Either extreme will not permit the anatomy to be sufficiently visualized (Fig. 1-21).

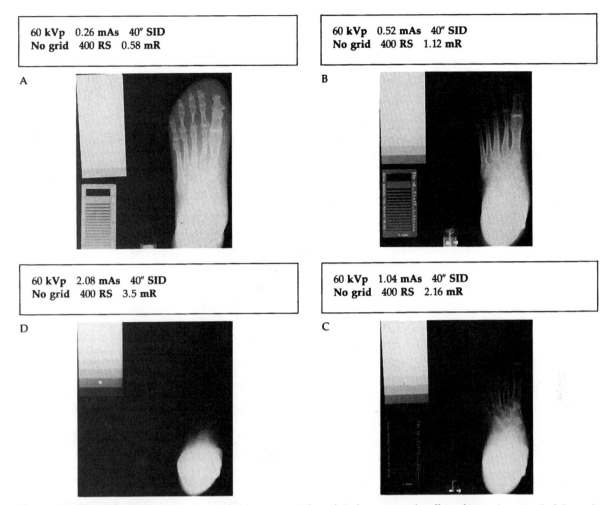

60 kVp 0.26 mAs 40″ SID
No grid 400 RS 0.58 mR

A

60 kVp 0.52 mAs 40″ SID
No grid 400 RS 1.12 mR

B

60 kVp 2.08 mAs 40″ SID
No grid 400 RS 3.5 mR

D

60 kVp 1.04 mAs 40″ SID
No grid 400 RS 2.16 mR

C

Figure 1-21 Effects of mAs changes on image density. Images **A** through **D** demonstrate the effect of increasing mAs. Each image is double the density of the previous one. *(From Carlton and Adler,[8] p. 363, with permission.)*

Radiographic Contrast

Radiographic contrast is the difference among various adjacent radiographic densities. Great variations among densities produces high contrast, and less variation produces low contrast. High or low contrast is not necessarily good or bad in itself. The purpose of contrast is to make anatomic detail more visible. So, in a chest radiograph, for example, low contrast is desired so as to visualize the very fine lung markings and the many shades of gray of the soft tissues of the heart and lungs (Fig. 1-22). In a skeletal radiograph, however, high contrast is often required to visualize cortical margins of bones clearly. The primary controlling factor for contrast is peak kilovoltage (kVp). The higher the kVp, the greater the energy of the x-ray beam, so that penetration occurs more uniformly through all tissue densities. The result is less variation in tissue absorption and low contrast among the radiographic densities on the radiograph. Conversely, the lower the kVp, the greater the variation in tissue absorption and the higher the contrast appears on the radiograph.

Voltage is also a secondary controlling factor for density. Higher kVp values result in a corresponding overall increase in density, decreasing the needed mAs. The relationship of mAs and kVp is balanced by the radiographer with the goal of reducing patient exposure to radiation while obtaining the best possible results in a radiograph. A general rule states that the highest kVp and lowest mAs that yield sufficient diagnostic information should be used on each radiographic examination.

Recorded Detail

Recorded detail is defined as the geometric sharpness or accuracy of the structural lines recorded on the radiograph. Recorded detail is also referred to as definition, sharpness, resolution, or simply detail. Lack of detail is known as blur or unsharpness. The primary controlling factor of detail is motion. Motion affects recorded detail because it does not allow sufficient time for an image to form. Unwanted motion may result from voluntary processes such as patient movement or breathing, involuntary processes such as the heartbeat or intestinal peristalsis, or vibration in the equipment (Fig. 1-23).

Other factors influencing detail are the *distances* between the beam source, patient, and image receptor and the *beam source size*. X-rays obey the common laws of light and projection, so the variables critical to the projected image are the beam source diameter, the distance between the beam source and the patient, and the distance between the beam source and the image receptor. These variables are adjusted to

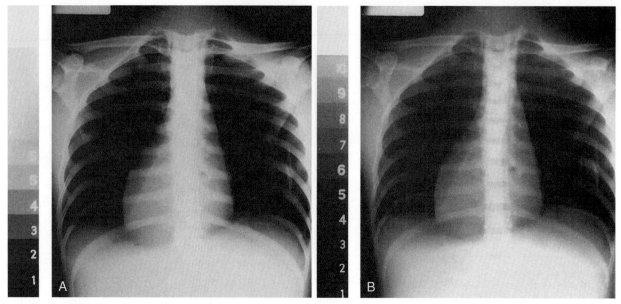

Figure 1-22 (A) High contrast, 50 kVp, 800 mA. **(B)** Low contrast, 110 kVp, 10 mA. *(From Bontrager,[15] p. 33, with permission.)*

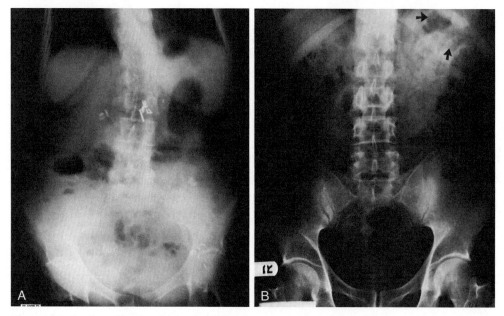

Figure 1-23 Detail can be blurred by either: **(A)** voluntary motion caused by breathing, or **(B)** involuntary motion from peristaltic action in the upper left abdomen. *(From Bontrager,[15] p. 34, with permission.)*

reduce the geometric blurring of the image as much as possible. With regard to the effect of distance on positioning, the viewer must be aware that the *closer an object is to the image receptor, the more sharply it is defined.* The chest radiograph, for example, is routinely done in a PA projection because the heart and lungs are located more anteriorly in the thorax, so this projection will place the heart and lungs closest to the image receptor. The lumbar spine, however, is routinely projected in an AP direction because this projection places the patient's spine closest to the image receptor. Additionally, the *portions* of the spine closest to the image receptor are most sharply defined, so the spinous processes are imaged with greatest clarity.

Radiographic Distortion

Radiographic distortion is the difference between the actual object being examined and its recorded image. This misrepresentation can be classified as either size or shape distortion (Fig. 1-24). Size distortion involves both elongation and foreshortening of the image. The primary factors controlling distortion are the distances between beam source, patient, and image receptor; the alignment of the body; and the position of the central ray.

With regard to distance, it has been common practice to use 40 inches as the distance between the beam source and the image receptor in most skeletal radiographs. The other

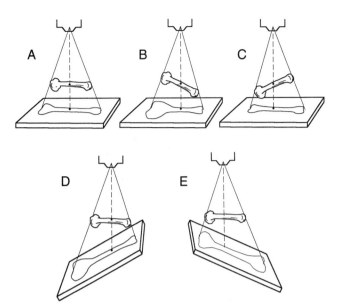

Figure 1-24 Foreshortening and magnification distortion caused by anatomic part and image receptor alignment. **(A)** Normal relationship between part and image receptor. **(B,C)** Foreshortening and magnification caused by changes in anatomic part alignment. **(D,E)** Elongation and magnification caused by changes in part/image receptor and central ray/image receptor alignment. *(From Carlton and Adler,[8] p. 422, with permission.)*

critical distance, that between the beam source and the particular structure in the patient being examined, varies. A calculation between these two distances gives the *magnification factor* of the image. Magnification is equal to the beam source–image receptor distance divided by the beam source–patient distance. This means that *the closer a structure is to the image receptor, the less magnification distortion occurs and the better the detail.* In viewing a radiograph and attempting to reconstruct the third dimension of depth perceptually, one must realize that subtle blurring and

magnification indicate that this portion of the structure is brought forward out of the plane of the radiograph, closer to the viewer, and sharp clarity indicates the portion of the structure farthest away from the viewer (Fig. 1-25).

Shape distortion results from unequal magnification of the structure being examined. The projected structure may appear *elongated*—of greater length and larger than the actual structure—*or foreshortened*—shorter than the actual structure and reduced in size (Fig. 1-26). Although adjustments are made to minimize distortion, the irregular planes of the skeleton, the distance between the skeleton and the image receptor, and the divergence of the beam always permit some degree of shape distortion to occur. The concept of beam divergence is basic to understanding how this distortion is created. Like projected light, x-rays emitted from the narrow focal spot diverge outward in straight lines to the patient and the image receptor. *Only at the central ray—the portion of the beam striking the structure and image receptor perpendicularly—is the image close to accurate.* The farther a structure is from the central ray, the greater its distortion because of increases in the angles of beam divergence. Additionally, the more inclined the structure, the greater the distortion. To diminish distortion, the radiographer centers the central ray over the area of interest and positions the body as parallel to the image receptor as possible. Correct body alignment results in less distortion and more "open" joint spaces. That is, the joint space itself is visualized and not superimposed by overlapping bone ends.

Electronic Image Processing

In the production of a radiographic image, the variables of density and contrast are adjusted as much as possible through mAs, kVp, and geometric properties to produce sufficient diagnostic detail on the radiograph. These adjustments are done prior to image acquisition. An advantage of computed or digital radiographs is that further technical alterations can be done after the radiograph is made, without having to repeat an exposure on the patient.

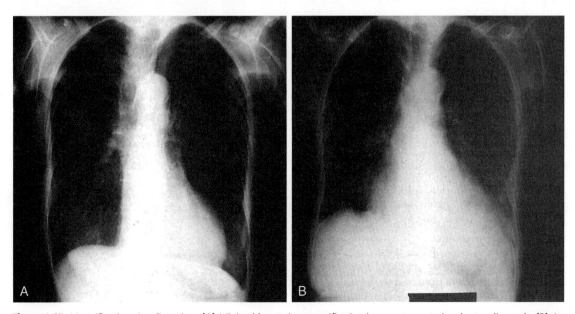

Figure 1-25 Magnification size distortion. **(A)** Minimal heart size magnification in a posteroanterior chest radiograph. **(B)** An anteroposterior projection of the same patient demonstrating greater heart size magnification. *(From Carlton and Adler,[8] p. 424, with permission.)*

CR centered

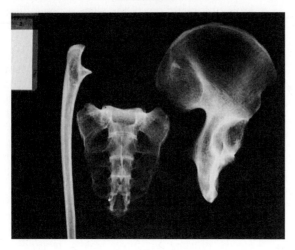

A

CR off-center to left

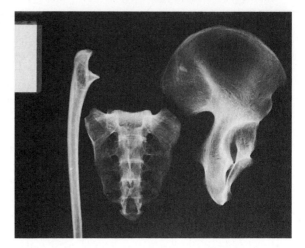

B

CR centered, but angled 25°

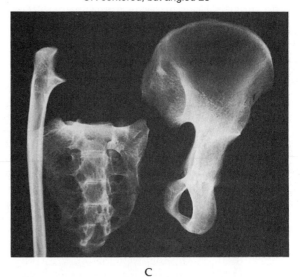

C

Figure 1-26 Shape distortion. **(A)** This radiograph was taken with a central ray perpendicular and centered to the center of the film. **(B)** This radiograph was taken with a central ray perpendicular to the film but off center to the left (away from the pelvis). The effect on distortion is not significant; however, changes in the image appearance are evident, particularly when studying the pelvis, which was farthest from the central ray. **(C)** This radiograph was taken with a central ray angle of 25 degrees and centered to the center of the film. Notice the significant distortion created by angling the central ray. *(From Carlton and Adler,[8] p. 425, with permission.)*

In general, postacquisition electronic processing is done to enhance contrast, density, and magnification. The viewer is able to alter contrast and adjust brightness to discern pathology better. The viewer is also able to magnify the image without loss of resolution (up to a maximum point).

It is interesting to recognize that the human visual range can see only 32 or fewer shades of gray. Most digital receptors are sensitive to the 1,000 shades of gray that are in the photon beam exiting the patient. The computer is able to store all 1,000 differences in density. Thus the computer can actually "see" densities beyond the range of human vision. By mathematically altering the image, the computer can bring these densities into our visual range. We can choose to display the range of densities that is most useful for us to identify specific anatomy. The range of densities displayed is described as a "window" (Fig. 1-27).

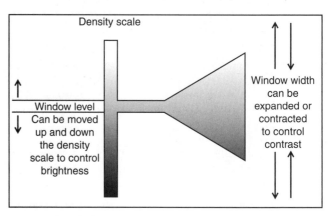

Figure 1-27 Each digital image is only a small "window" on the total data obtained by the computer. *(Adapted from Carlton and Adler,[8] p. 610.)*

Imaging windows have two parameters, which are chosen by the radiographer or radiologist to enhance diagnostic detail. The *window level* specifically controls image density. It is adjusted to the proper level to display diagnostically relevant information. There is a *direct* relationship between the window level and the image density. When the window level is increased, the image density (or darkness) also increases. Information outside the chosen window is lost from diagnosis. In some instances, then, more than one window is displayed and studied in order to visualize an appropriate range of densities fully. The *window width* controls the image contrast. There is an *inverse* relationship between window width and image contrast. A wide window *expands* the grayscale to display a large amount of data. A narrow window compresses the grayscale, which ignores a large amount of data but has the benefit of fine-detail visibility.

Although different electronic technologies presently do exist and others are in development, all share the advantages of improved image quality and the capability to improve the diagnostic utility of any study further through postacquisition processing. Postacquisition processing has reinforced the value and efficacy of conventional radiographs as the first-order diagnostic study in evaluation of the musculoskeletal system.

The Routine Radiographic Examination

When a patient is referred for radiographic assessment of an ankle, for example, the requisition or prescription form will request "ankle films," "ankle series," "ankle x-rays," "routine ankle films," "basic ankle views," or some similar phrase. Although all these phrases are different, they convey the same idea—that a radiographic examination of the ankle is requested to screen for possible abnormalities. Despite the variety of ways to ask for these radiographs, and the variety of patient complaints that instigate the need for radiographic assessment, the same initial radiographs will be made. In other words, the patient will receive a *routine radiographic examination*. The purpose of a routine (also called a *standard* or *basic*) examination is to provide the most visualization of anatomy with the least number of radiographs and thus to expose the patient to minimal radiation.

Routine radiographs serve as a basic assessment tool and screen for a significant portion of pathologies. The results of the routine radiographic examination may be one of the following:

1. *Positive* for the suspected clinical diagnosis, and thus serving to direct appropriate treatment
2. *Negative* for the suspected clinical diagnosis, thus directing appropriate treatment
3. *Negative* for one diagnosis but raising the index of suspicion for another diagnosis
4. *Inconclusive* requiring additional imaging to confirm or rule out a suspected diagnosis
5. *Wrong*

The possibility always exists for false positives, false negatives, the presence of early disease processes that do not show radiographic density changes until later stages, or errors in reader interpretation.

For example, consider the patient who is referred for radiographs of the ankle. The patient's chief complaint is chronic ankle pain. The clinician suspects either a soft tissue strain or some kind of bony involvement, such as a stress fracture, bone bruise, or degenerative arthritis. The radiographic examination is necessary to narrow the diagnostic possibilities and assist in determining correct treatment choices. The following are some possible scenarios, constructed to illustrate the potential outcomes of the initial routine radiographic examination:

1. *Positive for the suspected diagnosis:* The radiographs are positive for a stress fracture. No further imaging is needed. The ankle is immobilized, and the patient is instructed to return for follow-up radiographs in 4 weeks.
2. *Negative for the suspected diagnosis:* The radiographs are negative for fracture, pathology, and degenerative changes. No further imaging is needed. The patient is referred to physical therapy for conservative treatment.
3. *Negative for one diagnosis but raising the index of suspicion for another diagnosis:* The radiographs are negative for fracture and degenerative changes, but a radiolucent lesion characteristic of infection or osteonecrosis is identified. The patient is referred for an MRI and blood work.
4. *Inconclusive, requiring additional imaging:* The radiographs appear normal except for an inconclusive finding—is an this an avulsion fracture or a normal accessory ossicle? The radiologist recommends a CT exam.
5. *Wrong:* The routine films are negative for fracture or pathology. The patient undergoes physical therapy without improvement. The patient is reassessed with radiographs 1 month later. A stress fracture at the talar neck with diffuse talar osteonecrosis is now diagnosed. The patient is referred to orthopedics.

In the first four scenarios, the routine radiographic examination served its purpose by either defining a diagnosis, ruling out other diagnoses, or indicating a need for further workup. In the last scenario we are reminded of the limitations of the routine radiographic examination (or, in fact, of any diagnostic study). *If the results of any imaging studies do not fit the clinical symptoms, reassessment of the problem is needed.* This may include formulating a new differential diagnosis or utilizing other diagnostic tests.

The Radiologist as the Imaging Specialist[2,20,23]

Advancements in imaging technology, combined with widespread availability of advanced imaging modalities, has greatly expanded the armamentarium of the radiologist. The sometimes difficult process of diagnosis has been greatly facilitated by these advances. However, this rapid progress has made the determination of the *best* imaging diagnostic protocol for an individual patient increasingly complex. More than one imaging modality may be sensitive for a proposed diagnosis. The Americal College of Radiology provides evidence-based, clinical practice guidelines in the form of *appropriateness criteria* ratings for choices of imaging specific to pathology.[23] However, oftentimes, more than one imaging modality is given the same rating—that is, more than one modality can further the diagnostic process (Table 1-7).

Other factors must also be considered along with a pathology-specific sensitivity. Each imaging study will differ in tissue-specific sensitivity, structural clarity, radiation exposure, invasiveness, risk, and cost (Table 1-8). Thus, the

choice of imaging study and the *sequence* in which additional imaging studies are performed are critical to efficiently obtaining a comprehensive diagnosis, without redundant or extraneous studies being performed and with responsible awareness of the cost burden.

This modern and evolving situation of technological affluence continues to underscore the importance of (1) *the radiologist as the imaging specialist* who directs the diagnostic investigation in the most efficient manner and (2) *the place of conventional radiography* in the diagnostic investigation.

To paraphrase Adam Greenspan,[2] these are the objectives of the musculoskeletal radiologist:

1. To diagnose an *unknown* musculoskeletal disorder with *conventional radiography* before using advanced modalities, which are subsequently used only if conventional radiography is inconclusive.
2. To perform examinations in the proper sequence and know what to do next in the radiologic investigation.
3. To demonstrate the radiologic features of a known disorder, the distribution of the lesion in the skeleton, and its location in the bone.
4. To be aware of what specific information is important to the orthopedic surgeon.
5. To recognize the limits of noninvasive radiologic investigation and know when to proceed with invasive techniques.
6. To recognize lesions that require biopsy and those that do not ("don't touch" lesions).
7. To assume an active role in therapeutic management, such as performing image-guided procedures or interventional techniques.

Finally, two critical points must be stated for those clinicians involved in the patient's care. First, it is important that the radiologist is provided with sufficient patient history, clinical signs and symptoms, and results of other medical testing to direct an efficient diagnostic investigation. Second, the role of the radiologist and other health-care clinicians will never be minimized or rendered obsolete by the sophistication of modern imaging modalities. Technology is not infallible; false-negative and false-positive results do and will occur. *It is the clinician's responsibility to recognize that if the results of any imaging study do not fit the physical findings, further clinical evaluation and diagnostic investigation are warranted.*

Other Common Studies in Musculoskeletal Imaging[2,12–15,21]

Imaging studies can be grouped into two general categories: conventional radiography and related studies and advanced imaging. The category of conventional radiography includes contrast-enhanced radiographs and conventional tomography. These studies are modifications of basic x-ray technology. The broad category of advanced imaging includes different technologies. The development of these advanced modalities is interrelated with developments in computer science.

TABLE 1-7 ● *American College of Radiology Appropriateness Criteria*

Clinical Condition: Shoulder Pain

Radiologic Exam or Procedure	Appropriateness Rating	Comment
Variant 1: Acute trauma. Rule out fracture or dislocation		
X-ray, shoulder, AP external rotation and AP internal rotation views	9	
X-ray, shoulder, axillary, later, and/or scapular Y views	9	
CT, shoulder	1	
MRI, shoulder	1	
Arthrogram, shoulder	1	
Variant 2: Subacute pain. Rule out rotator cuff tear/impingement; radiographs normal.		
MRI, shoulder, routine	9	
US, shoulder	7	With appropriate expertise
Arthrogram, shoulder, with or without CT	5	If patient cannot have MRI or US expertise not available
CT, shoulder	1	
MRI, arthrogram	1	

Appropriateness criteria scale 1–9, with 1 = least appropriate and 9 = most appropriate. Available at http://www.acr.org. Updated 2008.

TABLE 1-8 ● *Comparison of Cost and Radiation Dose of Various Diagnostic Imaging Studies of the Lumbar Spine*

Examination	Average Combined Costs of Facility and Professional (Radiologist) Charges	Average Radiation Dose
Conventional radiographs (five views)	$450	2,000–3,000 mrad
Myelography	$1,200	2,000–3,000 mrad
Conventional tomography	$800	8,000–10,000 mrad
Computed tomography	$2,000	2,000–4,000 mrad
Magnetic resonance imaging	$3,000	No radiation dose
Bone scan, whole skeleton	$1,400	700 mrad

Average costs, in U.S. dollars, 2009.

Contrast-Enhanced Radiographs

In contrast-enhanced radiography a *contrast medium* (or simply, the *contrast*) is injected or ingested into the body before a radiograph is taken. The purpose of contrast-enhanced studies is to improve visualization by increasing radiographic contrast in areas with minimal inherent contrast. Contrast media may be radiolucent (*negative contrast,* such as air), radiopaque (*positive contrast,* such as barium sulfate or iodide solutions), or a combination of the two (*dual contrast,* such as barium sulfate plus air; see Fig. 1-9). Depending on the purpose of the study, images may be recorded as static radiographs, monitored by fluoroscopy, or recorded as moving images.

Contrast media studies are commonly used in all areas of medicine. Examples include *angiography*—the injection of contrast into the blood supply of an organ to demonstrate obstructions or other abnormalities—and *arteriography*—the injection of contrast into a specific artery to demonstrate blood flow. Numerous other contrast studies, specific

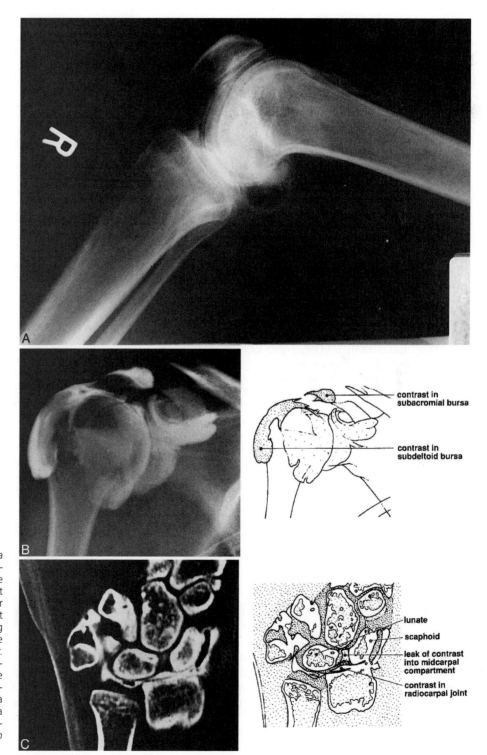

Figure 1-28 Examples of *contrast media* studies of synovial joints. **(A)** Negative-contrast study of the knee. Note that the full extent of the capsule is illustrated as it is distended with contrast. **(B)** Shoulder arthrogram. After injection of contrast into the glenohumeral joint, there is filling of the subacromial-subdeltoid bursae complex, indicating rotator cuff tear. *(From Greenspan,[2] p. 2.5, with permission.)* **(C)** Coronal CT arthrogram of the wrist demonstrates a subtle leak of contrast from the radiocarpal joint through a tear in the scapholunate ligament, a finding not detected on routine arthrographic examination of the wrist. *(From Greenspan,[2] p. 2.6, with permission.)*

contrast in subacromial bursa

contrast in subdeltoid bursa

lunate

scaphoid

leak of contrast into midcarpal compartment

contrast in radiocarpal joint

to each organ, exist, such as the *barium swallow* studies of the upper gastrointestinal system to evaluate dysphagia; *cholecystography* of the gallbladder; *sialography* of the salivary glands; *sinographs* of the sinus tracts; and *urograms, pyelograms,* and *cystograms* of the kidneys and bladder. All contrast media studies are invasive and thus carry an amount of risk to the patient. Some contrast studies have been replaced by noninvasive studies such as CT, MRI, and ultrasound (US).

Examples of contrast media studies utilized in musculoskeletal radiology are *arthrography* and *myelography.*

Arthrography

Arthrography is a contrast media study of a joint and its soft tissue structures. Contrast material is injected into the joint space, distending the capsule and outlining internal tissues (Fig. 1-28). Arthrography can effectively demonstrates abnormalities of the synovium, soft tissues, articular cartilage, and capsule of the joint.

A limitation of arthrography is that the images are not multiplanar and may vary in clarity of anatomic detail. However, arthrography can also be used in conjunction with other advanced imaging modalities to provide more information than is possible with a single modality. Examples of this include *arthrotomography (arthrography combined with tomography), CT arthrography (arthrography combined with CT), MR arthrography (arthrography combined with MRI),* and *digital subtraction arthrography (subtract the digitally acquired preinjection image).*

Myelography

Myelography is a contrast media study of the spinal cord, nerve root, and dura mater (Fig. 1-29). Contrast is injected into the subarachnoid space and mixes with the cerebrospinal fluid to produce a column of radiopaque fluid. The puncture site is usually at L2–L3 or L3–L4 for the lumbar exam, and C1–C2 for the cervical exam. The fluoroscopic table on which the patient is positioned is tilted until the contrast flows under the influence of gravity to the specific spinal level being evaluated. Images are recorded via static radiographs.

It is common to perform a CT scan while the contrast is still localized in order to visualize greater anatomic detail in cross section. This combination of modalities is referred to as a *CT myelogram.* Abnormal results of a myelogram may reveal a ruptured intervertebral disk, spinal cord compression, spinal stenosis, intravertebral tumor, obstruction in the spinal canal, or nerve root injury.

Conventional Tomography

Conventional tomography, also known as *body section radiography,* is the radiographic evaluation of one predetermined plane of the body (Fig. 1-30). This is accomplished by accessory equipment that allows the x-ray tube and film to move about a fulcrum point during a film exposure. The plane of the body that is level with the fulcrum will be in focus, with the rest of the body blurred by motion. Various *depths* of planes are imaged by preadjusting the fulcrum. The

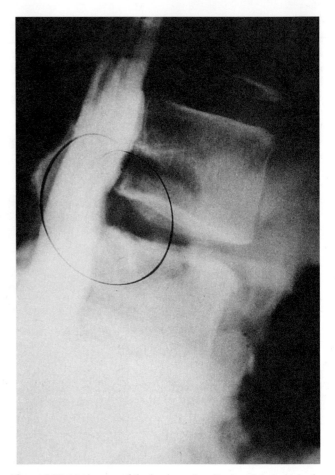

Figure 1-29 Myelogram of the lumbar spine. Contrast injected into the subarachnoid space mixes with cerebrospinal fluid to produce a column of radiopaque fluid. The *herniated disk* at L4–L5 protrudes posteriorly and causes an indentation of the column.

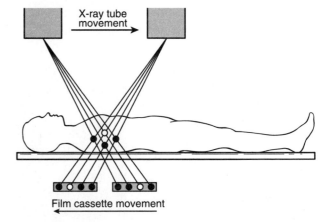

Figure 1-30 Principle of conventional tomography. The x-ray tube and the film move in opposite directions. The focal point (open circle) remains in sharp focus, whereas the other planes of the body (dark circles) are blurred by motion.

simplest tomography units use linear movement of the equipment; newly developed tomographic units employ multidirectional or trispiral movement of the x-ray tube. This allows for more uniform blurring of undesired structures and precise localization of lesions as small as 1 mm.

A major clinical application of tomography is in the evaluation of fractures (Fig. 1-31). Fractures of irregularly shaped bones such as the skull, the tibial plateau of the knee, or the cervical vertebrae may be difficult to visualize on plain films because of the depth of the structure or the amount of superimposition of adjacent structures. By imaging different depths of the bone, the extent of the fracture line can be determined. Additionally, tomography is used to assess healing of fractures. Whereas signs of healing may be obliterated on plain films by metallic fixation devices or callus formation, tomography can image *under* these obstructions. Other clinical applications include evaluating the extent of tumors within bone (Fig. 1-32).

A limitation of conventional tomography is that it cannot enhance detail; it is a process of controlled blurring. Patient and equipment motion variables can easily alter the image quality. Other disadvantages are insufficient soft tissue detail, difficulty in positioning a traumatized patient for various angles of projection, and high radiation doses. For these reasons, conventional tomography has, in many areas of clinical practice, been replaced by CT and MRI.

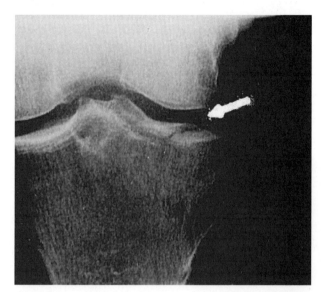

Figure 1-31 Tomogram of the knee. The arrow points to a tibial plateau fracture.

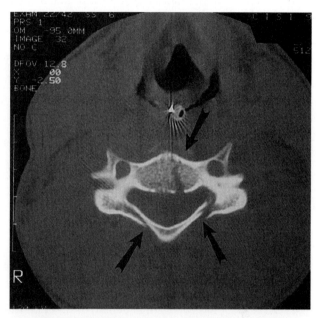

Figure 1-33 CT scan of fifth cervical vertebra. This axial view of C5 demonstrates a burst fracture of the vertebral body and both laminae.

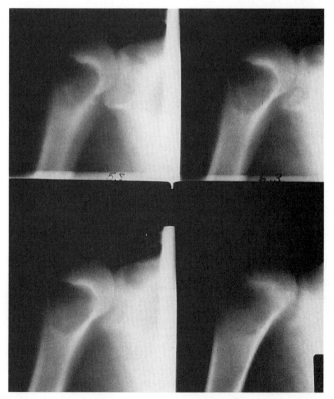

Figure 1-32 Tomograms of the shoulder. The extent of this chondroblastoma of the proximal humerus of a 15-year-old girl is evaluated by imaging successive depths through the bone. Numbers marked on the films (e.g., 5.8, 6.3) refer to millimeters of depth.

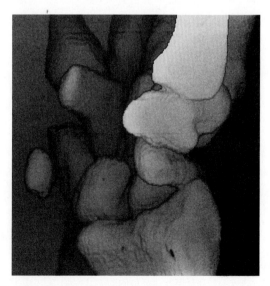

Figure 1-34 Three-dimensional CT reformation of the wrist. This oblique view of the wrist demonstrates a fracture through the waist of the scaphoid bone, complicated by avascular necrosis of the proximal fragment. *(From Greenspan,[2] p. 2.4, with permission.)*

Computed Tomography

Computed tomography (CT) merges x-ray technology with that of the computer. In CT, the x-ray beam and detector system is housed in a circular scanner and moves through an arc around the patient. The computer mathematically reconstructs an image based on the geometric plots where the measurements were taken. The shades of gray on a CT image are assigned by the computer to be specific to each tissue's exact radiation absorption properties. Thus CT identifies body structures with much greater sensitivity than conventional radiographs can.

Each image represents an axial cross-sectional slice of the body measuring 0.1 to 1.5 cm thick (Fig. 1-33). Additionally, computer software can reconstruct data obtained in the axial plane and reformat it to sagittal or coronal planes, or three dimensional images (Fig. 1-34).

CT is valuable in the evaluation of bone and soft-tissue tumors, subtle or complex fractures, intra-articular abnormalities, the detection of small bone fragments, and quantitative bone mineral analysis (important in the management of metabolic bone disorders). A disadvantage of CT is the *average volume effect*, which refers to the computer applying average values to a small volume of tissue and thus displaying it in one shade of gray even though it contains more than one type of tissue. This becomes important when normal and pathologic processes interface within a tissue (Fig. 1-35). See Chapter 4 for more on CT.

Nuclear Imaging

Nuclear medicine is a specialty that uses *radiopharmaceuticals* for diagnosis, therapy, and research. While most radiologic procedures diagnose disease based on the *structural*

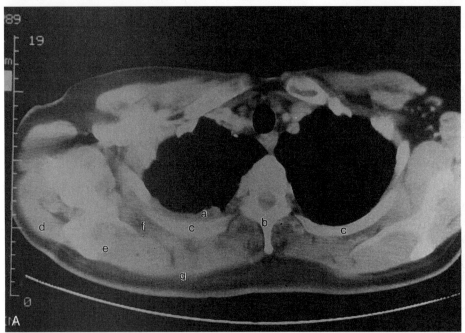

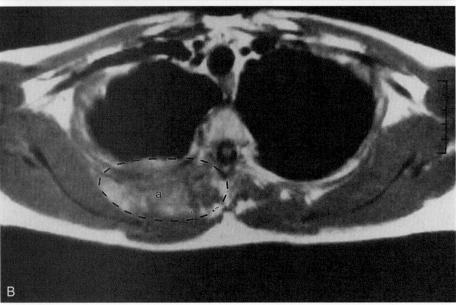

Figure 1-35 (A) Transverse axial CT image at the level of the fourth thoracic vertebra. The patient was a retired coal miner. Note pleural thickening caused by occupational hazards in the left lung (a). The patient's chief complaint was left scapular and radiating left upper extremity pain. This image is negative for pathological disease. See Figure 1-36B for further evaluation results. Note (b) vertebral spinous process, (c) rib, (d) infraspinatus muscle, (e) supraspinatus muscle, (f) subscapularis muscle, (g) trapezius. *(From Richardson and Iglarsh,[16] p. 685, with permission.)* **(B)** Transverse axial MRI at the level of the fourth thoracic vertebra. Note the large expanse of *lung tumor* invading the subscapularis muscle (a). This tumor was not detectable on the CT scan of the same patient in Figure 1-36A. *(From Richardson and Iglarsh,[16] p. 685, with permission.)*

changes of anatomy, nuclear imaging studies diagnose disease based on the *physiological* or *functional* changes of the tissue or organ.

Radiopharmaceuticals are made up of two parts—the pharmaceutical, which is targeted to a specific organ, and the radionuclide, which emits gamma rays. *Technetium-99m* (^{99m}Tc) is the radionuclide used in most nuclear imaging. The radiopharmaceuticals, also known as radioactive *tracers,* are introduced into the body via injection, ingestion, or inhalation. These tracers are absorbed by the specific organ in varying amounts, based on the levels of metabolic activity within the tissue. Pathologies or other changes in metabolism are identified by variations in the uptake of the tracer. The gamma rays emitted from the patient's body are detected by a *gamma* or *scintillation camera,* which transforms the rays into images that are recorded on the computer or film.

Methods of Imaging

Several methods of imaging are used in nuclear imaging. These include the following:

- *Static imaging (planar imaging).* A single "snapshot" images the distribution of the tracer within a part of the body. AP, lateral, and obliques images are often obtained. Examples include bone scan images, lung scans, and thyroid scans.
- *Whole-body imaging.* An entire anterior or posterior image of the body is made by passing the gamma camera over the body. Whole-body imaging is used primarily in bone scans.
- *Dynamic imaging.* Images are acquired in a timed sequence to display the flow of the tracer in an organ. This type of imaging is used in cardiac, hepatobiliary, and gastric studies.
- *Single photon emission computed tomography (SPECT).* This three-dimensional imaging technique produces thin slices of images similar to CT. Data can be reconstructed by the computer in multiple planes and several formats. SPECT has revolutionized nuclear medicine by increasing sensitivity, specificity, and ability to localize small abnormalities. It is used to study bone, cardiac perfusion (as in the thallium stress test), the brain, and the liver.
- *Positron emission tomography (PET).* These unique images are acquired by measuring positron emissions from tracers made from the basic elements of biological substances. The predominant tracer used is *fluorodeoxyglucose (FDG),* a glucose analogue. FDG is metabolized similarly to the naturally occurring glucose without altering metabolic equilibrium. This permits visualization of normal and abnormal biological function of cells. PET can image metabolism at a molecular level not possible with other nuclear studies. It is used in cardiology to study blood flow and perfusion, in neurology to study dementias and diseases of the central nervous system, and in oncology to detect and stage tumors.
- *PET/CT and SPECT/CT.* Images can be acquired by coupling the functional imaging capabilities of SPECT or PET with the excellent anatomical imaging of CT. Images from each modality are coregistered during the image

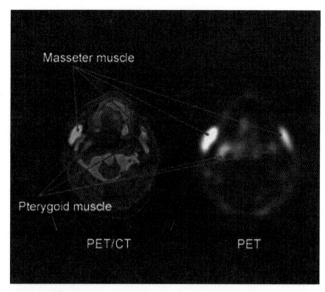

Figure 1-36 PET/CT scan, axial view at C1–C2. On the right is the PET scan; on the left is the combined PET/CT scan. Note an incidental but interesting teaching point: The patient was chewing bubblegum during injection and distribution of FDG. Note the physiological increased uptake in the muscles of mastication. As seen in this patient, the uptake is asymmetric because he habitually chews harder on one side of the mouth; those muscles are metabolizing glucose at a greater rate. *(Image courtesy of GE Healthcare at http://www.medcyclopaedia.com.)*

acquisition process, requiring the patient to undergo only one procedure (Fig. 1-36). The improved ability to localize lesions from CT enhances the diagnostic interpretation of the PET or SPECT images.

Radionuclide Bone Scan

Nuclear imaging of the skeleton is referred to as a bone scan or bone scintigraphy. Radiopharmaceuticals concentrate differently in normal versus pathological bone. Information is gained by viewing where and how much the radiopharmaceuticals have concentrated in the body. Abnormal conditions generally show an *increased* uptake of the radiopharmaceuticals and image as black areas or *"hot spots"* on the scan. Normal bone appears transparent and gray, with the exception of some structures that under normal conditions do show increased uptake (such as the growth plates in children or the sacroiliac joints). In general, a bone scan designates areas of *hyperfunction,* or *increased mineral turnover* (Fig. 1-37).

A bone scan is best described as a sensitivity test, an early indicator of increased bone activity. Bone scans are most valuable in confirming the presence of disease and demonstrating the distribution of disease in the skeleton. Indications for bone scans include the evaluation of subtle fractures, primary and metastatic tumors, various arthritides, infections, avascular necrosis, metabolic bone disease, or any *unexplained bone pain.*

The major limitation of bone scans is the lack of specificity in the differential diagnosis of disease. It is not possible to distinguish among the various processes that can cause increased uptake. Thus, a bone scan is not useful as

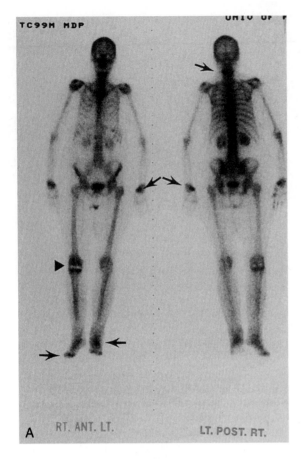

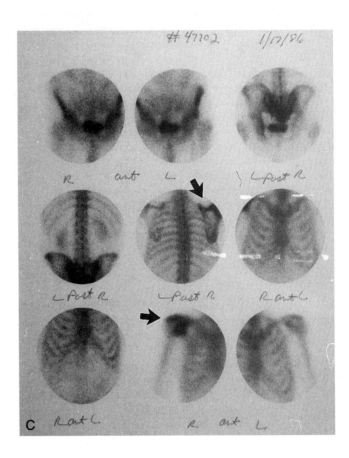

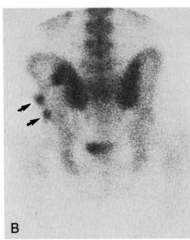

Figure 1-37 (A) Whole-skeleton bone scan. Diagnosis for this patient was degenerative joint disease in multiple sites (see arrows indicating increased uptake in the cervical spine, wrist, ankle, and toes). The arrowhead indicates a total joint prosthesis at the knee. **(B)** Bone scan of the pelvis. This patient suffered a contusion to the gluteus medius muscle during injury in a football game. In this case the increased uptake was an early indication of myositis ossificans developing in the muscle. *(From Richardson and Iglarsh,[16] p. 684, with permission.)* **(C)** This bone scan shows increased uptake at the right scapula and right shoulder area. In this case these findings demonstrated metastatic bone cancer. *(From Richardson and Iglarsh,[16] p. 646, with permission.)*

an independent study; rather, the results of other clinical evaluations are correlated with the bone scan to determine a diagnosis.

Magnetic Resonance Imaging

Magnetic resonance imaging (MRI) does not involve ionizing radiation; it produces information via the interaction of tissue with radio frequency waves in a magnetic field. The image obtained is based on a patient's re-emission of absorbed radio frequencies while in the magnetic field.

These images are reformatted to axial, sagittal, and coronal planes for viewing.

The musculoskeletal system is ideally suited to evaluation by MRI. The signal intensities from bone, muscle, articular cartilage, fibrocartilage, ligaments, tendons, vessels, nerves, and fat differ sufficiently to create high-quality images of anatomy. Additionally, pathological changes in different tissues can be highlighted through contrast manipulation. Thus, major uses of MRI in musculoskeletal radiology are in the evaluation of soft tissue trauma, internal joint derangement, and tumors (Fig. 1-38). See Chapter 5 for more on MRI.

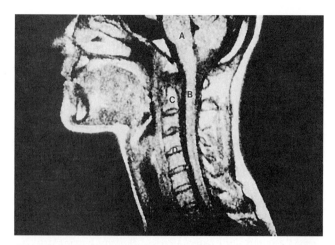

Figure 1-38 Magnetic resonance image of the cervical spine, sagittal view. No pathology is evident. Note pons **(A)**, spinal cord **(B)**, marrow of C2 vertebral body and dens **(C)**, and intervertebral disk of C4–C5 **(D)**.

Ultrasonography

Ultrasonography is the generation of anatomic images using reflected sound waves. As such, it is noninvasive and nonionizing. Images are based on the characteristics of tissue absorption of sound waves and reflection of sound waves at the interfaces between tissues of different acoustic qualities.

Although diagnostic ultrasound is well known for its use in obstetrics and abdominal evaluation, there is a growing interest in its use for the musculoskeletal system. Ultrasound is excellent for the diagnosis of lesions to muscles, tendons, and ligaments as well as the detection of cysts, soft tissue tumors, and the measurement of blood flow. A distinct advantage to ultrasound is that images can be made *during* the physical examination of tissues, such as during active muscle contractions, passive stretching, or traction, facilitating the detection of lesions. See Chapter 6 for more on ultrasound.

Interventional Techniques[24–28]

Interventional radiology (IR), also known as invasive or surgical radiology, is a subspecialty of diagnostic radiology in which radiologists diagnose and treat disease nonoperatively. Catheters, guide wires, needles, cannulas, balloons, stents, and other devices are placed under the guidance of imaging to perform procedures that are often alternatives to surgery. Fluoroscopy has been the most common modality used in IR since its origins over 50 years ago. Later developments in ultrasound and CT enabled more procedural advancements. More recently, MRI has been found to offer unique features that make it suitable for interventional purposes. These include no ionizing radiation to the patient or radiologist, identification of vascular structures without the need for contrast, and multiplanar imaging for three-dimensional localization of lesions and navigational control of instruments. Further development of MRI-compatible devices and equipment both inside and outside the magnetic field will advance the utility of MRI for IR.

Interventional procedures can be grouped into vascular and nonvascular procedures. Vascular procedures include angioplasty, vascular stenting, embolization, thrombolysis,

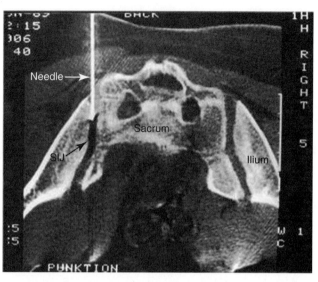

Figure 1-39 CT, axial view of bilateral sacroiliac joints. The patient is prone for this interventional procedure. The needle tip is in the left iliosacral joint space, ready for aspiration. Note the increased blackness in this joint space compared to the contralateral side, indicating the presence of fluid. *(Image courtesy of GE Healthcare at http://www.medcyclopaedia.com.)*

venous access, chemotherapy infusion, and vena cava filter placement. Nonvascular procedures include biopsies of lesions, abscess drainage, joint aspiration, abatement of pain, and screw placement (Fig. 1-39). Descriptions of some common IR procedures for the musculoskeletal system follow.

Epidural Steroid Injections

Epidural steroid injections of anesthetic and steroid medications are used to relieve pain in patients with spinal stenosis, disk herniation, or intractable neck or back pain of uncertain etiology by decreasing nerve root inflammation and swelling at the nerve–disk interface. This treatment may also help to delay or avoid surgical intervention and may give relief to patients who are not surgical candidates.

Prior to the procedure, all imaging studies of the spine are reviewed, with special attention to the level of the thecal sac in the sacrum for the sacral approach, the C7–T1 level for the cervical approach, and the size of the specific intralaminar spaces. Epidural injections may be administered at the sacral hiatus, at a lumbar interlaminar level, or at the C7–T1 interlaminar level. A local anesthetic is administered, first under the skin and then at the level of the periosteum. Under imaging guidance a needle is advanced into the epidural space, and its position is verified by injecting a small amount of contrast medium.

Spinal Nerve Blocks

Spinal nerve blocks can be used for therapeutic or diagnostic purposes. Diagnostically, these procedures are helpful in identifying the source of radicular pain, especially when prior imaging is inconclusive. After a nerve or joint is identified as the source of pain by "blocking" its transmission of pain via administration of an anesthetic to it, therapeutic steroids are then administered. Other techniques, such as radiofrequency ablation, may be considered for refractory cases. The four major types of nerve blocks include indirect, direct, facet joint, and common sympathetic nerve blocks.

Indirect nerve blocks are the epidural nerve blocks just described. In direct nerve root blocks, anesthetics are administered to the postganglionic portion of the nerve root sheath through a neural foramen. Facet joint nerve blocks are administered directly into a specific facet joint capsule or the sacroiliac joint. Common sympathetic nerve blocks include stellate ganglion blockade, celiac plexus blockade, lumbar sympathetic blockade, and impar ganglion (between the sacrum and the coccyx) blockade. These are usually performed for relief of intractable pain. All of these procedures include image-guided needle placement with contrast medium verification.

Radiofrequency Ablation

Radiofrequency ablation (RFA) is the selective destruction of nerve tissue to treat chronic pain disorders. This extreme treatment is preceded by diagnostic/prognostic nerve blocks to identify the spinal segment involved and to assess the potential benefit from the long-term resultant neurolysis. In general, the procedure involves thermal ablation from radio waves applied to the nerve via placement of a needle electrode under imaging guidance. Specific procedures include denervation of the medial branch of the posterior rami of the spinal nerve to treat cervical or lumbar facet joint arthropathy, denervation of the dorsal root ganglion for radiculitis or peripheral nerve lesions, and denervation of the stellate ganglion or sympathetic chain for complex regional pain syndrome, circulatory insufficiency, and hyperhidrosis.

RFA is also used in treating painful osseous metastases. Pain relief is thought to be due to destruction of secondary tumor cells and the effect of reducing tumor size, surrounding inflammatory reaction, and periosteal tension.

Discography

Discography is a method of correlating a patient's neck or back pain to internal disk morphology. Despite its controversial history, most agree that it remains the only imaging technique that provides both functional and anatomic information about a diseased disk and should be reserved for patients whose symptoms cannot be explained by noninvasive imaging.[26]

The process consists of placement of a needle into a disk, followed by injection of a small amount of contrast medium. A positive pain response that re-creates the patient's symptoms incriminates the disk as the source of pain.

Percutaneous Needle Biopsy of the Spine

Biopsy of spinal lesions is accomplished using imaging guidance and a system of needles and cannulas. Patients referred for biopsy often present with a chief complaint of back pain

and a lesion identified on prior imaging studies. Specific indications are focal vertebral column lesions, identification of the underlying pathology in a new fracture, malignant-appearing lesions, suspected osteomyelitis or discitis, and isolation of a suspected pathological organism.

Percutaneous Vertebroplasty, Kyphoplasty, and Cementoplasty

Percutaneous *vertebroplasty* is the image-guided injection of bone cement (methyl methacrylate) into the vertebral body to relieve intractable pain in patients with osteoporotic compression fractures, malignant vertebral destruction, aggressive hemangioma, benign tumors, or vertebral fracture associated with osteonecrosis. *Balloon kyphoplasty* is a similar treatment. Prior to the injection of bone cement, a balloon is inserted into the vertebra, inflated to restore vertebral body height, and then removed. The cement is injected to fill the space created by the balloon. Contraindications include the presence of infection, acute traumatic fracture, coagulopathy, radiculopathy, cord compression, or complete vertebral collapse.

Percutaneous *cementoplasty* is derived from vertebroplasty techniques. It is used primarily as a palliative treatment in cancer patients whose poor medical condition precludes surgery. Indications include osteolytic (bone-destroying) lesions at risk for fracture, unstable lesions that prevent weight-bearing, or painful lesions resistant to radiation or chemotherapy. Injection of cement into a fragile lesion consolidates it, which provides the structural strength to allow the patients to resume functional activities.

Automated Percutaneous Lumbar Diskectomy

Automated percutaneous diskectomy is performed with a specially designed probe that excises small pieces of nuclear material and removes them with aspiration. This procedure is used on individuals who have diagnostic evidence of an uncomplicated herniation contained within the annulus, symptoms of intractable discogenic or unilateral radicular pain, and failed conservative treatment. Relief is accomplished by internal decompression of the intervertebral disk. Contraindications include sequestered disk fragment, significant degenerative disease, spondylitic disease, spinal stenosis, and segmental instability.

Intradiscal Electrothermal Therapy

Intradiscal electrothermal therapy (IDET) is a minimally invasive procedure used to manage discogenic low back pain in patients who have not responded to conservative measures. IDET uses image-guided intradiscal delivery of thermal energy to the disk annular structure. Shrinking the disk substance in this manner purportedly promotes annular healing and granulation and also coagulates nerve tissue in the annulus to reduce pain. Contraindications include nerve root compression, extruded disk fragment, active infection, bleeding disorder, or severe degenerative disk disease. The efficacy of IDET has not been widely assessed in clinical trials, although initial studies show pain relief in patients with chronic unremitting low back pain.[27]

The Imaging Chain

The field of diagnostic radiology can only become more fascinating as the fusion of computer technology to radiography continues to evolve. The intersection of diagnostic radiology with rehabilitation can only produce more possibilities to enhance both patient evaluation and research in dynamic function and human movement.

The general principles of radiology covered in this chapter serve, we hope, as a foundation for the rehabilitationist to travel to unexplored areas in patient care. Along the journey, it is wise to remember the following:

1. *Humans play an important role in any imaging system.* A sophisticated imaging technology can be wasted by using an observer who cannot extract relevant diagnostic information from the image, whereas a relatively simpler technology may be adequate if the observer has the expertise to extract the required information from the image.
2. *Clinicians must always discriminate between imaging as a tool versus an answer.* The clinician bears the responsibility always to recognize that if the results of any

imaging study do not fit the physical findings, further clinical evaluation and diagnostic investigation are warranted.
3. *Imaging systems are only one link in a larger chain that starts and ends with the patient* (Fig. 1-40). Focusing on the characteristics of any technology should not distract us from the real reason we use imaging: *to achieve an optimal patient outcome.*

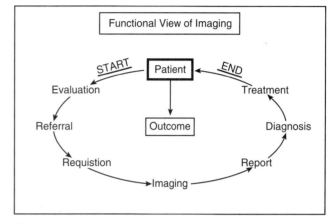

Figure 1-40 Diagnostic imaging is one link in a larger chain that starts and ends with the patient.

Summary of Key Points

1. Physical therapists and other clinicians involved in direct patient care will find it useful to study radiology to make their evaluation of the patient more comprehensive and to gather information from the image that may not be discussed on the radiologic report.

2. A radiograph is a recorded image of an anatomic part acquired by the passage of x-rays through the body. A conventional radiograph is a radiograph made without contrast enhancement or other equipment modification.

3. The conventional radiograph is generally the first diagnostic study to be done following the clinical examination. Conventional radiographs are the most efficient means of demonstrating a bone or joint abnormality.

4. The basic components of x-ray technology are the x-ray tube and the image receptor.

5. Three categories of image receptors used to capture the x-ray image are film/screen, fluoroscopy, and digital.

6. The shade of gray at any point in the image on the radiograph represents the sum of the radiodensities of the structures that the x-ray beam has passed through to reach that point. Radiodensity is determined by a structure's material composition and its thickness.

7. The tissues in the human body fall into four radiodensity categories: air, fat, water, and bone. Identification of anatomy is based on the contrast between these different densities.

8. An inverse relationship exists between the amount of radiodensity (absorption of x-rays) of an object and the radiographic density (amount of blackening) on film. Air images the blackest. Fat, water, and bone image in progressively lighter shades of gray. Contrast media such as barium image in bright white outline, and heavy metals image solidly white.

9. At least two images, as close to 90 degrees to each other as possible, are required to view all three dimensions of a structure. Remember the adage "one view is no view."

10. A routine radiographic examination evaluates a body segment via a standardized selection of positions and projections chosen to provide the greatest visualization with minimal radiation exposure. AP, lateral, and oblique projections compose most routine series.

11. The results of the routine radiographic examination direct treatment or nontreatment of the patient or serve as a departure point for additional studies that may be necessary to complete the diagnosis.

12. The quality of a radiograph is evaluated by four image quality factors: density, contrast, detail, and distortion.

13. The radiologist first attempts to diagnose unknown musculoskeletal disorders with the techniques of conventional radiography before employing more invasive or costlier advanced imaging techniques.

14. Interventional radiology is a subspecialty of radiology in which disease is diagnosed and treated nonoperatively.

15. Humans play a critical role in the imaging system by their interpretation of the image and by their correlation of clinical findings with imaging information. The clinician's responsibility is to recognize always that if the results of any imaging study do not fit the physical findings, further clinical evaluation and diagnostic investigation are warranted.

References

1. Venes, D (ed): Taber's Cyclopedic Medical Dictionary, ed. 20. FA Davis, Philadelphia, 2005.
2. Greenspan, A: Orthopedic Radiology: A Practical Approach, ed. 4. Lippincott Williams & Wilkins, Philadelphia, 2004.
3. Pflaum, R: Grand Obsession: Marie Curie and Her World. Doubleday, New York, 1989.
4. Goldsmith, B: Obsessive Genius: The Inner World of Marie Curie. WW Norton, New York, 2005.
5. Mould, RF: Century of X-rays and Radioactivity in Medicine. Institute of Physics Publishing, Bristol, England, 1994.
6. Thomas, A, and Isherwood, I (eds): Invisible Light: 100 Years of Medical Radiology. Blackwell Publishers, Oxford, England, 1995.
7. Adler, A, and Carlton, R: Introduction to Radiologic Sciences and Patient Care, ed. 4. WB Saunders, Philadelphia, 2007.
8. Carlton, R, and Adler, A: Principles of Radiographic Imaging, ed 3. Delmar Publishers, Inc., Clifton Park, NY, 2006.
9. Oakley, J: Digital Imaging: A Primer for Radiographers, Radiologists, and Health Care Professionals. Greenwich Medical Media, London, 2003.
10. Abdullah, BJ: What goes round comes round. Biomed Imaging Intervent J 2(1):e1, 2006.
11. Dreyer, K, and Hirschorn, D: PACS: A Guide to the Digital Revolution. Springer Science and Business Media, New York, 2006.
12. Hruby, W: Digital (R)evolution in Radiology: Bridging the Future of Health Care. Springer-Verlag, Vienna, 2006.
13. Lemke, HU, and Vannier, MW: Mission statement. Int J Comput Assist Radiol Surg 2, 2007. Accessed February 16, 2008 at http://springer.com/medicine/radiology/journal/11548.
14. Computed Radiography and Digital Radiography: A Technology Overview. Version 1.0 CD tutorial. Eastman Kodak Company, 2000.
15. Frank, E, Smith, B, and Long, B: Merrill's Atlas of Radiographic Positions and Radiologic Procedures, ed.11. Elsevier Health Sciences, Philadelphia, 2007.
16. Palmer, P, Holm, T, and Hanson, G: Radiology Worldwide—The WHO Approach. GE Healthcare, Bio-Sciences, Europe. Accessed March 12, 2008 at http://www.medcyclopaedia.com/Home/library/radiology/chapter05/5.
17. Standertskjold, C: Radiology in an International Perspective. GE Healthcare, Bio-Sciences, Europe. Accessed March 12, 2008 at http://www.medcyclopaedia.com/Home/library/radiology/chapter02.
18. Novelline, RA: Squire's Fundamentals of Radiology, ed. 6. Harvard University Press, Cambridge, MA, 2004.
19. Erkonen, W, and Smith, W: Radiology 101: The Basics and Fundamentals of Imaging, ed. 2. Lippincott Williams & Wilkins, Philadelphia, 2004.
20. Daffner, RH: Clinical Radiology: The Essentials, ed. 3. Lippincott Williams & Wilkins, Baltimore, 2007.
21. Bontrager, KL, and Lampignano, J: Textbook of Radiographic Positioning and Related Anatomy, ed. 6. Mosby, St. Louis, 2005.
22. Richardson, JK, and Iglarsh, ZA: Clinical Orthopaedic Physical Therapy. WB Saunders, Philadelphia, 1994.
23. Practice Guidelines and Technical Standards, 2008. American College of Radiology. Available at http://www.acr.org.
24. Williams, AL, and Murtagh, FR: Handbook of Diagnostic and Therapeutic Spine Procedures. Mosby, St. Louis, 2002.
25. Kastler, B: Interventional Radiology in Pain Treatment. Springer-Verlag, Berlin/Heidelberg, 2007.
26. Hodler, J, von Schulthess, GK, and Zollikofer, CL: Musculoskeletal Disease: Diagnostic Imaging and Interventional Technology. Springer, Italy, 2005.
27. Peh, WCG: Provocative discography: current status. Biomed Imaging Intervent J (1):e2, 2005.
28. Barna, S: Intradiscal Electrothermal Therapy. Article updated Feb 27, 2007. Accessed March 2008 at http://www.emedicine.com/NEURO/topic707.htm.
29. Burton, AW, and Hamid, B: Kyphoplasty and vertebroplasty. Curr Pain Headache Rep 12(1):22–27, 2008.

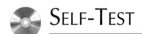 SELF-TEST

Radiograph A

1. Is *high* or *low radiographic contrast* evident between the soft tissues and bones?

2. Based on the type of radiographic contrast that was produced, do you think this film is intended to be a *chest film* or an *AP thoracic spine film*?

3. Is the film *positioned correctly* for viewing? What anatomic structure verifies this?

Radiograph B

4. Is this film *positioned correctly* for viewing? Why or why not?

5. Note the *foreign object*. What is its likely *material composition*?

6. Can you determine *where* in the patient's anatomy this object is located? Why or why not?

Radiograph C

7. Identify this *imaging study*.

8. What *mistake* was made during the radiographic examination?

Radiograph D

9. Use your knowledge of *form* to identify this common domestic pet. *Hint:* This lateral projection demonstrates a long flexible spine, tail, and small pelvis.

10. Use your knowledge of *radiographic densities* to infer why the pet's owner is distraught.

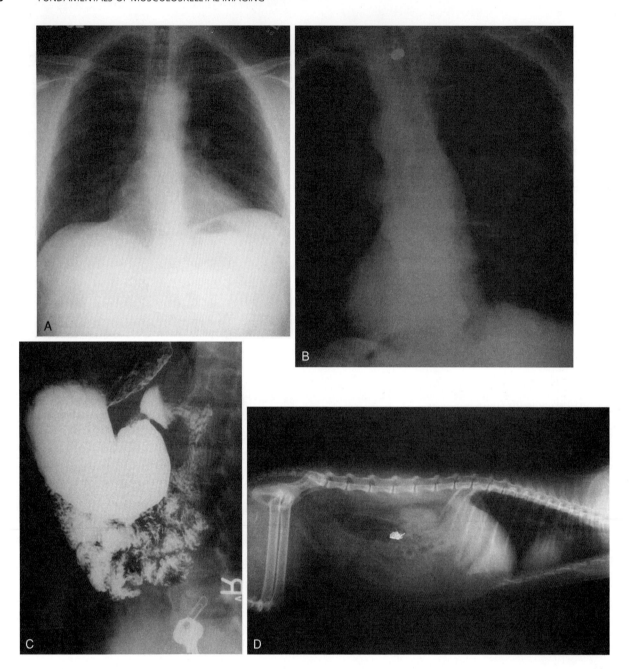

Chapter 2

RADIOLOGIC EVALUATION, SEARCH PATTERNS, AND DIAGNOSIS

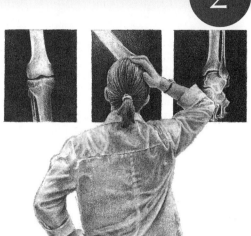

Where Does Radiologic Image Interpretation Begin?[1–14]

Radiologic image interpretation requires foundations in imaging technology, dimensional perceptions of anatomy, characteristic patterns of pathology, and an organized method of visually searching the image for abnormalities. A *search pattern* describes such a methodology.

Learning a tried and true search pattern is a good place to start looking at images in a meaningful manner. But it is wise to be a cautious learner. Strict application of an established search pattern might appear to make diagnosis easy to the novice. There are times when diagnosis is easy—a dislocated joint or a fractured bone is plain for anyone to see. Often, however, the variables of anatomic anomalies, complexity of multiple diagnoses, deviations in disease presentation, and insignificant findings that later prove significant (or the opposite) can make interpretation exceedingly difficult.

What Are the Pitfalls of Image Interpretation?

Errors! Nonradiologist interpreters of images should be aware studies show that 20% to 40% of statements made on radiologic reports by radiologists or radiology residents

were found to be erroneous, with many errors having life-threatening consequences.[1–5]

Errors can be classified as *errors of observation* or *errors of interpretation.*[6] Errors of observation can be linked to incomplete or faulty search patterns. Errors in interpretation can be linked to the practitioner's failure to link abnormal radiologic signs to relevant clinical data.

Be aware, however, that errors in reading images are inevitable and should not be confused with carelessness on the part of the reader.[7–9] Rather, errors are a consequence of the physiological process of perception, an unavoidable hazard of the human condition. And despite 21st-century advancements, technology has not solved but only displaced the problem of perceptual error to newer technologies. Attempts to identify factors that contribute to or reduce errors in reading images are ongoing. One factor known to reduce error is *collaboration between the clinican and radiologist.*

What Can the Nonradiologist Offer to Image Interpretation?

The nonradiologist can offer expertise from her or his own area of clinical specialty and *collaborate* with the radiologist and others involved in the patient's care to effect a positive patient outcome. An example of this is seen in the military's use of physical therapists as primary musculoskeletal screeners. A 1973 study of over 2,117 patients presenting with low back pain and screened by physical therapists demonstrated a *decrease* in radiologic examination by over 50%.[14] These physical therapists had sufficient additional training in basic radiology to assist them in discriminating which differential musculoskeletal diagnoses needed to be defined by radiology and which ones were inconsequential to radiologic examination. The significant factor was the physical therapist's specialty in musculoskeletal physical examination.

Where does radiologic interpretation begin for the non-radiologist? Chapter 1 covered fundamentals of x-ray technology and the perception of three-dimensional anatomy on a two-dimensional image. This chapter covers the fundamentals of a basic search pattern and describe the radiologic characteristics of some common pathologies that often appear in the patient population treated by rehabilitation clinicians. These fundamentals should promote an understanding of what radiology can offer, and they should facilitate interprofessional and intraprofessional communication about the patient. Professional collaboration to enhance the quality of patient care remains the singular most important goal.

Search Pattern: The ABCs of Radiologic Analysis[15–27]

A *search pattern* describes the methodology that one applies to look at an image in an organized fashion. Viewing the radiograph, expecting abnormalities to be conspicuous, is not enough. Consistent use of a search pattern helps to

TABLE 2-1 ● *ABCs Search Pattern for Radiologic Image Interpretation*

Division	Evaluates	Look For — Normal Findings	Variations/Abnormalities
A: Alignment	**General skeletal architecture**	• Gross normal size of bones • Normal number of bones	• Supernumerary bones • Absent bones • Congenital deformities • Developmental deformities
	General contour of bone	• Smooth and continuous cortical outlines	• Cortical fractures • Avulsion fractures • Impaction fractures • Spurs • Markings of past surgical sites
	Alignment of bones to adjacent bones	• Normal joint articulations • Normal spatial relationships	• Fracture • Joint subluxation • Joint dislocation
B: Bone Density	**General bone density**	• Sufficient contrast soft tissue shade of gray and bone shade of gray • Sufficient contrast within each bone, between cortical shell and cancellous center	• General loss of bone density resulting in poor contrast between soft tissues and bone • Thinning or absence of cortical margins
	Textural abnormalities	• Normal trabecular architecture	• Appearance of trabeculae altered; may look thin, delicate, lacy, coarsened, smudged, fluffy
	Local bone density changes	• Sclerosis at areas of increased stress, such as weight-bearing surfaces or sites of ligamentous, muscular, or tendinous attachments	• Excessive sclerosis • Reactive sclerosis that walls off a lesion • Osteophytes
C: Cartilage Spaces	**Joint space width**	• Well-preserved joint spaces imply normal cartilage or disk thickness	• Decreased joint spaces imply degenerative or traumatic conditions
	Subchondral bone	• Smooth surface	• Excessive sclerosis as seen in degenerative joint disease • Erosions as seen in the inflammatory arthritides
	Epiphyseal plates	• Normal size relative to epiphysis and skeletal age	• Compare contralaterally for changes in thickness that may be related to abnormal conditions or trauma
S: Soft Tissues	**Muscles**	• Normal size of soft tissue image	• Gross wasting • Gross swelling
	Fat pads and fat lines	• Radiolucent crescent parallel to bone • Radiolucent lines parallel to length of muscle	• Displacement of fat pads from bony fossae into soft tissues indicates joint effusion • Elevation or blurring of fat planes indicates swelling of nearby tissues
	Joint capsules	• Normally indistinct	• Observe whether effusion or hemorrhage distends capsule
	Periosteum	• Normally indistinct • Solid periosteal reaction is normal in fracture healing	• Observe periosteal reactions: solid, laminated or onionskin, spiculated or sunburst, Codman's triangle
	Miscellaneous soft tissue findings	• Soft tissues normally exhibit a water-density shade of gray	• Foreign bodies evidenced by radiodensity • Gas bubbles appear radiolucent • Calcifications appear radiopaque

ensure that everything possible to observe has been visually accounted for. Employing a search pattern is equivalent to gathering data—a critical step in the diagnostic process. A popular search pattern for musculoskeletal images exists in the form of the acronym *ABCs* (Table 2-1). This approach concisely organizes the essentials of radiologic analysis into four divisions:

A: Alignment
B: Bone density
C: Cartilage spaces
S: Soft tissues

These four divisions can be further subdivided into greater detail, as follows.

A: Alignment

Alignment analysis includes evaluation of each item in the following three lists.

1. General Skeletal Architecture

Assess gross normal size, appearance, and number of bones. Look for all of the following:

- *Aberrant size* of bones. Gross enlargement of bone is seen in conditions such as gigantism, acromegaly, or Paget's disease (Fig. 2-1). Grossly undersized bone may similarly be related to congenital, metabolic, or endocrine abnormalities.
- *Supernumerary bones.* For example, an extra navicular may be found among the tarsals, or an extra digit (polydactyly) may occur (Fig. 2-2).
- *Congenital anomalies.* Examples include a cervical rib or a transitional vertebra present at the lumbosacral junction.

- *Absence of any bones.* Bones may be missing as a result of amputation or congenital deformities (Fig. 2-3).
- *Developmental deformities.* Examples include scoliosis, genu valgum, and pronated feet.

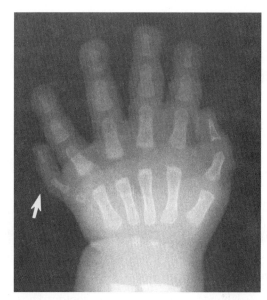

Figure 2-2 Polydactyly in a 10-month-old child. Note the extra sixth digit indicated by the arrow.

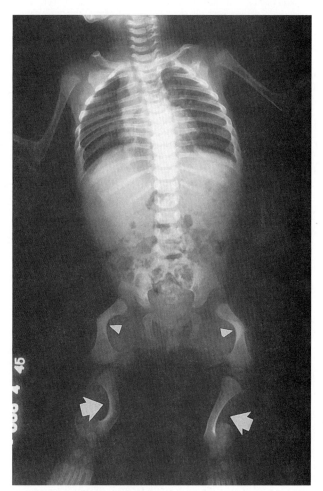

Figure 2-3 Congenital deformities in an 8-month-old girl include bowing of the femurs (arrowheads) and bowing of the tibias with absence of the fibulas (large arrows).

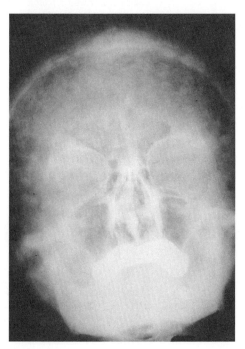

Figure 2-1 Paget's disease. The random proliferation of both osteoblastic and osteoclastic activity produces the curious fluffy sclerosis of the skull in this elderly man with Paget's disease. *(From Richardson and Iglarsh,[30] p. 644, with permission.)*

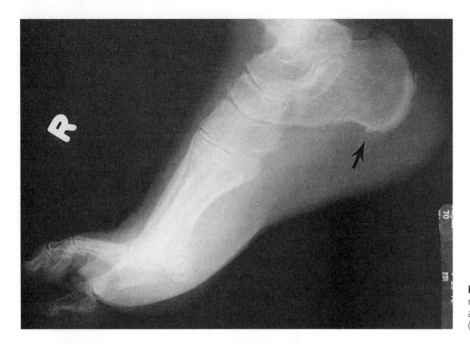

Figure 2-4 Heel spur is represented as a radiodense projection at the margin of the anterior inferior surface of the calcaneus (arrow).

2. General Contour of Bone

Assess each bone for normal shape and contour. Look for all of the following:

- *Internal or external irregularities.* These may be related to pathological, traumatic, developmental, or congenital factors.
- The *cortical outline* of each bone. The outline should be *smooth and continuous.*
- Any bony outgrowth of *spurs* at joint margins. These may be indicative of degenerative joint changes or may result from tension at areas of tissue attachment (Fig. 2-4).

- *Breaks in continuity of the cortex,* signifying cortical *fracture* (Fig. 2-5). Sharp angles in the cortex may be a sign of *impaction fracture* (Fig. 2-6). The sites of attachment of muscles, tendons, and ligaments are noted in trauma cases to evaluate for *avulsion fractures* (Fig. 2-7).[14]
- *Markings of any past surgical sites.* Examples include bone graft donation areas or drill holes for orthopedic appliances (Fig. 2-8).

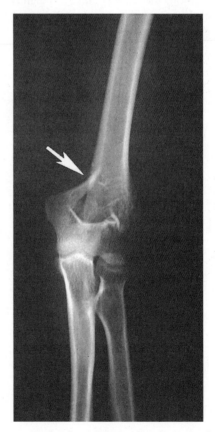

Figure 2-6 An example of an impaction fracture is seen in the *supracondylar* area of the distal humerus (arrow).

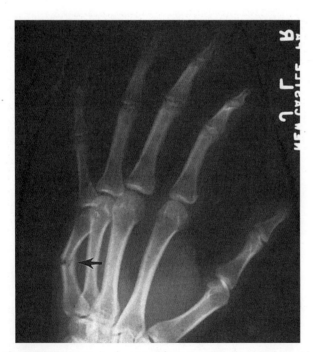

Figure 2-5 An example of a cortical fracture seen in the complete midshaft fracture of the fifth metacarpal (arrow). *(From Richardson and Iglarsh,[30] p. 681, with permission.)*

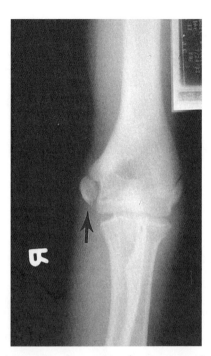

Figure 2-7 An example of an avulsion fracture is seen in this medial epicondyle avulsion of the distal humerus of a 10-year-old Little League pitcher. *(From Richardson and Iglarsh,*[30] *p. 663, with permission.)*

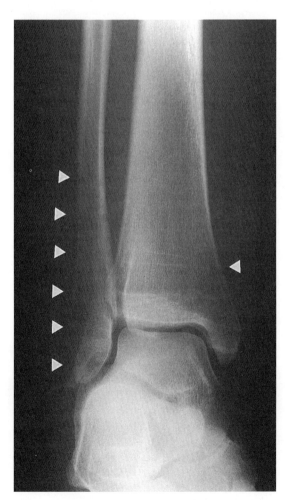

Figure 2-8 Note the odd appearance of old surgical sites as seen in the drill holes through the distal fibula and tibia of this patient, who had fixation screws removed after successful healing (arrowheads).

3. Alignment of Bones Relative to Adjacent Bones

Assess articulating bones for normal positional relationships. Look for the following:

- *Fracture,* which may disrupt joint articulations. Fracture is most often due to trauma.
- *Dislocation* of normal joint articulations. Dislocation is most often due to trauma but can be a consequence of advanced arthritides (Fig. 2-9).
- *Subluxation,* or partial dislocation, of joint surfaces. Common causes of joint subluxation include the inflammatory arthritides or degenerative joint diseases that erode articular cartilage and promote joint laxity (Fig. 2-10).

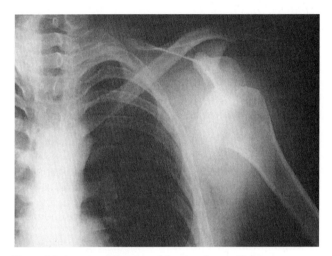

Figure 2-9 Anterior dislocation of the glenohumeral joint.

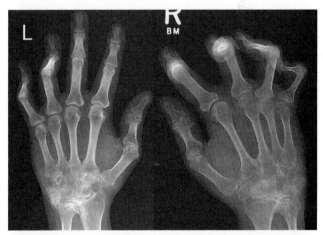

Figure 2-10 Advanced rheumatoid arthritis of the hands with joint subluxations. Posteroanterior (PA) views of the left and right hands show marked narrowing of the radiocarpal and intercarpal joints. Both wrists show ulnar carpal "drift" where the position of the scaphoid, normally projecting beyond the radial styloid, has rotated toward the ulnar side of the wrist. Other classic hallmarks of rheumatoid arthritis include symmetrical joint space narrowing, articular erosions, and periarticular osteoporosis. A boutonnière deformity (hyperextension at the distal interphalangeal joint with hyperflexion of the proximal interphalangeal joint) is present in the left fourth and fifth digits and the right second through fifth digits. *(Image courtesy of John C. Hunter, MD, University of California, Davis School of Medicine.)*

B: Bone Density

Bone density analysis includes evaluation of each item in the following three lists.

1. General Bone Density

Assess each bone for the shade of gray that represents normal density, which implies normal mineral content. Look for each of the following:

- *Sufficient radiographic contrast between the bone and the soft tissue.* Healthy bone and the soft tissue appear with clearly distinct shades of gray.
- *Sufficient contrast within the bone itself,* between the denser cortical shell of each bone and its relatively less dense cancellous bone center. Healthy cortex shows up with greater density than cancellous bone and appears as a white margin along bone shafts (Fig. 2-11).

Loss of this distinct cortical image and loss of contrast between bone and soft tissues indicate loss of bone mass. The degree of mineralization of bone is directly related to the patient's age, physiological state, and the amount of activity or stress placed on the skeleton. Certain diseases alter the mineral content of the skeleton. An overall increase in skeletal density is seen in some developmental bone disorders, such as osteopetrosis or osteopoikilosis (Fig. 2-12). An overall decrease in skeletal density is seen in osteoporosis and in the hypocalcification characteristic of osteomalacia (Fig. 2-13).

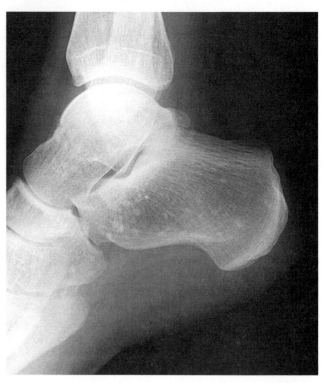

Figure 2-12 Osteopoikilosis is a benign bone disease characterized by spotty areas of calcification in bone, as seen in this lateral view of the foot. *(Image courtesy of John C. Hunter, MD, University of California, Davis School of Medicine.)*

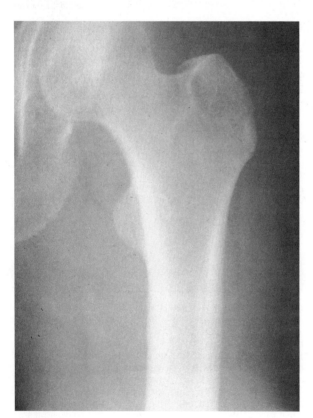

Figure 2-11 Normal proximal femur. Note in the image that healthy cortex is evident in the increased radiodensity of the margins of the femur, in contrast with the density of the medullary cavity.

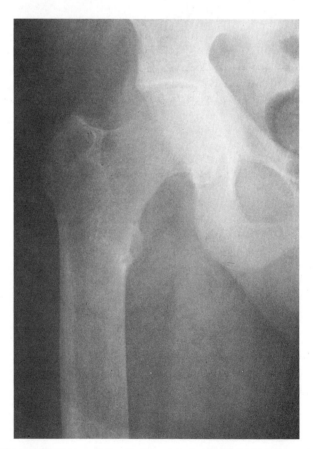

Figure 2-13 Osteomalacia, also known as "adult rickets," is a hypocalcification disorder. As seen in this proximal femur, the body is able to produce bone but is unable to calcify it. The result here is a very wide but porous femur. *(From Richardson and Iglarsh,[28] p. 642, with permission.)*

2. Textural Abnormalities

Assess the trabeculae for changes in appearance. When the mineralization of bone is altered, the appearance of the trabeculae is also altered. Altered trabecular appearance is often a radiologic hallmark in the diagnosis of disease processes. The image of the trabeculae is often described in terms likened to texture, such as *thin, delicate, coarsened, smudged,* or *fluffy.* Examples include the following:

- *Fluffy* trabeculae represent the random proliferation of both osteoblastic and osteoclastic activity, as seen in the skull of a patient with Paget's disease (see Fig. 2-1) and in hyperparathyroidism (Fig. 2-14).
- *Smudged* and indistinct trabeculae are a characteristic of osteomalacia (see Fig. 2-13).
- *Coarsening* of trabeculae is often seen in patients with chronic renal failure and osteoporosis. The accentuation of these trabeculae do not signify strength; rather, the loss of surrounding trabeculae cause the remaining trabeculae to appear prominent.
- *Lacy, delicate* appearance of trabeculae is secondary to thalassemia (Cooley's anemia) (Fig. 2-15).

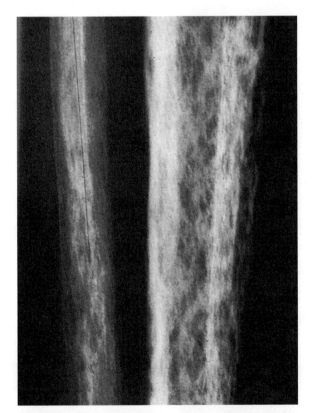

Figure 2-14 Hyperparathyroidism. A previously healthy 21-year-old man had been troubled for the preceding 18 months by increasing loss of strength in the lower extremities. Patient was found to have primary hyperparathyroidism secondary to a tumor of the parathyroid. Radiograph of his leg shows generalized skeletal changes with considerable decalcification of the bones and erosions of the cortex. *(From Eiken, M: Roentgen Diagnosis of Bones: A Self-Teaching Manual. FADLs, Forlag, AS, Copenhagen, 1975, p. 39, with permission.)*

3. Local Density Changes

Assess localized areas of density changes. Look for each of the following:

- *Sclerosis,* or normal local increases in bone density seen in areas subjected to increased physical stress, such as the weight-bearing areas of joints. These areas of localized sclerosis are actually signs of *repair*—extra bone is deposited to fortify bony architecture to withstand the forces of weight-bearing.

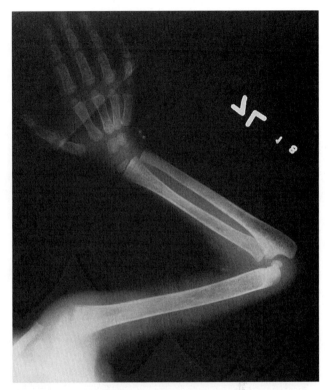

Figure 2-15 The lacy, delicate appearance of the trabeculae of the upper extremity of this child is secondary to thalassemia (Cooley's anemia).

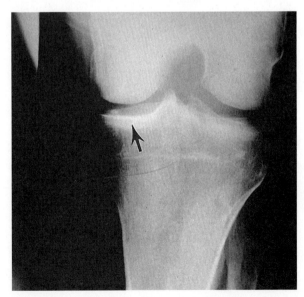

Figure 2-16 Degenerative joint disease of the knee. The arrow points to the sclerotic subchondral bone of the medial tibial plateau, which is a reparative response to the thinning of the articular cartilage.

- *Excessive sclerosis* may be evident in normal conditions, such as at the site of a healing fracture as callus is formed and new bone is remodeled. Excessive sclerosis may also be seen in abnormal conditions, as in the degeneration of an osteoarthritic joint (Fig. 2-16).
- *Reactive sclerosis* is present when the body acts to surround and contain a diseased area, such as a tumor or infection (Fig. 2-17).

C: Cartilage Spaces

The articular cartilage of joints and the cartilaginous intervertebral disks of the spine are not well demonstrated on plain films because of their water-like density. Cartilages and disks can be analyzed, however, by examining the space they occupy. Cartilage space analysis includes evaluation of the items on the following lists.

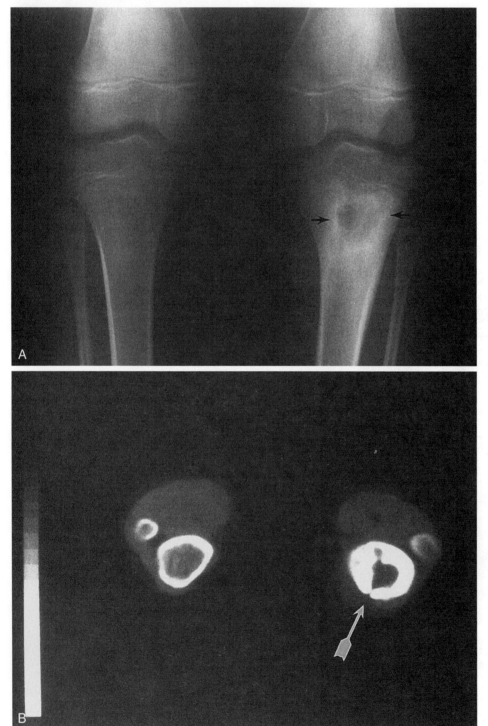

Figure 2-17 Osteomyelitis. **(A)** This 9-year-old girl had a 6-month history of progressive, enlarging soft tissue swelling at the left anterior proximal tibia. She was diagnosed with osteomyelitis of the proximal tibia. Note how the lesion is well circumscribed by the active sclerosis of bone in an attempt to surround and wall off the infected area (arrows). **(B)** The CT axial image further demonstrates the reactive sclerosis of the left tibia and also reveals a draining defect (white arrow), which formed to relieve the pressure of the pus, in the anterior tibia.

1. Joint Space Width

Assess joint spaces for normal thickness. Look for each of the following:

- A *well-preserved joint space* implies that the cartilage or disk is of normal thickness.
- A *decreased joint space* implies that the cartilage or disk is thinned down as a result of degenerative processes (Fig. 2-18).

Joint space is also referred to as the *potential space* or the *radiographic joint space*. The term *radiographic joint space* is specific in that it encompasses both the cartilage and any actual space present in the joint (such as the space due to skin traction when the patient is supine on the x-ray table). Evaluation of weight-bearing joints is best done *during weight-bearing* for accurate assessment of the articular cartilages, because this will eliminate any actual space from the image and present the true dimensions of the cartilage.

2. Subchondral Bone

Assess the subchondral bone (subjacent to the articular cartilage) for density changes or irregularities. Structural changes in the subchondral bone are significant in the radiologic diagnosis of different arthritides. Look for:

- *Increased sclerosis.* In the degenerative arthritides such as osteoarthritis, subchondral bone becomes increasingly sclerotic as new bone is formed to help withstand the increased stresses directed at it because of the loss of articular cartilage (Fig. 2-19).
- *Erosions.* In the inflammatory arthritides such as rheumatoid arthritis or gout, no reparative sclerosis is seen in the subchondral bone. Rather, erosions of the subchondral bone form radiolucent cysts (Fig. 2-20).

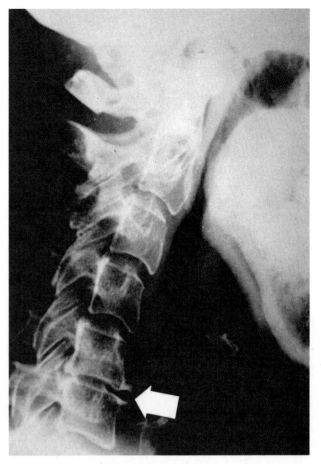

Figure 2-18 Degenerative disk disease of the cervical spine. This lateral view of the cervical spine shows the classic hallmarks of degenerative disk disease at C5–C6, including a narrowed joint space and osteophyte formation at the joint margins (arrow).

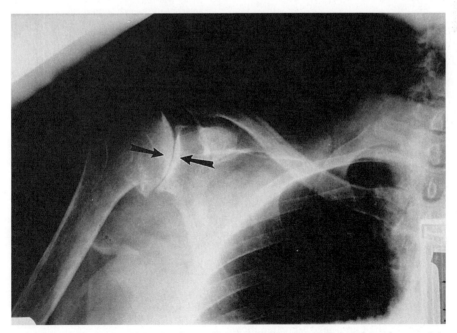

Figure 2-19 Osteoarthritis of the glenohumeral joint. Note the radiographic hallmarks of osteoarthritis, including decreased joint space, sclerotic subchondral bone (arrows), and osteophyte formation on the inferior joint margins. The severity of these degenerative changes is usually more common in weight-bearing joints. The arthritic changes here were probably accelerated by a prior trauma.

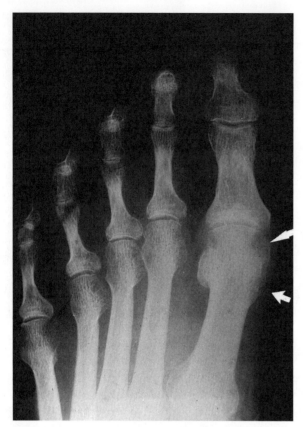

Figure 2-20 Gout at the first metatarsophalangeal joint. Joint erosions in gout and other inflammatory arthritides show no reactive subchondral sclerosis such as is seen in osteoarthritic conditions. Rather, erosions of the subchondral bone in knee inflammatory conditions form radiolucent cysts in the articular and periarticular regions (arrows).

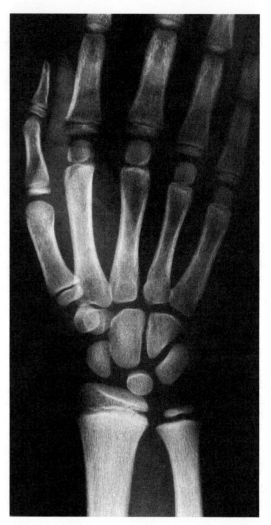

Figure 2-21 Normal radiographic appearance of hand of an 8-year-old child. The epiphyseal plates are evidenced by the radiolucent zones adjacent to the maturing epiphyses. The borders of epiphyses are normally bounded by a smooth margin with a band of sclerosis indicating increased bone activity. This is how they are distinguished from fracture fragments. Discriminating epiphyseal plate regions from fracture lines can at times be difficult; contralateral images may be needed for comparison purposes.

3. Epiphyseal Plates

Although the previous points were made in regard to joints, epiphyseal plates in a growing child are temporarily cartilaginous and thus fit into this category. Look for:

- The *position* of the epiphyseal plate as designated by the relationship of the ossified portion of the secondary epiphysis to the metaphysis (Fig. 2-21)
- The *size of the epiphyses* in relation to both skeletal maturity and chronological age
- A smooth margin at the *borders of the epiphyses,* with a band of sclerosis indicating increased bone activity associated with linear growth
- Disruptions in the epiphyseal plates from trauma or metabolic disease can be difficult to diagnose, and contralateral films may be needed for comparison.

S: Soft Tissues

Soft tissues do not image with specific distinction on conventional radiographs, because the densities of all soft tissues in the body are similar. Enough of an image is created, however, to permit observation of some extreme conditions. Soft tissue analysis includes evaluation of several types of tissue discussed in the following paragraphs.

1. Muscles

Assess the soft tissue image of muscles for:

- *Gross muscle wasting,* which may suggest a primary muscle disease, paralysis, inanition associated with severe illnesses, or disuse atrophy secondary to trauma (Fig. 2-22)
- *Gross swelling of muscles and soft tissues,* which may be indicative of inflammation, edema, hemorrhage, or tumor (Fig. 2-23).

2. Fat Pads and Fat Lines

Assess loss or displacement of fat lines or fat pads from their normal positions into the soft tissues. Such loss or displacement is usually due to swelling and is a clue to an adjacent abnormality. Examples include the following:

- Displacement of the pronator quadratus fat line at the wrist usually indicates a wrist fracture.

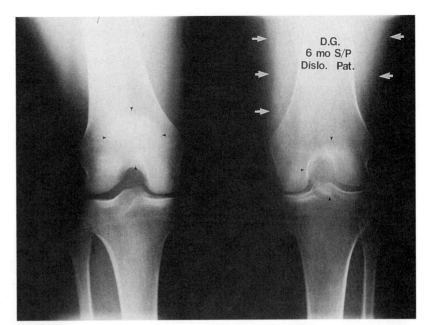

Figure 2-22 Disuse atrophy of the quadriceps secondary to traumatic patellar dislocation is evidenced by the shrunken appearance of the soft tissue outline of the thigh. Note the inferior position of the patella (patella baja) caused by quadriceps insufficiency.

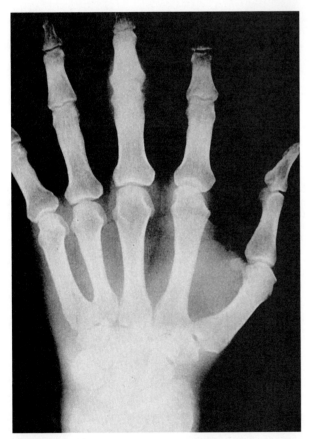

Figure 2-23 Rheumatoid arthritis of the hand. Note gross swelling of the hand and the proximal interphalangeal joint of the third digit, indicating an inflammatory phase. *(From American College of Rheumatology Clinical Slide Collection on Rheumatic Disease, 1991.)*

- Displacement of the fat pads at the elbow (from the olecranon fossa posteriorly and from the coronoid and radial fossae anteriorly) usually indicates gross effusion associated with fracture (Fig. 2-24).

3. Joint Capsules

Normally rather indistinct, joint capsules will become visible under abnormal conditions when *distended by effusion.* This is seen in exacerbations of arthritic conditions, infection, hemophilia, and in acute joint trauma.

Effusion from the trauma of an *intra-articular* fracture usually produces a *lipohemarthrosis* in the joint capsule. Lipohemarthrosis is the mixture of fat and blood from the marrow which enters the joint space through an osteochondral defect. Because fat is less dense than blood, it floats on the surface of blood. On a radiograph, this is referred to as a fat–fluid level or fat–blood interface (FBI sign). When seen on a radiograph, this sign is a strong indicator for a potentially overlooked intra-articular fracture (Fig. 2-25). (However, an even more specific finding of free fat in the joint is possible with advanced imaging. A third level of fluid, representing the mixed serum and synovial liquid, will be visible *between* the fat and blood layers on computed tomography [CT], magnetic resonance imaging [MRI], or ultrasound [US].)

4. Periosteum

Normally rather indistinct, the periosteum becomes evident in its response to abnormal conditions. Periosteal reaction (Fig. 2-26) is generally described as being one of four types, named by the characteristic radiographic images. Look for these types of periosteal reaction:

- *Solid:* This reaction indicates a benign process; seen in fracture healing and osteomyelitis.
- *Laminated or onionskin:* This reaction indicates repetitive injury, as in the battered child syndrome; it is also associated with sarcomas such as Ewing's sarcoma.
- *Spiculated or sunburst:* This reaction is almost always associated with malignant bone lesions, such as osteogenic sarcomas, and is less frequently seen in metastatic squamous cell tumors. The distinct appearance of the periosteum is due to the repeated breakthrough of the neoplastic process followed by new periosteal response.

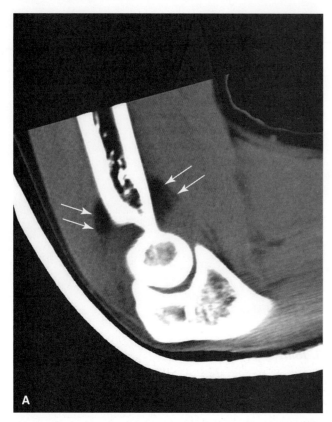

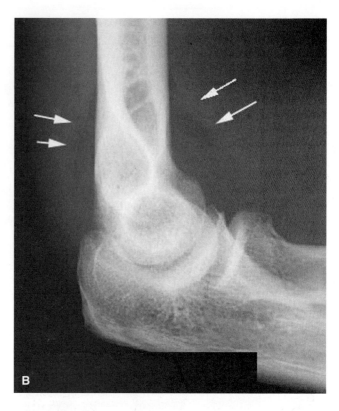

Figure 2-24 Positive *fat pad sign* or *sail sign* at the elbow. **(A)** CT sagittal view of the elbow demonstrating displaced fat pads as radiolucent triangular images present anteriorly and posteriorly to the humeral shaft (arrows). *(Image courtesy of http://www.radpod.org.)* **(B)** On radiograph, these displaced fat pads are also visible as radiolucent images in the soft tissues (arrows). The fat pads are displaced due to joint effusion, most commonly instigated by fracture, although other processes, such as infection, can produce gross effusion that displaces the fat pads.

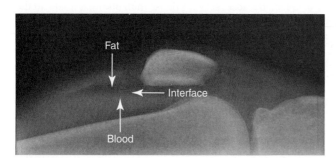

Figure 2-25 *FBI sign.* This non–weight-bearing, lateral view of the knee was made with a horizontal x-ray beam tangent to the fluid layers. Marrow fat and blood that seeped through the intra-articular tibial plateau fracture (not visible here) has accumulated in the suprapatellar area of the joint capsule and divided into layers because of differences in fluid density.

- *Codman's triangle:* A piece of periosteum elevated by abnormal conditions ossifies in a triangular shape. This may be present in a variety of conditions, including tumor, subperiosteal hemorrhage, and battered child syndrome.

5. Miscellaneous Soft Tissue Findings

Assess any miscellaneous findings within the soft tissue image. Look for the following:

- *Gas* in soft tissues is an indication of gas gangrene or trauma.

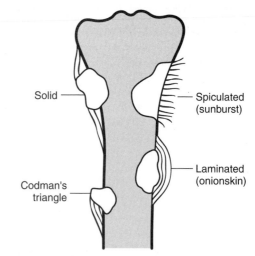

Figure 2-26 Periosteal reactions to abnormal conditions appear on radiograph in four characteristic images: solid, spiculated, laminated, or Codman's triangle. *(Adapted from Greenspan,[19] p. 551.)*

- *Calcifications* in soft tissues may be the result of old trauma whereby bloody hemorrhage has coagulated and calcified (Fig. 2-27). Additionally, calcifications occur in vessels and organs, for example, renal calculi, gallstones, or calcifications in the abdominal aorta.
- *Foreign bodies* (such as metal shards) may also be evident in the soft tissues.

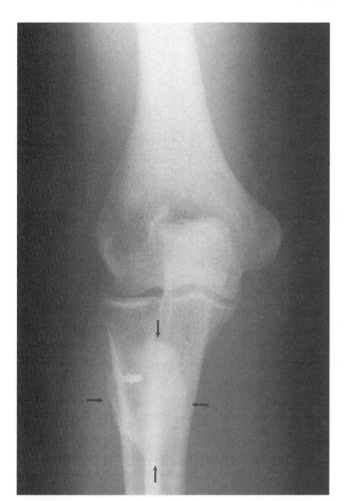

Figure 2-27 Myositis ossificans seen on the anteroposterior (AP) view of the elbow. Heterotopic bone developed in the soft tissues of the forearm of this 53-year-old man after a biceps tendon tear and repair with a mytex suture anchor. The boundaries of the abnormal bone tissue are indicated with arrows.

Distribution of the Lesion

The distribution of a lesion refers to how many locations in the body the lesion involves and is a significant clue to the etiology of that lesion. A lesion may be either:

- *Monostotic* or *monoarticular,* affecting only one bone or one joint
- *Polyostotic* or *polyarticular,* affecting multiple bones or multiple joints
- *Diffuse,* affecting all or nearly all bones or joints

Only two disease categories occur diffusely: neoplastic and metabolic (Table 2-2). The other categories occur in either monostotic/monoarticular or polyostotic/polyarticular patterns. Occasionally, however, metabolic disease may manifest itself in monostotic or polyostotic forms. Examples of pathology as related to distribution appear in Table 2-3.

TABLE 2-2 ● *Category of Pathology Related to Skeletal Distribution*

Category	Distribution		
	Monostotic/ Monoarticular	*Polyostotic/ Polyarticular*	*Diffuse*
Congenital	X	X	
Inflammatory	X	X	
Neoplastic	X	X	X
Metabolic	X	X	X
Traumatic	X	X	
Vascular	X	X	
Miscellaneous	(X)	(X)	

Radiologic Diagnosis of Skeletal Pathology[12,18,19,23,25]

A search pattern serves to gain data from the radiograph. Next, these data must be correlated with knowledge of the characteristic features of skeletal disease to lead the radiologist to a diagnosis.

The broad index of skeletal diseases can be organized for diagnosis by identifying the *category of pathology,* the *distribution of the lesion,* and *predictor variables* that characterize disease features.

Categories of Skeletal Pathology

There are six basic categories of pathology in the classification of skeletal diseases: *congenital, inflammatory, metabolic, neoplastic, traumatic,* and *vascular.* A seventh category, *miscellaneous or other,* is added to encompass any conditions that do not fall strictly into one category, such as *musculoskeletal infections* or *osteoarthritis.*

TABLE 2-3 ● *Examples of Pathology Related to Skeletal Distribution*

Category	Monostotic/ Monoarticular	Polyostotic/ Polyarticular	Diffuse
Congenital	Cervical rib	Cleidocranial dysostosis	
Inflammatory	Osteomyelitis, gout	Rheumatoid arthritis, gout	
Neoplastic	Any primary bone tumor	Myeloma	Metastases
Metabolic	Paget's disease	Paget's disease, fibrous dysplasia	Osteoporosis, osteomalacia
Traumatic	Single fracture	Multiple fractures, battered child	
Vascular	Legg-Calvé-Perthes disease	Avascular necrosis multiple sites	
Miscellaneous (osteoarthritis)	Osteoarthritis at first carpometacarpal joint	Osteoarthritis in all large weight-bearing joints	

Predictor Variables

Daffner[27] cites 11 predictor variables that may be applied to any bone or joint lesion to assist in making a diagnosis. These are the behavior of the lesion; the bone or joint involved; the locus within a bone; the age, gender, and race of the patient; the margin of the lesion; the shape of the lesion; involvement or crossing of a joint space; bony reaction (if any); matrix production by the lesion; soft tissue changes; and a history of trauma or surgery (Table 2-4).

Many of these predictor variables apply directly to the diagnosis of bone tumors. Specific diagnoses can at times still be difficult even if all of the predictor variables are applied; the information gained from conventional radiography, however, is usually sufficient for the radiologist to determine whether a lesion is *nonaggressive* (benign) or *aggressive* (malignant) and in need of biopsy.

Daffner's description of the predictor variables follows.

Behavior of the Lesion

Bone lesions are described as either osteolytic, meaning that bone has been destroyed by osteoclastic activity, or osteoblastic, meaning that new reparative or reactive bone is present. Occasionally, a mixture of the two processes may be present.

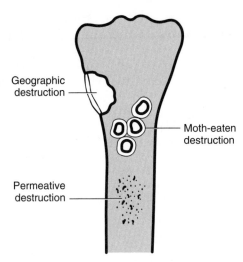

Figure 2-28 Different kinds of osteolytic lesions cause different types of bone destruction. The radiographic image that correlates with the pathologic process may be described as geographic, moth-eaten, or permeative. *(Adapted from Greenspan,[19] p. 550.)*

Osteolytic lesions take on three forms of destruction (Fig. 2-28):

- *Geographic destruction:* Large areas of bone are destroyed and appear as radiolucent lesions. Sharply defined borders suggest a benign lesion.
- *Moth-eaten appearance:* Several small holes throughout the bone appear similar to moth-eaten cloth. Ragged borders here suggest a malignant lesion.
- *Permeative destruction:* Very fine destruction of bone through the haversian system, sometimes requiring a magnifying lens to recognize on film. Poorly defined borders suggest a malignant lesion.

Bone or Joint Involved

Some diseases become manifest characteristically at specific bones or joints. Gout and rheumatoid arthritis, for example, appear primarily in the small joints of the hands and feet. Osteoarthritis commonly develops at the knees. Examples of other nonneoplastic and neoplastic diseases with predilection for certain areas are shown in Figure 2-29.

Locus Within a Bone

The site of the lesion within the bone itself is a significant clue to etiology. Certain tumors have a predilection for the bony shaft, whereas others favor the metaphyseal or epiphyseal regions. The arthritides have characteristic locations on the articular surfaces of bone. Osteoarthritis affects weight-bearing areas, whereas rheumatoid arthritis affects the entire joint surface.

Age, Gender, and Race

Age is a significant factor in predicting the type of malignant bone tumor as well as some benign tumors. See Table 2-5 for peak ages of various tumors.[17] In addition to age predominance, there is gender predominance (rheumatoid arthritis: female; Paget's disease: male) and race predominance in some diseases (sickle cell disease, thalassemia).

TABLE 2-4 ● *Predictor Variables for Bone and Joint Lesions*

1. Behavior of the lesion
  A. Osteolytic (or osteoclastic, bone destroying)
  B. Osteoblastic (reparative or reactive bone forms)
  C. Mixed

2. Bone or joint involved

3. Locus within a bone
  A. Epiphysis (or apophysis)
  B. Metaphysis (or equivalent)
  C. Diaphysis
  D. Articular surface

4. Age, gender, and race of patient

5. Margin of lesion
  A. Sharply defined (slow-growing lesion)
  B. Poorly defined (aggressive lesion)

6. Shape of Lesion
  A. Longer than wide (generally slow-growing lesion)
  B. Wider than long (generally aggressive lesion)
    a. Cortical breakthrough
    b. No breakthrough

7. Joint space crossed/joint space preserved

8. Bony reaction (if any)
  A. Periosteal
    a. Solid
    b. Laminated ("onionskin")
    c. Spiculated, sunburst, "hair-on-end"
    d. Codman's triangle
  B. Sclerosis
  C. Buttressing

9. Matrix production
  A. Osteoid
  B. Chondroid
  C. Mixed

10. Soft tissue changes

11. History of trauma or surgery

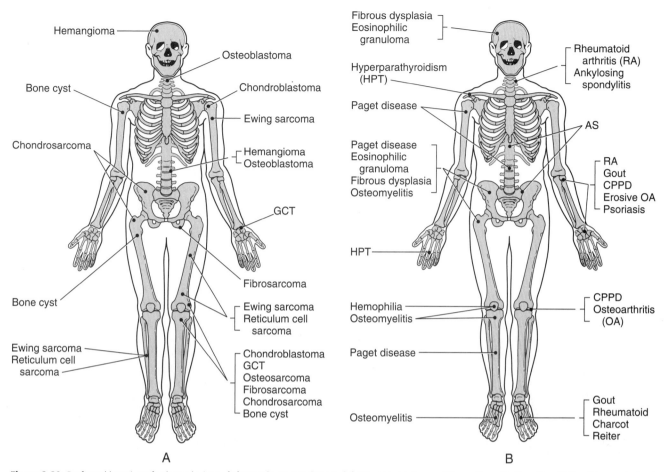

Figure 2-29 Preferred locations for bone lesions. **(A)** Neoplastic conditions. **(B)** Nonneoplastic conditions. *(From Daffner,[15] p. 288, with permission.)*

TABLE 2-5 ● *Peak Age Incidence of Benign and Malignant Tumors of Bone[19,33]*										
Histological Type	**Age**									
	0	**10**	**20**	**30**	**40**	**50**	**60**	**70**	**80**	**90**
Benign										
Osteochondroma		▓								
Bone cyst	▓	▓								
Giant cell tumor			▓	▓						
Endochondroma		▓	▓							
Fibrous dysplasia, polyostotic		▓	▓							
Osteoid osteoma		▓	▓	▓						
Osteoblastoma		▓	▓	▓						
Malignant, Primary (0.2% of all neoplasms)										
Osteosarcoma				▓	▓					
Ewing's sarcoma		▓	▓							
Chondrosarcoma					▓	▓	▓			
Chordoma					▓	▓	▓			
Malignant fibrous histiocytoma				▓	▓					
Malignant, Secondary (20–80% of organ cancers develop bone metastases)										
Metastatic from prostate, thyroid, breast, lungs, kidneys						▓	▓	▓	▓	

Margin of Lesion

In general, margins are either sharp and clearly defined or wide and poorly defined (Fig. 2-30).

- Sharp, clearly defined, sclerotic borders are characteristic of slow-growing or benign lesions. A *narrow zone of transition* is a phrase used to describe this type of border.
- Wide, poorly defined borders with minimal or absent reactive sclerosis are characteristic of fast-growing or malignant lesions.

This relationship is logical: In a slow-growing process, bone has time to wall the abnormal tissue off effectively with a border of new bone growth. In contrast, a malignant lesion or aggressive process progresses so rapidly that bone is unable to respond adequately.

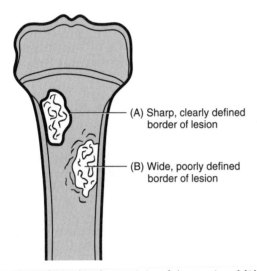

(A) Sharp, clearly defined border of lesion

(B) Wide, poorly defined border of lesion

Figure 2-30 Radiographic characteristics of the margins of **(A)** slow-growing, benign lesions versus **(B)** fast-growing, malignant lesions. *(Adapted from Greenspan,[19] p. 547.)*

Shape of Lesion

Like the margins, the shape of a lesion can help classify a lesion as aggressive or nonaggressive. In immature bone, lesions that are longer than are wide are likely to be benign, because the lesion has grown slowly along with the bone. By contrast, lesions that are wider than they are long and extending into the soft tissues are aggressive.

Joint Space Crossed

As a rule, tumors, benign or malignant, do not cross joint spaces or epiphyseal growth plates (Fig. 2-31). Infections, however, do cross joint spaces. Inflammatory processes are characteristic in that they cause destruction of bone on both sides of a joint (Fig. 2-32).

Bony Reaction

The responses of bone to lesion, trauma, or degenerative processes can include periosteal reaction, sclerosis, and buttressing.

Sclerosis is new bone growth established to fortify an area subjected to increased stress, as in the sclerosis of subchondral bone in osteoarthritis. Reactive sclerosis is the body's attempt to contain an area of abnormal bone (see the discussion of the margin of lesion above).

Buttressing is the formation of bony exostoses or osteophytes at joint margins, which serve to strengthen the architecture of the joint.

Periosteal reaction to a neoplasm is usually characterized as *interrupted* or *uninterrupted*. Interrupted periosteal response suggests malignant or nonmalignant but highly aggressive lesions. It may present in a sunburst or spiculated pattern, laminated or onionskin pattern, or a Codman's triangle, as commonly seen in the osteosarcomas. Uninterrupted periosteal response suggests benign processes and presents as

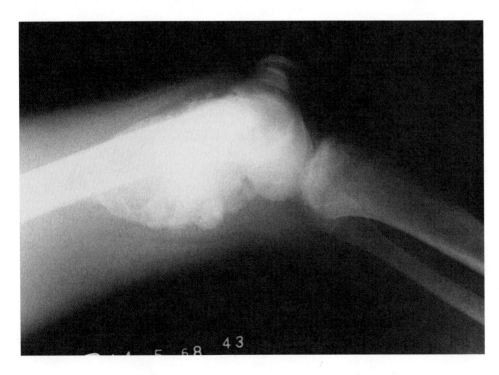

Figure 2-31 Osteosarcoma. This 16-year-old girl with a 3-month history of pain and swelling in her knee was diagnosed with an osteosarcoma of the distal femur. Note that this large tumor extends to the joint space of the knee *but does not cross it.*

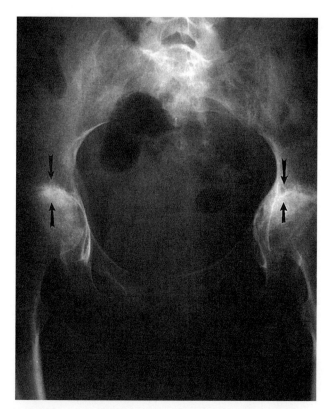

Figure 2-32 Advanced rheumatoid arthritis of the hip joints. Note that the destruction caused by rheumatoid arthritis involves the entire joint space and the bony regions on either side of the joint space.

a solid density, either longitudinal, undulated, or buttressing in pattern.

Matrix Production

Matrix is the intercellular tissue produced by some bone tumors. Tumor matrix is identified radiographically as chondroid (cartilaginous), osteoid (bony), or mixed, a combination of the two. Chondroid matrix appears as stippled, popcorn-like, or comma-shaped calcifications seen in tumors invading soft tissues. Osteoid matrix appears as white, cloud-like, fluffy density within the medullary cavity and in adjacent soft tissue, most often in osteosarcomas (see Fig. 2-31).

Soft Tissue Changes

Examining soft tissue density changes may provide clues to the underlying abnormality. All of these conditions alter the normal soft tissue outline and add density to the soft tissue image:

- Fractures and other trauma will have associated soft tissue edema, hemorrhage, or joint effusion.
- Displacement of fat pads and fat lines is also associated with trauma (see the previous "S" section in the discussion of the ABCs).
- Infections and inflammation also add density to the soft tissue image.
- Calcifications in soft tissues result from connective tissue disorders or old trauma.

- Tumor masses may develop in soft tissues or extend from adjacent bone or organs and become visible by the substance of their matrix or their disruption of normal soft tissue geography. Generally, benign tumors do not exhibit extension into the soft tissues. Extension of the mass through the cortex and into the soft tissues is typical of aggressive and often malignant tumors.

History of Trauma or Surgery

Because trauma represents the most common disorder of bone, a clear clinical history, including descriptions of any present or prior trauma, is a significant factor in the radiologic examination. Some traumatic conditions may have similar radiographic appearances to pathological processes. As Daffner[27] elaborates, a stress fracture may be misdiagnosed as a malignant bone tumor unless a specific history of pain related to activity and relieved with rest is elicited from the patient. Additionally, a history of past injury or surgery to a bone is necessary to account for the odd appearance of old surgical sites or remodeling deformities.

Radiologic Characteristics of Common Pathologies

A brief review of the radiographic characteristics of some of the more frequently encountered pathological conditions of the musculoskeletal system follows. Examples from the major pathological categories are presented, with the exception of *trauma* conditions, which are covered in the following chapter on fractures and additionally in each anatomic chapter, and *congenital* conditions, which are covered by body segment in each of the anatomic chapters.

In reading the descriptions of the radiologic characteristics of the following pathologies, the clinician should recognize how each feature can be associated with an ABCs search pattern or a predictor variable (Table 2-6). Furthermore, it should be noted how some radiographic features are unique to that diagnosis and how others are present in multiple conditions, necessitating differential diagnoses (Table 2-7).

Adult Rheumatoid Arthritis[12,18,19,23,25]

Rheumatoid arthritis (RA) is a progressive, systemic, inflammatory connective tissue disease affecting primarily the synovial joints, although it may involve nonarticular tissues including blood vessels, muscle, the heart, and lungs. It is the most common of the inflammatory arthritides. This disease is estimated to affect 3% of the populations of countries with temperate climates. Women are affected with three times greater incidence than men, and peak age at onset is between 35 and 40 years. The detection of specific antibodies or *rheumatoid factors* in the joint fluid or serum is significant in diagnosis.

RA is characterized by spontaneous exacerbations of bilateral and symmetrical joint inflammation, hyperplastic synovitis (pannus), resultant cartilage and bone destruction, and consequent loss of function. Early stages exhibit involvement of the small joints of the wrists, hands, and feet. Later stages exhibit various degrees of joint deformities, contractures, and ankylosis, affecting both small and large weight-bearing and non–weight-bearing joints (Fig. 2-33).

TABLE 2-6 ● *Radiologic Comparison of Rheumatoid Arthritis and Osteoarthritis*

	Rheumatoid Arthritis	**Osteoarthritis**
Clinical Signs and Symptoms	Pain, swelling, deformity, ↓ ROM	Pain, deformity, ↓ ROM
Typical Distribution	Bilateral involvement of synovial joints of hands, wrists, feet, hips, knees, or elbows or of the atlantoaxial joint	Unilateral involvement of synovial or cartilaginous joints of spine, hips, knees, first metatarsal, and phalanges
A: Alignment	MCP subluxation and ulnar deviation Swan-neck and boutonnière deformities of IPs Dislocations in later stages Acetabular protrusion at hip	Herberdens nodes at DIPs Bouchard's nodes at PIPs Valgus or varus deformities at knees Subluxations and joint misalignment
B: Bone Density	Periarticular rarefaction Generalized osteoporosis in late stages	Usually absence of osteoporosis
C: Cartilage Spaces	Symmetrical, concentric joint space narrowing Subchondral erosions Subchondral cysts	Asymmetric, irregular joint space narrowing Sclerotic subchondral bone Osteophytosis at joint margins Subchondral cysts Intra-articular loose bodies
S: Soft Tissues	Periarticular swelling Fusiform swelling	Joint effusion during acute exacerbations

DIP, distal interphalangeal joint; IPs, interphalangeal joints, MCP, metacarpophalangeal joint; PIP, proximal interphalangeal joint; ROM, range of motion.

TABLE 2-7 ● *Comparison of Characterisitics of the Arthritides: Inflammatory, Deposition, and Degenerative*[8,15]

	Peak Age Onset	Male:Female Ratio	Typically Affected Joints	Predominant Radiologic Findings
Inflammatory Arthritides				
AS	15–25	1–10:1	Symmetrical axial skeleton	Erosions, osseous proliferation, ankylosis
Juvenile RA	<16	1:1	Cervical, wrist	Periostitis, growth abnormalites, intra-articular fusion
Psoriatic arthritis	30–50	1:1	Asymmetrical axial skeleton, knee	Similar to AS and RA
RA	20–50	1:3	MCP, wrist	Periarticular swelling, rarefaction, articular erosion, pseudocysts, deformities
Reiter's syndrome	15–35	5:1	Feet and large LE joints, SIJ	Similar to RA
Scleroderma	20–50	1:3	Hand	Resorption of distal tufts, subcutaneous calcinosis
Systemic lupus erythematosus	20–40	1:9	Hand	Nonerosive, flexible deformities
Metabolic and Deposition Arthritides				
Gout	40–50	20:1	First MTP	Rarefaction absent, articular erosions more sharply defined
CPPD	Increases with age	1:1	Knee, wrist, MCPs, symphysis pubis	Chondrocalcinosis (calcification of cartilage), progressive joint degeneration; can mimic OA and gout
Degenerative Arthritides and Associated Conditions				
OA	>40 Radiographic evidence in all >65	Varies by skeletal region	Spine, hips, knees, first metatarsal, phalanges	Joint space narrowing, osteophytosis, subchondral sclerosis, subchondral cysts, intra-articular loose bodies, deformities
DISH	>40	M>F	Mid- to lower thoracic spine, lumbar spine, lower cervical spine	Flowing ossification of anterolateral aspects of at least four contiguous vertebral bodies, preservation of diskheight, absent sacrolilitis or ankylosis
Intervertebral disk herniation	25–45	M>F	L4–L5, C5–C6	Decreased diskheight, marginal osteophytosis
Neuropathic arthropathy (Charcot's Joint)	Secondary to impaired sensation; etiology dependent (diabetes, syringomyelia, syphilis, spinal cord trauma)		Hypertrophic form: spine, LEs Resorptive form: UEs	6 *D*s: *d*ense subcortical bone, *d*estruction of articular cartilage, and joint *d*ebris, *d*istension, *d*isorganization, *d*islocation Complete resorption of articular bone with sharp demarcation (pseudoamputation)
Spinal stenosis	40–50	M>F	Cervical and lumbar spines	Radiography of limited value except to evaluate related conditions (spondylolisthesis, Paget's disease)

AS, ankylosing spondylitis; CPDC, calcium pyrophosphate dihydrate crystal deposition disease; DISH, diffuse idiopathic skeletal hyperostosis; LE, lower extremity; MCP, metacarpophalangeal; MTP, metatarophalangeal joint; OA, osteoarthritis; RA, rheumatoid arthritis; SIJ, sacroiliac joint; UE, upper extremity.

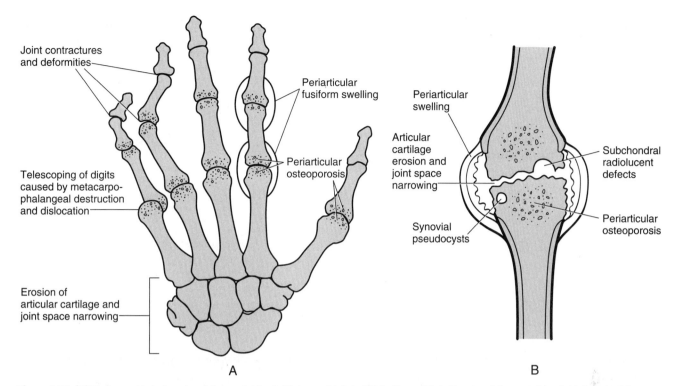

Figure 2-33 **(A)** Radiographic hallmarks of rheumatoid arthritis in small joints. **(B)** Radiographic hallmarks of rheumatoid arthritis in large joints.

The clinical features of RA are pain and swelling of the joints, limited range of motion (ROM), progressive deformities, and consequent loss of function.

Radiologic Features of Rheumatoid Arthritis

Early diagnosis and monitoring of the disease's progression have been demonstrated with advanced imaging studies. At present, conventional radiographs are most commonly used to characterize the effects of the disease.

Radiographic features characteristic of rheumatoid arthritis are described in the following paragraphs.

Soft Tissue Changes

The earliest sign of the disease is *fusiform periarticular swelling* of the small joints, representing a combination of joint effusion, tenosynovitis, and edema (see Fig. 2-23, Fig. 2-34). Swelling of both small and large joints continues to be evident throughout periods of exacerbations.

Articular Erosions

Articular erosions become apparent within the first 2 years of the disease, evidenced by altered joint congruity and altered joint surface topography (Fig. 2-35). The subchondral bone exhibits localized areas of resorption, appearing as *radiolucent defects.* Porous subchondral bone typically leads to the development of *synovial cysts* or *pseudocysts,* formed by intrusion of synovial fluid into periarticular bone. Reparative processes such as sclerosis are minimal or absent. Some sclerosis may be evident, however, if degenerative changes were pre-existing or superimposed on the underlying inflammatory condition.

Osteoporosis

Localized areas of decreased bone density, or *rarefaction,* appear in the early stages of RA at periarticular regions because of increased blood flow to the synovium. In later

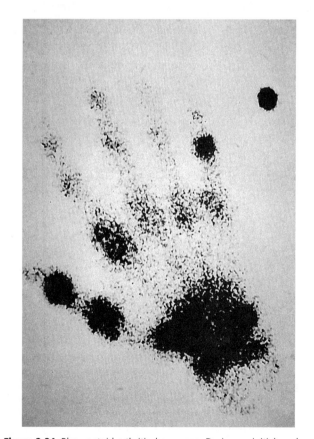

Figure 2-34 Rheumatoid arthritis, bone scan. During an initial workup on a young woman with complaints of bilateral hand pain, radiographs were negative for pathological changes, and laboratory findings were inconclusive. A bone scan was done to narrow the differential diagnosis further. The radiopharmaceutical technetium-99m was injected 2 hours before the scan. Note the abnormal uptake in the wrist, the distal interphalangeal joint of the fifth digit, the first and second metacarpophalangeal joints, and the interphalangeal joint of the thumb. This represents an inflammatory phase of the disease.

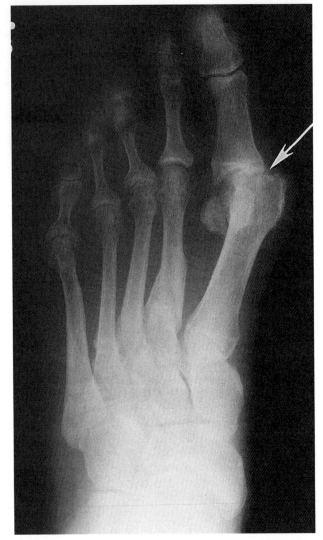

Figure 2-35 Rheumatoid arthritis of the foot. First metatarsopha-langeal joint shows severe *erosion* of the joint surface with *subluxation* of the metatarsal (arrow).

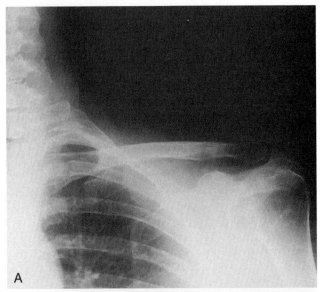

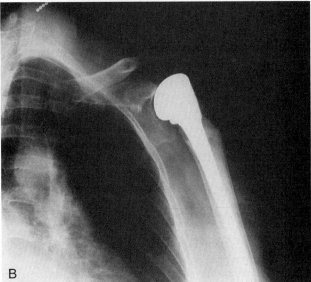

Figure 2-36 Advanced rheumatoid arthritis at the shoulder joint. **(A)** This anteroposterior view shows migration of the humeral head occurring as a result of articular erosion and associated rupture of the rotator cuff. **(B)** Postoperative film showing resection of humeral head and prosthetic replacement.

stages, generalized osteoporosis is evident as a result of inactivity (see Fig. 2-10).

Joint Space Narrowing

Erosion of articular cartilage results in *joint space narrowing*. Because the entire joint surface is affected in RA, narrowing is *concentric*. At the hip, concentric narrowing results in axial or medial *migration* of the femoral head, leading to *acetabular protrusion* (see Chapter 9), an outpouching of the acetabular cup caused by upward pressure from the femoral head into osteoporotic periarticular bone. At the shoulder, cephalad migration of the humeral head can occur as a result of articular erosion and associated rupture of the rotator cuff (Fig. 2-36).

Joint Deformities

Joint *subluxations* and *dislocations* occur secondary to a combination of capsular and ligamentous laxity, destruction of joint surfaces, and tendon rupture. *Flexion contractures* result from maintaining joints in a position of maximum capsular volume to gain pain relief from the pressure of joint swelling. Characteristic of, but not solely pathognomonic for, rheumatoid arthritis are the following deformities of the hands (see Fig. 2-10):

- *Swan-neck deformity:* hyperextension of the proximal interphalangeal joints with flexion of the distal interphalangeal joints
- *Boutonnière deformity:* the opposite configuration to swan-neck deformity—that is, flexion of the proximal interphalangeal joints with extension of the distal interphalangeal joints
- *Telescoping* or *main en lorgnette deformity:* the shortened appearance of the phalanges, caused by metacarpophalangeal joint destruction and dislocation
- Joint *ankylosis,* or bony fixation across a joint space, which is a relatively rare finding in adult rheumatoid arthritis but, when present, is most frequently encountered at the midcarpal articulations (Fig. 2-37).

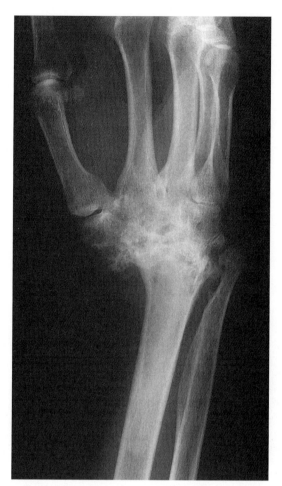

Figure 2-37 Advanced rheumatoid arthritis at the wrist. Note the diffuse ankylosis that has occurred throughout the carpals and radiocarpal joint. Note the marked erosion of the distal radius.

Joint deformities are also encountered at the feet. *Hallux valgus* and *hammer-toe* result from subluxations at the metatarsophalangeal joints of the great toe and remaining digits, respectively.

Changes in the Cervical Spine

RA is rare in other regions of the axial skeleton, but it affects the cervical spine in over half of patients within the first 10 years of disease onset. Erosion and narrowing of the apophyseal (facet) joints and intervertebral joints, leading to slight subluxations, are common findings. Life-threatening, however, is the subluxation of the atlantoaxial joint (C1–C2). This results from laxity in the transverse ligament of the atlas combined with erosive changes and superior migration of the odontoid process. Subluxation may occur in any direction, although anterior is most common. Diagnosis is made via *stress radiographs.* The cervical spine is radiographed at the end range of flexion, and again at the end range of extension. A standard measurement for assessing atlantoaxial anterior subluxation is an *atlantodental interface* that exceeds 3 mm. However, the degree of anterior subluxation has been shown to correlate poorly with neurological signs and cord compression. The poor correlation is in part due to the unknown thickness of the synovial pannus,

not visible on conventional radiographs. MRI is useful in determining true cord space. This segmental instability usually requires surgical intervention, because even minor trauma may result in fatal spinal cord compression (Fig. 2-38).

Osteoarthritis (Degenerative Joint Disease)[12,18,19,23]

Osteoarthritis (degenerative joint disease, osteoarthrosis, degenerative arthritis) is by far the most common type of arthritis. Some degree of osteoarthritis is evidenced radiographically in the majority of the population over age 65 in the United States. Osteoarthritis is characterized by degeneration of the articular cartilage and bony overgrowth at joint margins (Fig. 2-39). Clinical symptomatology, including pain, deformity, and loss of joint function, may range from absent or minimal to severe and necessitating surgical intervention. Osteoarthritis fits into the miscellaneous category of the pathological conditions as outlined earlier, since its etiology appears to be multifactorial and at times even obscure. Genetics, aging, gender, obesity, race, and mechanical trauma may all contribute to the condition.

Osteoarthritis is classified into two types—*primary* and *secondary.* Primary osteoarthritis is idiopathic, develops spontaneously in middle age, and progresses slowly as an exaggeration of the normal aging process of joints. (Some researchers question the validity of this classification, asserting that some type of mechanical deviation always precedes degeneration, even if subtle.) Secondary osteoarthritis, in contrast, develops at any age and is the result of a clearly defined underlying condition or precipitating injury.

Secondary osteoarthritis is the most common type of joint arthropathy. It is the result of any injury, disease, or deformity that damages the articular cartilage or disrupts optimal joint congruity and thereby alters normal arthrokinematics. Examples include inflammatory processes, joint infections, congenital deformities, major joint trauma such as torn menisci or torn ligaments, and microtrauma from repetitive occupational or athletic stresses. The secondary osteoarthritis that develops after *fracture,* caused by either an intra-articular extension of the fracture line or the altered surface kinematics from a malunion deformity, is commonly referred to as *posttraumatic arthritis.*

An interesting paradox can exist between the clinical presentation and the radiographic presentation of osteoarthritis: The severity of osteoarthritic findings demonstrated radiographically *does not always correlate with the clinical symptoms.* That is, a patient with significant osteoarthritic radiographic findings may experience relatively minor pain and loss of function, whereas a patient with minimal osteoarthritic radiographic findings may experience severe pain and impaired function. Thus it is important that therapeutic or surgical intervention be predicated upon the severity of pain and loss of joint function, not on the severity of the radiographic findings.

The clinical features of osteoarthritis are joint pain with movement or weight bearing. Acute exacerbations demonstrate temporary joint effusions. Joint deformities can

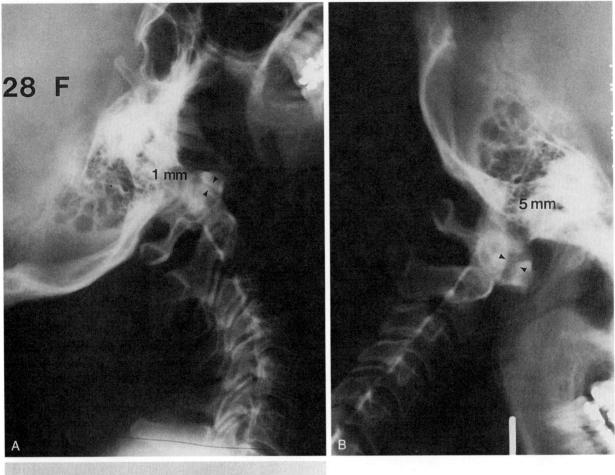

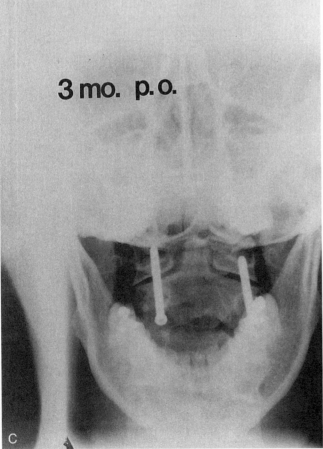

Figure 2-38 Instability of C1–C2 as demonstrated in this 28-year-old woman with rheumatoid arthritis. **(A,B)** On extension and flexion films the atlantodens interface is noted to gape from 1 to 5 mm. Normally this interface is to remain constant in any degree of flexion or extension. **(C)** Based on these findings, the patient underwent surgical fixation of the C1–C2 segment.

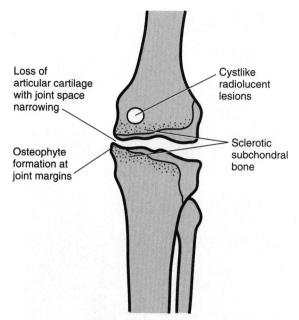

Figure 2-39 Radiographic hallmarks of osteoarthritis.

Loss of articular cartilage with joint space narrowing

Osteophyte formation at joint margins

Cystlike radiolucent lesions

Sclerotic subchondral bone

- Loss of normal elastic resilience
- Loss of support for collagen fibrils, rendering them more susceptible to joint friction
- A resultant acceleration of shedding of the cartilaginous surface layers with vertical splitting of deeper layers (fibrillation and fissuring).

Repair efforts are insufficient, and degeneration of the cartilage progresses, evidenced radiographically by diminution of the joint space (Fig. 2-40).

Subchondral Sclerosis

The reactive response of the subchondral bone to degeneration of the articular cartilage is a prominent feature of osteoarthritis (Fig. 2-41). The subchondral bone gradually becomes the weight-bearing surface. *Eburnation* describes the polished ivory appearance of the exposed surface of subchondral bone. In central areas of maximal stress and friction, the subchondral bone hypertrophies to the extent that it becomes radiographically more dense, or *sclerotic.* In areas of minimal stress, however, subchondral bone may atrophy, and loss of density, or *rarefaction,* may be evident.

Osteophyte Formation

A reparative response to articular cartilage loss is hypertrophy and hyperplasia at the peripheral margins of the joint. This formation of bony outgrowth is described as *osteophyte formation, bone spurs, osteoarthritic lipping,* or *osteophytosis.* Osteophytes may enlarge enough to impinge on adjacent tissues or restrict joint function.

Cysts or Pseudocysts

Excessive pressure, especially in weight-bearing joints, leads to microfractures of the trabeculae of subchondral bone. Intrusion of synovial fluid into the altered spongy

progress over time. Functional capabilites of the joint become increasingly limited.

Radiologic Features of Osteoarthritis

Radiologic features characteristic of osteoarthritis are discussed in the following paragraphs.

Joint Space Narrowing

The earliest biochemical change in osteoarthritis is loss of proteoglycan from the matrix of articular cartilage. The biomechanical consequences of this include the following:

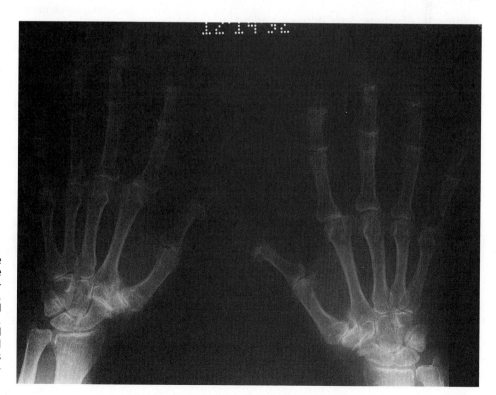

Figure 2-40 Osteoarthritis of the hands in a 75-year-old woman. The radiographic hallmarks of osteoarthritis, including joint space narrowing, sclerosis of the subchondral bone, and osteophyte formation at joint margins, is evident throughout the distal and proximal interphalangeal joints of all the fingers, the interphalangeal joints of the thumb, and the radial side intercarpal joints, bilaterally.

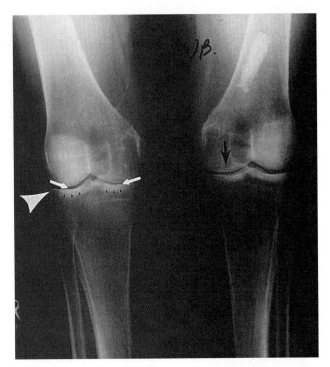

Figure 2-41 Osteoarthritis of the knees in a 66-year-old female. This film was taken under weight-bearing conditions. At the patient's right knee, osteoarthritis is evidenced by narrowed joint space (white arrows), osteophyte formation at the joint margins (large white arrowhead), and sclerotic subchondral bone (small black arrowheads) of both the medial and lateral tibial plateaus. At the patient's left knee, it is interesting to note that in the area of minimal weight-bearing stress the subchondral bone has lost density, and rarefaction is present on the medial aspect of the joint.

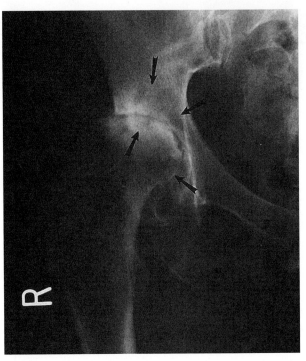

Figure 2-42 Severe osteoarthritis of the hip with pseudocysts. The radiolucent cystlike areas (arrows) are caused by intrusion of synovial fluid into areas of subchondral bone that have become weakened by microfractures.

bone forms cyst-like lesions, evident on radiographs as radiolucent areas (Fig. 2-42).

Additional Findings: Soft Tissue Swelling

Fragments of dead cartilage can dislodge into the joint, irritating the synovial membrane and causing acute inflammation and synovial effusion. The synovium may encapsulate this joint debris, thus enlarging and deforming the joint, as, for example, in Heberden's nodes in the distal interphalangeal joints (see Chapter 17).

Joint Deformities

Other joint deformities and joint misalignment can result from contractures (related to maintaining joints in positions of maximum capsular volume for pain relief) or from altered joint surface congruity (due to loss of articular cartilage). The knee, for example, can exhibit marked *genu valgum* (knock-knee) or *genu varum* (bowleggedness).

Osteoporosis[12,18,19,23]

Osteoporosis is a metabolic bone disease characterized by decreased osteoblastic formation of matrix combined with increased osteoclastic resorption of bone. The result is a *decrease in total bone mass and density.* However, while the *amount* of bone is insufficient, the bone itself remains normally mineralized.

The etiology of osteoporosis is widely varied. It may occur as a primary, age-related phenomenon or appear secondary to congenital or acquired underlying conditions (Table 2-8).[14] Osteoporosis may be one of the following:

- *Generalized,* involving the entire skeleton
- *Regional,* involving a limb or region of the skeleton
- *Localized,* involving only focal areas of bone

Conventional radiography is the most widely available method of evaluating osteoporosis, but it is insensitive to early stages of the disease: A 30% reduction in bone mass is required before density changes will be evident radiographically. Several other imaging modalities are sensitive to minute changes in bone density. These vary widely in cost, radiation dose, and availability. Dual-energy x-ray absorptiometry (DEXA) probably offers the greatest precision and lowest radiation dose and is the preferred diagnostic modality at present. See "Focus on DEXA Diagnosis of Osteoporosis" at http://www.fadavis.com/imaging.

On the conventional radiograph, the hallmark appearance of osteoporotic bone is increased *radiolucency.* This can lead to incorrect usage of the term *osteoporotic* as a radiologic *descriptor.* This usage is incorrect because it is usually impossible to distinguish on the basis of the radiogram between osteoporosis and the other potential causes of increased bone radiolucency. Compare the following three distinct clinical entities, which all present on the radiograph as radiolucent bone:

- *Osteoporosis:* deficient matrix, normal mineralization
- *Osteomalacia:* normal matrix, deficient mineralization (see Fig. 2-13)
- *Hyperparathyroidism:* normal matrix and mineralization, increased resorption (see Fig. 2-14).

TABLE 2-8 ● *Examples of Conditions Associated with Osteoporosis*

Generalized Osteoporosis (Most of Skeleton, Especially Axial Components Involved)

Endocrine
- Estrogen deficiency
- Hyperparathyroidism
- Hyperthyroidism
- Diabetes mellitus
- Pregnancy

Neoplastic
- Malignant bone disease
- Leukemia
- Lymphoma
- Metastatic disease

Iatrogenic
- Drug-induced
- Heparin
- Phenytoin (Dilantin)
- Steroids

Genetic
- Osteogenesis imperfecta
- Hemophilia
- Gaucher's disease

Deficiency States
- Anorexia
- Alcoholism
- Weight loss
- Malnutrition

Miscellaneous
- Involutional
- Senile osteoporosis
- Postmenopausal osteoporosis
- Paraplegia
- Weightlessness

Regional Osteoporosis (A Limb or Region of the Skeleton Involved)

- Migratory osteoporosis
- Transient osteoporosis
- Complex regional pain syndrome (formerly RSD)
- Paget's disease
- Disuse/pain

Localized Osteoporosis (Focal Involvement)

- Neoplasm
- Inflammatory arthritis

Therefore the term *osteoporosis* should not be used as a descriptor but only when appropriate as a *clinical diagnosis.* The appropriate descriptor of bone that appears abnormally radiolucent is *osteopenia,* which means "poverty of bone."

Clinical features of osteoporosis are the consequences that result from the disease: fractures and postural deformities.

Radiologic Features of Osteoporosis

Radiologic features characteristic to all forms of osteoporosis, regardless of etiology, are cortical thinning, osteopenia, trabecular changes, and fractures, discussed in the following paragraphs.

Cortical Thinning

The first sites affected by osteoporosis, as well as the ones that are best demonstrated radiographically, are the periarticular regions where the cortex is normally thinner. Loss of the cortical outline indicates loss of density. Along the shafts of the long bones, loss of density is also demonstrated by "thinning" of the cortices.

The normal amount of *cortical thickness* is an objective measurement and can be compared with normal standards or used as a baseline for subsequent studies in the same patient (Fig. 2-43A). Measured at the midpoint of a metacarpal shaft (usually the second or third), cortical thickness is simply the sum of the two cortices. This sum should equal approximately one-half the total diameter of the bone. Another measurement of density is the *index of bone mass,* which is simply the sum of the cortices divided by the total diameter (Fig. 2-43B).

Osteopenia

Osteopenia is the radiographic descriptor for increased bone radiolucency. Osteopenia is diagnosed by observing insufficent contrast between the soft-tissue shade of gray and the bone shade of gray. The term *rarefaction* is also used to describe periarticular, localized areas of decreased density.

Trabecular Changes

In osteoporosis, the trabeculae are diminished in number and thickness and so appear sparse, thin, and delicate. Observe the anteroposterior (AP) radiograph of the knee in a patient diagnosed with osteoporosis in Figure 2-44. Although the trabeculae appear accentuated, this is not because they are strong; rather, the resorption of surrounding trabeculae make the last few remining trabeculae appear prominent! Note also the effects of Wolff's law—the vertically oriented trabeculae are spared to the last to withstand the forces of weight-bearing.

Fractures

Increased incidence of fractures in patients with osteoporosis is directly related to the loss of bone mass and consequent loss of structural integrity. The most common sites of fracture in patients with generalized osteoporosis are the vertebral bodies, ribs, proximal humerus, distal radius, and proximal femur (Figs. 2-45 through 2-48). A cumulative effect of multiple vertebral body compression fractures is a characteristic *kyphotic deformity* of the spine, commonly seen in elderly women.

The Pathology Problem: Image Quality Versus Disease[30]

The characteristic demineralized appearance of osteoporotic bone can lead the novice to a logical question: How can I tell the difference between demineralized bone and poor image quality? This is the "pathology problem" that radiographers try to address for all disease processes. Radiographers must have an understanding of the patient's pathology and how it affects overall thickness and composition of body tissues in order to select the most appropriate technical exposure factors. Gathering data from the patient's requisition form, taking an adequate patient history, and observing the patient are essential responsibilities of the radiographer. In general, the radiographer classifies diseases

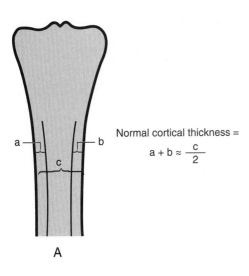

Normal cortical thickness =
$$a + b \approx \frac{c}{2}$$

A

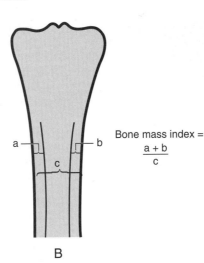

Bone mass index =
$$\frac{a + b}{c}$$

B

Figure 2-43 **(A)** Cortical thickness measurements are usually based on the cortices at the midshaft of the second or third metacarpal. Normally, the sum of the two cortex thicknesses should equal approximately one-half the overall diameter of the shaft. **(B)** Cortical thickness may also be expressed as an index of bone mass, which is the sum of the cortical thicknesses divided by shaft diameter.

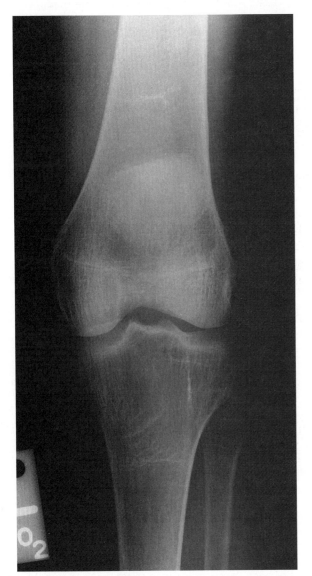

Figure 2-44 Osteoporosis is evident in this knee by the accentuation of the remaining trabeculae. The trabeculae have diminished in number and in thickness, and the remaining vertically oriented trabeculae stand out as thin, delicate line images.

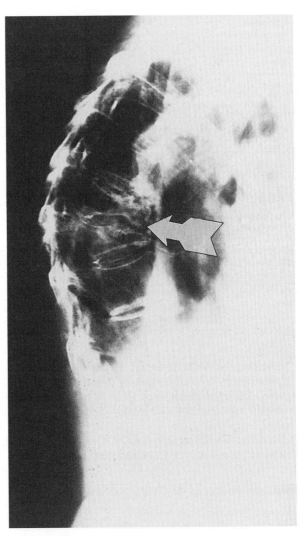

Figure 2-45 Osteoporosis of the spine with multiple compression fractures. The arrow points to the T8–T9 disk space, which is deformed by the collapse of these two vertebrae from multiple compression fractures. This 94-year-old woman has severe kyphosis of the thoracic spine (also known as a gibbous deformity) accentuated by vertebral collapse at multiple levels.

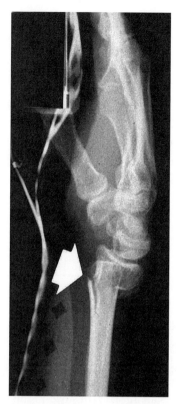

Figure 2-46 Distal radius fracture. This 54-year-old woman fell on an outstretched arm and sustained a fracture of the distal radius, commonly known as a Colles' fracture. There is a palmar apex of the fracture site with dorsal angulation. The osteoporotic changes present are difficult to visualize through the splint material.

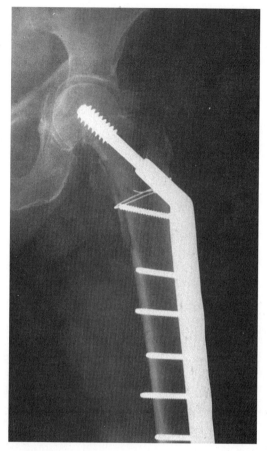

Figure 2-47 Intertrochanteric fracture of the left femur, fixed with compression plate and screws.

into conditions of additive or increased attenuation and destructive or decreased attenuation.

Additive conditions add density to the body. This, in turn, increases attenuation of the beam. These conditions require increased exposure to achieve proper density on the radiograph. Examples of additive conditions are acromegaly, chronic osteomyelitis, osteoblastic metastases, Paget's disease, and sclerosis. Destructive conditions decrease tissue density. These tissues attenuate less of the x-ray beam and require less exposure to achieve density on the radiograph. Examples of destructive conditions are osteoporosis, osteomalacia, osteolytic metastases, and hyperparathyroidism.

No magic technical formula exists for the radiographer to compensate for pathology. Too many variables exist—not the least of which are the significant differences between early and advanced stages of a disease. Thus, experience and judgment on the part of the radiographer factor into technical decisions. After the radiograph is made, the radiographer decides whether the radiograph is of *sufficient diagnostic quality*. Radiographs of poor image quality, with insufficient diagnostic detail, are discarded.

Conditions that are *unknown* prior to the radiographic exam may require additional exposures to produce

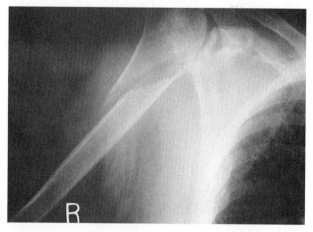

Figure 2-48 Spiral fracture through the surgical neck of the proximal humerus in a 62-year-old woman. Osteoporosis is evidenced by the thinning of the cortices along the shaft of the humerus.

radiographs of sufficient diagnostic quality. One of the advantages of digital over film radiography is the ability to adjust density after the exposure is made, thus negating the need for repeat exposures.

TABLE 2-9 ● *Musculoskeletal Infections*

Category	Common Route of Dissemination	Common Pathogen	Typical Region Affected	Radiologic Characteristics
Bone Osteomyelitis	Hematogenous	*Staphylococcus aureus*	Metaphyseal regions of long bones in children	● Soft tissue swelling 24–48 hours after onset ● Radiolucent lytic lesion in 7–10 days ● Sequestra and involucra in 6–8 weeks ● Draining sinus tracts
Joints Infectious or septic arthritis	Hematogenous	*Staphylococcus aureus*	Child: Hip, knee, elbow, intervertebral disks Adult: Hip, knee, shoulder, wrist, intervertebral disks	● Soft tissue swelling ● Joint effusion ● Periarticular rarefaction ● Joint space narrowing ● Subchondral bone erosion
Soft Tissues Cellulitis	Direct puncture of skin	*Clostridium novyi* and *Clostridium perfringens*	Feet	● Soft tissue swelling ● Radiolucent streaks or bubbles representing gas gangrene

Musculoskeletal Infections[19,31,32]

Infections of the musculoskeletal system can be divided into three categories (Table 2-9):

1. Infections of bone, *osteomyelitis*
2. Infections of joints, *septic* or *infectious arthritis*
3. Infections of soft tissue, *cellulitis* or *myositis*

The three basic mechanisms or routes that permit an infectious organism to gain entry are:

● *Direct implantation* from a puncture wound, open fracture, or operative procedure (Fig. 2-49)
● *Contiguous* from infection in adjacent soft tissues
● *Hematogenous,* via the bloodstream from a distant site of infection in the body

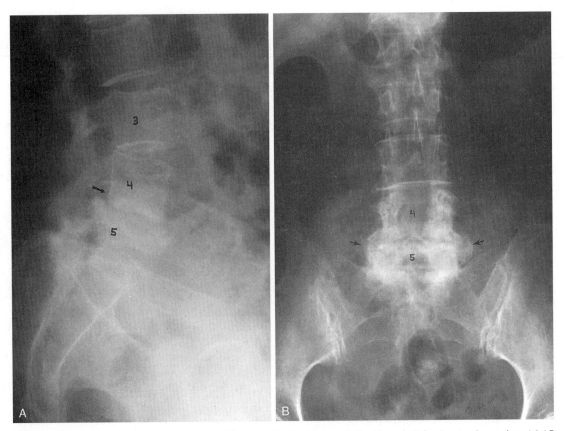

Figure 2-49 L4–L5 osteomyelitis. This 77-year-old woman had a history of L3, L4, and L5 laminectomies and an L4–L5 diskectomy secondary to radiculopathy and decreased bowel and bladder function. An infection developed postoperatively. **(A)** On the lateral film, an anterolisthesis of L4 on the eroded body of L5 is seen (arrow). **(B)** On the anterior posterior view, the sequestra are noted (arrows).

Bone and joint infections may present in acute, subacute, or chronic forms, defined by the intensity of the infectious process and the associated symptoms. Furthermore, bone and joint infections may be distinguished as either *pyogenic* (suppurative, or pus-producing) or *nonpyogenic* (nonsuppurative). The most common organism of pyogenic infection is *Staphylococcus aureus.* Nonpyogenic infections may be caused by *Mycobacterium tuberculosis, Treponema pallidum* (syphilis), and fungi.

General clinical signs and symptoms of musculoskeletal infection include pain, swelling, and tenderness in the affected joints and adjacent soft tissues. Fever, malaise, and weight loss may be present.

Radiologic Features of Osteomyelitis

Acute osteomyelitis is often pyogenic, resulting from hematogenous spread of the *S. aureus* organism. It most commonly presents in the long bones of children, with higher incidence in boys. The metaphyseal region is the primary site of involvement because of the unique blood supply of this region during growth. The radiologic features characteristic of acute pyogenic osteomyelitis are soft tissue swelling, lytic lesions, and sequestra with involucra, discussed in the following paragraphs.

Soft Tissue Swelling
The earliest signs of bone infection are soft tissue edema and *loss of tissue planes,* usually present within 24 to 48 hours after the onset of infection. The loss of tissue planes means a blurring of the normally sharp interface between tissues such as muscles and subcutaneous fat.

Lytic Lesion
A destructive lytic lesion, represented by an area of increased bone radiolucency, is visible within 7 to 10 days after the onset of infection. Progressive cortical and cancellous destruction occurs over the next 2 to 6 weeks (see Fig. 2-17).

Sequestra and Involucra
In 6 to 8 weeks after onset, *sequestra*—isolated segments of dead bone usually surrounded by pus—become apparent. A sequestrum is surrounded by an *involucrum,* an envelope of immature periosteal bone that also becomes infected. Draining *sinus tracts* (see Fig. 2-17) often are formed through the involucrum, and pus and small bits of the sequestrum may be discharged. At this stage, the condition is designated as *chronic osteomyelitis* (Fig. 2-50).

Radiologic Features of Infectious Arthritis

Infectious arthritis of the pyogenic type is seen predominantly in children and elderly individuals. Hematogenous dissemination is the most common route of infection. Although *S. aureus* is the most common causative agent, certain populations are predisposed to infection by other microbes. For example, individuals who abuse drugs intravenously are predisposed to *Pseudomonas aeruginosa* infections of the axial skeletal joints; infection of the

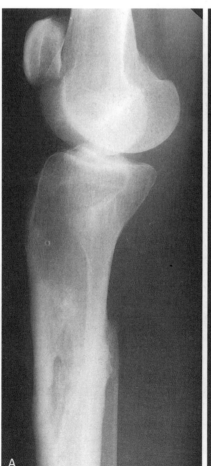
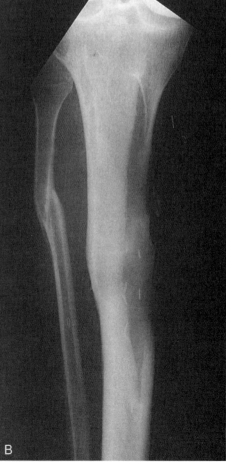

Figure 2-50 Chronic osteomyelitis of the tibia and fibula. This 44-year-old man developed osteomyelitis following a fracture. Involucrum **(A)** surrounds both the tibia and the fibula, seen on a lateral view of the leg. Patient received an extensive course of antibiotics and surgical debridement. **(B)** Resection of dead bone.

intervertebral joint is known as *diskitis* and is often associated with a vertebral body osteomyelitis (Fig. 2-51). *Salmonellae* commonly cause infectious arthritis in individuals with sickle cell disease. Additionally, conditions that lower resistance, such as prolonged adrenocorticosteroid therapy, may influence predisposition to infection.

Infections in prosthetic joints, although uncommon, lead to loosening, failure, and devastating degeneration of the remaining joint.

In children, the joints in which the metaphysis is entirely encapsulated—namely, the hip, elbow, and knee—are commonly affected (Fig. 2-52). Destruction of epiphyseal

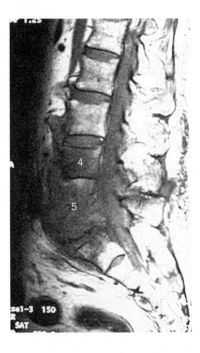
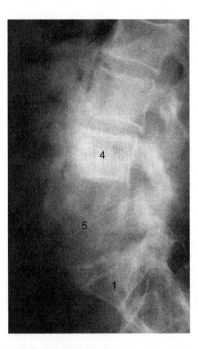

Figure 2-51 Osteomyelitis and diskitis of the spine secondary to intravenous drug abuse. This 44-year-old patient presented with complaints of low back pain. Sagittal MRI and lateral radiograph show complete destruction of the L5 vertebral body and extension of the infection across the disk spaces into the bodies of L4 and S1. *(Image courtesy of John C. Hunter, MD, University of California, Davis School of Medicine.)*

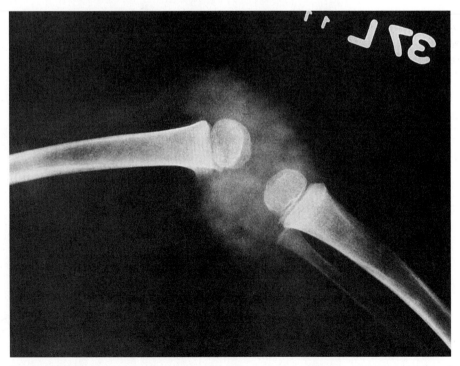

Figure 2-52 Infectious arthritis. This 3½-year-old toddler presented with a 3-month history of pain and swelling and with a visible lump on the knee. There was a history of frequent upper respiratory infections and pneumonia. Distension of the knee joint capsule with pus is evident. Note the absence of the image of the patella, which does not ossify until age 4.

plates, with resultant growth arrest, is a dreaded complication.

In adults, infectious arthritis may develop in any joint but is most common in the knee, hip, shoulder, and wrist, and some reports indicate an increase incidence in the spine secondary to intravenous drug abuse (Fig. 2-53). The radiographic features characteristic of pyogenic infectious arthritis are discussed in the following paragraphs.

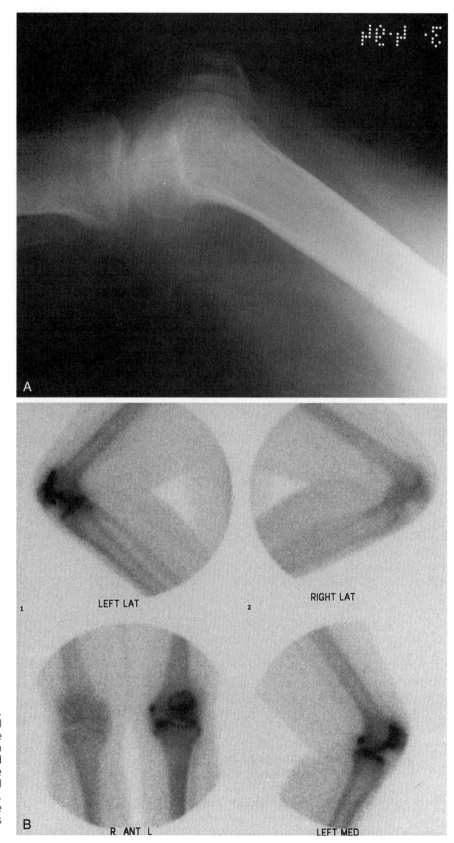

Figure 2-53 Infectious arthritis, bone scan. This 34-year-old man had a history of surgical debridement at the knee 1 year previously. He was re-evaluated for recurrent pain. **(A)** Plain film findings were suggestive of either mild osteoarthritis or infectious arthritis. **(B)** Bone scan showed increased uptake in the medial lateral compartment and patella of the knee. When these findings were correlated with the laboratory findings, a diagnosis of infectious arthritis was confirmed.

Soft Tissue Swelling

Early stages of joint infection are demonstrated by joint effusion and adjacent soft tissue swelling.

Periarticular Rarefaction

Radiolucency of bone at the periarticular regions is also an early radiographic finding.

Joint Space Narrowing

In later stages, destruction of articular cartilage on both sides of the joint will significantly narrow the joint space.

Subchondral Bone Erosion

As infectious arthritis involves all articular surfaces within the joint, erosion of subchondral bone will be evident on all joint surfaces.

Radiologic Features of Cellulitis

Cellulitis usually results from direct skin puncture, but it can also result from complications of systemic disorders such as diabetes. The most common infectious organisms are the gas-producing *Clostridium novyi* and *Clostridium perfringens.*

The radiographic features characteristic of cellulitis are discussed in the following paragraphs.

Soft Tissue Swelling

Cellulitis presents with soft-tissue edema and obliteration of fat and fascial planes.

Radiolucent Streaks or Bubbles

The gas-forming organisms may cause an accumulation of gas within the soft tissues, which is demonstrated on the radiograph as radiolucent bubbles or streaks. This is usually an indication of gas gangrene (Fig. 2-54).

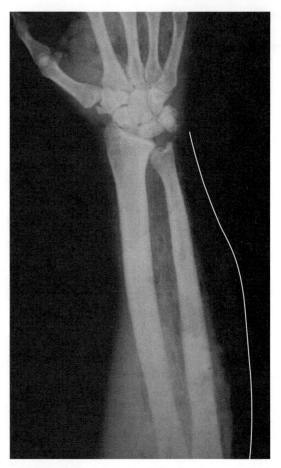

Figure 2-54 Gas gangrene and cellulits due to contamination by clostridium organisms. This AP radiograph of the forearm demonstrates the subcutaneous, linear, radiolucent collection of gas along the medial side of the forearm (line). *(Image courtesy of http://www .medcyclopaedia.com by GE Healthcare.)*

Bone Tumors[12,19,32–34]

Classification and Terminology

The term *tumor* refers to a mass of autonomous growth, an equivalent term being neoplasm. Tumors are generally divided into two categories: benign and malignant. Benign tumors usually are not recurrent or aggressive in bony destruction. Malignant tumors, in contrast, are aggressive and may produce local or remote metastases. Malignant tumors are thus further classified as primary, secondary (the result of a malignant transformation of a benign process), or metastatic. The incidence of primary bone tumors is only 0.2% of all neoplasms. In contrast, 20% to 80% of organ cancers will metastasize to bone (refer to Table 2-5). Specific histopathologic criteria additionally are applied in determining whether a tumor is malignant or benign.

Tumors are also classified by their tissue of origin (Table 2-10). Tumors that become manifest in bone may originate from bone, marrow, cartilage, fibrous tissue, or unknown tissues. Tumors that appear in soft tissues usually originate from fatty and fibrous tissues.

The terminology of tumor names can sometimes help identify the tissue of origin, and whether the processes are benign or malignant. The prefixes *osteo-, chondro-, fibro-, lipo-,* and *neuro-* identify tissue origin. The suffix *-oma* usually denotes benign processes. The suffix *-sarcoma* denotes malignant processes. For example, the *osteogenic benign tumors* are tumors originating from bone tissue, such as *osteoma, osteoid osteoma,* and *osteoblastoma.* Examples of malignant osteogenic tumors are the variants of *osteosarcoma.* Some obvious exceptions to the suffix clue are the malignancies *myeloma* and *neuroblastoma.*

Clinical Signs and Symptoms

Bone tumors may present with localized pain, tenderness, swelling, or a palpable mass. Fever, malaise, and weight loss may be present in some individuals. Less frequently, bone tumors are clinically silent and are detected on radiographs obtained for unrelated reasons. Pathological fractures, or fractures in bone that has been compromised by a pre-existing disease process (in this case, the tumor) can sometimes be the event that leads to discovery of a tumor.

Imaging of Bone Tumors

Conventional radiographs are the chief imaging modality for the initial assessment of bone tumors. The radiographic presentation defines the basic tumor category: The lesion is classified as either nonaggressive or aggressive. Conventional radiographs detail calcification, ossification, cortical

TABLE 2-10 ● *Classification of Tumors by Tissue of Origin*

Tissue Type	Tumors	Common Sites
Bone *(osteogenic tumors)*	**Benign**	
	Bone island	Femur, innominate, rib
	Osteoma	Skull, facial bone, paranasal sinus
	Osteoblastoma	Medullary lesion of spine, femur, tibia
	Malignant	
	Osteosarcoma	Femur, tibia, humerus
Marrow *(hematopoietic tumors)*	**Benign**	
	Giant cell tumor (<5% are malignant)	Femur, tibia, radius
	Malignant	
	Multiple myeloma	Vertebra, rib, innominate, femur
	Ewing's sarcoma	Femur, innominate, tibia
Cartilage *(chondrogenic tumors)*	**Benign**	
	Chondroma	Phalanges, humerus, wrist
	Chondroblastoma	Humerus, femur, tibia
	Osteochondroma	Humerus, femur, tibia
	Malignant	
	Chondrosarcoma	Humerus, innominate, femur
Nerves *(neurogenic tumors)*	**Benign**	
	Neurofibroma	Mouth, pleura, stomach
	Malignant	
	Neuroblastoma	Mediastinal, retroperitoneal
Fat *(lipogenic tumors)*	**Benign**	
	Lipoma	Femus, calcaneus, extremities
	Malignant	
	Liposarcoma	Buttocks, thigh, calf, retroperitoneal
Fibrous *(fibrogenic tumors)*	**Benign**	
	Fibrous dysplasia	Femur, tibia, skull
	Fibrous cortical defect	Femur, tibia
	Malignant	
	Fibrosarcoma	Femur, jaw, tibia
	Malignant fibrous histiocytoma	Femur, tibia, humerus
Unknown	**Benign**	
	Simple bone cyst	Humerus, femur
	Aneurysmal bone cyst	Metaphyses of long bones
	Malignant	
	Angioblastoma	Tibial diaphysis

destruction, and periosteal reaction. Tumors that demonstrate classic characteristic features of a nonaggressive lesion may lead to an immediate diagnosis, and no further imaging is required. Tumors that demonstrate ambiguous characteristics or aggressive characteristics require additional imaging. Usually the choice of which imaging modality to use next is dictated by the type of suspected tumor (Fig. 2-55).

MRI is useful for delineating bone marrow and soft-tissue involvement, and staging of tumors. CT is useful in assessing areas of complex anatomy and subtle cortical erosions and periosteal reactions. Radionuclide bone scans define the distribution of polyostotic pathology in the skeleton. While bone scans are nonspecific and highlight only variations in uptake of the tracer, this information can also be useful in some tumor diagnosis. Myeloma, for example, is one of the few tumors that *do not* exhibit increased uptake; a normal bone scan in this instance red-flags the possibility of myeloma. More recently, positron emission tomography (PET) scans

have been used to discriminate between indeterminant benign and malignant lesions, based on the uptake of 18-FDG (18-fluoro-2-deoxyglucose). Benign lesions generally have low FDG uptake, while highly metabolic malignant lesions show increased uptake. Because there are exceptions in the metabolic rates of benign tumors, the clinical value of PET in diagnosis is unclear. In treatment, 18-FDG PET has been used to assess the effectiveness of chemotherapy by comparing the tumor's uptake pre- and posttreatment. A decrease in uptake was associated with a good histological response.

Bone Biopsy

A biopsy is the surgical or percutaneous removal of suspect tissue for histological examination by a pathologist. In almost every circumstance a biopsy provides the most accurate diagnosis possible. A biopsy cannot, however, assess the rate of growth or aggressiveness of a tumor. Biopsy and imaging are complementary in the establishment of a diagnosis. Interestingly, laboratory values are often of little value in the diagnostic process, because benign and malignant tumors often demonstrate normal findings.

Radiographic Features of Tumors

Daffner's[18] 11 predictor variables, discussed earlier, define the characteristics of any lesion or tumor. Refer to Table 2-4 for predictor variables and the related text that elaborates on each point. Refer to Figure 2-29 for preferred locations of many common tumors and to Table 2-5 for peak age incidence of benign and malignant tumors.

An example of a benign tumor, a *chondroblastoma*, is seen in Figure 2-56. The most common primary malignant tumor of bone, an *osteosarcoma*, is seen in Figure 2-31. The second most common primary malignant tumor of bone, *Ewing's sarcoma*, is seen in Figure 2-57. One of the most common malignant soft tissue tumors that metastasize to bone is *rhabdomyosarcoma*, seen in Figure 2-58. An example of an organ cancer that metastasized to the spine is seen in Figure 2-59.

The Radiologic Report[12]

The written radiologic report serves the following purposes:

- It attempts to link the radiologic signs with the patient history and clinical examination findings.
- It provides a standard of comparison with previous or later radiologic examinations.
- It is a permanent record in case radiographs become lost or are not immediately available.
- It expedites the treatment regime by providing a résumé of important indications and contraindications for medical intervention.
- It can be utilized for research purposes.
- It facilitates interprofessional and intraprofessional communication.

Like any component of the medical record, the radiologic report is a reflection of the abilities and professionalism of the clinician. Unfortunately, the format and terminology of radiologic reports are not standardized. Wide variation exists in length and style of reporting.

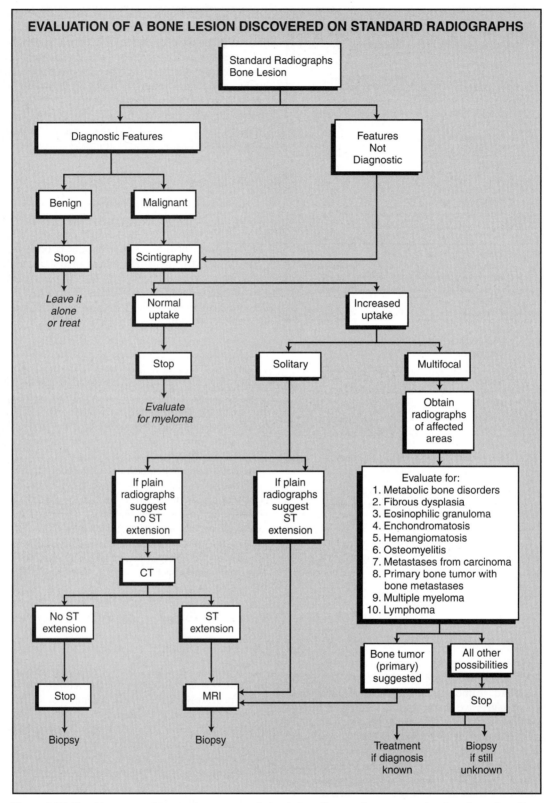

Figure 2-55 Algorithm to evaluate and manage a bone lesion discovered on conventional radiographs. *(From Greenspan,[19] p. 545, with permission.)*

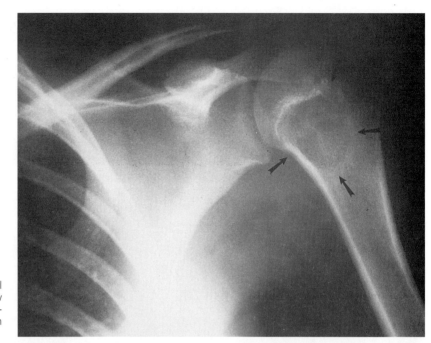

Figure 2-56 Chondroblastoma of the proximal humerus in a 15-year-old girl. Note the narrow zone of transition and well-defined sclerotic margin associated with slow-growing or benign tumors.

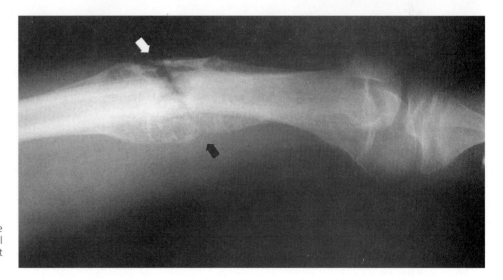

Figure 2-57 Ewing's sarcoma of the femoral shaft with a pathological fracture through the midshaft (arrows) in a 16-year-old boy.

In general, the radiologic report contains the following components:

- Heading
- Clinical information
- Findings
- Conclusions
- Recommendations (optional)
- Signature of radiologist

Heading

The heading of the radiologic report includes:

- Facility information: identification and address of facility, date of exam
- Patient information: name, age or date of birth, gender, case number

- Radiographic information: what anatomy part examined, and the number of views obtained

Variations in the headings for CT reports include:

- Levels imaged
- Whether slices are contiguous or interrupted
- Slice thickness
- Plane of imaging
- Angulation of gantry
- Reformatting
- Windows provided
- Use of contrast agent

Variations in the headings for MRI reports include:

- Area imaged
- Planes of imaging
- Imaging sequences

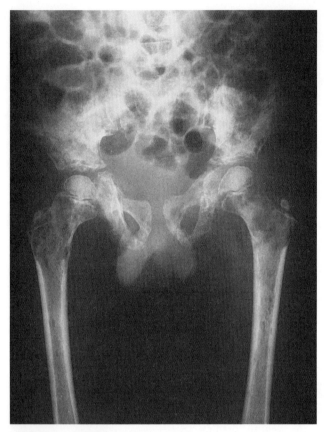

Figure 2-58 Diffuse lytic metastasis to bone secondary to rhabdomyosarcoma. Note the permeative destruction with poorly defined borders of the lesions, which is characteristic of an aggressive or malignant process.

Clinical Information

The *clinical information* section in the radiologic report includes a brief summary of relevant data in the history, physical exam, and laboratory studies. This information can include:

- Location, duration, onset, and symptoms
- History of injury
- Positive orthopedic or neurological tests
- Abnormal laboratory studies
- Abnormal physical examination findings

Findings

Findings make up the body of the report. This is presented in a narrative form with complete sentences, professional terminology, and absence of eponyms or jargon. The findings describe either radiologic abnormalities or normal appearance. Findings do not state a diagnosis, except in cases involving fractures or dislocations.

Findings may also be divided into paragraphs, reflecting the organization of the search pattern. The *ABCs* search pattern would result in four paragraphs with abnormalities grouped by these categories. For example, the first paragraph on *A: Alignment* would comment on any alignment abnormalities and provide roentgenometric lines, angles,

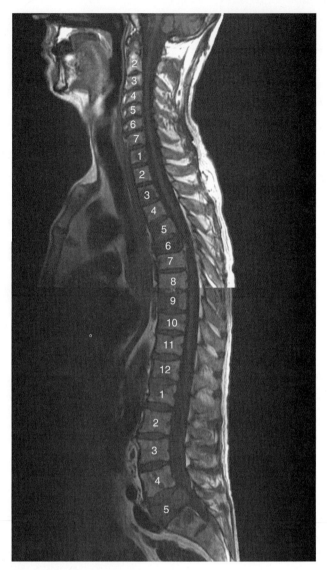

Figure 2-59 Lung cancer metastasized to the spine. Sagittal T1-weighted MRI shows multiple lesions, the largest at T6 where there is a collapse of the vertebral body and the tumor is impinging on the spinal cord, and also at L5 where an expansive tumor is impinging on the thecal sac. Further lesions are present in the vertebral bodies of T1, T3, T5, T9, T10, T12, L1, L4, and S1. *(Image courtesy of Nick Oldnall, http://www.xray2000.uk.co.)*

measurements, or positional terms to describe the abnormality. If no abnormalities existed in this category, it would be addressed with a statement such as "No abnormalities in alignment detected" or "Alignment of visualized osseous structures is within normal limits." Statements like these prove that the clinician actually evaluated this component.

Conclusions

This section may also be identified by other names including *Impressions, Diagnosis, Judgment, Interpretation,* or *Reading.*

This section is a point-by-point summation of the data presented in *Findings.* It is here that the conditions are labeled and diagnoses are reported. The diagnoses are reported in order of severity, beginning with the most serious condition. For example, "metastatic disease" would be listed before "degenerative joint disease." If the entire radiographic exam revealed no abnormalites, the conclusion may simply read "Radiographically negative."

Recommendations

Recommendations is an optional section that appears only if follow-up procedures are indicated. These recommendations are specific for the condition diagnosed or suspected. Recommendations may include additional conventional radiographs, optional projections or positions, other imaging modalities, laboratory evaluation, or referrals to other health-care providers.

Signature

All radiologic reports must be signed by the authors and include their professional credentials.

Radiologic Report Example

Heading:

Patient: Winnifred T. Pooh
Age/sex: 96 F
Case: # 061392
Imaging date: 01/31/10
Part: pelvis
Views: AP, recumbent

Clinical Information:

Fell at home 3 days ago. Presents with left hip pain.

Findings:

Sclerotic line is noted traversing femoral neck with cortical disruption at the medial aspect of the subcapital region. No displacement of femoral head or neck is visualized.

Osseous components of pelvis and proximal femurs exhibit generalized demineralization. No evidence of osteolytic disease is present.

Bilateral hips show moderately decreased joint spaces with sclerotic subchondral bone and minimal osteophytosis at joint margins. Sacroiliac joints and symphysis pubis are negative for abnormalities.

No abnormalities of soft tissues observed.

Conclusions:

1. Recent undisplaced impaction-type fracture of the left femoral neck
2. Generalized osteoporosis
3. Moderate osteoarthritic changes of the bilateral hip joints

Recommendations:

1. Immediate orthopedic referral for surgical consult.
2. Monitor for possible development of avascular necrosis of the femoral head.

Signature:

Christopher Robyn, MD

Summary of Key Points

1. *Remodeling* of bone, which occurs continuously throughout life, is directly related to *function*. To paraphrase Wolff's law, bone is deposited in the sites subjected to stress and resorbed in sites deprived of stress.

2. The essentials of radiographic analysis can be remembered with the acronym *ABCs*: alignment, bone density, cartilage spaces, and soft tissues.

3. There are six basic categories of pathology in the classification of skeletal diseases: congenital, inflammatory, metabolic, neoplastic, traumatic, and vascular. A seventh category, miscellaneous, encompasses those conditions that do not fall strictly into one category, such as osteoarthritis.

4. Radiographic diagnosis of skeletal pathology begins with (1) *defining the distribution of the lesion* and (2) *applying predictor variables to the lesion.*

5. *Predictor variables* are factors that further limit diagnostic choices. Daffner described 11 predictor variables: behavior of the lesion; the bone or joint involved; the locus within a bone; the age, gender, or race of the patient; the

margin of the lesion; the shape of the lesion; involvement of the joint space; bony reaction; matrix production by the lesion; soft tissue changes; and history of trauma or surgery.

6. Radiologic characteristics of *adult rheumatoid arthritis* are periatricular soft tissue swelling, articular erosions, minimal or absent reparative processes, concentric joint space narrowing, rarefaction of periatricular regions in early stages, generalized osteoporosis in later stages, and joint deformities.

7. Radiologic characteristics of *osteoarthritis* are joint space narrowing, sclerosis of subchondral bone, and osteophyte formation at joint margins.

8. Radiologic characteristics of *osteoporosis* are loss of cortical thickness, generalized osteopenia, and associated fractures. The most common sites for fracture are the vertebrae, proximal humerus, distal radius, and proximal femur.

9. *Infections of the musculoskeletal system* can be divided into infections of bone (*osteomyelitis*); infections of

joints (*septic* or *infectious arthritis*); and infections of soft tissues (*cellulitis, myositis*). The earliest radiographic feature of any infection is soft-tissue swelling.

10. *Bone tumors* are categorized as *benign* or *malignant*. They are futher categorized by their tissue of origin. Radiologic features that assist the radiologist in differentiating types of tumors include site of the lesion; margin of the lesion; whether the matrix is osteoid, chondroid, or mixed; the type of destruction (geographic, moth-eaten, or permeative); an interrupted or uninterrupted periosteal response; and the presence of a soft tissue extension of the lesion.

 Please refer to the text's enclosed CD-ROM for the American College of Radiology's current Musculoskeletal Appropriateness Criteria for the following topics: *Bone Tumors, Follow-up of Malignant or Aggressive Musculoskeletal Tumors, Soft Tissue Masses, Suspected Osteomyelitis in Patients With Diabetes Mellitus, Osteoporosis and Bone Mineral Density, and Metastatic Bone Disease.*

References

1. Christensen, E, et al: The effect of time search on perception. Diagn Radiol 138:361, 1981.
2. Doubilet, P, and Herman, P: Interpretation of radiographs: Effect of clinical history. Am J Roentgenol 137:1055, 1981.
3. Holman, BL, et al: Medical impact of unedited preliminary radiology reports. Radiology 191:519, 1994.
4. Rhea, J, et al: Errors of interpretation as elicited by a quality audit of an emergency radiology facility. Radiology 132:277, 1979.
5. Swensson, R, et al: Omissions in radiology: Faulty search or stringent reporting criteria? Radiology 123:563, 1977.
6. Peterson, CK: Factors associated with success or failure in diagnostic radiology. Master's thesis, University of Dundee Centre for Medical Education, Scotland, 1996.
7. Berlin, L: Accuracy of diagnostic procedures: Has it improved over the past five decades? Am J Roentgenol 188:1173–1178, 2007. Available at http://ajronline.org.
8. Goddard, P, et al: Error in radiology. Br J Radiol 74:949, 2001. Available at http://brj.birjournals.org/cgi/content/full/74/886/949.
9. Ashman, C, et al: Satisfaction of search in osteoradiology. 175:541, 2000. Available online at http://ajronline.org.
10. Fitzgerald, R: Radiological error: Analysis, standard setting, targeted instruction, and teamworking. Eur J Radiol 15; 8:1760, 2005. Available at http://www.springerlink.com/content/7ewte32mr7hell3k/
11. Berbaum, K, et al: Satisfaction of search in multitrauma patients: Severity of detected fractures. Acad Radiol 14:711, 2007. Available online at http://linkinghub.elsevier.com/retrieve/pii/S1076633207001390.
12. Marchiori, DM: Clinical Imaging with Skeletal, Chest, and Abdomen Pattern Differentials, ed. 2. Mosby, St. Louis, MO, 2004.
13. Taylor, JAM, et al: Interpretation of abnormal lumbosacral spine radiographs: A test comparing students, clinicians, radiology residents, and radiologists in medicine and chiropractic. Spine 20(10):1147, 1995.
14. James, JJ, and Stuart, RB: Expanded role for the physical therapist: Screening musculoskeletal disorders. Phys Ther Mag 55:121, 1975.
15. Novelline, RA: Squire's Fundamentals of Radiology, ed. 6. Harvard University Press, Cambridge, MA, 2004.
16. Bontrager, KL, and Lampignano, J: Textbook of Radiographic Positioning and Related Anatomy, ed. 6. Mosby, St. Louis, MO, 2005.
17. Frank, E, Smith, B, and Long, B: Merrill's Atlas of Radiographic Positions and Radiologic Procedures, ed.11. Elsevier Health Sciences, Philadelphia, 2007.
18. Daffner, RH: Clinical Radiology: The Essentials, ed. 3. Williams & Wilkins, Baltimore, 2007.
19. Greenspan, A: Orthopedic Radiology: A Practical Approach, ed. 4. Lippincott Williams & Wilkins, Philadelphia, 2004.
20. Sutton, D: Radiology and Imaging for Medical Students, ed. 7. Churchill Livingston, Edinburgh, Scotland, 1998.
21. Stoller, D: Pocket Radiologist Musculoskeletal, Top 100 Diagnoses. Saunders, Philadelphia, 2002.
22. Netter, FH: Atlas of Human Anatomy, ed. 4. Saunders, Philadelphia, 2006.
23. Yochum, TR, and Rowe, LJ: Essentials of Skeletal Radiology, ed. 3. Williams & Wilkins, Baltimore, 2004.
24. Nordin, M, and Frankel, VH: Basic Biomechanics of the Musculoskeletal System, ed. 3. Lippincott Williams & Wilkins, Philadelphia, 2001.
25. Salter, RB: Textbook of Disorders and Injuries of the Musculoskeletal System, ed. 2. Williams & Wilkins, Baltimore, 1983.
26. Brashear, HR, and Raney, RB: Shand's Handbook of Orthopedic Surgery, ed. 10. Mosby, St. Louis, MO, 1986.
27. Swain, JH: An Introduction to Radiology of the Lumbar Spine: Orthopaedic Study Course 94–1, Orthopaedic Section. APTA, Inc., LaCrosse, WI, 1994.
28. Richardson, JK, and Iglarsh, ZA: Clinical Orthopaedic Physical Therapy. Saunders, Philadelphia, 1994.
29. Costa, DN, Calvacanti, FA, and Sernik, RA: Sonographic and CT findings in lipohemarthrosis. Am J Roentgenol 188:W389, 2007. Available online at http://ajronline.org.
30. Carlton, R, and Adler, A: Principles of Radiographic Imaging, ed. 3. Delmar, Albany, NY, 2006.
31. Sheldon, H: Boyd's Introduction to the Study of Disease, ed. 11. Lippincott Williams & Wilkins, Philadelphia, 1992.
32. Dahnert, W: Radiology Review Manual, ed. 5. Lippincott Williams & Wilkins, Philadelphia, 2002.
33. Hodler, J, von Schulthess, GK, and Zollikofer, CL: Musculoskeletal Disease: Diagnostic Imaging and Interventional Technology. Springer, Italy, 2005.
34. Bernstein, J (ed): Musculoskeletal Medicine. American Academy of Orthopedic Surgeons, Rosemont, IL, 2003.

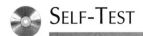 SELF-TEST

Radiograph A

1. Identify this *projection*.

2. A fracture has occurred through the shaft of the femur. What radiographic evidence leads you to believe that this is a *pathological fracture*?

3. Does the entire femur exhibit this radiographic evidence? Does the pelvis?

4. An intermedullary rod is present to unite the fracture gap. Does this appear to be the *first* internal fixation device used at this site?

5. Does the *hip joint* appear normal?

Radiograph B (same patient as radiograph A)

6. Identify this *projection*.

7. The fracture is noted. Identify two other abnormal features of the distal femur.

8. Would you categorize this pathology as probably being related to an *infection*, an *inflammatory process*, or a *neoplasm*? What radiographic evidence suggests a likely category?

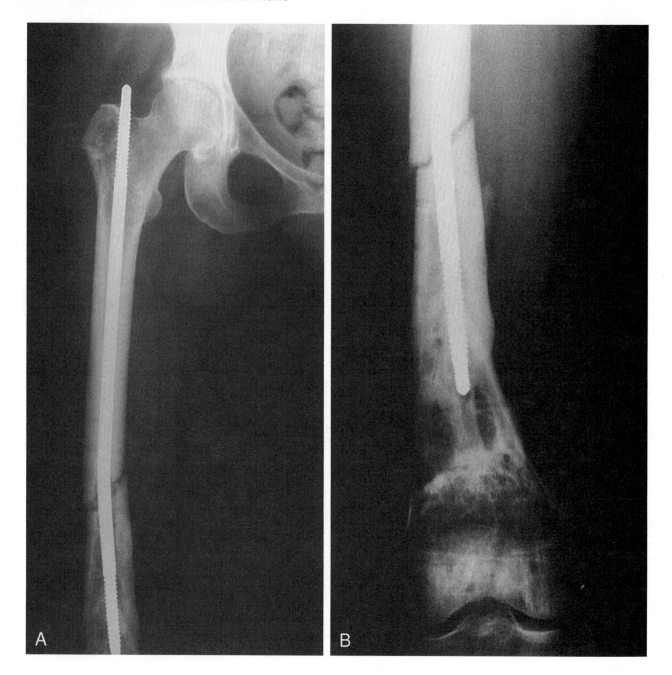

Chapter 3

RADIOLOGIC EVALUATION OF FRACTURE

mcKinnis 09

Trauma, the Most Common Disorder[1-3]

Trauma is the most common disorder of the musculoskeletal system evaluated by radiology. The fractures and dislocations that make up the majority of traumatic conditions are among the most frequently encountered patient problems in hospital emergency rooms, physicians' offices, and rural clinics. Rehabilitation clinicians are involved in many phases of trauma patient care, including clinical evaluation, postoperative care, the management of activities of daily living and ambulation, prevention of complications related to immobilization, and, finally, restoration of strength, range of motion, and functional abilities after healing.

The imaging of musculoskeletal trauma is dominated by conventional radiography. Conventional radiographs effectively evaluate most fractures and dislocations. In addition, computed tomography (CT) is used to help visualize areas of complex anatomy, and magnetic resonance imaging (MRI) is used in the assessment of soft tissue injury. In dealing with trauma, the task of the radiologist is threefold: (1) to diagnose and evaluate the characteristics of the fracture or dislocation, (2) to ensure that the clinical history and reported mechanism of injury match the injury pattern, and (3) to assess the results of treatment and to monitor the healing process and potential complications.

Trauma Radiology[4-17]

Rehabilitation clinicians who treat patients after trauma should be aware of what imaging was performed initially in the emergency department—this is referred to as the *primary trauma survey*. In some cases this is the only imaging that will be performed prior to rehabilitative treatment. In other cases, a *secondary* survey of follow-up imaging, or further imaging investigation, may be indicated to further the diagnostic process after the patient is clinically stable.

Imaging in the Primary Trauma Survey

The primary trauma survey is a protocol series of radiographs or advanced imaging that assist in screening and prioritizing a trauma patient's multiple injuries. For patients involved in high-velocity injuries (for example, motor vehicle accidents or falls from great heights) the trauma survey includes the following conventional radiographic projections:

- *Lateral cervical spine:* assess gross instability, fractures, dislocations
- *Anteroposterior (AP) chest:* assess for hemothorax, pneumothorax, pulmonary contusion
- *AP pelvis:* assess for fractures, hemorrhage

Possible additions to the trauma survey, as dictated by the injury pattern, clinical signs, and available imaging modalities, include:

- *FAST (focused abdominal ultrasound for trauma):* identify free fluid in the peritoneal cavity
- *CT of the head:* assess for intracranial bleeding
- *CT of the cervical spine:* further assess for fracture, especially craniovertebral and cervicothoracic areas difficult to see on lateral view
- *CT of the thorax, abdomen, and pelvis, with or without contrast:* identify injuries to abdominal and pelvic organs
- *Lateral thoracolumbar spine radiograph:* gross assessment of instability, fractures, and dislocations
- *Extremity radiographs:* identify fractures and dislocations

In some trauma centers, CT scanning performed for head, chest, abdominal, and pelvic injuries is also used, in place of radiographs, to screen for spinal fractures. Studies indicate this practice decreases assessment time, cost, and radiographic "misses" of fractures difficult to assess on plain radiographs. Current CT scanners are able to reconstruct spine images at the same time scans are obtained for the major organs. Thus, where available, CT is the definitive radiographic study in most patients with multiple trauma.[17]

The trauma survey is an assessment tool for life-threatening injuries and injuries of serious consequence. Although orthopedic conditions are not usually the priority in a major trauma case, there are some conditions that by themselves require urgent action to prevent serious complications. Fractures that can cause hemorrhage, fat embolism, or neurovascular damage warrant immediate treatment[2] (Table 3-1).

Radiographic Positioning for Trauma[18]

Adaptation of normal radiographic procedures is often necessary in trauma cases. In regard to high-velocity injury patients, the most critical skeletal region to assess is the cervical spine, because over half of all spinal cord injuries occur here. The patient will not be moved from a stabilized position until a lateral cervical spine projection is obtained and read. To achieve this projection, a horizontal x-ray beam is used. The central ray passes laterally through the cervical spine, parallel to the table, hence the phrase "cross-table lateral view." If vertebral alignment is abnormal, suspicion is raised for fracture, dislocation, and potential threat to

TABLE 3-1 • *Injuries Requiring Urgent Action*

Injury	Possible Complication	Comments
Fractures		
Pelvic fracture	Hemorrhage	Half of all pelvic fractures require transfusion
Femur fracture	Hemorrhage	Occurs with closed fractures
Multiple or crushing type fractures	Fat embolism	Develops 12–72 hours after fracture
Elbow fracture	Brachial artery injury	Associated with supracondylar fracture
Proximal humeral fracture	Axillary nerve injury	Paresthesias over deltoid
Dislocations		
Shoulder dislocation	Axillary artery injury Brachial plexus, axillary nerve injury	Arterial tears can be initially asymptomatic but later develop into occlusion.
Elbow dislocation	Brachial artery injury Median and ulnar nerve injury	Most nerve injuries are temporary neurapraxias; however, monitor sensory and motor exam distal to injury.
Hip dislocation	Femoral artery injury Femoral nerve injury	
Knee dislocation	Popliteal artery injury Peroneal nerve injury	

the spinal cord, usually necessitating further imaging with CT.

For fractures of the extremities, at least two views 90 degrees apart from each other are obtained. This ensures three-dimensional appreciation of the injury. All attempts are made to obtain an AP and a lateral projection, as these are the views with which clinicians are most familiar. Perfect positioning may not be possible, however, owing to obstacles such as first-aid splinting, severe pain, the potential for further injury if an extremity is forced to move, or an uncooperative patient. Two oblique views made at 90 degrees to each other may have to suffice. Furthermore, in adapting positioning to nonroutine conditions, the radiographer strives to maintain the perpendicular relationship of the x-ray beam to the anatomy and the image receptor. This relationship provides the most visualization and least distortion on the radiograph. Compromises in positioning that angulate the beam and result in distortion may have to be tolerated in some instances.

Radiologic evaluation of an extremity fracture must also include the joints adjacent to that bone. This is significant because many injury patterns involve associated fractures, subluxations, or dislocations at sites remote from the apparent primary injury.

What Is a Fracture?[19–24]

Biomechanics of Bone

Bone consists of cells embedded within an abundant extracellular matrix of inorganic minerals and organic collagen. Minerals in the matrix give bone its rigidity and strength, and the collagen gives it flexibility and resilience. The mix of the two types of bone tissue—cancellous and cortical—provides bone with optimal strength for its own weight.

The characteristics of bone classify it as a *viscoelastic* material. This means that bone will deform when physically loaded and then return to its original shape after loading ceases. How much load bone can withstand is dependent on many factors, including the geometric configuration of the bone, the physiological health of the bone, and the type and rate of loading. When the imposed load exceeds the bone's tolerance, the bone will fracture. Fractures may be caused by *direct trauma* or *indirect trauma*, according to whether a load was applied directly to the bone or applied at a distance from the bone and then transmitted to it.

A novice viewer of radiographs may be surprised to see the frequency of similar fracture patterns among patients. A patient's fracture configuration is rarely unique. Rather, the patterns in which fractures occur are predictable based on the viscoelastic properties of bone combined with the biomechanics of load. See Table 3-2 for a summary of

long-bone fracture patterns and their related appearances, precipitating forces, and soft-tissue hinge locations. The term *soft-tissue hinge* refers to the intact soft tissues adjacent to the shaft that serve as an aid in the reduction and stabilization of displaced fractures.

Definition of Fracture

A fracture is a break in the structural continuity of bone or cartilage. The words used to describe fractures in the radiologic report are anatomic and standardized terms. This formality is important because only then is the correct information accessible to all clinicians involved in patient treatment. *Eponyms* (e.g., *Colles' fracture*) are commonly used in verbal exchanges, but they are avoided in radiologic description because of their generality, lack of descriptive detail, and ease of misinterpretation.

A basic clinical distinction in defining fractures is whether or not the fracture site is exposed to the external environment. A *closed fracture* is one in which the skin and soft tissues overlying the fracture are intact (Fig. 3-1). An *open fracture* exists any time the skin is perforated, regardless of the size of the wound. In the past, the terms *simple* and *compound* were employed; however, due to ambiguous usage (for example, *compound* was sometimes used as the equivalent of *comminuted*), they are no longer in use in diagnostic coding terminology.

Elements of Fracture Description[1,21–27]

Description of fractures on the radiology report is not standardized, and wide variations exist in style, length, and format. The clinical management of fractures begins with proper identification and description. Greenspan[1] identifies

TABLE 3-2 ● *Summary of Long Bone Fracture Biomechanics*			
Mechanism of Injury	**Fracture Pattern Appearance**	**Location of Soft Tissue Hinge**	**Appearance**
Direct Force			
Tapping	Transverse	Concavity	
Crushing	Comminuted	Destroyed	
Penetrating:			
Low velocity	Comminuted	Variable	
High velocity	Comminuted	Destroyed	
Indirect Force			
Bending	Transverse	Concavity	
Torsion	Spiral	Vertical segment	
Compression + bending	Oblique–transverse or butterfly	Concavity or side of butterfly	
Compression + Bending + Torsion	Oblique	Concavity (often destroyed)	
Traction	Avulsed fragment	Slack ligament	

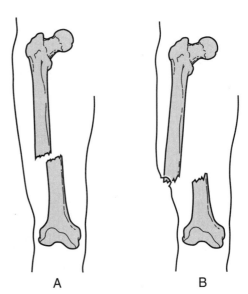

Figure 3-1 (A) A *closed* fracture does not communicate with the external environment. **(B)** An *open* fracture denotes an opening in the skin, and the fracture site is susceptible to infection from the external environment.

seven elements that might be included in a complete radiologic description of fractures:

1. The anatomic *site* and *extent* of the fracture
2. The *type* of fracture, whether *complete* or *incomplete*
3. The *alignment* of the fracture fragments
4. The *direction* of the fracture line
5. The presence of *special features* of the fracture, such as *impaction* or *avulsion*
6. The presence of *associated abnormalities,* such as joint dislocations
7. The *special types* of fractures that may occur as a result of *abnormal stresses* or secondary to *pathological processes* in the bone, such as *stress fractures* or *pathological fractures*

Explanations of these seven points follow.

Anatomic Site and Extent of the Fracture

Establishing the location of a fracture requires points of reference (Fig. 3-2). The *shafts* of long bones are divided into thirds. Fractures may be present at the *proximal, middle,* or *distal thirds* of the shaft or at the *junction* of these regions, for example, at the junction of the middle and proximal thirds. The ends of long bones are designated as the *distal* or *proximal* end, and each end is divided into *extra-articular* and *intra-articular* portions (Fig. 3-3). The intra-articular portions are the joint surface areas. Fractures may *extend intra-articularly* from an extra-articular region (Fig. 3-4).

Reference points for flat or irregularly shaped bones may be noted as either the *intra-articular* or *extra-articular* regions. Additionally, all bones may be referenced by standard anatomic landmarks or parts, such as the *surgical neck of the humerus,* the *intertrochanteric region of the femur,* the *supracondylar area of the distal femur,* or the *medial malleolus of the distal tibia.*

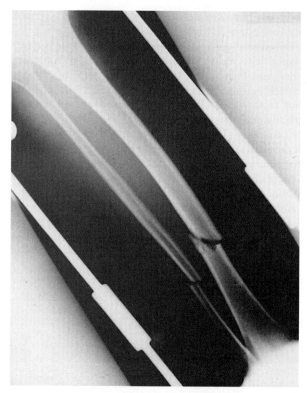

Figure 3-3 Bilateral shaft fracture of the right lower leg. These fractures are described as complete fractures occurring at the junction of the middle and distal thirds of the shafts. The fracture line is oblique in the fibula and is oblique in the tibia with comminution. In both fracture sites, some degree of apposition remains between the fragments, so they are described as minimally displaced, with slight lateral angulation of the distal fragments.

Type of Fracture: Complete or Incomplete

A *complete fracture* is a fracture in which all cortices of the bone have been disrupted (Fig. 3-5). In a complete fracture, what was once one bone is now *two fragments* (Fig. 3-6). If a fracture has more than two fragments, it is classified as a *comminuted* fracture.

An *incomplete fracture,* by contrast, has only one portion of the cortex disrupted (Fig. 3-7). Generally, incomplete fractures are relatively stable and will maintain their position indefinitely *if no subsequent stresses are placed on them.* Incomplete fractures are seen predominantly in short bones, irregularly shaped bones, and flat bones. There are some types of incomplete fractures that occur exclusively in children; these are discussed under "Incomplete Fractures" in the following section.

Alignment of Fracture Fragments

Further description of a fracture includes identifying the position of one fracture fragment in relationship to the other fracture fragment. Common practice is to describe the position of the *distal fragment* in relation to the *proximal fragment.* Many terms are needed to express this relationship accurately.

Position refers to the relationship of the fragments to their normal anatomic structure. Loss of position is *displacement.*

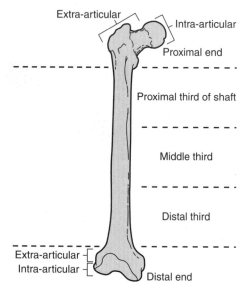

Figure 3-2 Location reference points on long bones.

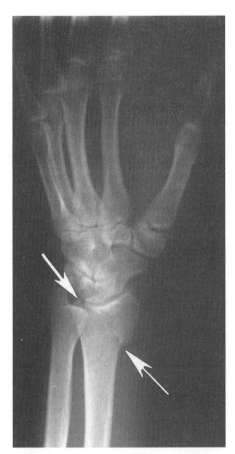

Figure 3-4 Intra-articular fracture of the distal radius. The arrows mark the extent of the fracture line. The fracture line is oblique, extending from the metaphysis on the radial side of the bone to the intra-articular surface. The fracture is complete, with minimal displacement and minimal angulation.

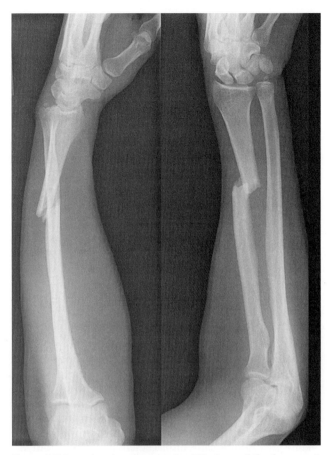

Figure 3-6 Lateral and posteroanterior (PA) views of the forearm. A complete fracture is present at the junction of the middle and distal third of the radius. The fracture line is oblique. The distal fragment is displaced dorsally and laterally. There is disruption of the distal radioulnar joint, most obvious by the dorsal displacement of the distal ulna as seen on the lateral view. This combination of injuries results from a fall on an outstretched hand and is known by the eponym Galeazzi's fracture. *(Image courtesy of John C. Hunter, MD, University of California, Davis School of Medicine.)*

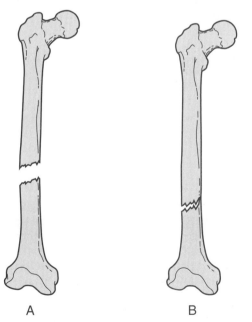

A   B

Figure 3-5 **(A)** Complete fracture. All cortical margins are broken, and now there are two fracture *fragments*. **(B)** Incomplete fracture. One cortical margin remains intact.

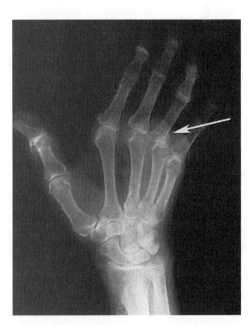

Figure 3-7 Incomplete fracture at the base of the proximal phalanx of the fourth digit, or ring finger. Note the abnormal position of the metacarpophalangeal joint, indicating possible subluxation or dislocation. Note also the great amount of soft-tissue swelling and edema.

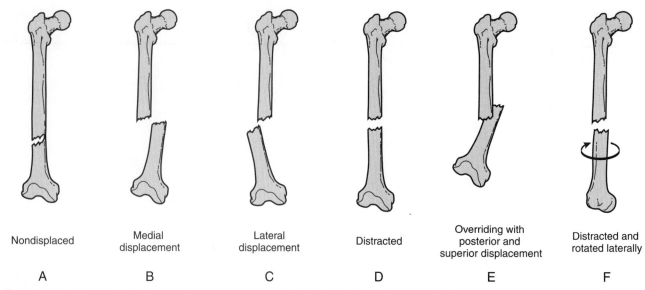

Nondisplaced	Medial displacement	Lateral displacement	Distracted	Overriding with posterior and superior displacement	Distracted and rotated laterally
A	B	C	D	E	F

Figure 3-8 (A–F) The *position* of fracture fragments may be described by how the *distal* fragment displaces in relationship to the *proximal* fragment.

Fractures are *displaced* if there is some loss of *apposition* or contact between the broken surfaces of the fragments. The direction of displacement (of the distal fragment) may be *medial, lateral, anterior, posterior, superior,* or *inferior* (Fig. 3-8). The amount of displacement is quantified with terms such as *one cortex width, one-half shaft width,* or *full shaft width*. Additionally, displacement may result from *distraction, overriding,* or *rotation* of the fracture fragments. *Nondisplaced* fractures, by contrast, have some degree of contact remaining between the fracture fragments.

Alignment is the relationship of the longitudinal axis of one fragment to the other. Fracture fragments are said *to be in alignment* when the longitudinal axes of both fragments line up in tandem or in parallel (Fig. 3-9). Deviations from alignment are the result of *angulation* of the fracture fragments. Angulation may be described by either (1) the direction of angular displacement of the distal fragment in relationship to the proximal fragment (e.g., *medial angulation of the fracture site [medial apex] with lateral angular displacement of the distal fragment*) or (2) the direction of the *apex* of the angle formed by the fracture fragments (e.g., *volar apex with dorsal angulation of the distal fragment*).

Direction of Fracture Lines

The *direction* of the fracture line is described in reference to the longitudinal axis of a long bone. Fracture lines in irregularly shaped bones are referenced by the cortices. Fracture lines can be *transverse, longitudinal, oblique,* or *spiral* (Fig. 3-10).

A *transverse* fracture line, the result of a bending force, occurs at right angles to the longitudinal axis or cortices of a bone. A *longitudinal* fracture line is approximately parallel to the shaft.

An *oblique* line represents a diagonally oriented fracture, the result of the combined forces of compression, bending, and torsion. A *spiral* line represents a fracture that spiraled around the long axis due to a torsional force. At first glance, spiral and

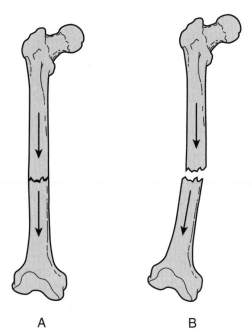

A	B

Figure 3-9 Alignment is the relationship of the longitudinal axes of the fracture fragments. **(A)** Fracture is in good alignment. **(B)** Fracture is poorly aligned, as the distal fragment is angulated.

oblique fracture lines appear similar on radiographs. Spiral fractures can be identified, however, by a vertical segment and sharp jagged edges. A spiral fracture may disrupt more surface area than an oblique fracture, but it actually has advantages in healing. The configuration of the fragments fit together with greater stabilization and promote faster healing.

A *comminuted* fracture does not always have a clear direction, because this term refers to any fracture with more than two fragments. A commonly occurring comminuted fracture pattern is the *butterfly fragment,* a wedge-shaped fragment split from the main fragments, secondary to the

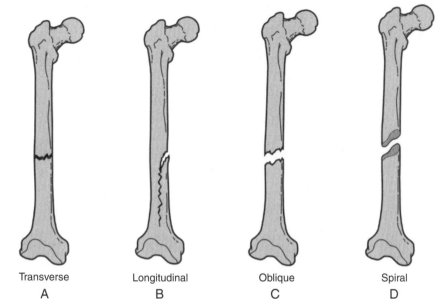

Transverse

A

Longitudinal

B

Oblique

C

Spiral

D

Figure 3-10 (A–D) Directions of fracture lines are described in reference to the longitudinal axis of the bone.

combined forces of compression and bending. *Segmental* fractures are also comminuted fractures. In these the bone is segmented by more than one fracture line (Figs. 3-11, 3-12).

Comminuted fractures generally are the result of extremely high energy loads, such as crushing forces in motor vehicle accidents. The term *comminuted* is used to describe any fracture with more than two fragments—be it 20 or 200. A variety of methods exist to document the *amount* of comminution: percentages, centimeter measurements, or descriptions using the terms *minimal, moderate,* or *severe* are all in use.

On the radiograph, fracture lines are evident by their radiolucency. This radiolucency is the result of (1) the extent of acute hemorrhage into the fracture site and (2) any actual space that may exist between the fragments. The amount of space will be related to the amount of displacement of the fracture fragments.

Presence of Special Features

Special features of fractures are *impaction* and *avulsion* (Fig. 3-13). Fractures of the epiphysis and *epiphyseal plates* are special features of fractures in children and will be discussed in that section.

Impaction Fractures

Impaction fractures result from compression forces related to axial loading. In this injury, bone is driven into itself. The trabeculae telescope or enmesh into each other. This occurs predominantly in areas of cancellous bone, because its porous architecture permits the compression necessary to allow impaction. Some degree of natural stability is produced with impaction fractures, and this, combined with the close contact of the fragments, is advantageous for fracture healing.

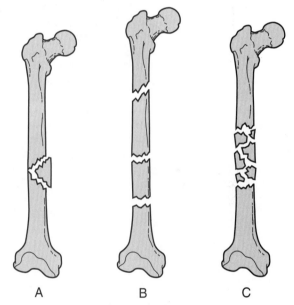

A

B

C

Figure 3-11 *Comminuted* fractures are fractures with more than two fragments. Some frequently occurring comminuted fracture patterns are **(A)** the wedge-shaped or butterfly pattern, **(B)** a two- or three-segmented level fracture. **(C)** Other fractures with multiple fragments, be it several or several hundred, are still described as comminuted.

Two forms of impaction are *depression fractures,* in which the surface of one bone is driven into the surface of another, and *compression fractures,* in which both surfaces of a bone are forced together. For example, a *depression fracture of the tibial plateau* results from the impacting force of the architecturally stronger arch of the distal femoral condyle into the relatively weaker flat tibial plateau. A *compression fracture of a vertebral body,* on the other hand, results from axial loading of the spine, which compresses the vertebral body between superior and inferior adjacent vertebrae (Fig. 3-14).

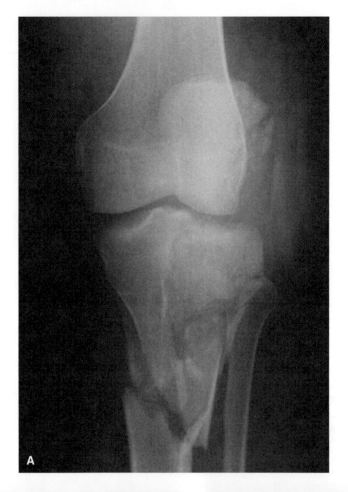

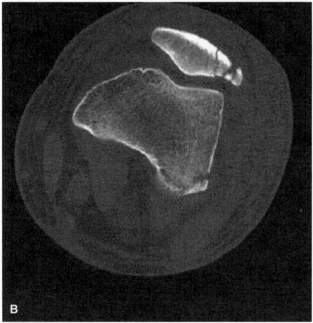

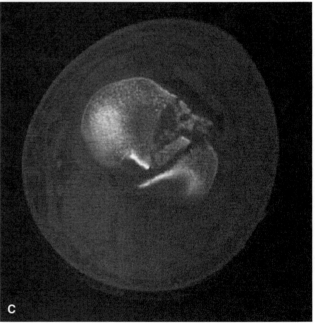

Figure 3-12 **(A)** AP radiograph of the knee. Comminuted fractures are visible at the proximal tibia and patella. **(B)** Axial CT demonstrating comminution of the patella and posterolateral femoral condyle. **(C)** Axial CT demonstrating comminution of the proximal tibia. *(Image courtesy of John C. Hunter, MD, University of California, Davis School of Medicine.)*

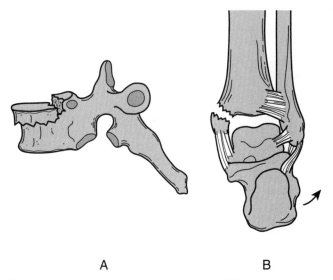

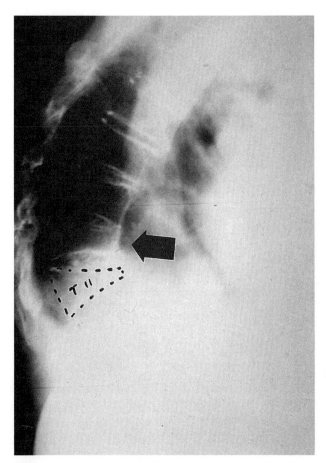

On the radiograph, impaction fractures are *radiodense* as a result of the increased density of the enmeshed trabeculae.

Avulsion Fractures

Avulsion fractures are the result of tensile loading of bone. Fragments of bone are avulsed, or pulled away from the main body of bone, via active contraction of a muscle or passive resistance of a ligament against a tensile force. Avulsion fractures occur at bony prominences, which serve as attachment sites for muscles, tendons, and ligaments. Avulsion fractures are descibed by anatomic landmarks—for example, *an avulsion of the calcaneal tuberosity at the attachment of the calcaneal tendon* (Fig 3-15).

On the radiograph, avulsion fractures will be *radiolucent* as a result of hemorrhage and actual space between the fragment and the main body of bone.

Associated Abnormalities

Abnormalities associated with fractures are varied. *Subluxations* and *dislocations* of related joints are probably the most common injuries associated with fracture (Fig. 3-16). Involvement in nearby soft tissues is also common, such as disruptions of the joint capsules, the ligaments, the interosseous membrane between the long bones of the forearm, or the tibiofibular syndesmosis. Some soft tissue disruption can be suggested on the conventional radiograph but requires further imaging for specific diagnosis.

Figure 3-13 Special features of fractures include **(A)** impaction, seen, for example, in a compression fracture of a vertebral body, or **(B)** avulsion, as seen in a medial malleolar avulsion during an eversion force trauma at the ankle.

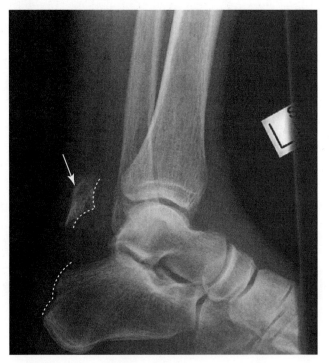

Figure 3-14 Multiple compression fractures of the thoracic spine. Severe osteoporosis is a striking feature. Much of the cortical outline of the vertebral bodies is no longer apparent because of bony demineralization, so the shape of the bodies is deduced primarily from the remaining fibrous disk spaces. The large arrow marks T10, which has collapsed from multiple compression fractures and is deformed into a wedge shape. T11 is similarly deformed but is largely obscured by the soft tissues.

Figure 3-15 Lateral view of the foot with an avulsion fracture of the calcaneal tuberosity. The avulsed fragment (arrow) has moved superiorly as the now unattached tendon has recoiled. Dotted lines indicate normal contact areas of fragment to main body of bone. (*Image courtesy of Laughlin Dawes, MD.*)

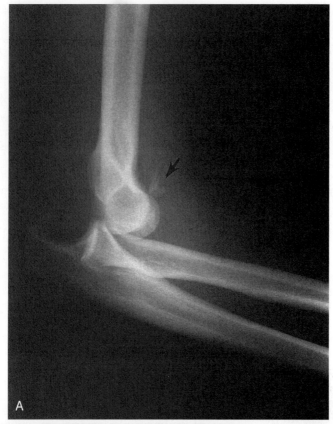

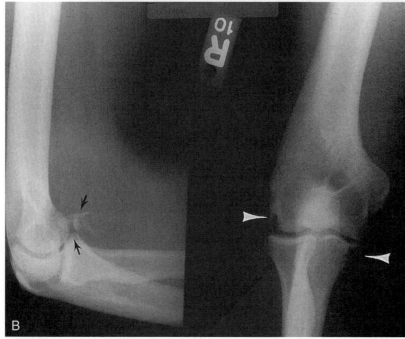

Figure 3-16 Posterior dislocation of the elbow with associated fractures. This 39-year-old man injured his elbow in a fall from a skateboard. **(A)** Lateral view of the elbow before reduction demonstrates the posterior position of the radius and ulna in relationship to the distal humerus. The black arrow marks a fracture fragment in the anterior soft tissues. **(B)** Lateral and **(C)** anteroposterior films made after reduction show good positioning of the joints and multiple fracture fragments in the soft tissue (arrows). Note the gross soft tissue swelling of the arm visible on the lateral view.

Fractures Due to Abnormal Stresses or Pathological Processes

Stress Fractures

Stress fractures are also known as microfractures, fatigue fractures, and insufficiency fractures. Stress fractures occur in two ways. The first mechanism is repetitive minor trauma to otherwise normal bone. Chronic high-frequency, low-level loading does not allow bone sufficient time to heal and remodel. Such stress fractures are found most frequently in the lower extremities; the predominant example is stress fractures of the metatarsals associated with prolonged walking, marching, or running. The second mechanism that produces stress fractures is normal loading on abnormal bone. The most common example is vertebral body fractures in elderly women with osteoporosis.

Imaging Considerations for Stress Fractures

On the radiograph, obvious stress fractures appear as irregular localized areas of increased radiodensity, representing the bone's ongoing attempts at repair (Fig. 3-17). However, stress fractures can be difficult to diagnose on radiograph as initial radiographs often appear normal. A fracture line or periosteal reaction may not be evident for up to 6 weeks. Thus radiography is useful when positive, but generally has low sensitivity.

Radionuclide bone scanning is highly sensitive for stress fractures but lacks specificity and the ability to visualize fracture lines directly. MRI provides a highly sensitive and specific evaluation for bone marrow edema and periosteal reaction as well as detection of subtle fracture lines. Current American College of Radiology (ACR) guidelines recommend MRI for the diagnosis of extremity stress fractures.[27]

Pathological Fractures

Pathological fractures are fractures that occur in bone that has been structurally weakened by a pathological process (Fig. 3-18). The pathology that induces the susceptibility of

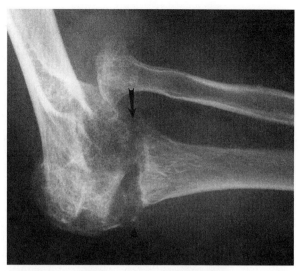

Figure 3-18 Pathological fracture through the distal third of the olecranon in a 26-year-old man. The underlying pathology is osteogenesis imperfecta, a disease characterized by abnormal maturation of collagen, affecting both intramembranous and enchondral bone formation. Note the diffuse decrease in bone density, pencil-thin cortices, flared metaphyses, and cystic appearance of the proximal ends of the radius and ulna.

bone to fracture may be systemic or localized in origin (Figs. 3-19A,B). Systemic processes may be congenital (osteogenesis imperfecta, osteopetrosis) or acquired (osteoporosis, Paget's disease). Some local processes are tumors, infections, disuse, or sequelae of irradiation.

Periprosthetic Fractures

Fractures occurring in association with prosthetic joint replacement are known as periprosthetic fractures.

Fractures can occur intraoperatively during the surgical preparation of the site or the insertion of the prosthetic components. More frequent is the occurrence of fractures around the prosthetic components several years postoperatively. The precipitating risk factors are variable and differ between joints. Risk factors include loosening of the components, cortical thinning, necrosis at the cement–bone interface, and osteoporosis.

Bone Graft Fractures

Fractures through large-segment allografts usually occur spontaneously 2 to 3 years after implantation and are not related to trauma. The most frequent sites of fracture are the distal femur, proximal tibia, and distal tibia. The occurrence is as high as 40% and increases four- to fivefold in patients with related plate fixation or adjuvant chemotherapy. The fractures generally occur through defects in the bone graft (screw holes) or areas where revascularization and host–tissue ingrowth are absent. Treatment by immobilization is ineffective; revision with allografts, autografts, intramedullary fixation, or prosthetic replacement is necessary. Good results are expected in 50% to 80% of patient cases.

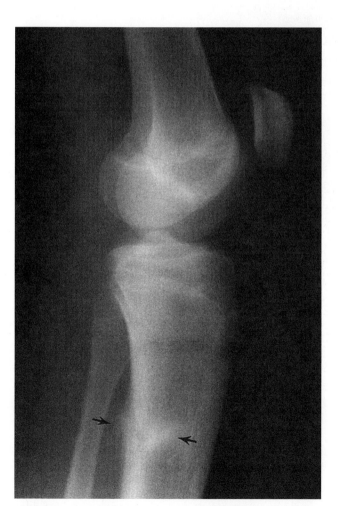

Figure 3-17 Stress fracture in the proximal third of the tibial shaft of a 15-year-old male runner. Arrows mark the zone of increased radiodensity representing bony response to repetitive trauma.

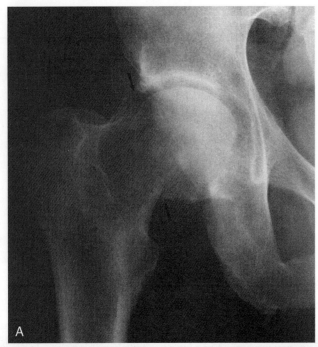

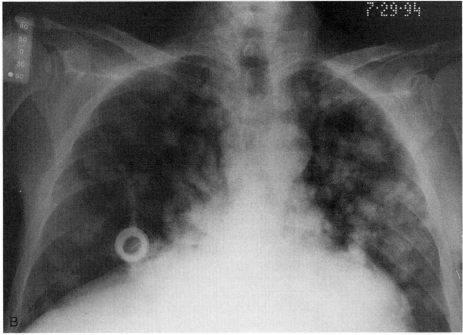

Figure 3-19 Pathological fracture of the femoral neck. **(A)** Arrows mark the extent of the fracture line. Demineralization of the femur is evident by the thinning of the cortices. **(B)** The underlying pathology is lung cancer, revealed in the abnormal densities of the chest film.

Fractures in Children[1,20–25,28,29]

Fractures in growing bone have unique patterns of injury and present special problems in diagnosis, treatment, and healing. Although the primary advantage of fracture in immature bone is rapid healing and great ability to remodel, the primary concern is the potential for disruption of growth.

Location Description

The location of fractures in the long bones of children is generally described by the region of development (Fig. 3-20). *Diaphyseal* fractures involve the central shaft, *metaphyseal* fractures involve the expanding end, *physeal* fractures involve the epiphyseal growth plate, and *epiphyseal* fractures involve the epiphysis.

Difficulties in Assessment of Immature Bone

The radiographic diagnosis of adult fractures can be complicated by anatomic features that resemble fracture. Children's fractures can be even more complicated by the additional presence of epiphyseal growth plates, dense growth lines, secondary centers of ossification, and large nutrient foramina, all of which may be confused with fracture lines (Table 3-3). For this reason, *comparison films* of the

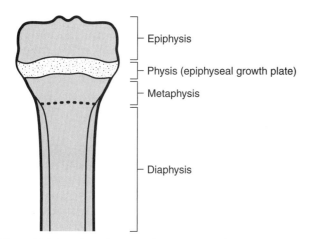

Figure 3-20 Location reference points on growing bone.

Epiphysis
Physis (epiphyseal growth plate)
Metaphysis
Diaphysis

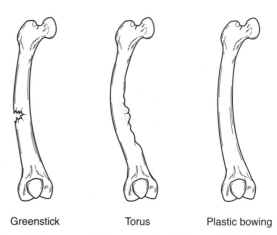

Greenstick   Torus   Plastic bowing

Figure 3-21 *Incomplete* fractures in children exhibit characteristics unique to the structural architecture of growing bone.

TABLE 3-3 ● Conditions That Look Like Fractures on Radiograph but Are Not

Condition	Example
Accessory bones	Found frequently in foot, less often in wrist and shoulder
Epiphysis	Multiple ossification centers, giving some epiphyses a comminuted appearance
Juxta-articular calcification	Calcium deposits at tendon insertions
Multipartite conditions	Bi- or tripartite patella, bipartite scaphoid
Nutrient foramina	Oblique radiolucency in shafts of long bones
Sesamoids	Metacarpal and metatarsal heads, fabella, pisiform

uninvolved extremity are sometimes needed to assist in diagnosis. An additional difficulty in radiographically examining immature bone is that only the ossified portions of bone have sufficient radiographic density to be imaged. The preformed cartilage model is not imaged. Normal position is assessed by evaluating spatial relationships of the visible ossified portions, using line measurements, angles, and distances correlated to chronological and skeletal age.

Elements of Fracture Description

Greenspan's seven elements of radiologic description of fractures, listed earlier, are the same for children as for adults. Additions within this list include describing (1) the patterns of incomplete shaft fractures, seen predominantly in children, and (2) the special features of fractures of the epiphysis and ephiphyseal plate. Descriptions of these points follow.

Incomplete Fractures

Incomplete fractures of the shafts of long bones in children are classified as the following (Fig. 3-21):

Greenstick fracture: This term has become almost standardized in usage, because it accurately depicts the appearance of this incomplete fracture: The *shaft is fractured on the tension side,* while the *cortex and periosteum remain intact on the compression side* (Fig. 3-22). Because this intact cortical

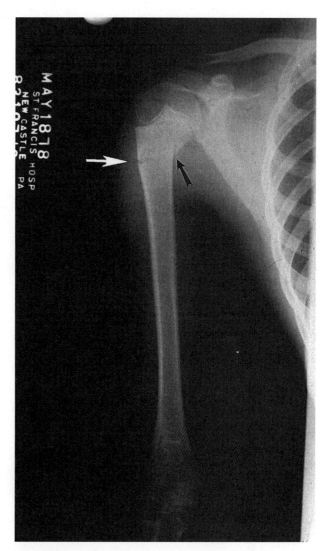

Figure 3-22 Greenstick fracture of the surgical neck of the humerus in a 13-year-old boy. The white arrow points to the incomplete transverse fracture line on the lateral aspect of the humerus. The black arrow points to an associated fracture on the medial aspect of the humerus, proximal to the greenstick fracture.

bone is often *plastically deformed* or *bowed,* an angular deformity is common, sometimes necessitating conversion to a complete fracture to reverse the deformity.

Torus fracture: This term is also common and describes an *impaction fracture that results in buckling of the cortex.* This pattern occurs predominantly at the metaphyseal regions, which are predisposed to a compressive response because of the amount of cancellous bone and newly remodeled trabecular bone present. Occasionally, this type of fracture is seen in adults if an underlying pathology exists (Fig. 3-23).

Plastic bowing: This is a result of the unique biomechanical nature of developing bone. When longitudinal compression forces imposed on a naturally curved, tubular growing bone exceed the point in which *elastic recoil* returns the bone to its prior position, that bone will become *plastically deformed* or *bowed.* Plastic bowing means that even when the force is removed, the bone remains bowed. Plastic bowing is a type of incomplete fracture, as microscopic fatigue lines, or *microfractures,* are evident in plastically deformed bone. Note that with additional increased force, bone would continue to weaken and eventually fail or fracture. It is reasonable to assume, then, that plastic bowing is a component of all fractures of childhood.

The younger the child, the more likely plastic bowing is to occur. It is particularly common in the fibula and the ulna. Additionally, a common injury pattern is *bowing in one bone combined with greenstick type of fracture in the paired bone*—for example, bowing of the fibula with fracture of the tibia or bowing of the ulna with fracture of the radius. In some cases the bowed bone must be clinically fractured in order to reverse the deformity and allow healing of both bones to proceed in good alignment.

Epiphyseal Fractures

Fractures involving the epiphyseal plate (also referred to as the physis, physeal region, or physeal growth plate) have been estimated to account for 15% to 20% of all fractures in children. An increased incidence of physeal fractures occurs at the onset of puberty, hypothesized to be related to biomechanical and structural weakness of the physeal cartilage during this stage of growth. Additionally, boys seem to be affected with greater frequency than girls, possibly related to a higher propensity for injury and to growth plates that remain open longer. Accurate diagnosis is critical, because the chosen treatment must strike the delicate balance of assisting healing without disrupting subsequent growth. The most commonly used method of radiographically identifying the varieties of epiphyseal fractures is the Salter–Harris classification system of types I through V (Fig. 3-24), with later additions made to this system by Rang and Ogden, types VI through IX.

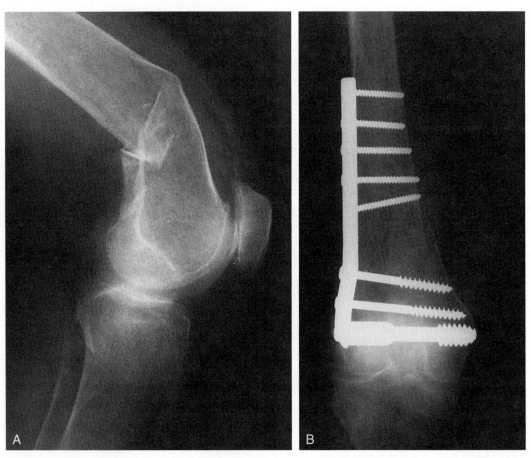

Figure 3-23 Buckle fracture of the distal femur. **(A)** The unusual buckle configuration of this fracture in a 56-year-old woman is secondary to decalcification of the skeleton as related to osteomalacia. It has the characteristics of torus fractures in children: a buckling of the cortex in the metaphyseal region. **(B)** Postoperative film demonstrating open reduction and internal fixation of the fracture site.

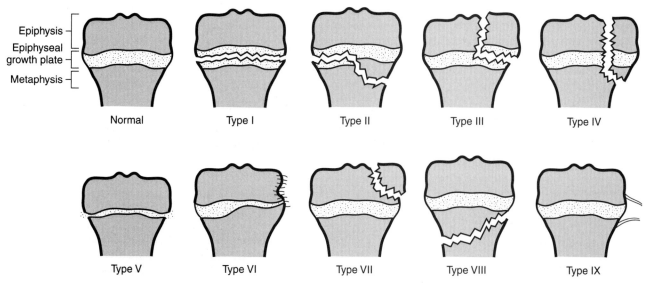

Figure 3-24 Schematic of the Salter–Harris classification of epiphyseal fractures, types I through V, with later additions made by Rang and Ogden, types VI through IX. Type II is the most common injury pattern.

Salter–Harris Classification of Epiphyseal Fractures

- *Type I:* The fracture line extends through the physis, separating and displacing the epiphysis from the normal position. This type is common in younger children and is associated with birth injuries. Prognosis is usually good for normal growth, but this can depend upon the amount of displacement.

- *Type II:* The fracture line extends through the physis and exits through the metaphysis, creating a triangular wedge of metaphysis that displaces with the epiphysis. This is the most common type and occurs most frequently in children over 10 years of age (Fig. 3-25). Prognosis is usually good for normal growth, but this can depend upon the amount of displacement.

- *Type III:* The fracture line extends from the joint surface through the epiphysis and across the physis, resulting in a portion of the epiphysis becoming displaced. Partial growth arrest is a possibility, and surgical fixation may be warranted.

- *Type IV:* The fracture line extends from the joint surface through the epiphysis, physis, and metaphysis, resulting in one fracture fragment. Partial growth arrest is possible, and surgical fixation may be necessary.

- *Type V:* The fracture is a crush type of injury that damages the physis by compression forces. It is difficult to diagnose this injury in acute stages. Eventual growth arrest may be the only clue that this injury occurred. Two nontraumatic causes of this type of injury are infection and epiphyseal avascular necrosis (AVN), which may cause dissolution of cartilage cells with resultant growth arrest.

- *Rang's type VI:* This injury involves the *perichondrial ring* or the associated periosteum of the physis. While little or no damage occurs directly to the physes, the reparative process at the periosteum may cause an osseous bridge to develop between the metaphysis and the epiphysis, arresting growth and leading to angular deformity.

- *Ogden's types VII, VIII, and IX:* These perichondral fractures do not directly involve the physis but may subsequently disrupt the physeal blood supply and result in

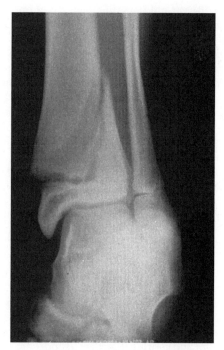

Figure 3-25 Salter–Harris type II fracture of the distal tibia. The fracture line extends through the physis and exits through the metaphysis, creating a triangular wedge of metaphysis that is displaced with the epiphysis.

growth disturbances. Type VII is an osteochondral fracture of the articular portion of the epiphysis, type VIII is a fracture of the metaphysis, and type IX is an avulsion fracture of the periosteum.

Healing Factors

As in the adult, fracture healing can be divided into three sequential, partially overlapping phases: the inflammatory phase, the reparative phase, and the remodeling phase. In children, the remodeling phase is much more extensive and physiologically more active than the comparable phase in adults. The remodeling phase is further complicated by the effects of the physeal growth plate and its response to changing joint reaction forces and biomechanical stresses, which can alter angular growth dynamics.

Remodeling Considerations

Children's fractures do not always remodel with acceptable results. The remodeling capacity of a deformity is dependent on three basic factors:

- The skeletal age of the child
- The distance of the fracture site from the growth plate
- The severity of displacement of the fragments

Skeletal Age of the Child

The criteria for acceptable fragment alignment after closed reduction is based on anticipated remodeling capabilities. Remodeling in general may be expected in children with 2 or more years of remaining skeletal growth. However, this is not always a favorable scenario. For example, the growth potential in two 10-year-old boys differs greatly if one boy has a skeletal age of 8 and the other a skeletal age of 12. The child with less skeletal maturity has more years available to remodel prior to closure of the growth plate; that is advantageous. However, in the event of partial growth arrest, more time is also available to develop deformity. In contrast, the boy with greater skeletal age has fewer years available to remodel prior to growth plate closure; that is a disadvantage. However, in the event of partial growth arrest, he also has less time to develop deformity. When the growth plates are closed, the deformity cannot continue to develop.

Remodeling, in general, is not something that can be relied upon. Every effort is made to obtain as near normal anatomic alignment as possible in reduction.

Distance From the Growth Plate

In some bones and some fracture configurations, remodeling fares better closer to the physeal growth plate. The growth plate has the pability to realign and assume a more normal growth pattern. For example, a fracture at the distal radius epiphysis will facilitate realignment in the growth plate, resulting in progressive metaphyseal remodeling. As the child grows, the deformed region migrates further away from the joint and continues further remodeling.

Severity of Displacement of the Fragments

Remodeling is definitely not expected to help in certain fracture configurations or in the presence of severe displacement. Surgical fixation of some type is required in the following fractures: displaced intra-articular fractures, significantly displaced fractures at the midshaft of bone, displacement of a fragment at right angles to the normal plane of movement, rotational deformities, and displaced fractures crossing a physeal growth plate.

Anticipating Future Longitudinal Growth

Potential for limb length inequality consequent to trauma is a primary concern in the management of children's fractures. Limb length inequality can also be a consequence of congenital or acquired conditions. When future longitudinal growth is anticipated accurately, the result of any corrective surgery for bone shortening, overgrowth, growth plate arrest, or amputation is enhanced.

Published charts and graphs based on selected populations estimate the percentage contributed by each physis to the relative longitudinal growth of a long bone. While it is recognized that wide variations exist, these percentages serve as a reasonable guide to the average growth pattern and show a range of normal dimensions per skeletal age and gender.

Skeletal Maturity

When graphs are used for the prediction of growth and proper timing of surgery, the role of skeletal maturity is taken into account. Skeletal maturity is measured by skeletal age. Like other morphological ages (biological age, dental age, sexual age), skeletal age differs from chronological age. Studies on variations in skeletal age relative to chronological age have shown diverse influences on skeletal maturation, including gender, environment, and genetic regulation.

The most popular method of assessing skeletal maturity has been the comparison of a series of radiographs of typical age and gender groups. The *Greulich and Pyle*[27] reference atlas contains hundreds of chronologically ordered radiographs of the hand and wrist to use for comparison purposes in defining skeletal age. Errors in such inspectional methods are known and other methods have been explored. Radiographic measurement of the actual size of various bones and assessment of ossification centers that have formed or fused are other methods.

The onset of adolescence is established by the appearance of ossification at the crest of the ilium. This radiographic indicator is present within 6 months of menarche, at approximately age 13 in girls. In boys an analogous skeletal maturation is present about 1½ years later. Complete ossification along the iliac crest generally coincides with the completion of longitudinal growth in the arms and legs. Additional height may still be contributed by the continued longitudinal development of the thoracolumbar bodies through the third decade.

Reduction and Fixation of Fractures[1,2,22–26]

Although the fundamental principles of fracture reduction and fixation are beyond the scope of this text, a brief discussion introduces terms that may appear in the radiographic report.

Reduction

Once a fracture has occurred and the fragments are identified on radiograph as *displaced*, restoration of the fragments to their normal anatomic positions, or *reduction*, is attempted. Reduction is not necessary if the fragments show an insignificant amount of displacement. Reduction may be accomplished in two ways: closed reduction and open reduction.

Closed Reduction

During closed reductions of fractures, no surgical incisions are made. Rather, fragments are physically guided back into position via manipulation, traction, or a combination of both. In most fractures a soft tissue hinge will be present between the bone ends. This hinge will lie in the concavity of a transverse or oblique fracture or in the vertical segment of a spiral fracture. This soft tissue hinge is the linkage that allows the fracture to be reduced, and under appropriate tension it will stabilize the fracture after reduction (Fig. 3-26).

Open Reduction

Open reductions of fractures surgically expose the fracture site. Some possible indications for open reductions are the following:

- Closed methods have failed.
- Closed methods are known from experience to be ineffective (as in fractures of the femoral neck).
- Articular surfaces are fractured and displaced, and perfect alignment is necessary for joint function.
- Fracture is secondary to metastasis (open reduction may allow quicker pain relief and return home).
- There is an associated arterial injury (open reduction may be needed for protection of arterial repair).
- Multiple injuries are present (open reduction may afford ease of nursing care, transportation, and prevention of complications).
- Continued confinement to bed is undesirable (geriatric patients, especially, suffer less complications with the earliest possible return to ambulation).
- The cost of treatment may be substantially reduced (earlier discharge from hospital and earlier return to work).

Fixation

Fixation is the method of maintaining fracture fragments in position after reduction in order to achieve healing. *All fractures benefit from fixation*—immediately to provide pain

TABLE 3-4 ● *Benefits of Immobilization*
Provides considerable pain relief
Protects adjacent structures from additional injury
Prevents loss of anatomic position of fragments
Permits healing to proceed to successful union

relief and, over time, to promote healing (Table 3-4). The goals of fixation are the following:

1. To avoid further compromise of the injured soft tissues
2. To maintain the length of the bone, especially in the lower extremities
3. To produce alignment of the fragments and particularly of the joints

Fixation is of two types. *External fixation*, as with plaster cast immobilization or splints, is used to maintain closed reductions. Open reductions utilize *internal fixation*, which employs orthopedic appliances such as pins, wires, plates, screws, and rods. The combination of open reduction and internal fixation is often referred to by the abbreviation *ORIF*. Bone grafts can also be thought of as a form of internal fixation. Additionally, methods of internal and external fixation and their devices may be combined. Examples of fixation are seen in Figure 3-27.

Stress Sharing/Shielding

Fixation devices can also be classified as stress sharing or stress shielding. A stress-sharing device permits some transmission of load across a fracture site. This controlled stress facilitates healing via the phenomenon of Wolff's law. Without mechanical stress, immobilized bone will undergo periosteal and subperiosteal resorbtion. Stress-sharing devices are the most common type used for fixation. Examples are casts, rods, pins, wires, and external fixators.

Stress-shielding devices shield the fracture completely from mechanical stress and transfer imposed forces to the fixator device. Surgical plates are an example. The healing time is prolonged, and the rehabilitation plan is modified accordingly.

Fracture Healing[1,18,20,21,25]

Fracture healing begins shortly after the fracture occurs. The mechanism of healing is not uniform and differs somewhat between cortical bone, cancellous bone, and bone that has been surgically compressed and fixated.

Cortical Bone Healing

Briefly, cortical bone fractures heal by the formation of new bone or *callus* bridging the fracture gap (Fig. 3-28). This is achieved by a reaction of the periosteum and endosteum with organization and ossification of the acute fracture hematoma. New bone is initially deposited on either side of the fracture site, several millimeters away from the actual fracture line, and then proceeds toward the gap, eventually linking together and forming a collar of external *primary callus*. This randomly organized immature bone is gradually replaced by *secondary callus* via the resorptive activity of the

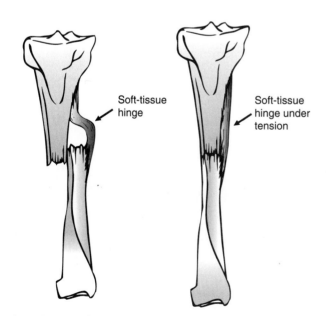

Figure 3-26 A soft-tissue hinge is the linkage that allows fractures to be reduced to nearly normal alignment.

Soft-tissue hinge

Soft-tissue hinge under tension

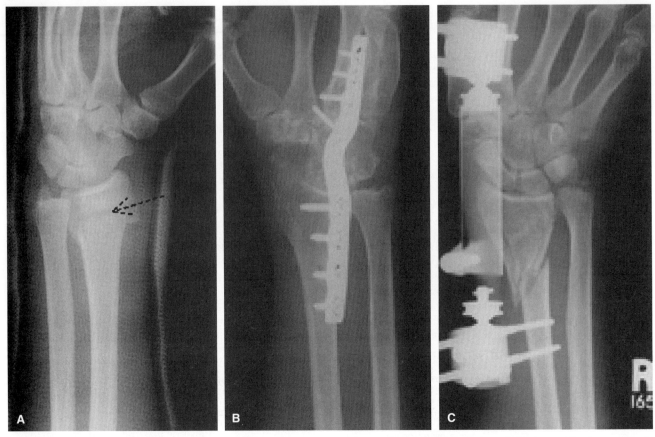

Figure 3-27 Three types of fixation. **(A)** *External fixation:* a plaster cast immobilizes a distal radius fracture (arrow). **(B)** *Internal fixation:* a dynamic compression plate used for wrist arthrodesis. **(C)** *Combination of internal and external fixation:* standard uniplanar external fixator used for treatment of a comminuted distal radius fracture. Pins are anchored into the second metacarpal and radial shaft. An ulnar styloid fracture is also present. *(Image courtesy of Mihra Taljanovic, MD, University of Arizona Radiology.)*

osteoclasts combined with osteoblastic deposition of new bone. The secondary callus now becomes organized in response to the mechanical stresses of normal function, in accordance with Wolff's law.

Remodeling of fractures is a complex biophysical event and is the most easily seen manifestation of Wolff's law. The end result of remodeling is one or the other of the following:

1. A bone returned to its original form.
2. A bone altered so that it may best perform the function demanded of it.

Interestingly, radioisotope studies have shown that increased activity in a fractured bone lasts much longer than had previously been thought. In humans, there is increased activity for 6 to 9 years after a tibial fracture.

Cancellous Bone Healing

Cancellous bone fractures unite with little or no callus formation. Healing occurs via direct osteoblastic activity at the fracture site, also referred to as *creeping substitution.* This method of healing requires that the fracture fragments be in close contact with each other. If approximation cannot be achieved, hematoma fills in the gap, and healing proceeds by callus formation.

Surgically Compressed Bone Healing

Surgically compressed and fixated bone heals via direct osteoblastic activity with little or no periosteal reaction or callus formation (Fig. 3-29). Additionally, immediate remodeling occurs as bone deposition and resorption continue simultaneously as a result of osteoblastic and osteoclastic cell activity.

Radiologic Evaluation of Healing

Some terms that describe the radiographic evidence of fracture healing are the following:

- *Formation of callus:* Radiodense periosteal and endosteal lines bridge the fracture gap (Fig. 3-30A).
- *Primary bone union:* Healing of a fracture occurs by trabecular new bone, without callus formation (because apposition is perfect).
- *Early union:* A trabecular pattern appears across the fracture line.
- *Clinical union:* Callus is seen uniting the fracture site, yet a radiolucent band remains between the fracture fragments, suggesting that the repair lacks normal strength (Fig. 3-30B).

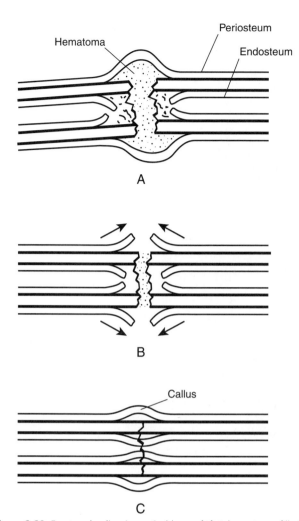

Figure 3-28 Fracture healing in cortical bone. **(A)** A hematoma fills in the fracture site after the periosteum and endosteum rupture. **(B)** Periosteal and endosteal response results in bone deposition that proceeds toward the fracture. **(C)** A collar of callus surrounds the fracture site and will progressively remodel over time. *(Adapted from Schultz,[24] p. 25.)*

- *Radiographic union:* A dense bridge of periosteal and endosteal callus unites the fracture site.
- *Established union:* Cortical structure and remodeling begin to appear.
- *Remodeling:* Trabeculae become reorganized along lines of weight-bearing stress.
- *Fibrous union:* Fracture site is clinically stable and pain free, with no evidence of the fracture line repair remaining (Fig. 3-30C).

Time Frame for Fracture Healing[2,22,25,26]

The time frame for complete fracture healing is divisible into three phases, which overlap somewhat. The *inflammation* phase occupies approximately 10% of total healing time, the *reparative* phase approximately 40%, and the *remodeling* phase approximately 70%.

The actual number of weeks or months over which these three phases can extend is influenced by innumerable factors. The process of healing can be affected by almost any endogenous or exogenous factor that influences the

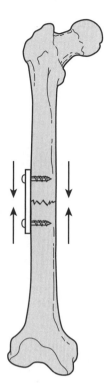

Figure 3-29 Fracture healing on compressed and surgically fixated bone occurs via direct osteoblastic activity, with little or no periosteal reaction or callus formation.

metabolic function of cells. In clinical practice, however, fracture healing appears to proceed with a certain degree of predictability and is modified by relatively few influences. The majority of nonoperative extremity fractures, for example, heal in between 4 and 8 weeks (Table 3-5).

Factors That Influence Rate of Fracture Healing

The following factors can influence the rate of fracture healing.

Age of the Patient

Generally, the younger a patient, the more rapidly fractures heal. The positive bone balance state of growing children contributes to rapid healing and excellent remodeling capabilities. Additionally, the periosteum in children is thick and loosely attached to the shafts of bones and thus is less likely to tear during fracture. Its presence acts as an aid in maintaining reduction and readily supplies critical vascular support to the repair process. In contrast, the periosteum of adult bone is relatively thin and firmly attached to the shaft, usually tearing during fracture.

Degree of Local Trauma

Greater local trauma at the fracture site and in adjacent soft tissues delays fracture healing. More tissues involved in the injury diffuse the cellular repair effort to many different fronts. Greater displacement of the fracture fragments also is known to delay fracture healing.

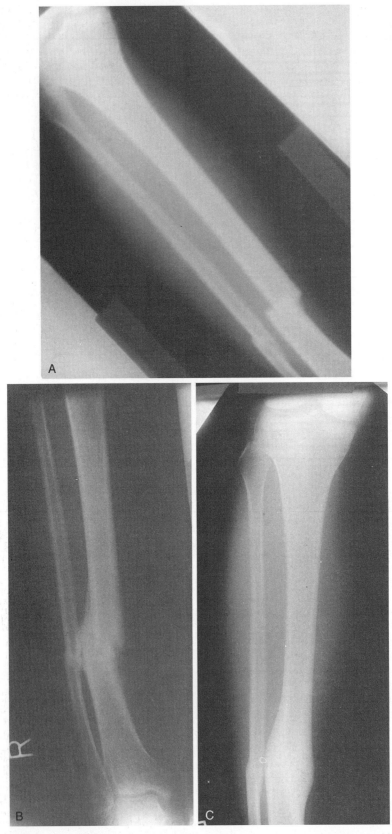

Figure 3-30 Successful healing of both bone fractures of the lower leg in a 17-year-old girl. **(A)** Emergency room film made after a sled-riding accident. The fracture is located at the junction of the distal and middle thirds of the shafts of the tibia and fibula. In both bones, the fracture fragments are overriding and displaced laterally. Good alignment exists. **(B)** Follow-up films 3 weeks later through plaster show formation of callus bridging the fracture gap. **(C)** Follow-up films 1 year later show good progression of remodeling and no evidence of the fracture lines remaining.

TABLE 3-5 ● Healing Time of Nonoperative Fractures

Fracture	Median Healing Time in Weeks	Recommended Length of Immobilization in Weeks
Proximal phalanx	4.1	4
Middle phalanx	3.7	4
Distal phalanx	4.4	3
Metacarpal	4.9	4
Scaphoid	7.7	6–12
Distal radius	5.6	6
Distal radius and ulna	6.7	6
Clavicle	3.9	4–6
Fibula	5.9	7–8
Metatarsal	5.9	4–6
Toes	3.6	3–4

Adapted from Eiff.[2]

Degree of Bone Loss

Loss of bone substance or excessive distraction of the fragments compromises the ability of the cells to bridge the fracture site and contributes to delay in healing.

Type of Bone Involved

Cancellous bone unites rapidly, but only at points of direct contact. Cortical bone unites by two mechanisms, depending on local conditions. A rigid immobilized site with contact of fragment ends will heal faster than a poorly immobilized site with displacement.

Degree of Immobilization

The degree of immobilization, along with the amount of soft tissue trauma, is of paramount importance in fracture healing. Inadequate immobilization leads to delayed union or to nonunion. If movement persists during the repair process, a cleft or false joint (pseudoarthrosis) can develop between the fragment ends.

Infection

When infection is imposed on a fracture or results in a fracture, healing will be delayed or may not happen at all, as the local cell response will be mobilized toward containing or eliminating the infection.

Local Malignancy

Unless the malignancy is treated, fractures through a primary or secondary malignant tumor will not heal significantly, even though microscopic evidence of callus may be present.

Nonmalignant Local Pathological Conditions

Fractures through nonmalignant but abnormal bone may heal, but in some instances (such as Paget's disease or fibrous dysplasia) healing may be delayed or may not happen at all.

Radiation Necrosis

Bone that has been irradiated heals much more slowly and in some cases fails to unite because of local cell death, thrombosis of vessels, and fibrosis of the marrow, all of which interfere with the ingrowth of capillaries necessary for repair.

Avascular Necrosis

Normally, healing occurs from both sides of a fracture site. If one fragment is rendered avascular, healing must proceed from only one side and thus is delayed. If both fragments have disrupted vascularity, the chances of healing are minimal.

Hormones

Corticosteroids are powerful inhibitors of the rate of fracture healing. Growth hormones are potent stimulators of fracture healing.

Exercise and Local Stress About the Fracture

Bone formation is stimulated by forces acting across the fracture site, and weight-bearing techniques are used to take advantage of this fact. Appropriate stress, however, is not to be confused with imposing unwanted motion at a fracture site, which can result in delayed union.

Radiologic Examination Intervals During Fracture Healing

Intervals for radiographic examination during fracture healing vary according to (1) the potential for fragments to become displaced and (2) the need for monitoring any of the complications discussed in the preceding section.

The least amount of radiographic monitoring is appropriate in a nondisplaced, uncomplicated, closed fracture immoblized in a cast. In this case, the patient would have initial radiographs to diagnose and direct treatment and then none further until the cast was removed, approximately 6 weeks later, to document radiographic evidence of successful healing.

Displaced fractures may be radiographed several days after initial treatment to verify maintenance of fragment alignment. Fractures that are known to have potential alignment problems or high risk for complications will require more frequent monitoring by radiology. These cases may have radiographs made in 1-, 2-, or 4-week intervals during the course of immobilization.

Complications in Fracture Healing[1–3,20–26]

Complications at Fracture Site

The following are some terms that describe complications of fracture healing, and are evidenced radiographically. (Table 3-6).

TABLE 3-6 ● *Complications of Fractures*

Life-Threatening Conditions
Hemorrhage
Fat embolism
Pulmonary embolism
Gas gangrene
Tetanus

Complications in Associated Tissues
Arterial injury
Nerve injury
Compartment syndrome
Infection
Tenting of skin
Significant soft tissue damage

Complications of Bone at Fracture Site
Delayed union
Slow union
Nonunion
Malunion
Pseudoarthrosis
Osteomyelitis
Avascular necrosis

Late-Effect Complications
Complex regional pain syndrome
Limb length discrepancy

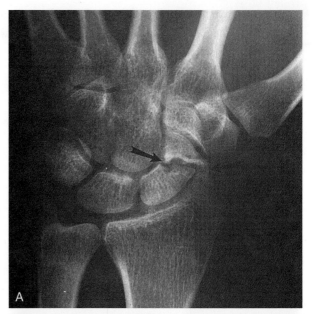
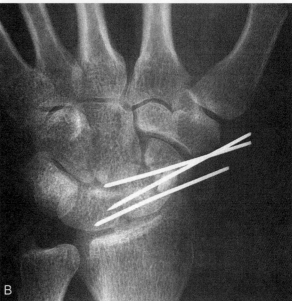

Delayed Union

Delayed union is present in any situation where a fracture fails to unite in the time frame usually required for union. Yet although fracture healing is delayed, the process of cellular repair is present and will continue on to complete union, provided that the adverse factors that are delaying the union are removed and no additional stresses are imposed. Causes of delayed union may be disrupted vascularity, infection, inadequate or interrupted immobilization, unsatisfactory reduction, severe local trauma, loss of bone substance, or wide distraction of fragments.

Slow Union

Slow union is known to occur in many fractures, even when ideal conditions are present. The rate of union, although slow, may be average or normal given the significant factors involved, such as patient age and fracture site. Thus, slow union is distinct from delayed union, which is a pathological state.

Nonunion

Nonunion exists when there is a failure of the fracture fragments to unite and the processes of bone repair have ceased completely (Fig. 3-31). The factors contributing to delayed union, if left unchecked, will cause nonunion. The radiographic appearance of nonunion shows persistence of the fracture line, sclerosis and rounding off of the fragment

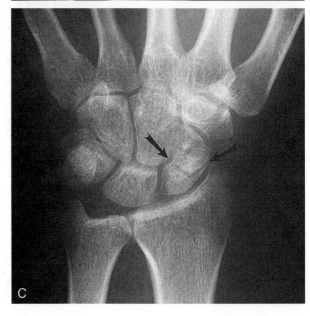

Figure 3-31 Fracture through the waist of the scaphoid. **(A)** Arrows mark the fracture site. **(B)** The fracture was internally fixated with three pins. This follow-up film made 2 months after surgery shows no indication of fracture healing. The radiolucent line representing the fracture site remains unchanged. The pins were subsequently removed. **(C)** Follow-up film made 6 weeks after metal removal shows a nonunion of the scaphoid.

ends, and occlusion of the medullary canal. Callus and bony bridging are absent.

Malunion

This occurs when the fracture has successfully united but a degree of angular or rotary deformity exists. If the deformity causes significant functional problems, surgery may be warranted for correction.

Pseudoarthrosis

This condition, also known as "false joint," refers to an abnormal condition at the fracture site associated with nonunion (Figs. 3-32 and 3-33). In nonunion the fragment bone ends are usually connected by dense fibrous or fibrocartilaginous tissue. Sometimes, however, a false joint may form between the ends and be surrounded by a bursal sac containing synovial fluid.

Osteomyelitis

Osteomyelitis after fracture is the result of contiguous dissemination of a pathogen from an open fracture or surgical fixation. The long bones of the extremities are most often involved. Chronic osteomyelitis is difficult to eradicate, and surgical débridement is often necessary.

Avascular Necrosis

Avascular necrosis (aseptic necrosis, ischemic necrosis, osteonecrosis) exists when the blood supply to a bone or segment of a bone is compromised, leading to localized bone death. The initial stages of avascular necrosis are not evident on plain films, but in later stages increased density is present (Fig. 3-34). See "Focus On Avascular Necrosis" at http://www.fadavis.com/imaging.

Late-Effect Complications of Fracture

Complex Regional Pain Syndrome

Complex regional pain syndrome (CRPS) denotes a wide variety of regional, posttraumatic, and neuropathic chronic pain conditions. Other names associated with this condition are *causlagia, posttraumatic dystrophy, shoulder-hand syndrome,* and *Sudek's atrophy.* This syndrome was formerly

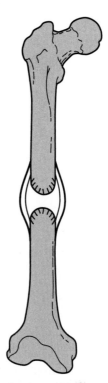

Figure 3-32 A pseudoarthrosis, or "false joint," is an abnormal condition at a nonunion fracture site, where by a bursal sac surrounds the fracture site.

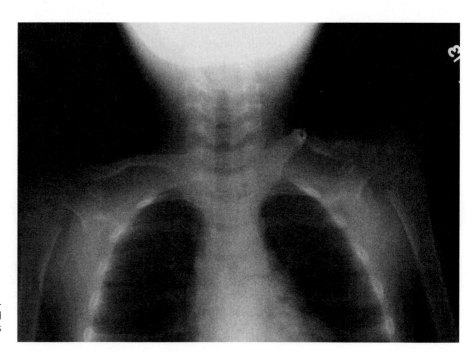

Figure 3-33 Pseudoarthrosis of the left clavicle, 1½ years after fracture, in a 5-year-old girl. The nonunion of the fracture site has resulted in the formation of a "false joint."

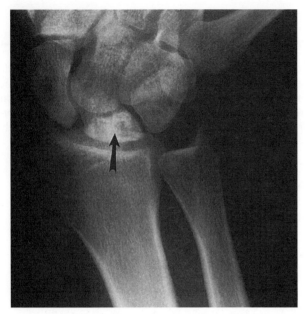

Figure 3-34 Avascular necrosis of the lunate in a 25-year-old man. The increased density of the lunate represents the body's attempt to revascularize and produce new bone.

known as reflex sympathetic dystrophy syndrome (RSDS), because it was theorized to be due to a sympathetically maintained reflex arc. Recent evidence indicates that the sympathetic nervous system is not necessarily involved in every case of CRPS. No single concept of pathogenesis has been proven at this time.

CRPS is divided into types 1 and 2. The distinguishing characteristic of type 2 is the presence of a major peripheral nerve injury. Otherwise, both types have identical clinical features, which are predominantly pain, hyperesthesia, and tenderness. Additional features can be grouped into three stages of progression. Not all patients, however, experience this order of progression. Stage 1 lasts 1 to 3 months and is characterized by constant, burning, aching pain out of proportion to the initial injury. Stage 2 lasts 3 to 6 months and is characterized by cold, glossy skin, limited range of motion, and diffuse bone demineralization seen on radiographs. Stage 3 is characterized by progressive atrophy of skin and muscle, joint contractures, and marked segmental demineralization on radiograph.

Diagnosis is predicated on clinical presentation only. Sympathetic nerve blocks can relieve pain and narrow the diagnosis to RSDS. Generally, diagnostic testing is performed only to rule out other causes of pain in the extremity.

The primary goals of treatment are to control pain and preserve function. Physical therapy is one of the few modalities that have been shown to be effective in treating CRPS. Adequate analgesia is necessary to permit the patient to participate fully in rehabilitation.

Bone Length Discrepancy

Some fracture healing can result in unacceptable shortening of bone length. "Unacceptable" shortening can mean significant functional loss, cosmetic deformity, or risk for degeneration and loss of adjacent joint function. At risk are fractures that are severely comminuted or have a complete loss of a segment of bone (such as those secondary to a gunshot wound). Late complications, such as infection, nonunion, or malunion, also present risk for loss of bone length. Surgical techniques that lengthen bone can be applied during the acute phase of healing or as a delayed procedure.

External fixation devices are the cornerstone of bone lengthening surgery. The basic components are percutaneous transfixing pins attached to an outrigger frame. This results in an effect that is a compromise between definitive skeletal pin traction and internal fixation. These devices stabilize the fracture fragments in alignment while at the same time permit bone growth to fill in a gap. In general, external fixators are temporary devices; after sufficient length is obtained, the external hardware is removed and the fracture site is stabilized with internal fixation (Fig. 3-35).

Associated Complications in Other Tissues

Soft Tissue Injuries

The severity of soft tissue injuries associated with fracture range from mild edema to gross disruption of cartilaginous, capsular, ligamentous, and muscle tissue. Open fractures, in general, suffer more soft tissue damage than closed fractures. Injury results from the external trauma as well as the displaced fragments, which can tear tissue from the inside. Closed fractures can also have significant soft tissue injury; this is usually seen in fracture–dislocation cases that disrupt joint-stabilizing tissues. Closed fractures, if severely angulated, may cause a tenting of the skin, in which a fragment protrudes from under the skin, like a tent pole. This can produce localized ischemia, break down viable skin tissue, and convert a closed fracture into an open fracture.

Arterial Injury

Arterial injuries are associated with a small percentage of fractures. Supracondylar fractures of the distal humerus present risk of occlusion to the brachial artery. Dislocations are more frequently the cause of vascular injury; the elbow and knee are most susceptible to vascular insult. In regard to knee dislocations, some treatment protocols advise arteriograms after reduction, regardless of normal pulses, to detect initially asymptomatic intimal tears that may develop into complete occlusion.

Eiff[2] advises primary care providers to minimize adverse outcomes of arterial injuries by following these guidelines:

1. Assess distal circulation in all patients with a fracture or dislocation. Slowed pulse, pallor, and slow capillary refill (more than 3 seconds) are signs of arterial injury.
2. Assess circulation *as soon as possible,* prior to radiographic examination.
3. When dislocations and fractures are accompanied by absence of pulse, and orthopedic care is not readily available, primary care providers should attempt reduction. In many cases, the artery is kinked rather than torn. If the limb is pulseless, much is to be gained and little lost by attempted reduction.

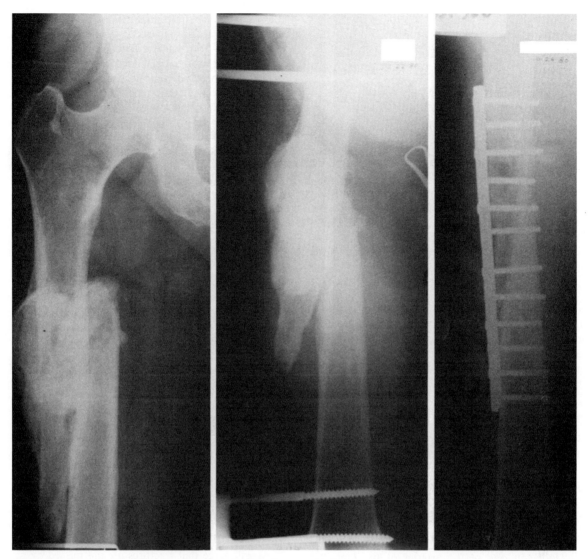

Figure 3-35 The use of the Wagner device for gradual lengthening. This 44-year-old man fractured his femur when he overturned a tractor. He was treated at a military installation by a cast-brace. After removal of the cast-brace he developed pain in his thigh but kept walking anyway. He was seen by four orthopedists for disability evaluation, all of whom reported different leg length discrepancies, which they believed to be due to shortening with malunion. **(Left)** This x-ray shows the man had no union at all. **(Center)** The limb was pulled out to length gradually by a Wagner apparatus. **(Right)** Internal fixation by a sideplate device after the femur had been pulled out to the desired length. The internal fixation is necessary to close the skin, allow healing of the fragments in normal alignment, and promote progressive ambulation without the hindrance of the external device.

Nerve Injury

Fortunately, most nerve injuries associated with fractures and dislocations are temporary neurapraxias that result from stretching of the nerve; these resolve spontaneously over time. Many patients experience temporary paresthesia due to soft tissue edema; this is also benign and self-limited.

More serious nerve injuries are associated with open fractures and penetrating injuries. Fractures near the elbow and knee are most often involved, as are dislocations of the hip, knee, and shoulder. Open exploration and nerve repair are often necessary in such cases.

Compartment Syndrome

A compartment syndrome is defined as a condition in which the circulation and function of tissues within a closed space are compromised by increased pressure within that space. Compartment syndrome was first documented by Richard von Volkmann in his classic paper of 1881. He observed ischemic muscle necrosis in a limb that progressed to paralysis and contracture due to being "too tightly bandaged." The condition that bears his name, Volkmann's ischemia, refers to increased pressure within the fascial compartment of the forearm. Despite different names that exist for the many different etiologies or locations, the underlying features of any compartment syndrome are essentially the same.

The classic signs of impending compartment syndrome are the "five Ps." Arranged in their most common order of appearance, the "five Ps" are *pain, pallor, paresthesia, paralysis,* and *pulselessness* (Table 3-7). These are not, however, always all present. Each sign must be evaluated and interpreted with the overall clinical picture.

TABLE 3-7 ● *Symptoms of Compartment Syndrome: The 5 Ps*	
Pain	Deep, poorly localized
Pallor	Distal to compartment
Paresthesia	Of sensory nerve passing through compartment
Paralysis	Permanent damage likely
Pulselessness	

Life-Threatening Complications

A minority of fractures have life-threatening consequences. The key to the management of these conditions is early recognition and prompt treatment. Life-threatening conditions that can occur with fracture include hemorrhage, fat embolism, pulmonary embolism, gas gangrene, and tetanus.

Hemorrhage

Hemorrhage is the most common life-threatening condition associated with fracture. One-half of all pelvic fractures result in blood loss sufficient to require transfusion. Closed femoral fractures can also result in significant hemorrhage. Generally, however, open fractures result in greater blood loss because the tamponade effect of the surrounding soft tissue is absent.

Fat Embolism

Fat embolism in single fractures is rare, but when it does occur it is usually associated with long-bone fractures in young adults or hip fractures in the elderly. Studies have shown the greatest risk of fat embolism is related to multiple fractures sustained in motor vehicle accidents and battlefield injuries, with mortality from respiratory failure as high as 50%. Crushing-type fractures allow fat from bone marrow to enter the veins in the form of globules, which eventually lodge in one of the arteries of the lung. Fat embolisms generally develop 12 hours postfracture but can appear up to 72 hours postfracture. Symptoms are similar to those of pulmonary embolism in the early stages. Clinical signs also include fever, hypoxia, confusion, restlessness, changing neurological signs, urinary incontinence, and a petechial rash across the chest and in the conjunctiva.

Pulmonary Embolism

The immobilization, decreased activity, and soft tissue injury associated with fracture slows the bloodstream and increases the risk of venous thrombosis. A thrombus always has the potential to detach and enter the bloodstream as an embolus. The classic signs of pulmonary embolism are sudden onset of dyspnea and anxiety, with or without substernal pain. The hallmark of treatment of thromboembolic disease is prevention via prophylactic blood thinners and physical measures (compression garments, elevation, and range-of-motion and mobility exercise as appropriate).

Gas Gangrene

Gas gangrene after a fracture is almost always associated with a deep penetrating injury to muscle. The *Clostridium* group of organisms responsible for this condition are found in the intestinal tracts of humans and animals. The risk of contamination is always present because these organisms are found everywhere—from barnyards to hospital operating rooms. Initial symptoms are pain, edema, and an exudate of thin, dark fluid. The fluid and bubbles of foul-smelling gas, produced from fermentation of muscle sugars, spread along muscle sheaths, separating them from muscle, and can be physically pressed up and down the length of the muscle. The fluid is highly toxic, and the condition can rapidly progress to toxemia and death. Prophylactic antibiotics are given routinely in cases of deep penetrating tissue injuries. If gangrene does develop, surgical intervention to remove necrotic tissue is necessary.

Tetanus

Open fractures can also be contaminated by *Clostridium tetani,* commonly found in soil fertilized with horse manure. The resulting infection stays localized in the wound and, in this respect, is the opposite of the clostridial infection causing gas gangrene. However, it produces toxins more virulent than the most deadly snake venom. Within 7 to 10 days, the toxin gradually passes along nerves from the wound to the spinal cord, anchoring onto motor neurons. Stimulation of the motor nerves causes rigidity and convulsions. The jaw muscles are involved earliest, hence the name "lockjaw."

Tetanus antitoxin is usually given prophylactically in cases of street accidents or contaminated wounds.

Commonly Missed Fractures[31–61]

Why Are Fractures Missed on Radiographs?[31–40]

Most will agree that fractures *are not* missed by patients—acute pain is a reliable indicator. Fractures *are* missed by clinicians who read radiographs. (It is a mistake to assume that a radiologist has read every patient's images—the majority of acute care hospitals do *not* have radiologist interpretation available 24 hours a day, 7 days a week.) Retrospective studies performed by radiologists have shown that radiographic errors made by various emergency department physicians can be linked to one or more of the following factors:

1. Failure to order radiography
2. Failure to recognize fractures on the radiograph
3. Subtle fractures that may not be evident on initial radiographs
4. Presence of multiple injuries
5. Inadequate patient history

This known diversity in error source serves to emphasize the significance of the *clinical evaluation* and application of a conservative *rule of treatment* as a critical safety net in the acute management of injuries.

Importance of the Clinical History and Evaluation

Trauma almost always precipitates a fracture, and this information should be disclosed in the history. Knowing the mechanism of injury is usually helpful in identifying potential fracture sites. There are instances, however, when a history is not helpful. Sometimes the fractures may result from relatively minor cumulative stresses that are not recognized by the patient as such (as in stress fractures). Sometimes the patient may be physically, mentally, or emotionally unable to give a clear history. And sometimes the details of the trauma may be withheld by the patient for personal reasons.

The clinical evaluation for fracture does not usually suffer the same ambiguities as the history. *Acute point tenderness* to palpation over the fracture site is both a reliable perception of the patient and a reliable clinical sign of fracture. Furthermore, a clinician may apply joint-specific *clinincal decision rules (CDRs)* to help decide whether to order radiography or not. CDRs are well-substantiated lists of clinical patient factors that have a strong predictive value for whether a patient has a fracture or not. The application of CDRs helps to ensure that injuries requiring definition by radiography *do* get imaged and to prevent unnecessary radiography for injuries whose outcome is *unaffected by imaging*. See Chapter 18 for more on CDRs.

Rule of Treatment in Fracture Management

If the clinical evaluation and/or radiographic findings are ambiguous, the clinician should apply the general *rule of treatment* for fracture management: *If it acts like a fracture but radiographs are negative, treat it as a fracture (immobilize!) and reevaluate with radiographs in 1 to 2 weeks.* If a fracture is present, it will announce itself on the follow-up radiograph by localized density changes at the fracture site. If a fracture is not present, the patient has only suffered minor inconveniences. The good sense of this fracture management principle avoids the detrimental possibilities of an unstabilized fracture and the reality of malpractice actions. Errors on the side of caution rarely have adverse outcomes.

Which Fractures Are Missed?

Clinicians should be aware of the fractures that occur with statistical frequency, as these will lend themselves to statistical "misses." The literature calls attention to commonly missed fractures and the radiographic signs that can assist in identifying subtle fractures (see Table 3-8).

Commonly Missed Fractures of the Spine[41–49]

The most common site of traumatic injury in the cervical spine is C1–C2, followed by injuries at C6–C7. The reported frequency of missed injuries in the cervical spine varies from 4% to 30%. The most common reason cited for error is inadequate radiographic exam—the anatomy is not well visualized at the craniovertebral and cervicothoracic junction on routine radiographs. A delay in identifying cervical spinal fractures puts the patient at risk for progressive instability and permanent neurological sequelae.

In the thoracic and lumbar spine regions, osteoporotic vertebral body fractures often go undetected by clinicians and are underdiagnosed by radiologists. Delay in pharmacological therapy increases the risk for future fractures of the spine and hip.

Commonly Missed Fractures of the Upper Extremity[50–54]

The scaphoid is the most often fractured carpal bone, and its miss rate on conventional radiographs is the highest. This miss rate is partly due to the fact that radiographs can appear normal up to 20% of the time.[51] The rule of treatment dictates a thumb spica cast or splint to all injured wrists with anatomic snuffbox tenderness, regardless of positive or negative radiographic findings.

At the elbow, radial head fractures can be difficult to visualize, but they have an advantage of being associated with a reliable radiographic soft tissue sign. A displaced fat pad is highly correlated with radial head fractures. The classic appearance of a triangular radiolucency anterior to the distal humerus led to the term *sail sign* to describe displacement of the anterior fat pad.

Other frequently missed fractures share the same mechanism of injury: a fall on an outstretched hand. These include fractures of the *triquetrum* and fracture–dislocation combination injuries of the forearm and wrist.

In fracture–dislocation injury patterns, errors can occur when only the predominant injury and not the associated injury is noted. Examples include *distal radius fracture with scapholunate dissociation, distal radial fracture with distal radioulnar joint dislocation* (Galeazzi's fracture), and *proximal ulnar fracture with radial head dislocation* (Monteggia's fracture).

Commonly Missed Fractures of the Lower Extremity[31–36,38,54–61]

Femoral neck fractures are the most commonly missed hip fracture. Missed hip fractures that are initially *nondisplaced* are very likely to become *displaced*. The potential for vascular disruption and avascular necrosis of the femoral head is significant; history of a fall and painful weight bearing dictate conservative treatment regardless of negative radiographic findings.

At the knee, common fracture sites include the tibial plateau and avulsions at the lateral tibial plateau (Segond fracture) often associated with anterior cruciate tears. CT is indicated when radiographic findings are negative and clinical presentation is positive. Subtle fractures of the patella are best seen on the tangential "sunrise" view.

The calcaneus is the most commonly fractured tarsal bone and has a "miss rate" in some studies of 10%.[39] A key in detection of subtle fractures is visualizing the *Boehler angle* on the lateral view. Calcaneal fractures have a 10% association rate with thoracolumbar fracture. Patients whose mechanism of injury includes an axial load when landing on the heels should have spinal imaging as well as calcaneal films.

A summary of these and other fractures commonly missed on conventional radiographs is presented in Table 3-8.

TABLE 3-8 ● *Commonly Missed, High-Risk Fractures on Radiographs*[14–30]

Bone	Mechanism of Injury	Comments
Spine		
C1–C2 fractures C6–C7 fractures	Falls or motor vehicle accidents	● Radiographic clues to instability include segmental kyphosis, loss of lordosis, anterior soft tissue swelling, antero/retrolisthesis; best imaged with CT
Vertebral body fractures secondary to osteoporosis	Increased incidence in postmenopausal females with age, with or without trauma	● Loss of vertebral body height that exceeds 20%
Wrist		
Scaphoid fracture	Fall on an outstretched hand	Consider obtaining additional scaphoid views since routine radiographs often appear normal
Triquetrum fracture	Fall on an outstretched hand	Triquetrum fractures are most easily seen on lateral view as this is the most dorsal carpal bone
Galeazzi Fracture (distal third of radius fracture with disruption of distal radioulnar joint)	Fall on an outstretched hand with forearm pronation	PA view: Ulnar styloid fracture may be seen with widening of distal radioulnar joint Lateral view: Ulna does not overlie radius and ulnar styloid is not aligned with dorsal triquetrum
Distal radius Fx + carpal injury	Fall on an outstretched hand	Distal radius fracture sometimes associated with findings of scapholunate dissociation
Elbow		
Monteggia Fx (proximal ulna fracture with radial head dislocation)	Fall on an outstretched hand with rotational forces	● Obvious proximal ulna fracture ● Misalignment of radiocapitular line
Radial head	Fall on an outstretched hand	● Cortical break in the radial head may be very subtle or absent in a nondisplaced Fx ● Large anterior fat pad (Sail sign); any posterior fat pad sign
Hip		
Femoral neck	Direct trauma, as from a fall	*Note:* Some patients can bear weight despite a Fx ● Look for cortical disruption or impacted hyperlucency ● See loss of smooth cortical transition from femoral neck to head as well as trabecular disruption
Acetabulum	Direct contact with femoral head, as in "dashboard" injuries	● Anterior acetabular Fx is revealed by a break in the iliopubic line ● Posterior acetabular fracture is shown by a break in the ilioischial line, looking behind the superimposed femoral head ● Additional oblique views help for initially negative standard view films
Pelvis		
Sacrum	Fall from a height, motor vehicle accident	● Note subtle break in smooth sacral arcuate lines ● Pelvic outlet views improve visualization of the sacrum and rami
Pelvic ring Fx	Motor vehicle accidents, pedestrian accidents, fall from height	Look for multiple injuries due to the inflexible ring structure of the pelvis; watch for rami fracture and sacroiliac dissociation
Knee		
Tibial plateau Tibial spine	Valgus force with axial load, such as strike by car bumper	Two views provide only 85% sensitivity; oblique views increase sensitivity
Segond fracture (small proximal lateral tibial avulsion Fx)	Internal rotation and varus stress	May be accompanied by other injuries: ● ACL tear (75%–100%), medial and lateral menisci tears (66%–70%), fibular head avulsion fracture ● MRI is needed to evaluate the ACL and possible injuries to menisci and other structures
Patella	Motor vehicle injuries, direct fall onto the knee	● Assessed with axial patellofemoral "sunrise" view ● Lateral view is best to detect transverse fractures
Maisonneuve fracture (proximal fibula fracture with distal tibiofibular disruption)	Abduction and external rotation of the ankle	Requires AP view of the knee as well as AP view of the ipsilateral ankle
Foot		
Calcaneus	Fall on the heels from a height	● A Boehler angle of less than 25° suggests a Fx ● Consider obtaining a "calcaneal view" (long axial view) ● Often requires CT imaging to assess fragments and intra-articular extension
Talus	Excessive dorsiflexion of the ankle	Can find subtle cortical break on lateral view
Thoracolumbar Fx + calcaneus Fx	Jump from a height transmits force from heels to spine	● These two fractures have a 10% association rate ● Ensure both thoracolumbar and calcaneal studies are evaluated

ACL, anterior cruciate ligament; AP, anteriorposterior; CT, computed tomography; Fx, fracture; MRI, magnetic resonance imaging.

Summary of Key Points

1. The task of the radiologist who evaluates trauma is twofold: (1) to diagnose the physical characteristics of the fracture or dislocation and (2) to assess and monitor the results of treatment.

2. A *fracture* is a break in the continuity of bone or cartilage. A *closed* fracture does not break the skin surface. An *open* fracture communicates with the external environment through a tear or perforation in the skin.

3. *Fracture description includes seven elements:* anatomic site and extent of the fracture, incomplete versus complete fracture pattern, alignment of fragments, direction of fracture line, special features such as impaction or avulsion, associated abnormalities such as joint dislocation, and special types of fractures due to abnormal stresses or underlying pathology such as stress fractures or pathological fractures.

4. Location of fractures in children named by the region of development: the *diaphysis, metaphysis, epiphyseal growth plate,* and *epiphysis.*

5. Unique patterns of *incomplete fractures* in immature bone include: *greenstick, torus,* and *plastic bowing.*

6. The *Salter–Harris* classification system describes patterns of injury to the epiphyseal growth plate and surrounding bone.

7. Fifteen to twenty precent of childhood fractures involve the *epiphyseal region.* Accurate diagnosis is critical to preventing growth arrest. Salter–Harris type II is the most common injury pattern.

8. The capacity of immature bone to *remodel* deformities depends on skeletal maturity, fracture displacement, and distance of the fracture from the growth plate.

9. *Skeletal age* is a measurement of skeletal maturity. Skeletal age assists in anticipating longitudinal growth, remodeling potential, and treatment options.

10. Fracture fragments are guided back to their best possible anatomic position by either *closed reduction* (manipulation, traction) or *open reduction* (surgical exposure of the fracture site).

11. Fractures are immobilized to facilitate the healing process by either *external fixation* methods (splints, casts) or *internal fixation* methods (pins, wires, compression plates, and screws). At times a combination of the two methods is used.

12. Fractures may heal by the formation of *callus* or by direct osteoblastic activity, referred to as *creeping substitution.*

13. *The time frame for healing is influenced by several factors* including patient age; degree of tissue trauma; fracture site and configuration; type of bone; degree of immobilization; presence of infection, malignancy, avascular necrosis, pathological process, or radiation necrosis; corticosteroids; exercise and local stress about the fracture.

14. Complications at a fracture site include *delayed union, slow union, nonunion, malunion, pseudarthrosis,* and *avascular necrosis.*

15. Complications of fractures in associated tissues include *arterial injury, nerve injury,* and *compartment syndrome.*

16. Late-effect complications of fractures include *complex regional pain syndrome* and *bone length discrepancy.*

17. *Life-threatening complications of fractures* include hemorrhage, fat embolism, pulmonary embolism, gas gangrene, and tetanus.

18. *Commonly missed fractures* are due to either (1) failure to obtain radiographs, (2) failure to recognize fractures on the radiograph, or (3) occult fractures that are difficult to see on conventional radiographs.

19. *A basic principle of fracture management is* that if it seems like a fracture but radiographs are normal, treat it as a fracture with immobilization, and reradiograph in 1 to 2 weeks to verify.

20. The use of *eponyms* (e.g., *Colles' fracture, hip pointer*) to describe orthopedic trauma has historic roots and newer terms (e.g., *keyboard wrist*) continue to be generated today. Although eponyms serve as a type of orthopedic verbal shorthand, they should always be avoided in radiologic description because of their anatomic inexactness.

21. *Professional collaboration* can enhance patient outcome, as illustrated in a case study where *the absence of collaboration had serious negative consequences.*

 Please refer to the text's enclosed CD-ROM for the American College of Radiology's current Musculoskeletal Appropriateness Criteria for the following topics: *Stress/Insufficiency Fractures, Including Sacrum, Excluding Other Vertebrae.*

CASE STUDY

Avulsion Fracture in a Ballet Dancer

This case study, condensed and retold with permission from Quarrier and Wightman,[62] exemplifies the difficulty of diagnosis complicated by (1) failure to link radiologic evidence with clinical presentation and (2) failure of interprofessional communication regarding clinical and radiologic evidence. It is an unfortunate example of how the good intentions of health-care professionals resulted in an astonishing amount of irrelevant imaging and invasive procedures and prolonged a patient's pain and disability.

History of Injury

An 18-year-old preprofessional female ballet dancer was referred to physical therapy with chronic left hip pain of undiagnosed origin. An original injury occurred when the patient was 15 years old. It was described as a groin pull during ballet class. The sharp intermittent pain in the left groin was exacerbated with activity and during menstruation.

Initial Differential Diagnoses

During the prior 3 years, various physicians considered a range of diagnoses, including ovarian cyst, ligamentous sprain, fibrositis, synovitis, spastic colon, ureteral dysfunction, inguinal hernia, abdominal epilepsy, somatoform pain disorder, psychosomatic disorder, inflammatory bowel disease, gastroenteritis, endometriosis, rectus femoris strain with psoas avulsion, acetabular labral tear, and iliopsoas tendinitis.

Initial Imaging

To assist in the differential diagnosis, a series of diagnostic tests were performed over this time period. These included pelvic and abdominal sonograms, blood analysis, upper/lower gastrointestinal series, intravenous pyelogram, Meckel's diverticulum nuclear imaging scan, CT of abdomen/pelvis, laparoscopy, groin exploratory surgery, hip radiographs, sigmoidoscopy, bone scan, MRI of pelvis/hip, nerve block, and electroencephalogram. All testing was negative, and no confirmed diagnosis was made. Two radiologic reports described an *"insignificant secondary bony ossicle at the lesser trochanter."*

Treatment

The patient had to stop dance and eliminate the possibility of a career in dance. Years of unsuccessful interventions were tried, including anti-inflammatory medications, acupuncture, Rolfing, myofascial release, psychological counseling, biofeedback, chiropractic, and physical therapy. The referring physician desired to exhaust all forms of conservative treatment before possibly making a diagnosis of endometriosis with the possibility of hysterectomy. Four physical therapy evaluations were performed, and each therapist documented psoas involvement.

This brings us to the patient in therapy at age 18. Therapeutic measures applied to a dysfunctional hip failed to relieve pain, and she was referred to an orthopedic surgeon specializing in the hip. Arthroscopic surgery was performed on the suspicion of a labral tear. After normal findings, a second surgery was suggested for joint arthrotomy to recess the rectus tendon head and remove scar tissue. The patient declined.

Additional Imaging

At this point, frustration led the patient to terminate all therapy and medical intervention for 1½ years until an injury from a fall generated new radiographs of the hip, which were reported as normal. The insurance-recommended physician referred the patient to a sports medicine physician, who reevaluated the radiographs. The ossicle at the lesser trochanter, first reported 6 years earlier as "insignificant," was finally recognized by this physician as significant, and surgical excision was recommended.

Outcome

A 1- by 0.5-cm avulsed ossicle, entirely loose and embedded in the iliopsoas tendon near its insertion in the lesser trochanter, was removed.

After struggling with hip pain for over 6 years, undergoing major invasive procedures, and fearing the possibility of hysterectomy, this 21 year old was finally pain free and returned to normal activity, including recreational dance.

Discussion

Why Did No One Make the Correct Diagnosis?

Let's look at how many professionals had the correct information but did not make the correct diagnosis. At least three radiologists identified the ossicle. At least four physicians (orthopedic surgeon, primary care physician, gynecologist, and internist) were aware of the radiologic report. A total of five different physical therapists identified psoas involvement. Everyone documented and no one really communicated! The significance of the ossicle as a probable avulsion fracture eluded all but the sports medicine physician.

CRITICAL THINKING POINT

The physical therapists did not have training in radiologic interpretation and could not link the radiographic finding with their knowledge of functional anatomy. Conversely, the physicians, who did not have training in functional anatomy, could not link the clinical findings with the radiologic evidence. The absence of professional collaboration resulted in extensive costs, pain, disability, and loss of a potential career for this young patient.

References

1. Greenspan, A: Orthopedic Radiology: A Practical Approach, ed. 4. Lippincott Williams & Wilkins, Philadelphia, 2004.
2. Eiff, MP, et al: Fracture Management For Primary Care, ed. 2. WB Saunders, Philadelphia, 2003.
3. Hoppenfeld, S, and Murthy, VL: Treatment and Rehabilitation of Fractures. Lippincott Williams & Wilkins, Philadelphia, 2000.
4. Dries, D, and Perry, J: Initial evaluation of the trauma patient. Emedicine, 2007. Available at http://www.emedicine.com/med/TOPIC3221.HTM
5. Helling, T, Wilson, J, and Augustosky, K: The utility of focused abdominal ultrasound in blunt abdominal trauma: A reappraisal. Am J Surg 194(6):728, 2007.
6. Torretti, JA, and Sengupta, DK: Cervical spine trauma: Review article. Indian J Orthop 41(4):255, 2007.
7. Brandt, MM, Wahl, WL, Yeom, K, Kazerooni, E, and Wang, SC: J Trauma 56(5):1022, 2004.
8. Wilson, A, and Walsh, M: Clinical review: ABC of emergency radiology, major trauma. BMJ 330:1136, 2005.
9. Diaz, JJ, et al: Practice management guidelines for the screening of thoracolumbar spine fracture. J Trauma 63(3):709, 2007.
10. Kaur, S, et al: Lumbar spine plain film in blunt trauma: Is it necessary if an abdominal and pelvis CT are obtained? Am J Roentgenol 188:A16, 2007.
11. Bell, RM: Clearing the cervical spine. Tutorial. Available at http://www.swsahs.nsw.gov.au/livtrauma/education/x-ray/cspline.asp. Accessed April 25, 2008.
12. Hoffman, JR, et al: Selective cervical spine radiology in blunt trauma: Methodology of the national emergency x-radiography utilization study. Ann Emerg Med 32(4):461, 1998.
13. Hendey, GW, et al: Spinal cord injury without radiographic abnormality: Results of the National Emergency X-ray Utilization Study in blunt cervical trauma. J Trauma 53(1):1, 2002.
14. Kanz, KG, et al: Priority-oriented shock trauma room management with the integration of multiple-view spiral computed tomography. Unfallchirurg 107(10):937, 2004.
15. Berry, GE, et al: Are plain radiographs of the spine necessary during evaluation after blunt trauma? Accuracy of screening torso computed

tomography in thoracic/lumbar spine fracture diagnosis. J Trauma 59(6):1410, 2005.

16. Quencer, R, Nunez, D, and Green, B: Controversies in imaging acute cervical spine trauma. Am J Neuroradiol 18:1866, 1997.

17. Brown, CV, et al: Spiral computed tomography for the diagnosis of cervical, thoracic, and lumbar spine fractures: Its time has come. J Trauma 58(5):890, 2005.

18. Drafke, MW, and Nakayama, H: Trauma and Mobile Radiography, ed. 2. FA Davis, Philadelphia, 2001.

19. Nordin, M, and Frankel, VH: Basic Biomechanics of the Musculoskeletal System, ed. 3. Lippincott Williams & Wilkins, Philadelphia, 2001.

20. Daffner, RH: Clinical Radiology: The Essentials, ed. 3. Williams & Wilkins, Baltimore, 2007.

21. Whiting, W, and Zernicke, R: Biomechanics of Musculoskeletal Injury, ed. 2. Human Kinetics, Champaign, IL, 2008.

22. Koval, KJ, and Zuckerman, JD: Handbook of Fractures, ed. 3. Lippincott Williams & Wilkins, Philadelphia, 2006.

23. Gustilo, RB: The Fracture Classification Manual. CV Mosby, St Louis, MO, 1991.

24. Schultz, RJ: The Language of Fractures, ed. 2. Williams & Wilkins, Baltimore, 1990.

25. Beaty, J, and Kasar, J (eds): Rockwood and Wilkins' Fractures in Children, ed. 6. Lippincott Williams & Wilkins, Philadelphia, 2005.

26. Bucholz, RW, Heckman, J, and Court-Brown, C (eds): Rockwood and Green's: Fractures in Adults, ed. 6. Lippincott Williams & Wilkins, Philadelphia, 2005.

27. Practice Guidelines and Technical Standards, 2008. American College of Radiology. Available at http://www.acr.org.

28. Greulich, WW, and Pyle, SI: Radiographic Atlas of Skeletal Development of the Hand and Wrist, ed. 2. Stanford University Press, Stanford, CA, 1999.

29. Gilsanz, V, and Ratib, O: Hand Bone Age: A Digital Atlas of Skeletal Maturity. Springer, New York, 2004.

30. Sheldon, H: Boyd's Introduction to the Study of Disease, ed. 11. Lippincott Williams & Wilkins, Philadelphia, 1992.

31. Kachalia, A, et al: Missed and delayed diagnoses in the emergency department: A study of closed malpractice claims from four liability insurers. Ann Emerg Med 49(2):196, 2007.

32. Wei, CJ, et al: Systematic analysis of missed extremity fractures in emergency radiology. Acta Radiol 47(7):710, 2006.

33. Lin, M: Pitfalls in orthopedic radiographic interpretation. Mediterranean Emergency Medicine Conference. 2003. Available at http://www.emcongress.org/handouts/lin_handout.pdf. Accessed September 27, 2003.

34. Espinosa, JA: Reducing errors made by emergency physicians in interpreting radiographs: Longitudinal study. BMJ 320(7237):737, 2000.

35. Guly, HR: Diagnostic errors in an accident and emergency department. Emerg Med J 18(4):263, 2001.

36. Massachusetts College of Emergency Physicians: Module 6: Fractures. Risk Management Course. Available at http://www.macep.org/practice_information/rm /rm_module6.htm. Accessed August 28, 2004.

37. John, H, et al: Fatigue fracture: R frequently overlooked injury? Helvetica Chirurgica Acta 60(4):551, 1994.

38. Gagliardi, JA, Nunberg, SM, Fisher, T: Fracture detection: A possible method to aid in diagnosis and improve reporting accuracy. RadiologyWeb, 2001. Available at http://www.radiologyweb.com_direction/ii/01apr/jg-ii-mar01.

39. Freed, HA, and Shields, NN: Most frequently overlooked radiographically apparent fractures in a teaching hospital emergency department. Ann Emerg Med 13(10):900, 1984.

40. Moore, MN: Orthopedic pitfalls in emergency medicine. South Med J 81(3):371, 1988.

41. Lenchik, L, Rogers, L, Delmas, P, and Genant, H: Diagnosis of osteoporotic vertebral fractures: importance of recognition and description by radiologists. Am J Roentgenol 183:949, 2004.

42. Barrett, TW, et al: Injuries missed by limited computed tomographic imaging of patients with cervical spine injuries. Ann Emerg Med 47(2):129, 2006.

43. Bernstein, MR, Mirvis, SE, and Shanmuganathan, K: Chance-type fractures of the thoracolumbar spine:imaging analysis in 53 patients. Am J Roentgenol 187:859, 2006.

44. Levi, AD, et al: Neurologic deterioration secondary to unrecognized spinal instability following trauma—a multicenter study. Spine 31(4):451, 2006.

45. Sava, J, et al: Thoracolumbar fracture in blunt trauma: Is clinical exam enough for awake patients? J Trauma 61(1):168, 2006.

46. Dai, LY, et al: Thoracolumbar fractures in patients with multiple injuries: diagnosis and treatment—A review of 147 cases. J Trauma 56(2):348, 2004.

47. D'Costa, H, et al: Pitfalls in the clinical diagnosis of vertebral fractures: a case series in which posterior midline tenderness was absent. Emerg Med J 22(5):330, 2005.

48. Harris, RD, and Harris, JH, Jr: The prevalence and significance of missed scapular fractures in blunt chest trauma. Am J Roentgenol 151(4):747, 1988.

49. Ferrar, L, Jiang, G, Adams, J, and Eastell, R: Identification of vertebral fractures: An update. Osteoporosis Int 16:717, 2005.

50. Stanley, BG, and Tribuzi, SM: Concepts in Hand Rehabilitation. FA Davis, Philadelphia, 1992.

51. Waeckerle, JF: A prospective study identifying the sensitivity of radiographic findings and the efficacy of clinical findings in carpal navicular fractures. Ann Emerg Med 16(7):733, 1987.

52. Shearman, CM, and el-Khoury, GY: Pitfalls in the radiologic evaluation of extremity trauma: Part I. The upper extremity. Am Fam Physician 57(5):995, 1998.

53. Welling, RD, et al: MDCT and radiography of wrist fractures: Radiographic sensitivity and fracture patterns. Am J Roentgenol 190:10, 2008.

54. Moser, T, et al: Wrist ligament tears: evaluation of MRI and combined MDCT and MR arthrography. Am J Roentgenol 188:1278, 2007.

55. Shearman, CM, and el-Khoury, GY: Pitfalls in the radiologic evaluation of extremity trauma: Part II. The lower extremity. Am Fam Physician. 57(6):1314, 1998.

56. Parker, MJ: Missed hip fractures. Arch Emerg Med 9(1):23, 1992.

57. Ray, JM, and Hendrix, J: Incidence, mechanism of injury, and treatment of fractures of the patella in children. J Trauma 32(4):464, 1992.

58. Yamamoto, LG: Sunrise view of the knee. Radiology Cases in Pediatric Emergency Medicine, Volume 6, Case 8. Kapiolani Medical Center for Women and Children. University of Hawaii John A. Burns School of Medicine, 2008. Available at http://www.hawaii.edu/medicine/pediatrics/pemxray/v6c08.html.

59. Fayad, LM, et al: Distinction of long bone stress fractures from pathological fractures on cross sectional imaging: how successful are we? Am J Roentgenol 185:915, 2005.

60. Nork, SE: Percutaneous stabilization of U-shaped sacral fractures using iliosacral screws: Results and early results. Session I—Pelvic trauma. 1998. Available at http://www.hwbf.org/ota/am/ota98/otapa/OTA98104.htm. Accessed October 6, 2003.

61. Kim, MY, et al: Transverse sacral fractures: Case series and literature review. Can J Surg 44:359, 2001.

62. Quarrier, NF, and Wightman, AB: A ballet dancer with chronic hip pain due to a lesser trochanter bony avulsion: The challenge of a differential diagnosis. J Orthop Sports Phys Ther 28(3):168, 1998.

63. Kilcoyne, RF, and Farrar, E: Handbook of Radiologic Orthopedic Terminology. Yearbook Medical Publishers, Chicago, 1986, p 25.

SELF-TEST

1. Identify the *two projections* of this patient's lower leg.

2. Describe the *anatomic site* of the fracture.

3. Is the fracture *complete* or *incomplete*?

4. Describe the alignment of the fracture fragments in regard to *angulation* and *displacement*.

5. Describe the *direction of the fracture line*.

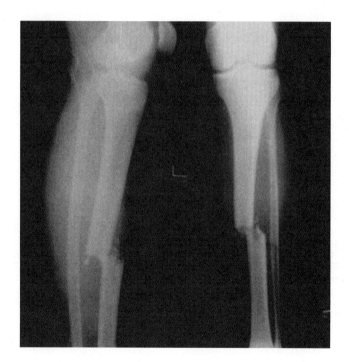

APPENDIX: FRACTURE EPONYMS

The use of eponyms to describe fracture anatomy and orthopedic trauma has historic roots and certainly predates the discovery of x-rays a century ago. Many current eponyms have survived for decades or longer, and newer eponyms continue to appear. As stated earlier, eponyms are usually avoided in radiographic description because of their general characteristics, anatomic inexactness, or ease of misinterpretation. Additionally, some terms have acquired new meanings over the years, and some have always been controversial. However, the use of eponyms survives because they serve as a convenient type of orthopedic short-hand. Kilcoyne and Farrar[61] have compiled an extensive list of common orthopedic eponyms, and it is reproduced here with some additions.

Anterior malleolus fracture: An uncommon fracture of the anterolateral margin of the distal tibia at the site of attachment of the anterior tibiofibular ligament. This fracture fragment is also known as the "tubercle of Chaput."

Aviator's astragalus: A variety of fractures of the talus that include compression fractures of the neck, fractures of the body or posterior process, or fractures with dislocations.

Backfire fracture: See *Chauffeur fracture.*

Bado: A classification of Monteggia-type fractures based on the direction of dislocation of the radial head.

Bankart lesion: A detached fragment from the anteroinferior margin of the glenoid rim; it is seen with anterior shoulder dislocations.

Barton fracture: Intra-articular fracture of the rim of the distal radius. It may involve either the dorsal or volar rim.

Baseball finger: Hyperflexion injury to the distal interphalangeal joint, often associated with a dorsal avulsion fracture of the base of the distal phalanx; it is also called "dropped" or "mallet" finger.

Basketball foot: Subtalar dislocation of the foot.

Bennett fracture: Intra-articular avulsion fracture subluxation of the base of the first metacarpal. The fracture produces a small volar lip fragment that remains attached to the trapezium and trapezoid by means of the strong volar oblique ligament while the shaft fragment is displaced by proximal muscle pull.

Bennett fracture, "reverse": Intra-articular fracture subluxation of the base of the fifth and/or fourth metacarpal.

Boot-top fracture: Fracture of the midportion of the distal third of the tibia and fibula, as caused by a fall while on skis with attached boots.

Boutonnière deformity: Hyperflexion of a proximal interphalangeal joint of a finger due to disruption of the central slip of the extensor tendon.

Boxer's fracture: Fracture of the neck of the fifth metacarpal with dorsal angulation and often volar displacement of the metacarpal head.

Boyd classification (Boyd-Griffin classification): A classification of intertrochanteric hip fractures.

Buckle fracture: See *Torus fracture.*

Bumper fracture: Compression fracture of the lateral tibial plateau, often associated with avulsion of the medial collateral ligament of the knee; it is also called "fender fracture."

Bunkbed fracture: Intra-articular fracture of the base of the first metatarsal in a child.

Burst fracture: Severe comminution of a vertebral body, usually secondary to axial loading, sometimes with a rotatory component. Frequently there is a sagittal fracture through the body plus fractures in the posterior elements; this pattern is often seen with unstable spinal fractures.

Butterfly fragment: Comminuted wedge-shaped fracture that has split off from the main fragments; this implies high velocity of trauma from a direction opposite the fragment.

Chance fracture: A flexion distraction injury that results in compression of the vertebral body. Posteriorly there may be ligament disruption without fracture, and the disk–annulus complex may be disrupted. Alternatively, there may be transverse noncomminuted fractures of the vertebral body and neural arch. Described by G. Q. Chance in 1948, it is also known as "lap-type seat belt" fracture.

Chauffeur fracture: Intra-articular oblique fracture of the styloid process of the distal radius. It is so named because a person attempting to start an early automobile engine with a hand crank could suffer this fracture if the engine backfired; hence it is also called a "backfire fracture" or "lorry driver fracture." It is also called a "Hutchinson" fracture.

Chisel fracture: Incomplete intra-articular fracture of the head of the radius extending distally about 1 cm from the center of the articular surface.

Chopart fracture–dislocation: Fracture–dislocation of the talonavicular and calcaneocuboid joints. The name is derived from F. Chopart's (1743–1795) description of an amputation through these midtarsal joints.

Clay shoveler's fracture: Avulsion fracture of the spinous process of one or more of the lower cervical or upper thoracic vertebrae, most commonly at C7. More than one vertebra may be involved.

Coach's finger: Dorsal dislocation of a proximal interphalangeal joint.

Colles' fracture: Transverse fracture of the distal radial metaphysis proximal to the joint with dorsal displacement of the distal fragment and volar angulation. The ulnar styloid may also be fractured. Described by C. Pouteau in 1783 and again by A. Colles in 1814, it is also known as a "Pouteau fracture" or "Pouteau–Colles fracture."

Colles' fracture, "reverse": See *Smith fracture.*

Contrecoup injury: Injury on the side opposite the impact point.

Cotton fracture: See *Trimalleolar ankle fracture.*

Dashboard fracture: Fracture of the posterior rim of the acetabulum caused by impact through the knee, driving the femoral head against the acetabulum. It is frequently associated with a posterior cruciate ligament injury, a femoral shaft fracture, or patellar fracture.

de Quervain fracture: Fracture of the scaphoid with volar dislocation of a scaphoid fragment and the lunate.

Desault dislocation: Various dislocations of the distal radioulnar joint.

Descot fracture: A fracture of the "third malleolus" (that is, the posterior lip of the tibia).

Die punch fracture: A spectrum of intra-articular fractures of the distal radius resulting from impaction of the lunate, as can result from the axial loading of a closed-fist punch.

Dome fracture: A fracture involving the weight-bearing surface of the acetabulum or the upper articular surface of the talus.

Drawer syndrome: Severing of anterior or posterior cruciate ligaments at the knee.

Dropped finger: See *Baseball finger.*

Dupuytren fracture: Fracture of the fibula 2½ inches above the tip of the lateral malleolus caused by a pronation-external rotation injury. It is associated with tear of the tibiofibular ligaments and the deltoid ligament (or fracture of the medial malleolus).

Duverney fracture: Isolated fracture of the iliac wing.

Essex-Lopresti fracture: Comminuted fracture of the head of the radius with dislocation of the distal radioulnar joint.

Fender fracture: See *Bumper fracture.*

Ferguson–Allen classification: A type of spinal fracture classification based on the number of columns fractured.

Fielding–Magliato classification: A classification of subtrochanteric hip fractures based on the distance from the lesser trochanter (I–III).

Flail chest: An effect produced when several consecutive ribs are broken in more than two places. That section of the chest now functions independently, in opposition to the rest of the chest and normal breathing. Also called paradoxical breathing.

Frykman classification: A classification of distal radius fractures based on involvement of the radiocarpal/radioulnar joints with or without ulnar styloid fracture.

Galeazzi fracture: Fracture of the radius at the junction of the middle and distal thirds with associated dislocation or subluxation of the distal radioulnar joint. Also called a "reverse Monteggia fracture."

Gamekeeper's thumb: Partial or total disruption of the ulnar collateral ligament at the metacarpophalangeal joint of the thumb. It may also have an avulsion fracture from the base of the proximal phalanx.

Garden classification: A classification of femoral neck fractures, described by R. S. Garden in 1963. Types I, II, III, and IV are based on the displacement present.

Gosselin fracture: A V-shaped fracture of the lower third of the tibia that extends distally into the tibial plafond.

Greenstick fracture: An incomplete fracture of the shaft of a long bone, with disruption on the tension side and plastic deformation on the compression side.

Hangman's fracture: Traumatic spondylolisthesis with fracture through the pedicles or lamina of C2 secondary to a distraction–extension force.

Hawkins sign: Radiolucent line in the dome of the talus, indicating that the talus fracture will heal without osteonecrosis. This subchondral osteoporosis can develop only if the blood supply of the talus is intact.

Hawkins types: A classification of talar fracture–dislocations.

Henderson fracture: See *Trimalleolar fracture.*

Hill-Sachs lesion: Posterolateral defect of the humeral head caused by anterior shoulder dislocation and "implosion" fracture.

Hill-Sachs lesion, "reverse": Anterior defect of the humeral head secondary to posterior shoulder dislocation.

Hip pointer: An impaction fracture of the superior iliac wing.

Hoffa fracture: Coronal fracture of the medial femoral condyle.

Holstein-Lewis fracture: Fracture of the humerus at the junction of the middle and distal thirds where the radial nerve is tethered by the lateral intermuscular septum. Thus, it is associated with radial nerve palsy.

Horseback rider's knee: Dislocation of the fibular head (as caused by a bump against the gatepost).

Hutchinson fracture: See *Chauffeur fracture.*

Jefferson fracture: A burst fracture of the ring of the atlas, with fractures both anterior and posterior to the facet joints. It is secondary to an axial load on top of the head. There are usually four breaks in the ring and lateral spread of the lateral masses.

Jones fracture: A term sometimes applied to both extra- and intra-articular fracture of the base of the fifth metatarsal.

Kocher fracture: Intra-articular fracture of the capitellum of the humerus.

Kohler's disease: Fracture of the tarsal navicular with aseptic necrosis (in children).

Lauge-Hanson classification: A classification of ankle fractures, based on the mechanism of injury.

Laugier fracture: Fracture of the trochlea of the humerus.

LeFort fracture (fibula): See *Wagstaffe-LeFort fracture.*

Lisfranc fracture–dislocation: Fracture–dislocation through the tarsometatarsal joints, commonly associated with disruption of the second tarsometatarsal joint and lateral dislocation of the second through fifth tarsometatarsal joints. It may also show other patterns of tarsometatarsal disruption. It is named for J. Lisfranc's (1790–1847) description of an amputation through the tarsometatarsal joints.

Little Leaguer's elbow: Avulsion of the medial epicondyle of the elbow secondary to valgus stress.

Lorry driver fracture: See *Chauffeur fracture.*

Maisonneuve fracture: Fracture of the proximal third of the fibula with tearing of the distal tibiofibular syndesmosis and the interosseous membrane. It may also have fracture of the medial malleolus or tear of the deltoid ligament.

Malgaigne fracture (of humerus): Extension-type supracondylar fracture.

Malgaigne fracture (of pelvis): Fracture–dislocation of one side of the pelvis. This is an unstable injury, with two vertical fractures produced by a vertical shear force. The anterior fracture is in the superior and inferior rami of the pubis, and the posterior fracture or dislocation is in the ilium, the sacrum, or the sacroiliac joint. This makes the lateral fragment (containing the acetabulum) unstable.

Mallet finger: See *Baseball finger.*

March fracture: Stress or fatigue fracture of the metatarsals, as sometimes suffered by military recruits after long marching. (Other bones may have stress or fatigue fractures.)

Mason classification: A classification of radial head fractures based on the amount of articular surface involved (types I–IV).

Mechanical-bull thumb: Fracture at the base of the first metacarpal.

Midnight fracture: Oblique fracture of the proximal phalanx of the fifth toe.

Monteggia fracture: Fracture of the proximal third of the ulna with an anterior dislocation of the radial head. Other types of ulnar shaft fractures and radial head dislocations are sometimes included. These fractures are classified by J. L. Bado as follows: I: ulnar shaft fracture with anterior radial head dislocation; II: ulnar shaft fracture with lateral radial head dislocation; III: ulnar shaft fracture with posterior radial head dislocation; IV: both forearm bones fractured with radial head dislocation.

Monteggia fracture, "reverse": See *Galeazzi fracture.*

Montercaux fracture: Fracture of the fibular neck associated with diastasis of the ankle mortise.

Moore fracture: Colles' fracture of the distal radius with fracture of the ulnar styloid and dorsal subluxation of the distal ulna.

Mouchet fracture: Fracture of the capitellum of the humerus.

Nightstick fracture: Single bone fracture of the ulnar shaft due to a direct blow without disruption of the interosseous membrane or either of the radioulnar joints.

Nursemaid's elbow: Dislocation of the radial head in a toddler with an intact annular ligament. It is difficult to prove with x-ray, because the radial head may not be ossified. The dislocation may be reduced by supination during the x-ray examination.

Parachute jumper injury: Anterior dislocation of the fibular head.

Paratrooper fracture: Fracture of the distal tibial and fibular shafts.

Pauwels classification: A classification of fractures of the proximal femoral neck. Types I, II, and III designate the angle of the fracture.

Pelvic ring fracture: Fracture involving at least two parts of the pelvic circumference.

Piedmont fracture: Oblique distal radius fracture without disruption of the distal radioulnar joint. It is difficult to control by closed means. It was described at a Piedmont Orthopaedic Society Meeting.

Pilon fracture: Comminuted, intra-articular fracture of the distal tibia with a long oblique component, secondary to axial loading (*pilon* = French for "pestle," "rammer") and impaction of the talus into the tibial plafond.

Pipkin classification: A classification of fibular head fractures based on the amount of head fractured (I–III).

Plafond: The articular surface (*plafond* = French for "ceiling") of the distal tibia.

Posada fracture: Transcondylar fracture of the distal humerus with anterior flexion of the condylar fragment and posterior dislocation of the radius and ulna.

Pott fracture: A misnomer applied to bimalleolar fractures of the ankle; originally used to describe an abduction injury with fracture of the distal fibula and disruption of the medial ankle ligaments.

Pouteau fracture: See *Colles' fracture.*

Rolando fracture: Severely comminuted form of Bennett fracture through the base of the first metacarpal.

Salter–Harris classification: A classification of growth plate injuries. Stage I = epiphyseal plate fracture; II = I + metaphyseal fragment (Thurston–Holland sign); III = I + epiphyseal fragment; IV = II + III; V = I + severe comminution.

Seat belt fracture: See *Chance fracture.*

Segmental fracture: Fracture dividing the long bone into several segments.

Segond fracture: Avulsion fracture of the lateral tibial condyle at the site of attachment of the iliotibial band on Gerdy's tubercle. It is often associated with anterior cruciate ligament (ACL) injury.

Shepherd fracture: Fracture of the lateral tubercle of the posterior process of the talus, described by F. Shepherd (1851–1929). The fragment may simulate an os trigonum.

Sideswipe elbow fracture: Comminuted fracture of the distal humerus. It may include fracture of the radius and ulna.

Sinegas classification: A classification of acetabular fractures.

Ski boot fracture: See *Boot-top fracture.*

Ski pole fracture: Fracture of the base of the first metacarpal. It may be intra-articular.

Smith fracture: Transverse fracture of the distal radial metaphysis with anterior displacement of the distal fracture fragment. The fracture may be intra-articular. It is also called "reverse Colles" or "reverse Barton" or "Smith–Goyrand" fracture.

Sprinter's fracture: Fracture of the anterosuperior or anteroinferior spine of the ilium with a fragment of bone being avulsed by sudden muscular pull.

Stieda fracture: Avulsion fracture of the medial femoral condyle at the origin of the tibial collateral ligament. The term "Pellegrini–Stieda disease" describes ossification in the tibial collateral ligament at the margin of the medial femoral condyle from chronic trauma.

Straddle fracture: Bilateral fractures of the superior and inferior pubic rami.

Swan neck deformity: Hyperextension of the proximal interphalangeal joint of the finger secondary to disruption of the volar plate or contracture of the intrinsic muscles.

Teardrop fracture: Comminuted vertebral body fracture with a displaced anterior fragment. It is caused by an axial compression force with flexion of the midcervical spine. The same term sometimes is applied to an extension injury. It implies possible instability with posterior displacement of the vertebral body producing spinal cord damage.

Terry Thomas sign: Scapholunate dissociation, seen on the posteroanterior (PA) view of the wrist. The gap in the proximal carpal row is similar to the gap-tooth smile of this famous British actor.

Thurston–Holland sign: A metaphyseal fragment observed in association with an epiphyseal fracture (Salter–Harris II fracture).

Tillaux–Kleiger fracture: Intra-articular fracture of the anterolateral part of the distal tibial epiphysis (tubercle of Chaput) in children aged 12–14 years.

Toddler's fracture: Spiral fracture of the tibia, usually in a 2- to 3-year-old child.

Tongue fracture: Horizontal fracture of the posterosuperior surface of the calcaneus.

Torus: Compression fracture of a long bone in or near the metaphysis. It is usually an incomplete fracture and occurs in young children. It is derived from the Greek term for the "bulge" in an architectural column.

Trimalleolar fracture: Fracture of the medial and lateral malleoli and the posterior articular lip of the distal tibia. This fracture is also called a "Cotton fracture" or "Henderson fracture"; various calcaneus fractures were described by F. J. Cotton and F. F. Henderson in 1916. The term *trimalleolar* was coined by Henderson.

Triplane fracture: Fracture of the distal tibia involving the growth plate in early adolescence. It is of the Salter–Harris IV type.

Tubercle of Chaput: The anterior tubercle of the distal tibia where the anterior tibiofibular ligament attaches.

Turf toe: Hyperextension injury to the capsule of the first metatarsal phalangeal joint.

Wagon wheel: Traumatic separation of the distal femoral epiphysis.

Wagstaffe–LeFort fracture: Avulsion of the distal fibula at the site of attachment of the anterior inferior tibiofibular ligament.

Walther fracture: Transverse ischioacetabular fracture. The fracture line passes through the ischiopubic junction, the acetabular cavity, and the ischial spine.

Weber classification: A classification of ankle fractures.

Whiplash: Injury to the cervical spine whereby the mechanism resembles the motion of the end of a whip being cracked. Hyperflexion and/or hyperextension of the neck can result in a range of injuries from soft tissue strain to vertebral fractures.

Wilson fracture: Fracture of the volar plate of the middle phalanx of a finger.

Chapter 4

COMPUTED TOMOGRAPHY

Hilmir Agustsson, MHSc, DPT, MTC, CFC

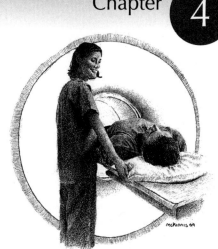

Computed Tomography

Computed tomography (CT) merges x-ray technology with the computer to provide detailed digital cross-sectional images of the body relatively free from superimposition of the different tissues.

History

CT, which revolutionized the ability to visualize soft tissues, was invented in 1972 by Godfrey Hounsfield, a British engineer, of EMI Laboratories. Hounsfield was awarded the Nobel Prize in medicine in 1979 for his invention. His work was based on mathematical formulas developed by Alan Cormack, which were used for reconstruction of the images from digital signals.

The first scanners were dedicated to scanning the head, but larger scanners, accommodating the whole body, were introduced in 1976 and became widely available during the 1980s. In the early years, acquiring the CT image data took hours and reconstruction of the image took days, but advancements in computer technology have decreased image acquisition time to where it is possible to collect the information needed for imaging the entire chest in seconds. The amount of information collected, and with it detail and clarity, has also increased dramatically. The first scanners had an image matrix of only 80 by 80 (6,400) data points, whereas modern scanners may have a matrix of 1,024 by 1,024 pixels, or 1,048,576 data points.

Principles of CT

CT is based on some of the same imaging principles as conventional radiography. CT employs x-rays that are attenuated by body tissues. The radiodensities of the body tissues are represented in the image as shades of gray. The main difference between the two modalities is that CT creates images based on cross-sectional (axial) slices, created by up to 1,000 projections from different angles.

Elements of a CT Scanner

The following description refers to spiral/helical scanners, which are now most commonly used (Fig. 4-1). A CT scanner has three components:

- The gantry, into which the patient slides during the examination
- The operator's console
- The computer(s)

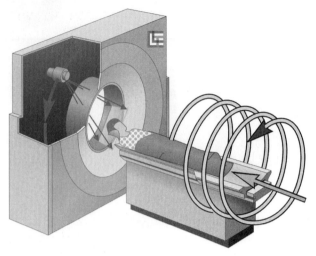

Figure 4-1 Spiral scanning. The patient's table moves continually during the examination while the x-ray tubes moves in continuous circles around the patient, projecting to stationary detectors.

The Gantry

The gantry contains the x-ray tube, its high-voltage generator, a collimator assembly, a detector array, and a data acquisition system.

The X-Ray Source

CT employs a high-intensity x-ray tube in order to provide uniform penetration of the tissues and reduce attenuation by bone relative to soft tissue.

The Collimators

The fan-shaped x-ray beam must be tightly collimated. The collimators are apertures through which the x-rays pass on the way to the patient and serve the following functions:

● Control radiation scatter
● Create a narrow, fan-shaped beam of x-rays, determining the field of view
● Determine the slice thickness

The Detectors

X-rays are attenuated by body tissues and then exit the patient's body as remnant radiation, similarly to conventional radiography. Up to 1,000 detectors are arranged in an array, encircling the patient, for the purpose of measuring this remnant radiation. Modern units commonly have 4 to 16 rows of detectors.

The Data Acquisition System

The data acquisition system amplifies the signal from the detectors. The incoming signal is in the form of a varying electrical current, known as an analog signal. The data acquisition system converts it from analog to digital form and then sends it to the computer.

The Operator Console and CT Computer

The operator console is the desk from which the CT technologist controls the scanning process and selects slice thickness, reconstruction algorithms, and other specifications.

Making the CT Image

Scanning Process

Prior to CT scanning, a *scout image*, which is a two-dimensional digital radiograph, is produced by the CT scanner. This is done for the purpose of localizing the structures to be scanned. Following this, the scanning starts.

In earlier generations of CT scanners, the x-ray tube moved circumferentially around the patient to complete a set number of projections. Once the circle is completed, the table, with the patient, is advanced for a new slice, with a resultant delay between scans. The movement of the tabletop is referred to in terms of *pitch*. Pitch represents the ratio of tabletop movement, during one 360-degree x-ray tube rotation, to slice thickness. In single-detector-row spiral CT, a pitch of 1 means that the tabletop moves a distance equal to the slice thickness for each rotation; a pitch of 2 means that the tabletop moves twice the distance of the slice thickness, with the result of poorer coverage of the scanned area; a pitch of 1/2 means that the "slices" are partly overlapping.

Modern spiral scanners do not have that stop-and-go action but move continuously during the examination process. Thus, the resulting slice is not axial but helical, with data collected by multiple detector rows simultaneously. These multiple-detector-row scanners, or *multislice CT (MSCT)* scanners, represent a major advance in the ability to acquire large volumes of data with high accuracy and short imaging times. In this *volumetric scanning*, images are no longer limited to the axial plane but can be constructed in any plane, or even three-dimensionally, without loss of spatial resolution (Fig. 4-2).

Converting the Data

While scanning for each slice, the fan-shaped beam of x-rays produces projections from multiple angles. These projections provide enough data to calculate the radiodensities for each cubic millimeter or less within the slice. These radiodensities are converted by computer from digital signals into a matrix. Each cell of the matrix is a *pixel* (picture element). Each pixel is assigned a shade of gray, which represents the radiodensity of that cell of the matrix, expressed in terms of *Hounsfield* units.

A matrix is transformed into an image by a mathematical process called back projection. After the image is created, it can be manipulated in the computer's software for the purpose of improving contrasts or modifying the window. This phase of image reconstruction is referred to as postprocessing.

Different Forms of CT

Some of the "variants" of CT scanning include three-dimensional CT, CT myelography, and cone beam CT.

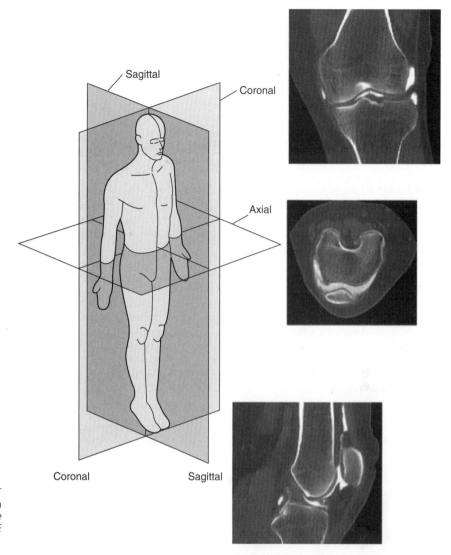

Figure 4-2 Orthogonal planes employed in CT and MRI. The imaging examples are from a CT arthrography study of the knee. *(Source of image: http://www.medcyclo.com by GE Healthcare.)*

Three-Dimensional CT

One of the advantages to volumetric scanning is the ability to create three-dimensional (3D) presentations of body parts that can be rotated in "in space" on the computer screen; a process called multiplanar reconstruction (MPR).

Viewing images in 3D makes it possible to convey complex anatomic information in a manner not previously possible (Fig. 4-3). It is safe to say that the full impact of this technology has not been realized. It presents the radiologist, and other clinicians used to two-dimensional imaging studies, with many challenges. These images are not adequately viewed in the printed format (hard copy); they reveal their potential only when viewed in the digital format (soft copy), using software that allows free 3D rotation of the examined body part.

CT Myelogram

With the advent of CT and later magnetic resonance imaging (MRI), it seemed that myelography might be replaced; partly because of its invasive nature, requiring the injection of contrast material into the subarachnoid space. Today the

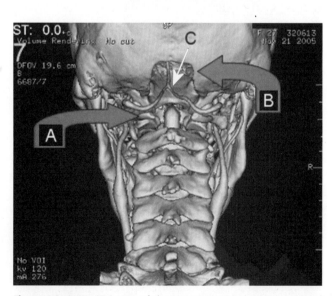

Figure 4-3 A 3D CT image of the posterior cervical spine; a coronal view, taken following surgery for Chiari malformation, aimed at relieving pressure off the vertebral artery. The posterior arch of the arch of atlas has been removed **(A)**, and so has a part of the occipital bone **(B)**. The vertebral arteries are visible, merging to form the basilar artery **(C)**.

pendulum seems to have partly swung back, but now myelography is most commonly performed with CT; not conventional radiographs. Using CT, the radiodense column created by contrast material in the spinal fluid can be visualized in every plane while simultaneously gathering accurate information about what structures impinge on the thecal sac and nerve roots (Fig. 4-4). CT myelography is better able to distinguish between osteophytes, ligament infolding, and annular material than is MRI. Where there is history of symptomatic lumbar stenosis, CT myelography is considered the definitive preoperative investigation.[1]

Other possibilities remain largely unexplored. Owing to its superior speed of image acquisition, CT lends itself to semidynamic studies of spinal cord impingement in every plane.[2] This approach can accurately identify the structures responsible for impingement as well as the conditions under which impingement occurs.

Cone Beam Computed Tomography (CBCT)

Whereas conventional scanners use a collimated beam paired with detectors while the patient is continuously moved through a gantry, CBCT acquires all the data in a single sweep of the scanner employing a large, cone-shaped x-ray beam matched with a flat-panel detector for volume acquisition of data (Fig. 4-5).

Thus, images in a CBCT scanner are not constructed from a large number of slices but rather based on one volume of data. This allows shorter scanning times and lower radiation exposure. Furthermore, the spatial resolution is greater than with conventional scanners.[3] CBCT scanners have been used in areas suited for this type of scanning, such as dentistry—including imaging of the temporomandibular joint—and imaging of the breast.[4]

Viewing CT Images

After the image has been acquired, it can be printed as a "hard copy" on film or paper. Increasingly, however, "soft copy" images are viewed online via *picture archiving and communication systems (PACS)*.

Radiodensities

Like conventional radiographs, CT images reflect the radiodensities of the tissues interposed between the x-ray tube and the detectors. The resultant shades of gray, which represent various tissue radiodensities, are similar to those of conventional radiographs. However, in the CT image, unlike the conventional radiograph, the shades of gray accurately reflect the radiodensity of the tissue, relatively free from the

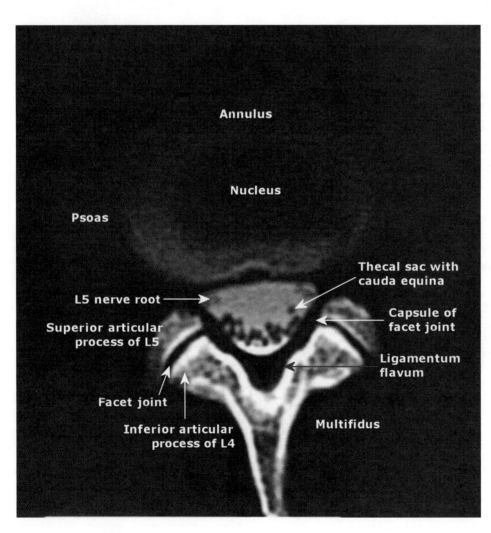

Figure 4-4 CT myelogram at the level of the L4–L5 intervertebral disk and facet joint. The L4 nerve exits above the level displayed in the image.

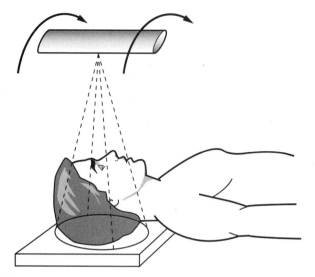

Figure 4-5 Drawing of a cone beam scanner as used in dentistry.

superimposed radiodensities of other tissues (Fig. 4-6). Generally speaking, dense structures appear white or have a light shade of gray, whereas less dense structures appear dark, just as they would on conventional radiographs. This fact differentiates the CT image from the MR image, in which dense structures typically appear black or dark gray.

The Image

In the CT image, radiodensities of the tissues are relatively but not completely free from superimposition. The residual superimposition is due to the fact that CT slices are not infinitely thin. A pixel in the image does not represent just a surface area (as it would in a photograph) but rather a slice

anywhere from 0.1 to 10 mm thick. The product of the pixel and slice thickness is referred to as a *voxel*. A single voxel may contain different tissues.

Volume Averaging

If the voxel contains different tissues, its radiodensity represents the average value for the radiodensities of the tissues contained in that voxel. In an area where, for example, a tendon attaches to bone, a voxel may contain both osseous and tendinous tissue. The radiodensity of this voxel will therefore represent the sum of the densities of tendon and bone (Fig. 4-7). This phenomenon, called volume averaging, can result in loss of contrast resolution. This can be partly solved with thinner slices; thin slices are less affected by volume averaging and therefore have better contrast. They, however, contain less information, which can result in loss of image quality (see below, under "Slice Thickness").

Viewing the Patient's Images

An axial image, representing a transverse slice (e.g., a CT image of the lumbar spine), is displayed as if the patient were in the supine position and the viewer looking in a caudocephalad direction, looking upward at the anatomic structures from below. Sagittal images are viewed from the left toward the right.

Viewing the CT images requires good knowledge of cross-sectional anatomy; there often is not much in the image to orient the viewer, although viewing adjacent slices helps.

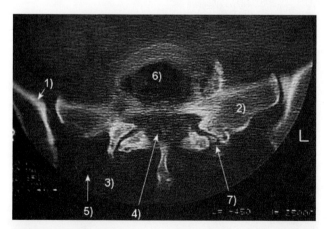

Figure 4-6 Radiodensities in a CT image. This axial CT image of the L5–S1 joint demonstrates the various radiodensities. Cortical bone (1) appears white, but the cancellous bone of the sacral ala (2) gray. The paraspinal muscles (3) have a slightly darker shade than the cerebrospinal fluid (4), and the intervening fat planes (5) are still darker. Note the radiolucent gas in the disk (6). This byproduct of degenerative changes in the disk is called the "vacuum sign." These signs frequently show up on lateral radiographs of the lumbar spine as horizontal streaks of radiolucency, but on a CT image this gas appears black, as it can be seen without superimposition of other structures. Another point of interest in this image: There is an ossicle in the left facet joint (7). *(Image courtesy of A. Graham-Smith, MD.)*

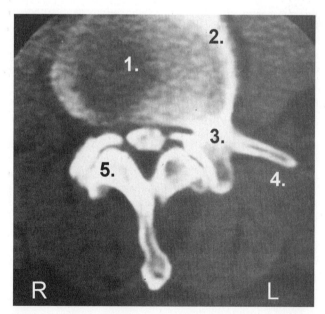

Figure 4-7 Volume averaging in an axial CT myelogram at the L4–L5 intervertebral joint. Note that since the patient is "viewed from below," the patient's right side (R) is to the left in the image. The slice is made through the L4–L5 disk (1) and a part of the endplate of L5 (2). The patient was in an oblique position, or laterally flexed to the left, during the examination, with the result that the vertebral endplate, pedicle (3), and transverse process (4) of the L5 vertebra are visible on the patient's left but not on the right. Therefore the left part of the intervertebral space shows volume averaging of the radiodense endplate and the superior aspect of the disk. Note the radiodense articular processes of the right facet joint (5). *(Image courtesy of A. Graham-Smith, MD.)*

Keep in mind that although image examples in any publication are presented as single images, the person reading CTs or MRIs scrolls through numerous contiguous images. These slices are identified in terms of slice numbers that correspond to the scout image. Sometimes the scout image appears as a small locator image inserted into the image for each slice.

Selective Imaging—Windowing

By selecting the radiodensities displayed in the image (windowing) the operator can determine what tissues are emphasized. *Windowing* refers the range of radiodensities displayed in an image. Consider that humans can distinguish only 32 shades of gray, whereas the computer can distinguish hundreds of shades of gray and can select which of these shades to display. Because of the limited capacity of human vision, many structures with different radiodensities appear as one shade of gray, making it impossible to distinguish between them.

The cervical spine can be taken as an example. A CT image includes numerous radiodensities, from the radiolucent air in the trachea to the radiodense cortical bone of a spinous process. If an image window is set to display the entire range of radiodensities, each of the 32 shades of gray visible to the human eye represents a wide range of radiodensities in one shade of gray. With this window setting, it may not be possible to distinguish between fat and muscle, because their radiodensities are too similar. Displaying a narrower range of radiodensities is useful for distinguishing between various soft tissues, such as fat and muscle.

CT has the ability to choose the range of radiodensities displayed and thereby make it possible to distinguish between tissues of similar densities, such as gray matter and white matter in the brain. To achieve this goal, a narrow window setting is chosen, with a central value representing the average attenuation of brain tissue. This value is called the "level" of the window.

Bone Window Versus Soft Tissue Window

It is common practice to refer to window levels in general as bone windows or soft tissue windows (or bone or soft tissue algorithms), depending on which tissues are emphasized (Fig. 4-8). This is a simple way of indicating the range of densities displayed. For instance, a CT image made for the purpose of viewing musculature, soft tissues, or viscera will be displayed using a soft tissue window (Figs. 4-8 and 4-9). The window is chosen following the image acquisition, unlike the corresponding process in MRI, of selecting "sequences," which are chosen prior to the imaging process itself.

Quality of the Image

In CT, image quality is primarily described in terms of contrast resolution and spatial resolution. But whereas radiolucency and contrast in conventional radiographs is partly decided by prior to imaging milliampere (mA) and megavolt (MV) settings, CT scanning employs preset mA and MV settings, and contrast and density are determined during postprocessing.

Contrast resolution is the ability to distinguish between tissues that have similar radiodensities. It is possible to have too much contrast; an image with high contrast resolution is similar to a grainy photograph; it is easy to see contrasts in it, but visible detail may be limited. *Spatial resolution* refers to the visible details in the image. Good spatial resolution allows for distinction between small objects with high contrast. The following factors improve spatial resolution:

- Large matrix size
- Small field of view
- Thin slices

A large matrix size means that more pixels are available to display the sampled tissue; a small field of view means that a smaller tissue sample is being shown by the available pixels. Image quality is inversely proportional to pitch, because the amount of information, on which the quality of the image depends, is related to slice overlap, which decreases with increasing pitch values.

Factors Degrading Image Quality

Known examples of image degradation are referred to as imaging artifacts.[5] These include hardening, streak artifacts, and motions artifacts:

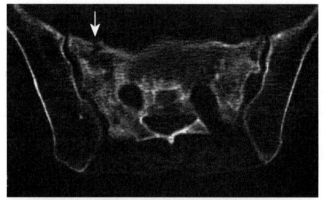
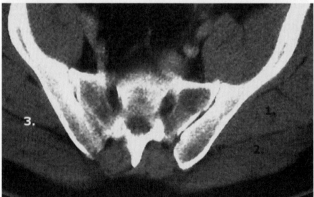

Figure 4-8 Sacrum and ilia; bone window (top) and soft tissue window (bottom). The bone window setting clearly demonstrates the sacral insufficiency fracture (arrow) and distinguishes the architecture of cancellous and cortical bone. The soft tissue setting allows us to distinguish between the gluteus medius (1) and maximus (3) and also to visualize the fat plane between the two (3). However, since the radiodensities of both cortical and cancellous bone are for the most part greater than the greatest densities imaged with this window, the bones appear very bright, with the associated difficulties in distinguishing their architecture. (*Source of image: http://www.medcyclo.com by GE Healthcare.*)

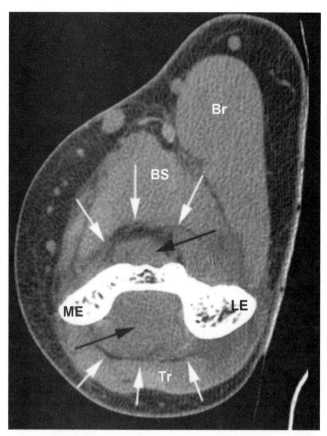

Figure 4-9 Axial CT scan of the left elbow; soft tissue window. A young woman who fell on the outstretched hand sustained a radial head fracture (not seen in image). The joint capsule is distended with effusion (black arrows) and the anterior and posterior fat pads are lifted out of their normal positions in the olecranon fossa and coronoid fossa. This axial slice is made just proximal to the slightly flexed elbow and shows the medial epicondyle (ME), lateral epicondyle (LE), brachialis (BS), brachioradialis (Br), and triceps (Tr). *(Image courtesy of John C. Hunter, MD, University of California, Davis School of Medicine.)*

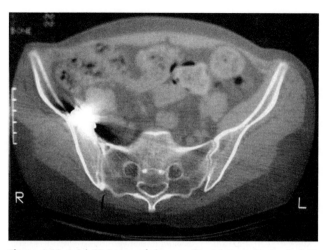

Figure 4-10 Axial CT image of the sacroiliac joints at the level of S2 showing artifacts related to the presence of metal; in this case surgical fixation hardware in the right sacroiliac joint. *(Image courtesy of A. Graham-Smith, MD.)*

in the image. Thin slices present other problems. They require greater radiation to produce the same image quality, increase the duration of the examination, and also increase the number of slices required per area, thus further increasing the total radiation dose. Thus the slice thickness chosen is a compromise between the need for good spatial resolution, and the need for moderate radiation and short examination time. Slice thickness for musculoskeletal CT can vary from 0.5 to 2 mm (for small joints) to 2 to 3 mm (for the pelvis).

Clinical Uses of CT

CT represented tremendous progress from conventional radiography. Furthermore, it has numerous advantages over other advanced imaging methods.

What Does CT Image Best?

For evaluating bone, CT is usually the imaging modality of choice. At present:

1. CT is best for identifying subtle fractures and/or complex fractures (Fig. 4-11).
2. CT is best for evaluating degenerative changes, such as spinal arthritic changes.
3. CT may be the first imaging choice in serious trauma, since multiple injuries to both osseous and soft tissue structures can be determined from one imaging series.
4. CT excels in the evaluation of spinal stenosis (Fig. 4-12), especially if performed as CT myelography.
5. Combined with a diskogram, it may give invaluable information on the condition of the intervertebral disk (Fig. 4-13).
6. CT is the best modality for the evaluation of loose bodies in a joint.
7. CT is less time-consuming than MRI or ultrasound.

● *Hardening:* As the photons in the x-ray beam pass through structures such as the skull, the beam becomes "harder," since lower-energy photons are absorbed more readily. This can lead to dark bands in the image between areas of great radiodensity.
● *Artifacts associated with metals:* Metals can lead to streaking artifacts, which may present as bright lines in the image, extending radially from the interfering metal (Fig. 4-10).
● *Motion artifacts:* Patient movements can lead to shading or streaking in the image. The risk of motion artifacts is reduced with faster scanning times.

Slice Thickness

Slice thickness is chosen to achieve a desired level of accuracy. During scanning of the lungs, a slice thickness of 8 mm may be used, whereas for the wrist, a slice thickness of 0.5 to 2 mm may be used. Thinner slices are typically used in areas of rapidly changing anatomy. There is, however, a limit to how far spatial resolution can be improved by using thinner slices. With thinner slices, the imaged volume is smaller, which results in less radiodensity and increases the "noise"

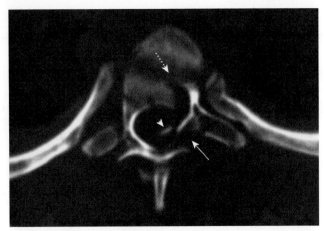

Figure 4-11 Complex fracture of a thoracic vertebra. There is a fracture through the left lamina (arrow) resulting in impaction of the pedicle into the vertebral body (dotted arrow). Note the free fragment in the spinal canal (arrowhead). *(Source of image: http://www.medcyclo.com by GE Healthcare.)*

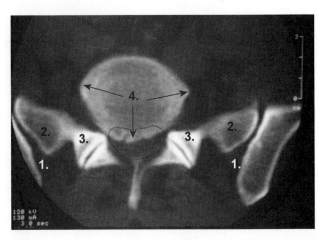

Figure 4-12 Narrowing of the spinal canal and intervertebral foramina at the L5–S1 joint of a patient complaining of right leg pain: (1) Sacroiliac joints, (2) Sacral ala. (3) Hypertrophied superior articular processes of S1, causing narrowing of the intervertebral foramina. (4) Vertebral body of S1, with large osteophytes on the lateral and posterior margins (arrows). The dotted line shows the normal outlines of the spinal canal. *(Image courtesy of Cliff Spohr, MD.)*

8. CT allows for accurate measurements of osseous alignment in any plane.
9. CT is usually less expensive than MRI.
10. CT is less problematic for patients with claustrophobia.

Many uses of 3D imaging have been discussed in the literature.[6] An example of the clinical usefulness of this method from the perspective of the physical therapist is the evaluation of malunion after fracture healing. The rehabilitation of patients with malunion can be complicated and associated with considerable movement abnormalities. The therapist benefits tremendously from having the ability to view the postfracture shape and position of related joints. Therapists can, furthermore, use 3D reconstructions that

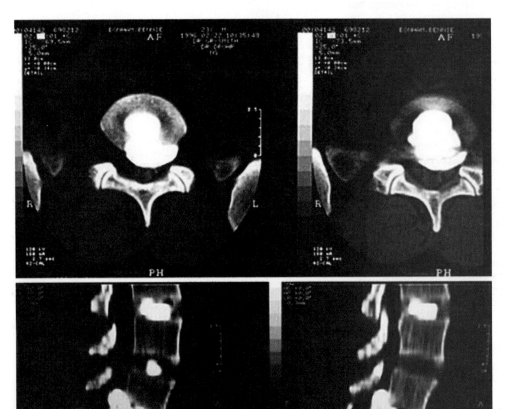

Figure 4-13 Axial CT diskogram showing a large disk herniation at L5–S1 extending into the left L5 foramen. Paracentral sagittal reformatting shows the extruded material creeping up behind the L5 vertebra as well spondylolisthesis at this level. *(Image courtesy of A. Graham-Smith, MD.)*

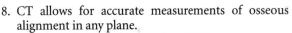

display both bones and tendons, to improve their understanding of alignment and joint configurations, including possible interferences with tendon movements over osseous surfaces (Fig. 4-14).[7]

What Are the Limitations of CT?

CT has limited capabilities for determining the histological makeup of the imaged tissues because it identifies tissues primarily on the basis of radiodensity. Different tissues may be assigned the same shade of gray if their radiodensities are similar. For example, a tumor that has the same radiodensity as the muscle surrounding it may be missed because the computer assigns the same shade of gray to the tumor as to the muscle. The relatively high radiation exposure associated with CT is also a limitation.

Summary and Future Developments

It is claimed that the performance of CT scanners has doubled every 2 years over the last 25 years, largely owing to the developments in computer power.[8] Thus further developments are certain and may include improved capabilities for the evaluation of soft tissue structures as well as continued increases in the speed of image acquisition.

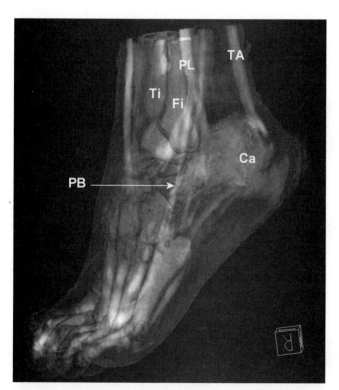

Figure 4-14 A 3D reformatted CT image of the lateral left ankle. The tibia (Ti), fibula (Fi), calcaneus (Ca), Achilles' tendon (TA), and tendons of peroneus longus (PL) and peroneus brevis (PB) are clearly visible. Images such as these well demonstrate interference with movements of tendons over areas of healed fractures or degenerative changes. *(Source of image: http://www.medical.siemens.com.)*

At present, CT is the modality of choice for detailed imaging of cortical and trabecular bone. In addition, the capability of CT to scan large volumes of tissue in very short periods of time has made CT the modality of choice for cardiac and pulmonary imaging.

Neuroimaging

Neuroimaging, or imaging of the brain, can be described in terms of *structural* imaging and *functional* imaging. Structural imaging, demonstrating the macroanatomy of the brain, is used in the diagnosis of injury and disease. Functional imaging, which displays the activity of the brain based on metabolic activity, is employed in research of the function of the brain and to diagnose diseases and lesions that are too small to be detected in terms of structural changes.[9]

History

In the beginning of the 20th century, the brain was imaged indirectly by radiography combined with invasive procedures, including *ventriculography,* the injection of air into the ventricular system of the brain, and later by *cerebral angiography,* which could demonstrate the blood the vessels in and around the brain. In the 1970s, CT scanning revolutionized neuroimaging. The value of CT for neuroimaging was further augmented in the 1980s when it was combined with nuclear medicine to create single photon emission computed tomography (SPECT) and positron emission tomography (PET), employing radioactively labeled chemicals for functional imaging of the brain. When MRI arrived on the scene, it offered even greater anatomic detail, although with longer imaging times.

CT Versus MRI

At present, because of its short scanning times, CT is considered the modality of choice for neuroimaging in acute settings. The "head CT" is a standard protocol in trauma for the immediate assessment of intracranial bleeding.

However, MRI plays a significant role in neuroimaging. MRI can detect changes in fluid content, ischemia, edema, and hemorrhage more accurately than CT can. Furthermore, *functional MRI (fMRI)* can display changes in blood flow based on the paramagnetic properties of hemoglobin or through the use of contrasts. fMRI has become the key method in mapping neuronal activity in the brain.

Apart from its uses in research, fMRI is increasingly used for diagnostic purposes. Owing to its sensitivity to changes in blood flow, it can demonstrate ischemia associated with stroke immediately following its occurrence, when differential diagnosis between ischemic stroke and cerebral hemorrhage is crucial. Furthermore, once it has been decided that the patient is suffering from stroke, fMRI can assist in staging the disease, which is crucial in deciding pharmaceutical treatment.

CT and MRI Characteristics of the Brain

The CT and MRI characteristics of the brain are similar to their musculoskeletal imaging characteristic (see Chapter 5, Fig. 5-15).

In the CT image, the gray matter of the brain is more radiodense, and thus brighter, than the white matter. The cerebrospinal fluid (CSF) is more radiolucent (darker) than both the white and the gray matter (Fig. 4-15). The bones of the cranium appear bright and the subcutaneous fat dark.

On T1 MRI, the gray matter gives rise to lower signal intensity (darker) than the white matter and the subcutaneous fat is bright. On T2 images, signals from fat and water are different from those in T1 images; the gray matter gives rise to higher signal intensity (brighter) than white matter and the CSF gives the highest signal and is bright white. The bones of the cranium are dark on all MRI sequences.

CT Exam: Six Brain Images

The brain may be scanned in all three orthogonal planes. Axial slices, made in the oblique axial plane, anteriorly and superiorly directed, are most often employed for diagnostic purposes. Coronal slices, however, offer the best view of the ventricular system, and sagittal slices best show the spinal cord, medulla, pons, and midbrain.

A typical axial CT examination with 2-mm slice thickness may involve 50 to 100 images. For the scope of this book, only six axial images that can be considered representative are shown. As a memory aid, these slices are referred to as "The Cross," "The Star," "Mr. Happy," "Mr. Sad," "The Worms," and "The Coffee Bean."[10] Figures 4-15 to 4-20 provide this basic overview of the CT and MRI anatomy of the brain.

Common Cerebral Pathologies

The most common cerebral pathologies involve either ischemia or hemorrhage.

1. Ischemic stroke
   - Caused by emboli, vasospasm, loss of cardiac output, or atherosclerosis.
   - Lesions may be small and round.
   - Lesions are frequently located in the brainstem, basal ganglia, or thalamus.
   - In thrombosis in a large vessel, the vessel itself may be more radiodense and thus brighter on CT than the surrounding brain tissue (Fig. 4-21).
   - The cerebral lesions are dark, because of the ensuing edema.
   - On T2 MRI, the edema associated with the death of brain tissue gives rise to a brighter signal (Fig. 4-22).
2. Cerebral hemorrhage/hematoma
   - Caused by the rupture of a blood vessel.
   - On CT in the acute stage, the parenchyma is bright and, if there is blood in the CSF, its radiodensity is also increased (Fig. 4-23).
   - In the subacute phase, the hemorrhagic area becomes less radiodense on CT than the surrounding brain matter.
   - MRI
     ○ Acute hemorrhage shows high signal intensity on T1 and low intensity on T2 images, but may show high signal intensity on T2 in cases of pronounced edema (Fig. 4-24).
     ○ Chronic hemorrhage has high signal intensity on T2 but low on T1.

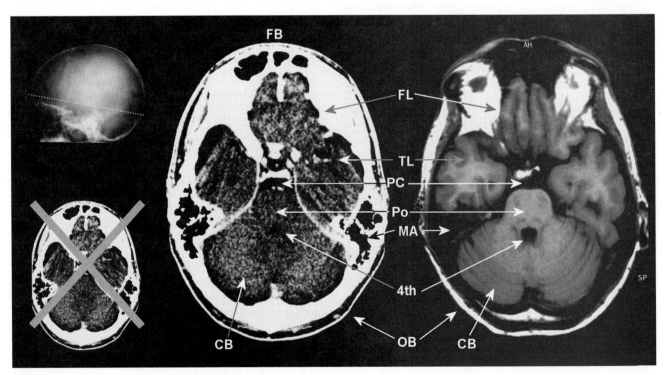

Figure 4-15 CT and T1 MR images, first slice; "the cross." Note the frontal bone (FB), frontal lobe (FL), temporal lobe (TL), pontine cistern (PC), pons (Po), mastoid air cells (MA), fourth ventricle (4th), occipital bone (OB), and cerebellum (CB). (*Source of images: http://www.medcyclo.com by GE Healthcare.*)

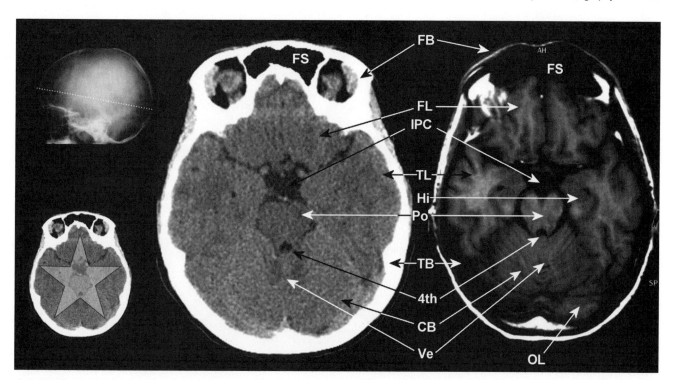

Figure 4-16 CT and T1 MR images, second slice; "the star." Note that this is where the circle of Willis is located. Observe the frontal bone (FB), frontal sinus (FS), frontal lobe (FL), interpeduncular cistern (IPC), temporal lobe (TL), hippocampus (Hi), pons (Po), temporal bone (TB), fourth ventricle (4th), cerebellum (CB), and vermis (Ve). *(Source of images: http://www.medcyclo.com by GE Healthcare.)*

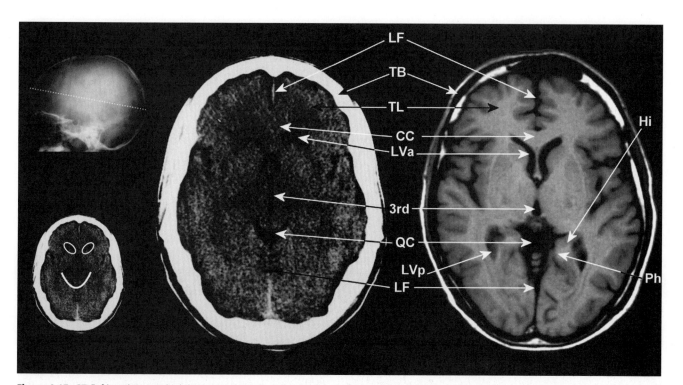

Figure 4-17 CT (left) and T1 MR (right) images, third slice; "Mr. Happy." Observe the longitudinal fissure (LF), anterior horn of the lateral ventricle (LVa), third ventricle (3rd), quadrigeminal cistern (QC), temporal lobe (TL), corpus callosun (CC), hippocampus (Hi), parahippocampal gyrus (Ph), temporal bone (TB), and posterior horn of the lateral ventricle (LVp). *(Source of images: http://www.medcyclo.com by GE Healthcare.)*

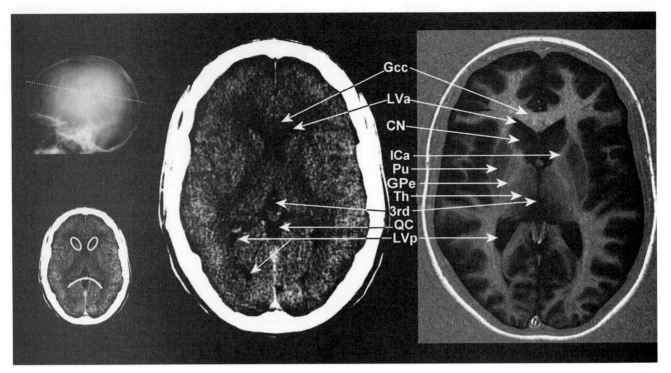

Figure 4-18 CT and inversion recovery MR images, fourth slice; "Mr. Sad." Observe the genu of the corpus callosun (Gcc), anterior horn of the lateral ventricle (LVa), caudate nucleus (CN), anterior internal capsule (ICa), putamen (Pu), globus pallidus externus (GPe), thalamus (Th), third ventricle (3rd), quadrigeminal cistern (QC), and posterior horn of the lateral ventricle (LVp). *(Source of images: http://www.medcyclo.com by GE Healthcare.)*

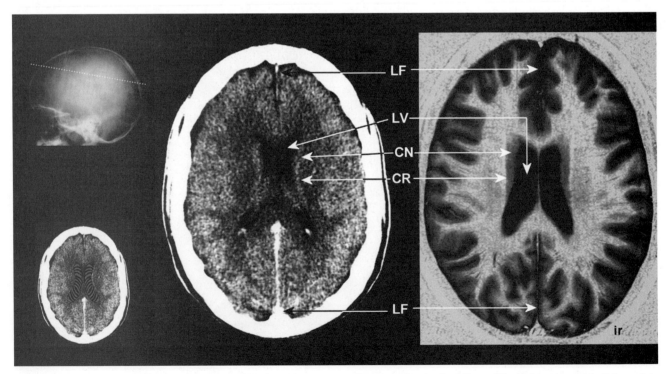

Figure 4-19 CT and inversion recovery MR images, fifth slice; "the worms." Observe the longitudinal fissure (LF), the lateral ventricle (LV), caudate nucleus (CN), and corona radiata (CR). *(Source of images: http://www.medcyclo.com by GE Healthcare.)*

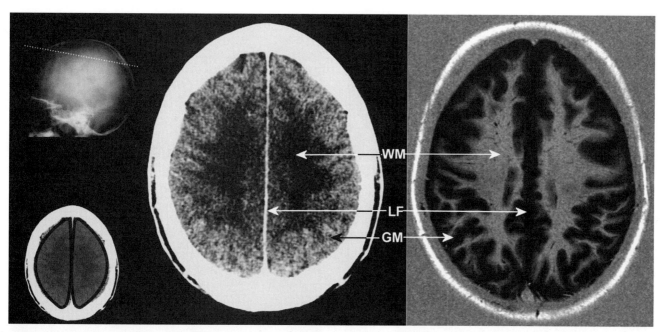

Figure 4-20 CT and inversion recovery MR images, sixth slice; "the coffee bean." Observe the white matter (WM), longitudinal fissure (LF), and gray matter (GM). *(Source of images: http://www.medcyclo.com by GE Healthcare.)*

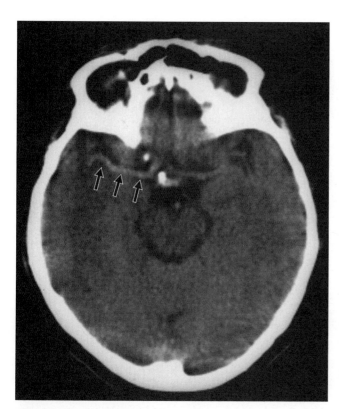

Figure 4-21 Acute stroke (2 hours postinfarct). CT without contrast demonstrates a thrombosis in the right middle cerebral artery (arrows). *(Source of image: http://www.medcyclo.com by GE Healthcare.)*

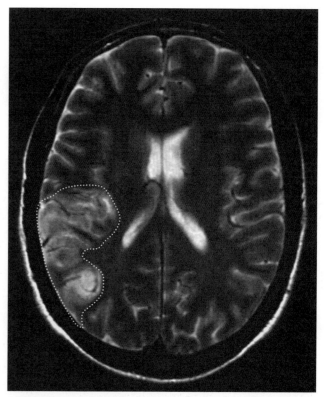

Figure 4-22 The same patient as in Figure 4-21. A T2-weighted MRI 12 hours later shows increased signal intensity (brighter image) in the area of the infarct (dotted area). *(Source of image: http://www .medcyclo.com by GE Healthcare.)*

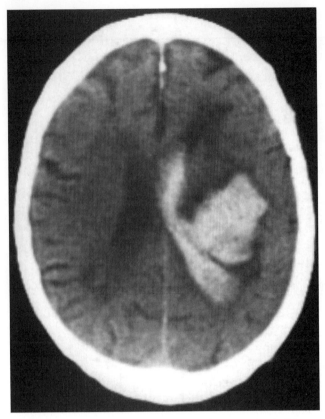

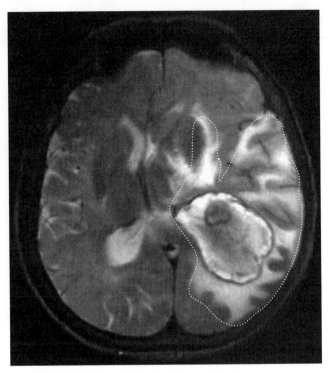

Figure 4-24 The same patient as in Figure 4-23 at 2 weeks postinsult. A T2-weighted MRI shows increased signal intensity in the hematoma and the area surrounding it (dotted area). Note the considerable swelling resulting in a shift of the longitudinal fissure and midline over to the right. *(Source of image: http://www.medcyclo.com by GE Healthcare.)*

Figure 4-23 Cerebral hematoma 5 hours after a stroke. A CT scan shows increased radiodensity of blood in the left basal ganglia as well as intraventricular bleeding. *(Source of image: http://www.medcyclo.com by GE Healthcare.)*

Summary of Key Points

1. The images are axial slices, based on multiple radiographic projections from different angles.

2. Modern CT scanning collects volumetric data and allows display in any plane.

3. Images display the radiodensities of the tissues.

4. Slices can contain different tissues within single pixels, giving rise to volume averaging.

5. Three-dimensional CT and CT myelography are valuable variants of CT.

6. By setting the radiodensities (windowing), it is possible to select what tissues are best displayed.

7. Thinner slices and smaller pixels improve spatial resolution.

8. Thicker slices and larger pixels improve contrast resolution.

9. CT has the advantage of fast scanning, thin slices, and superior osseous detail but the disadvantage of relatively high radiation.

10. Modern neuroimaging consists of CT, MRI, and variants of the two employed to depict metabolic activity.

11. CT is the modality of choice for neuroimaging in acute settings and in case of trauma.

12. Imaging characteristics of the brain for CT and MRI follow patterns familiar from musculoskeletal imaging, based on cell density, fat, and fluid content.

References

1. Saifuddin, A: The imaging of lumbar spinal stenosis. Clin Radiol 55:581, 2005.
2. Yamazaki, T, Suzuki, K, Yanaka, K, and Matsumura, A: Dynamic computed tomography myelography for the investigation of cervical degenerative disease. Neurol Med Chir (Tokyo) 46:210, 2006.
3. Patel, S, Dawood, A, Ford, TP, and Whaites, E: The potential applications of cone beam computed tomography in the management of endodontic problems. Int Endod J 40:818, 2007.
4. Hussain, AM, Packota, G, Major, PW, and Flores-Mir, C: Role of different imaging modalities in assessment of temporomandibular joint erosions and osteophytes: a systematic review. Dentomaxillofac Radiol 37:63, 2008.
5. Barrett, JF, and Keat, N: Artifacts in CT: Recognition and avoidance. Radiographics 24:1679, 2004.
6. Pretorius, ES, Fishman, EK: Volume-rendered three-dimensional spiral CT: Musculoskeletal applications. Radiographics 19:1143, 1999.
7. Choplin, RH, Farber, JM, Buckwalter, KA, and Swan, S: Three-dimensional volume rendering of the tendons of the ankle and foot. Semin Musculoskel Radiol 8:175, 2004.
8. Prokop, M: New challenges in MDCT. Eur Radiol 15:E35, 2005.
9. Muir, KW, Buchan, A, von Kummer, R, et al: Imaging of acute stroke. Lancet Neurol 5:755, 2006.
10. Hugue Ouellette, H, and Tetreault, P: Clinical Radiology Made Ridiculously Simple. Miami, FL: Medmaster, 2000.

SELF-TEST

Image A

These are axial CT images at the L5/S1 level. The images are made 9 mm apart.

1. What are the structures marked 1 to 4?

2. Contrast the "joints" marked 5 and 6.

3. Which image is more caudal (distal)? How can you know?

Image B

These Images are an external rotation, AP radiographs of the left shoulder and axial CT images through midglenoid level.

4. What are the tissues and/or structures numbered 1 through 8?

5. What abnormality do you see in these images? Does it look like a benign or malignant process?

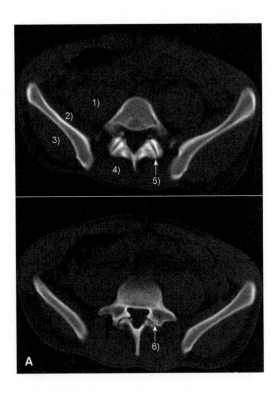

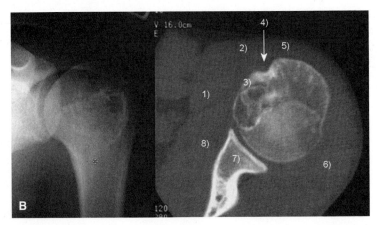

(Images courtesy of John C. Hunter, MD, University of California, Davis School of Medicine.)

Chapter 5

MAGNETIC RESONANCE IMAGING

Hilmir Agustsson, MHSc, DPT, MTC, CFC

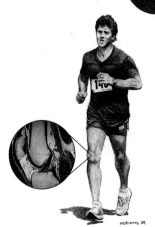

mcKinnis 09

CHAPTER OUTLINE

Magnetic Resonance Imaging

Magnetic resonance image (MRI) is a cross-sectional imaging technology that uses a magnetic field and radiofrequency signals to cause hydrogen nuclei to emit their own signals, which then are converted to images by a computer.

History

MRI presents a radical departure from imaging methods based on the absorption of x-rays (conventional radiography and computed tomography [CT]) or reflection from tissues (ultrasound). The magnetic resonance phenomenon has been known since the 1940s. Initially employed to determine the structures of molecules, it was discovered by Felix Bloch and Edward Purcell, two American scientists, who were awarded the Nobel Prize in physics in 1952 for their discovery. In 2003, Paul C. Lauterbur and Sir Peter Mansfield were awarded the Nobel Prize in medicine for their contribution to the development of MRI for medical purposes.

Principles of MRI

Simply stated, MRI is based on measurements of energy emitted from hydrogen nuclei following their stimulation by radiofrequency signals. The energy emitted varies according to the tissues from which the signals emanate. This allows MRI to distinguish between different tissues.

The Magnetic Resonance Phenomenon

Magnetic resonance is the process by which nuclei, aligned with an external magnetic field, absorb and release energy. Many molecules display magnetic resonance, but for all practical purposes MRI is based on signals from hydrogen nuclei in water molecules. Because these nuclei consist of only a proton, the hydrogen nucleus is referred to simply as the proton in the context of MRI.

Alignment of Protons in an External Magnetic Field

The process of image acquisition begins by placing the patient in the scanner, which contains coils that produce an extremely strong magnetic field. In the magnetic field, protons line up like tiny bar magnets, either in the direction of the magnetic field or in the opposite direction.[1] There is a slight difference between the number of protons lining up parallel with the magnetic field and the number lining up in the opposite direction. This difference gives rise to net magnetization, parallel with the external magnetic field, referred to as *longitudinal magnetization.*

Altering the Alignment of Protons

A pulse of radiofrequency (RF) waves is applied at right angles to the longitudinal magnetization. This pulse alters the alignment of the protons to a transverse plane, and the energy absorbed in the process brings them to a higher energy state; transverse magnetization (Fig. 5-1).

Realignment and Decay

Following the RF pulse, the protons realign with the main magnetic field, frequently aided by a 180-degree RF pulse, applied at point in time midway between the 90-degree pulses. As the protons realign, the energy they absorbed while being displaced out of alignment is released. This induces a current in a receiver coil and gives rise to the data that are the basis of MRI.

The T1 and T2 Phenomena

The T1 and T2 phenomena, which occur simultaneously, are different processes related to the return of the protons to alignment with the main magnetic field. Following the RF pulse, two things happen:

1. The protons gain longitudinal magnetization or realign with the magnetic field.
2. The protons lose their transverse magnetization.

Although these two events may appear to be two sides of the same coin, they are different processes and help MRI differentiate among various tissue types and disease processes.

The return to longitudinal magnetization is called T1 recovery. During T1 recovery, protons lose energy to the surrounding molecules. The time of return differs for different tissues, and the faster this recovery (shorter T1), the stronger the resulting signal from the protons of that tissue.

The relaxation of transverse magnetization toward equilibrium is called T2 decay. The transverse magnetization decays because of the loss of phase coherence, owing to interaction between protons. Note that the slower this decay, the stronger the signal that is recorded near the end of this process (Fig. 5-2).[2]

T1- and T2-Weighted Imaging

In MRI, tissue contrast in images is created on the basis differences in T1, T2, and proton density (number of hydrogen nuclei) in the different tissues by employing different

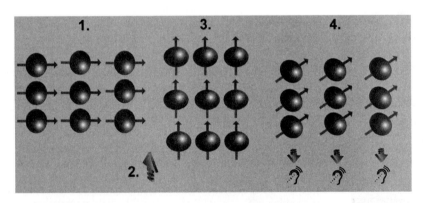

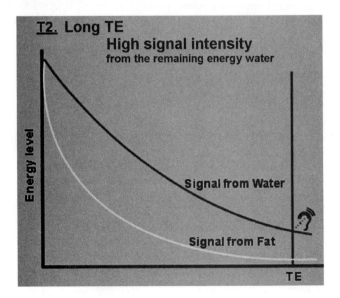

Figure 5-1 Displacement and gradual realignment of protons. In this image, the protons are aligned with the main magnetic field (1) when a RF pulse is applied at right angles (2), resulting in an altered alignment of the protons. After the cessation of the RF pulse, the protons gradually return to alignment with the main magnetic field (3).

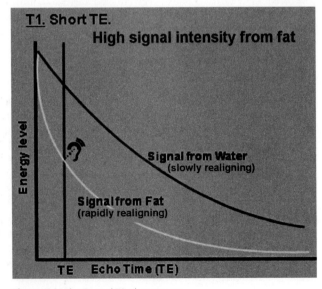

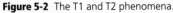

Figure 5-2 The T1 and T2 phenomena.

sequences that target these phenomena. The concept "sequence" refers to imaging protocols characterized by the timing of events during image acquisition. Two parameters are most important for creating contrast in the image—time to repetition (TR) and time to echo (TE):

- TE is the time at which the signal is captured.
- TR is the time at which the RF pulse is repeated to again displace the protons.

The difference between T1 and T2 imaging lies in their different TE and TR values. The values for TE and TR, as well as other relevant imaging parameters (see below, under "Imaging Sequences"), are always stated in the MR image. This allows the reader to determine the sequence employed.

T1-Weighted Imaging

T1 imaging is characterized by short TR and TE times. Thus the signal is caught early, at a time when the difference in relaxation characteristics for fat and water is most noticeable and tissues that rapidly recover their longitudinal magnetization, such as fat, give rise to high signal intensity (create a bright image). When short TE is employed, tissues that are slow to regain longitudinal magnetization, such as tissues with high free-water content, render low signal intensity (see Fig. 5-2). These tissues appear dark on T1 weighted images.

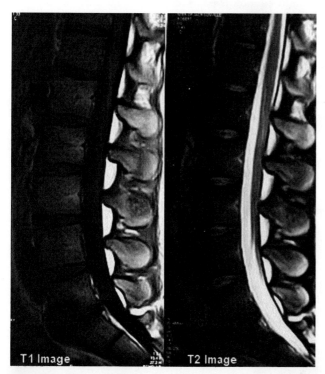

Figure 5-3 Differences between T1 and T2 imaging. *T1 image*: Bone marrow gives rise to relatively high signal intensity. Cerebrospinal fluid (CSF), giving rise to low signal intensity, is black in the image, and the fluid-saturated intervertebral disks are dark. Note the intermediate signal intensity of the spinal cord and cauda equina when contrasted with CSF. *T2 image*: The CSF shows high signal intensity and, with the exception of the degenerated L5–S1 disk, the intervertebral disks give rise to fairly high signal intensity. Note the anterior herniation of the L5–S1 disk. The signal intensities from the adjacent area of bone edema anteriorly in the L5 and S1 vertebrae are different on T1 and T2. The edema shows increased signal intensity on the T2 image relative to the surrounding cancellous bone. *(Image courtesy of A. Graham-Smith, MD.)*

T2-Weighted Imaging

Long TR and TE times characterize T2 imaging. Because in T2-weighted imaging the signal is measured late in the decay process, tissues that are most reluctant to give up energy are selectively imaged. Free water is slow to give up its energy and consequently renders high signal intensity on T2 sequences. Fat, which gives up its energy rapidly, gives rise to low intensity on T2.

The Difference Between T1- and T2-Weighted Imaging

T1 and T2 are complementary but different methods. T1 images are made when much of the energy from the RF pulse remains in the tissues, while the T2 image is made at low energy levels. Therefore T2 images are grainier and display less spatial resolution (Fig. 5-3).

The difference between T1 and T2 can be summarized as follows:

- T1 imaging measures energy from structures such as fat, which give up energy rapidly, early in the process of longitudinal remagnetization. T1 imaging provides images of good anatomic detail, displaying the tissues in a fairly balanced manner.
- T2 imaging measures energy late in the decay of transverse relaxation and selectively images structures that do not readily give up energy, such as water. It is particularly valuable for detecting inflammation.

Image Information and Protocols

Image Information

Like a radiograph, each MR image slice displays, in the corners of the image, two categories of information: personal and technical. The patient information includes name, date of birth, case number, date of examination, facility, and body part being examined. The technical information indicates the sequence used (often only by stating values for TR and TE), the size of the field of view, and slice thickness in millimeters. Other letter combinations refer to the number of the slice within the series of slices being displayed. This information differs for each MRI scanner manufacturer, and the technical data displayed on an image may not be consistent between facilities.

Protocols

The term *protocol* refers to a combination of sequences performed during a MRI procedure for the body part being examined. There are no "standard" protocols for MRI examination; the combination of sequences used depends on the body part and the suspected pathology. In view of the time-consuming nature of MRI, it is neither practical nor necessary to employ a high number of sequences for each orthogonal plane. When avascular necrosis is suspected, a protocol for imaging the hip may look like this:

1. Coronal T1, non–fat-saturated
2. Coronal short tau inversion recovery imaging (STIR)
3. Axial T1, non–fat-saturated
4. Axial T2 fast spin echo
5. Sagittal T2, fat-saturated

There are two main categories of MRI sequences; the spin-echo (SE), such as T1 and T2 imaging, and the gradient-echo (GRE) sequences. A multitude of variations of each of these sequences have been devised (Fig. 5-4).

Sequences

SE Sequences

The imaging methods described above constitute the most commonly used imaging sequences; the so-called SE sequences. They are characterized by a 90-degree pulse flip, followed by T1 relaxation and T2 decay, aided by a 180-degree rephasing pulse. Numerous variants have been created by the manufacturers of MRI equipment, but in today's radiographic literature, SE imaging sequences are increasingly referred to simply as T1- or T2-weighted, with the specific parameters stated. Still, some commonly named variants must be discussed.

Fast SE

Conventional SE sequences take very long to execute, but the efficiency of the imaging process has been increased using fast, or turbo, SE sequences. In fast SE imaging, the 90-degree pulse is followed by multiple 180-degree pulses. This results in imaging that is twice as fast as conventional SE or, alternatively, allows acquisition of several images in the same slice position without increasing imaging time.

Proton Density (PD)

When a long TR and a short TE are used, the contrast in the MR image is primarily due to the difference in proton density; tissues with high-density of protons give rise to higher signal intensity. Imaging based on these parameters is referred to as proton density imaging. It has the following properties:

1. TR is long (more than 2,000 ms) and TE is short (20 to 30 ms).
2. Images are based on measurements of proton density and are similar in appearance to T1 images, but with greater anatomic detail (see Fig. 5-4).

Inversion Recovery Sequences

Conventional inversion recovery is an SE sequence in which a 180-degree preparatory pulse is used to flip the net magnetization vector to the opposite direction, and cancel out signals from selected entities, such as water. Following this the 90-degree RF pulse is applied, and the SE sequence continues. The interval between the 180-degree pulse and 90-degree pulse is referred to as time to inversion (TI). This inversion time affects the signals from different tissues; changing this parameter allows suppression of signals from fat and water. The inversion recovery sequences can provide a strong contrast between tissues with different T1 relaxation times, but has the disadvantage that imaging times are longer. Short tau inversion recovery imaging (STIR) is the most common example of inversion recovery sequences.

In STIR, the inversion recovery pulse is used to cancel out the signal from fat, to make its signal intensity even smaller than it is in T2 weighted images. Therefore STIR sequences excel in depicting bone marrow edema, which is useful in the detection of pathologies. STIR has the following properties:

1. TR is long but TE is short, although slightly longer than in T1 or proton density sequences.
2. Images are similar to T2 images, with even greater emphasis on fluid-rich structures.
3. Resolution is poor, relative to conventional SE or PD images (see Fig. 5-4).

GRE Sequences

GRE imaging has characteristics that are very different from spin echo imaging. In a GRE sequence, the RF pulse applied only partly flips the net magnetization vector into the transverse plane; anywhere from 0 to 90 degrees (variable flip angle). This sequence allows reformatting to any imaging plane, not limited to the orthogonal planes and thus is frequently used to image complex anatomy.

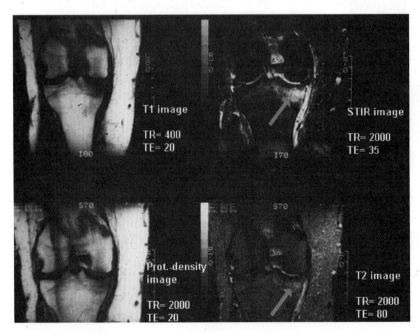

Figure 5-4 Differences between four commonly used sequences displaying a fracture of the medial tibial plateau. Note that the associated marrow edema has the lowest signal intensity in the T1 image, intermediate signal intensity on T2, and high signal intensity on the STIR image. Signal intensity from fat decreases in the same order. Note that the synovial fluid is clearly visible both in the T2 and STIR images. *(Image courtesy of Cliff Spohr, MD.)*

GRE has the following properties:

1. Fast image acquisition
2. High resolution and thin slices
3. High contrast (depending on parameters) between fluid and cartilage

Use of Contrasts

Frequently MRI diagnostics can be improved using intravenous gadolinium-containing contrast agents. Gadolinium is a paramagnetic metal ion, which can be used both for regular MRI applications (Fig. 5-5), magnetic resonance angiography (MRA), and MR arthrography.

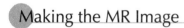

Making the MR Image

The MR imaging unit is specifically designed to measure the processes associated with magnetic resonance in the tissues.

The Elements of an MRI Scanner

The elements of the MRI scanner are the main magnet, the gradient coils, the RF coils, the workstation, and the computer(s) (Fig. 5-6).

The Magnet

The magnet of the conventional MRI scanner resides within a gantry, large enough for the human body and the necessary receiver coils. Open scanners, where the patient is not fully surrounded by the magnet, are also common (discussed below). However, for the purpose of this discussion, conventional scanners are described. Typically the magnet has a field strength of anywhere from 0.3 to 3 tesla. For comparison, 1 tesla equals 20,000 times the strength of the earth's magnetic field.

Gradient Coils

Three gradient coils, one for each of the orthogonal planes, are located within the core of the MRI unit. The gradient coils produce sequential variations in the main magnetic field that are used for providing spatial information.

RF Coils

The RF coils serve two purposes:

1. Transmit the RF pulses that alter the alignment of the protons
2. Receive the signals emitted from the protons

The body coil, which encircles the patient within the gantry, is used for reception when larger areas, such as the

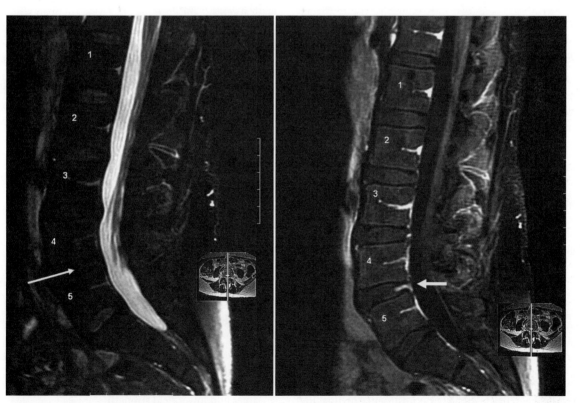

Figure 5-5 Evidence of repair of the annulus in a 50-year-old woman with a history of microdiskectomy at L4–L5. The sagittal T2-weighted image to the left shows a horizontal cleft in the posterior annulus. Note that the signal intensity from the cleft is similar to that of the well-hydrated nuclei above. This could point to nuclear material leaking outward. However, a fat-suppressed T1 image with gadolinium enhancement (right) shows high signal intensity in the cleft, while nuclei remain dark. This points to vascularization associated with repair of the annulus.

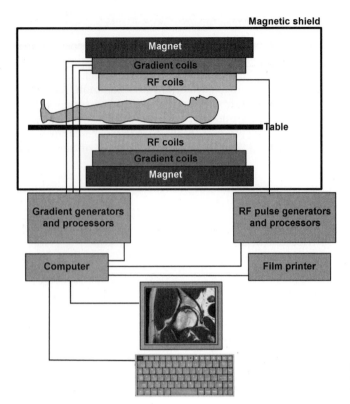

Figure 5-6 Elements of an MRI scanner. The computer controls the function of the gradient coils and the RF coils as well as receiving and processing signal from the RF coils.

pelvis, the lumbar spine, or both hips, are imaged. However, it is too large to allow adequate resolution for smaller joints. Therefore specialized limb coils are employed as receivers when viewing smaller joints.

The Workstation and Computer

At the workstation, the imaging protocols are selected by the MRI technologist or radiologist prior to imaging, according to diagnostic needs. The computer directs the scanning process, converts data from the RF coils, and reconstructs images.

Open Scanners

Open MRI scanners were developed for the examination of the extremity joints and to allow imaging of patients who, owing to claustrophobia or obesity, could not be imaged in conventional scanners (Fig. 5-7). Some variations include semiopen scanners, having a short bore with flared ends, and upright scanners (see below).

The advantages of open scanners include the following:

- Greater ability to scan claustrophobic or obese patients
- Reduction of scanning noise
- Possibilities of performing tests or procedures during scanning

The disadvantages of open scanners include the following:

- Lower field strength, requiring adjustments of imaging sequences
- Lower signal-to-noise ratio
- Longer scanning times

Upright Scanners[3,4]

Upright (positional) MRI scanners are increasingly used in the clinical setting and in research. These are open scanners that allow tilting of the MRI units for the exam to be performed in the upright position, sitting or standing (Fig. 5-8). This allows the spine and other joints to be placed in whatever position is desired, bearing weight or not.

The advantages of upright scanners include the following:

1. The ability to examine the spine under weight-bearing conditions, which may facilitate the ability to detect the following:
   - Protrusions
   - Intradiscal herniations
   - Spinal stenosis
   - Position-dependent instability of the spine
   - Nerve root impingements, since placing the spine in a weight-bearing position narrows the spinal canal and spinal foramina
2. Ability to scan patients who are too large to fit into the bore of the magnet or must be scanned in the upright position because of conditions such as congestive heart failure or severe thoracic kyphosis.[5]

The disadvantages of upright scanners include the following:

- Longer scanning times; up to three times longer than with conventional high-field scanners
- Possible image degradation due to the longer scanning times and lower field strength
- Placement of the patient in a painful position, which may lead to increased patient movement during the examination, thus degrading image quality

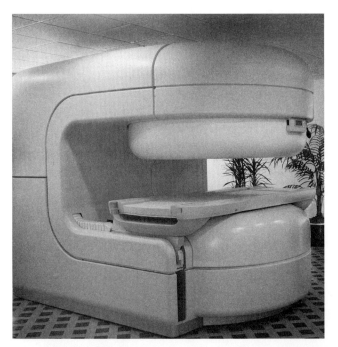

Figure 5-7 Open scanner. Instead of placing the patient inside the bore of the gantry, the patient is placed on a table, which slides under the magnet from the side.

Viewing MR Images

MRI, like CT, produces gray-scale images of the tissues. These images represent slices; the pixels on the monitor display a volume of tissue, as in CT scanning. Coronal images are viewed from the front, as if facing the patient, and axial images are viewed from below. Sagittal images are viewed from left to right for either side of the body.

Imaging Characteristics of Different Tissues

Different tissues display different imaging characteristics on T1 and T2 images; comparison of the two is often used for evaluating disease processes and trauma. Frequently disease processes that give rise to low signal intensity on T1 imaging give rise to high signal intensity on T2 (see Fig. 5-3).

The Language of the MRI Report

Whereas radiographic reports identify anatomy and pathology by variations in radiodensity, descriptions of structures and pathology, as viewed on MRI, relate signal intensities emanating from the tissues. To understand the MRI report, it is imperative to be familiar with signal intensities of normal tissues in T1- and T2-weighted images as well as the signal intensities associated with common pathologies.

Imaging Characteristics of Different Tissues

What follows is a brief discussion of the T1 and T2 imaging characteristics of various tissues. For an overview of signal intensities, view Table 5-1 and compare with Figure 5-9.

- Fat gives rise to high signal intensity on T1-weighted images and low to intermediate signal on T2.
- Free water gives rise to high signal intensity on T2-weighted images and very low signal on T2.
- Tendons, ligaments, and menisci show low signal intensity on all sequences.

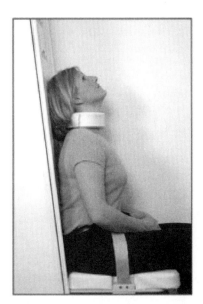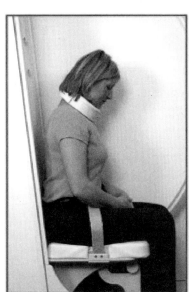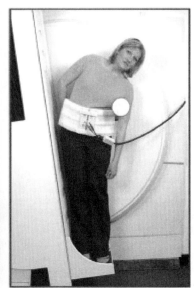

Figure 5-8 Open, upright scanner. The magnets of the upright scanners have an open configuration. Note the receiver coils around the patient's neck during full extension and flexion of the cervical spine, as well as the coil around the patient's waist for imaging lumbar lateral flexion. *(Source of image: Fonar; http://uprightmrinews.com.)*

- Cortical bone displays very low signal intensity on all sequences.
- Red (hematopoietic) marrow displays intermediate signal intensity on T1, whereas yellow marrow has high signal intensity.[6]

- Muscles exhibit intermediate signal intensity on both T1- and T2-weighted images, although the signal intensity is slightly lower on T2.
- Cartilage gives rise to intermediate signal intensity on both T1- and T2-weighted images.

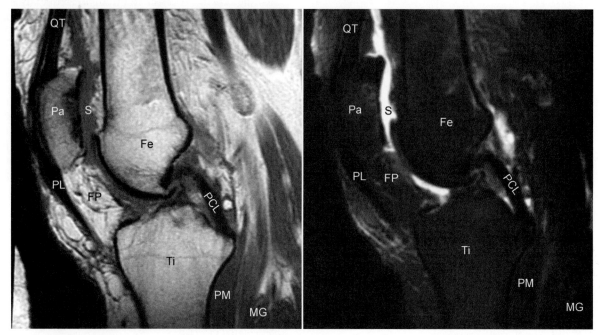

Figure 5-9 T1 (left) and T2 (right) images of a knee of a patient with chondromalacia patellae. Contrast the two and compare T1 and T2 characteristics listed in Table 5-1. These are midsagittal slices of the knee, showing the quadriceps tendon (QT), patella (Pa), synovial fluid (S), femur (Fe), posterior cruciate ligament (PCL), patellar ligament (PL), infrapatellar fat pad of Hoffa (FP), tibia (Ti), popliteus muscle (PM), and medial head of gastrocnemius (MG). *(Image courtesy of John C. Hunter, MD, University of California, Davis School of Medicine.)*

TABLE 5-1 ● *Imaging Characteristics of MRI*

	T1-Weighted Signal Intensity	T2-Weighted Signal Intensity
Normal Tissue		
Cortical bone/calcium	Very low	Very low
Cartilage	Intermediate	Low–intermediate
Red marrow	Intermediate to low	Intermediate
Fat/yellow marrow	High	Intermediate
Ligament and tendons	Low	Low
Muscle	Intermediate	Intermediate
Fluid: CSF, synovial fluid	Low	High
Disease/Disorder		
Inflammation	Low	High
Synovial hypertrophy	Low to intermediate	Intermediate to high
Acute hemorrhage	High	Intermediate to low
Subacute hemorrhage	Intermediate to high	Intermediate to high
Chronic hemorrhage	Variable	High
Soft tissue calcifications	Low	Low
Soft tissue tumors	Low	High
Bone tumors	Variable	Variable
Chondromalacia	Decreased; cartilage hyperplasia	Increased signal
Acute fractures	Low, with a dark band	High, with a dark band
Stress fractures	Low, with a dark band	High, with a dark band
Early avascular necrosis	Low	Intermediate to high
Later avascular necrosis	Low (in subchondral band)	High (in subchondral band)

Abnormal Findings and Pathology

Disease processes are typically associated with increased concentration of free water. Consequently there is often decreased signal intensity on T1- and increased signal intensity on T2-weighted images, although this rule has exceptions:

1. Hemorrhage:
   - Acute hemorrhage shows high signal intensity on T1- but may show low to moderate signal intensity on T2-weighted images; this, however, may vary according to the amount of accompanying edema.
   - Subacute hemorrhage shows moderate to high signal intensity on both T1- and T2-weighted images.
   - Chronic hemorrhage shows variable signal intensity on T1- but high signal intensity on T2-weighted images.
2. Inflammation and other pathology that increases the free-water content of tissues displays decreased signal intensity on T1- but increased signal intensity on T2-weighted images.
3. Proliferated synovium associated with rheumatoid arthritis (synovial hypertrophy) gives rise to intermediate to high signal intensity (Fig. 5-10).
4. Muscle atrophy is often associated with infiltration of the substance of the muscle by fat and fluid, with increased signal intensity on both T1- and T2-weighted images (Fig. 5-11).
5. Soft tissue calcifications contain little or no free water; consequently they display low signal intensity on both T1- and T2-weighted images.
6. Soft tissue tumors typically have high free-water content, exhibiting low signal intensity on T1- but high signal intensity on T2-weighted images.
7. Bone tumors have various signal intensities depending on the tissue from which they arise and whether they are osteogenic or osteolytic in nature.
8. Acute fractures are displayed as straight or serpiginous (worm-like) lines of low signal intensity on both T1- and T2-weighted images. These lines are typically surrounded by marrow edema, which exhibits low signal intensity on T1- but high signal intensity on T2-weighted images.
9. Stress fractures may display as bone bruises, with low signal intensity on T1- but high signal intensity on T2-weighted images before a fracture line is visible (see below, "Clinical Thinking Point 2: MR Imaging of Stress Fractures").

Image Quality

The quality of MRI and CT images depends on many of the same parameters, such as field of view and pixel size. There are, however, a few differences.

Intrinsic and Extrinsic Factors

The most important intrinsic factor in image creation, other than T1 and T2 times, is proton density.[7] A low number of protons, as seen in cortical bone, gives rise to low signal intensity, resulting in a dark image on all pulse sequences. Structures with low proton density may, however, be imaged successfully if they are surrounded by other structures with higher signal intensity.

The most important extrinsic factors have to do with the choice of imaging sequence. The strength of the magnet also affects quality; other things being equal, higher magnetic

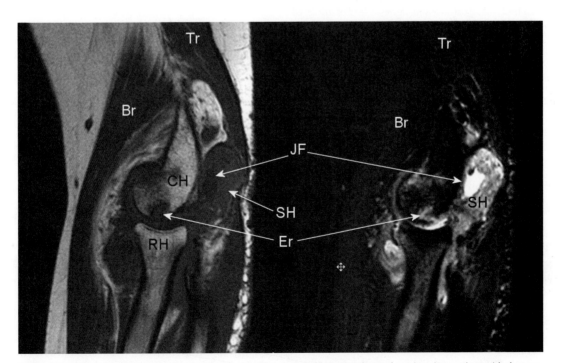

Figure 5-10 Signal intensities associated with inflammation, synovial hypertrophy, and erosions in a patient with rheumatoid arthritis. The joint fluid (JF) displays dark in the T1 image (left) but bright in the T2 image (right). The synovial hypertrophy (SH) and fluid-filled joint erosions (Er) give rise to low to intermediate signal on T1 image but a bright signal on T2. This slice, from the lateral aspect of the joint, shows the brachialis (Br), triceps brachii (Tr), capitulum of the humerus (CH), and radial head (RH). *(Image courtesy of John C. Hunter, MD, University of California, Davis School of Medicine.)*

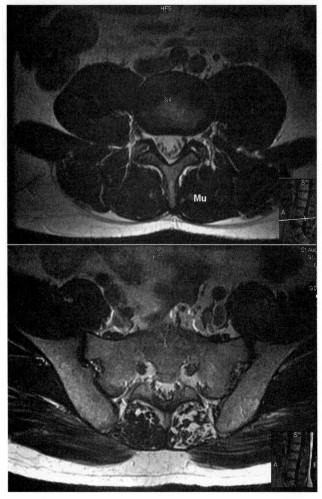

Figure 5-11 Severe atrophy of the multifidus muscle following laminectomy at the L4–L5 level. The upper slice is made at the level of the L3–L4 disk, showing normal appearance of the multifidus muscle (Mu); the lower image is made at the level of S1. Note the "moth-eaten" appearance of the left multifidus, which has lost most of its muscle substance.

field strengths improve image quality. Paramagnetic agents, such as gadolinium, can enhance the image and render inflammation visible on T1 sequences.

Clinical Uses of MRI

What Does MRI Image Best?

- MRI is very sensitive for detecting changes and variations in bone marrow. This is important in the diagnosis of bone tumors, stress fractures, and avascular necrosis.
- MRI excels in the display of soft tissue detail. It is widely used in the diagnosis of sports injuries because of its ability to differentiate between the different soft tissues and distinguish partial tears of tendons and ligaments from complete tears.
- In some cases, MRI has replaced invasive diagnostic procedures such as arthroscopy, as in the detection of meniscal tears.

- MRI is the best modality for differential diagnosis between disk herniations and other causes of nerve root impingement (Fig. 5-12).
- MRI has the ability to stage neoplasms in bone and soft tissues as well as evaluate the extent of tissue invasion, prior to surgery.[8] It is more sensitive than bone scan for detecting bone metastases, although bone scan is more effective as a screening technique.

What Are the Limitations of MRI?

The limitations of MRI lie in imaging of cortical bone because of its low signal intensity. Other limitations of MRI include the following:

- Length of time needed to produce an image
- High cost

Contraindications and Health Concerns

The magnetic field of the MRI unit is strong enough to lift oxygen containers off the ground and into the bore of the magnet. Consequently, metals, from implants to industrial shards or bullets, may present problems when brought into the proximity of the MRI magnet.

- Ferromagnetic surgical clips can be displaced. In the case of brain aneurysm clips, such displacement can cause fatal hemorrhage.
- Orthopedic hardware can cause image distortion, but it generally does not represent a health hazard.

Other concerns are the following:

- Pacemakers may malfunction within or near the magnetic field.
- Claustrophobia, which affects about 10% of patients.
- The need to sedate patients (such as children) who may not be able to stay still for the duration of the examination.

MR Arthrography

MRI arthrography, which has been increasingly used in the last 10 years, combines elements of the standard arthrogram with MRI.[9] This method is most often used in the investigation of labral tears of the hip and shoulder and for the investigation of ligament tears in the wrist and ankle. Most commonly, the radiologist adds small amounts of gadolinium into the iodine contrast for injection into the joint. The gadolinium renders a bright signal, which allows the radiologist to see small defects in the capsule, articular surfaces, ligaments, or labra.

MR Myelography[10]

The term *MRI myelography* may give rise to misunderstanding; implying the use of contrast materials, as used in CT myelogram. However, MRI myelography is simply the study of the spinal canal and subarachnoid space using high-resolution MRI with strong T2-weighting; a noninvasive approach where no contrast material is injected into

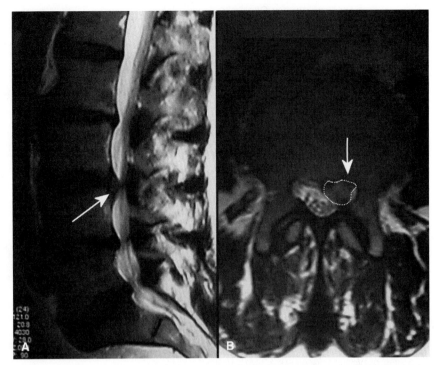

Figure 5-12 Lumbar disk herniation superimposed on pre-existing spinal stenosis in an elderly man. **(A)** Left paracentral sagittal T2 image showing considerable stenotic changes, mostly due to annular protrusions of the lowermost three intervertebral disks. Additionally a fairly large disk protrusion is seen at, and below, the L3–L4 intervertebral space. **(B)** An axial T2 image demonstrates that the protrusion fills the left lateral recess of the spinal canal.

the cerebrospinal fluid. This technique largely allowed the dicontinuation of conventional radiographic myelography.

Comparison of MRI and CT

Imaging Characteristics

Even though MRI and CT are frequently employed for similar purposes, they are based on very different principles. CT creates images based on the radiodensities of the tissues but MRI creates images based on energy emitted from hydrogen protons in water or soft tissues. Consequently, tissue characteristics are very different on CT and MR images. Structures that appear bright on radiographs and CT typically appear dark on MRI (Fig. 5-13).

Advantages and Disadvantages of MRI

MRI is often compared and contrasted with CT, as these are competing methods. The advantages of MRI over CT are:

- Greater contrast resolution for soft tissue imaging
- Greater ability to image organs surrounded by dense bone structures
- No ionizing radiation
- Less risk of missing disease processes, since processes missed by one sequence are often picked up using another sequence

The advantages of CT over MRI scanning are:

- Less expense
- Greater availability
- Faster imaging times
- Less operator time involved in selecting imaging parameters
- Thinner slices

- Less loss of image quality owing to motion
- Greater power of resolution when imaging cortical bone
- Easier imaging of individuals with metal implants

Clinical Thinking Points

Many clinical conditions that previously were not diagnosed have come to be recognized because of the possibilities offered by MRI. Many of those hold special interest for the physical therapist. Two such conditions are bone bruises and stress fractures.

Clinical Thinking Point 1: Bone Bruise—The Footprint of Injury[11]

Bone marrow contusions are frequently identified with MRI following musculoskeletal injury. These are injuries that typically do not involve permanent changes to osseous structures.

Bone marrow contusions, which have aptly been called the "footprints of injury," may be the result of traction injury to ligaments, such as injury to the medial ligament during valgus stress on the knee. This traction on the ligament can lead to injury of underlying bone. Bone marrow contusions may also result from direct blows to the bone or from compression forces at the joint surfaces during injury, as compression of the lateral joint surfaces of the knee during valgus stress.

Frequently an injury that is not visible on radiographic examination or CT is discovered because it leaves a "footprint" in the form of bone marrow edema visible on MRI. A good example is transient patellar dislocation. It is now thought that most cases of lateral patellar dislocation involve transient dislocations that are spontaneously reduced; an injury that may

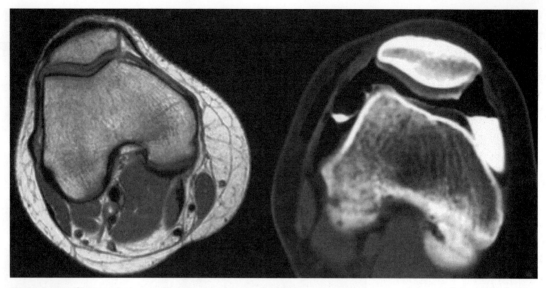

Figure 5-13 Differences between CT and MR images. To the left is an axial T1 MR image of the patellofemoral joint, but to the right an axial CT arthrogram (note the bright contrast medium in the medial joint space). The bony cortex appears bright on CT but dark on MRI. Fat is dark in the CT image but bright in the T1 MR image. The dense soft tissues of the capsule and patellar retinacula appear fairly bright on CT but dark on the MR image. Furthermore, note the superior ability of MRI for the imaging of soft tissue. *(Source of image: http://www.medcyclo.com by GE Healthcare.)*

result in limited MRI evidence of soft tissue damage. However, this injury results in bone marrow edema, bright on T2-weighted images and dark on T1, in the inferomedial aspect of the patella and the anterior aspect of the lateral femoral condyle. Patterns of marrow edema indicate occult injury and elucidate the forces involved, helping predict what soft tissue damage is likely (Fig. 5-14).

Clinical Thinking Point 2: MR Imaging of Stress Fractures[12]

Stress fractures, which most commonly involve the bones of the lower extremity, are the result of repeated subliminal trauma. This process starts with accelerated turnover and remodeling of bone, which may progress to a stress fracture if the stress continues.

The various imaging modalities have their advantages and disadvantages. Conventional radiography, the most commonly used imaging tool for diagnosing suspected stress fractures, may not detect a stress fracture until 4 to 6 weeks after clinical suspicion arises—that is, once considerable fracture healing has taken place. Consequently the majority of stress fractures are overlooked on initial radiographs. Early diagnosis, however, is of paramount importance, since more advanced stress fractures are associated with a longer recovery time. Furthermore, a stress fracture can, with continued activity, progress to a full-blown, displaced fracture. Femoral neck fractures are the most serious examples of this.

Radionuclide bone scan has long been claimed to be the gold standard for the diagnosis of stress fractures, but while its sensitivity is close to 100%, its specificity is low, since it only identifies pathological processes on the grounds of increased metabolic activity. Furthermore, it is a time-consuming investigation that is associated with considerable radiation. Lately, both CT and MRI have been shown to be as sensitive as bone scan or more so, and far more specific. This is exemplified by stress fractures of the navicular, where CT is the most accurate

diagnostic modality, and in femoral neck fractures, where MRI is the most sensitive method.

MRI clearly demonstrates the reactions that precede stress fractures; the resorption and replacement of bone. This metabolic activity is accompanied by local hyperemia and edema in bone marrow and periosteum. Initially, bone marrow changes are visible only on MRI sequences that are especially sensitive to inflammatory changes, such as STIR; but as the stress reactions become more severe, these changes give rise to the typical high signal intensity on T2-weighted images and a decreased signal on T1. Once the stress reaction progresses to stress fracture, a fracture line can be seen as a band of low signal intensity (Fig. 5-15).

MRI has the value, over the other imaging modalities, of being able to demonstrate the often considerable soft tissue abnormalities adjacent to the fractured bone. These abnormalities include inflammation of adjacent muscle, giving rise to high signal intensity on T2-weighted images.

MRI investigations of the progression of stress fractures have revealed that not all stress reactions visible on MRI give rise to stress fractures. Painful bone marrow edema and hemorrhage, presumably due to extensive microfractures in cancellous bone, may not progress to full-blown stress fractures. Frequently, stress reactions seen on MRI are not even symptomatic. They may simply signal early stress response to exercise or represent a chronic condition, as in the case of professional ballet dancers who were all found to have an area of bone marrow edema in the neck of the talus, asymptomatic in many cases and in none associated with impairment.[13]

Summary and Future Developments

MRI is still the overall best imaging method for viewing soft tissue detail, although CT is gaining ground. The problems of long imaging times are being addressed with faster sequences.

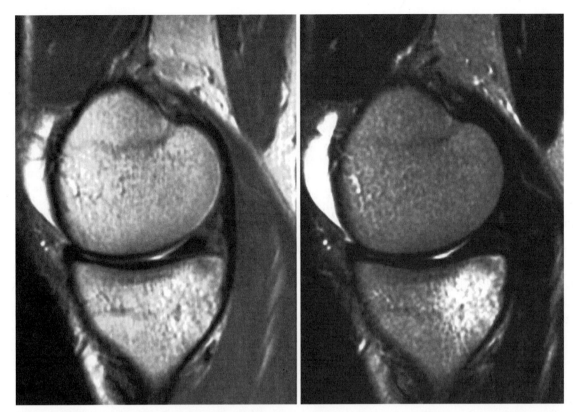

Figure 5-14 Bone bruise in the medial tibial plateau of a young man who sustained a pivot-shift injury (external rotation) while the knee was in a flexed position, resulting in compression to the medial side of the joint. A sagittal proton-density image (left) shows a slightly altered trabecular pattern in the posterior aspect of the medial tibial plateau; while the T2-weighted shows increased signal intensity within this part of the marrow. *(Source of image: http://www.medcyclo.com by GE Healthcare.)*

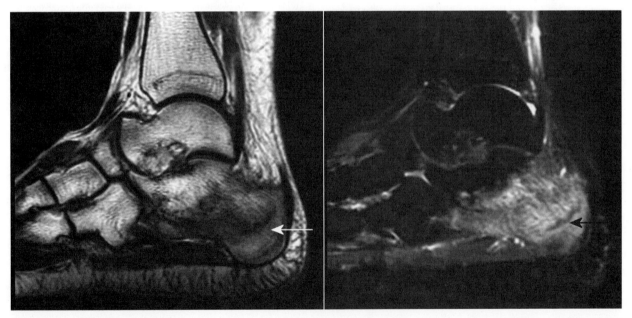

Figure 5-15 Stress fracture of the calcaneus in a 23-year-old female runner. The posteroinferior half of the calcaneus shows an area of decreased signal intensity on T1 (left); a slightly larger area of significant increase in signal intensity is seen on T2. Both images show an oblique line of low signal intensity on extending across the posterior talus, representing the fracture line. *(Image courtesy of John C. Hunter, MD, University of California, Davis School of Medicine.)*

The development of open scanners and faster acquisition times has not only solved the problem of claustrophobia but also opened the possibility of interventional imaging. With the use of open scanners, it is possible to image joints during movement, even applying resistance. This technique has been applied to the study of arthrokinematics of the spine, allowing visualization of segmental spinal motion.[14]

Summary of Key Points

1. MR images are made on the basis of energy emitted by protons during their re-alignment with the main magnetic field.

2. Diagnosis is often based on the differences between T1-weighted and T2-weighted images.

3. T1-weighted images demonstrate great anatomical detail and tend to highlight structures rich in fat, while T2-weighted images are grainier and emphasize structure with high free-water content and inflammation.

4. Sequences, such as SE Sequences (T1 and T2, as well as proton density) and GRE sequences, are different methods for capturing the MR signal.

5. Protocols refer to the choice of imaging planes and combinations of sequences used for certain clinical conditions.

6. Contrasts (e.g., gadolinium) can be used intravenously for the purpose of highlighting structures or pathology with rich blood supply, or be used in intra-articular injections (MR arthrography).

7. Open and upright scanners reduce the problem of claustrophobia and offer the possibility for imaging in a weight-bearing position, but are associated with lower field strength and longer imaging times.

8. Structures of high density, like cortical bone, ligaments, menisci, and tendons, are dark (have low signal intensity) on all MRI sequences, while most other structures show different signal intensities on T1-weighted images, as compared to T2.

9. MRI excels at detecting changes in bone marrow, displaying soft tissue detail, and demonstrating areas of inflammation.

10. Advantages of MRI over CT include no use of ionizing radiation, greater contrast resolution, and greater ability to image structures surrounded by bone.

11. Disadvantages of MRI include long imaging times and expense.

References

1. Elster, AD, and Burdette, JH: Questions and Answers in Magnetic Resonance Imaging, ed 2. Mosby, St. Louis, MO, 2000.
2. Bitar, R, Leung, G, Perng, R, et al: MR pulse sequences: What every radiologist wants to know but is afraid to ask. Radiographics 26:513, 2006.
3. Alyas, F, Lee, J, Ahmed, M, et al: Upright positional MRI of the lumbar spine. Clin Radiol 63:1035, 2008.
4. Chung, YN, Chou, CN, Lan, HC, and Ho, WH: Kinematic patellar tracking from MR images for knee pain analysis. Comput Biol Med 37:1653, 2007.
5. Skelly, AC, Moore, E, and Dettori, JR: Upright MRI Effectiveness of Upright MRI for Evaluation of Patients with Suspected Spinal or Extra-Spinal Joint Dysfunction. Health Technology Assessment Program, Olympia, WA, 2007.
6. Porter, BA, and Deutsch, AL: Marrow. In Deutsch AL, Mink JH (eds): MRI of the Musculoskeletal System: A Teaching File, ed 2. Lippincott-Raven, Philadelphia, 1997.
7. Kneeland, JB: Magnetic resonance imaging of the musculoskeletal system. Part 1. Fundamental principles. Clin Orthop 321:274, 1995.
8. van der Woude, HJ, Bloem, JL, and Pope, TL Jr: Magnetic resonance imaging of the musculoskeletal system. Part 9. Primary Tumors. Clin Orthop 347:272, 1998.
9. Steinbach, LS, Palmer, WE, and Schweitzer, ME: Special focus session. MR arthrography. Radiographics 22:1223, 2002.
10. Nagayama, M, Watanabe, Y, Okumura, A, et al: High-resolution single-slice MR myelography. AJR Am J Roentgenol 179:515, 2002.
11. Sanders, TG, Medynski, MA, Feller, JF, and Lawhorn, KW: Bone contusion patterns of the knee at MR imaging: footprint of the mechanism of injury. RadioGraphics 20:135, 2000.
12. Moran, DS, Evan, RK, and Hadad, E: Imaging of lower extremity stress fracture injuries. Sports Med 38:345, 2008.
13. Elias, I, Zoga, AC, Raikin, SM, et al: Bone stress injury of the ankle in professional ballet dancers seen on MRI. BMC Musculoskel Disord 9:39, 2008.
14. McGregor, AH, Anderton, L, Gedroyc, WM, et al: Assessment of spinal kinematics using open interventional magnetic resonance imaging. Clin Orthop 392:341, 2001.

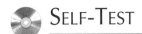

SELF-TEST

Image A

These are midsagittal images of the lumbosacral spine.

1. What is the condition of the intervertebral disks in these images?

2. How would you describe the vertebral end plates?

3. What is the phenomenon marked 1) in the image?

4. What is the phenomenon marked 2)?

Image B

These are sagittal images through the lateral condyle of the knee.

5. What are the tissues/structures numbered 1 through 10?

6. What similarities and differences between T1 and T2 help you identify the tissues?

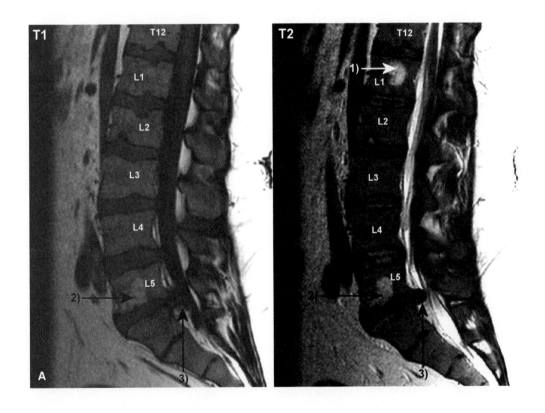

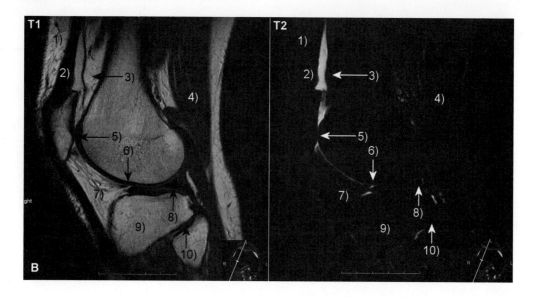

Chapter 6

DIAGNOSTIC ULTRASOUND

Hilmir Agustsson, MHSc, DPT, MTC, CFC

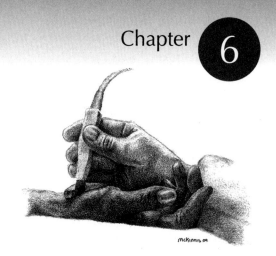

mcKinnis 09

Diagnostic Ultrasound

Diagnostic ultrasound is a cross-sectional imaging method based on sound waves reflected off tissue interfaces. Ultrasound predates computed tomography (CT) and magnetic resonance imaging (MRI) for pelvic and abdominal soft tissue imaging and, in the last 30 years, has been increasingly employed in imaging of the musculoskeletal system.

History

Diagnostic ultrasound has its origins in sonar (sound navigation and ranging), a technique developed as a navigational tool for submarines and the detection of objects under water. Ultrasound was employed in an unsuccessful attempt to locate the wreck of the *Titanic* in 1912 and was widely used in the submarine warfare of World War I (1914–1918).[1]

Medical use of diagnostic ultrasound started in the 1940s, and in the early 1950s the ability to detect lumps in breast tissue was demonstrated. Although ultrasound was the first technique available for accurate diagnosis of soft tissue lesions, it was not until the 1980s that ultrasound gained widespread acceptance for the evaluation of the musculoskeletal system.

The Unique Position of Diagnostic Ultrasound

The interpretation of CT, MRI, and, to a large degree, conventional radiographs has been the domain of radiologists. These imaging studies are typically read as static images, after being created. Diagnostic ultrasound, however, is a dynamic imaging modality, applied to the patient in real time, as a part of the clinical examination. This approach requires continuous modification of the imaging process based on the imaging findings and, furthermore, allows the application of physical examination techniques during the imaging procedure. As a consequence, nonradiologist health-care providers have welcomed this modality as a part of clinical practice.[2] At the same time, ultrasound has not been widely embraced by radiologists.

Principles of Diagnostic Ultrasound

Diagnostic ultrasound can be defined as the generation of images using reflected ultrasound and measuring the difference between emitted and received ultrasound.

147

Diagnostic Ultrasound Equipment

The ultrasound unit consists of a pulser, ultrasound transducer, scan converter, and monitor (Fig. 6-1).

The Pulser

The ultrasound pulser produces waves of electrical energy in the frequency range of 2 to 15 MHz. This frequency is referred to as the *base frequency.* The pulser delivers 1,000 to 5,000 bundles of waves at this base frequency per minute to the ultrasound transducer at (pulse repetition frequency). Between these bundles there is "silence." Thus, sound waves are emitted for only about 1% of the examination time; the transducer acts as a receiver for the reflected sound waves 99% of the time.

The Ultrasound Transducer

The ultrasound transducer converts the electricity from the pulser into sound energy, delivers the ultrasound to the tissues, receives the reflected waves, and converts those waves back to electrical signals. The transducer used for diagnostic ultrasound contains an array of crystals. These arrays can be of linear or curvilinear; musculoskeletal ultrasound typically employs a linear array, while transducers used for pelvic and abdominal investigations employ a curved array (Fig. 6-2).

The Scan Converter and Monitor

The scan converter is a computer that changes the incoming signal from an analog signal to a digital matrix, allowing it to be displayed as an image. The converter also amplifies the

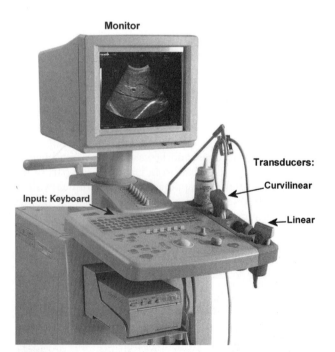

Figure 6-1 Ultrasound equipment. Note the different shapes of the transducers.

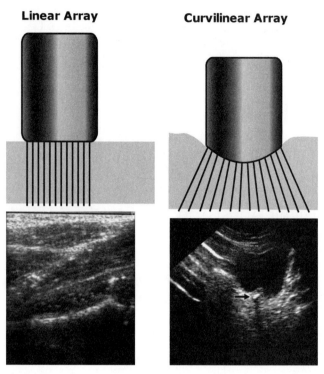

Figure 6-2 Linear and curvilinear transducers. The linear array transducer (left) displays the anterior hip with a field of view as wide as the transducer itself. Using a curved array transducer (right), the field of view widens as the distance from the transducer increases, producing images where deep structures are imaged disproportionally larger than superficial structures. The image shows a calculus in the bladder (arrow). Note the acoustic shadow (dark line) deep to it.

signal and performs functions aimed at increasing the signal-to-noise ratio. Most monitors display 256 shades of gray, but Doppler imaging employs color monitors.

Ultrasound Physics

Ultrasound consists of longitudinal waves transmitted from the transducer to the tissues of the body. Because the sound waves represent mechanical forces, they require matter for propagation.

Production

Electrical charges applied to a crystal cause deformation of the crystal according to the reversed piezoelectric effect. The current from the pulser oscillates at the base frequency and it gives rise to a wavelike motion of the crystal at the same frequency as the applied current. The wavelike motion forms the ultrasound beam that is transmitted in the soft tissues of the body.

Reception

The waves reflected from the body tissues cause the transducer crystals to deform, which in turn gives rise to electrical charges on the opposing surfaces of the crystal; negative or positive, depending on which way the crystal is deformed. This creation of electricity, on the basis of deformation of a crystal, is called the piezoelectric effect. This electricity forms the data from which an image is constructed.

The Ultrasound Beam

Each ultrasound wave represents a pressure cycle on the longitudinal axis of the beam. The waves of each cycle travel away from the ultrasound crystal in the form of oscillations of positive (compression) and negative pressure (rarefaction).

Beam Characteristics

The ultrasound intensity varies across the transverse dimension of the beam, with the greatest intensity at the center of the beam. The sides of the beam are not parallel; the beam first converges, then spreads. The zone along the beam where it is narrowest is called the focal zone. Larger transducers, with lower frequency, have a more distant focal zone.

Interaction Between Ultrasound and Tissues

Ultrasound is mechanical energy. Some energy gets reflected back to the transducer, and some energy is absorbed by the tissues and converted into thermal energy. The energy level of diagnostic ultrasound, however, is not high enough to cause measurable rise in tissue temperature. Attenuation of ultrasound takes place through absorption, reflection, refraction, and scattering (Fig. 6-3).

Absorption

Absorption is responsible for most of the attenuation of ultrasound. Absorption is the result of intermolecular friction, which converts the mechanical energy of ultrasound waves to heat.

Reflection

Ultrasound imaging is based on reflected sound. When sound is transmitted from one type of tissue to another type that has different resistance to the passage of sound waves (acoustic impedance), some of the sound waves get reflected at the interface between the two tissues. The amount of reflection is determined by (1) the degree to which the tissues reflect sound waves (echogenicity); (2) the difference in acoustic impedance of the two tissues forming the interface—large differences result in more reflection; (3) the smoothness of the reflecting interfaces—smooth reflectors, such as the liver and diaphragm, reflect more; and (4) the angle of reflection—the more the angle deviates from the perpendicular, the less energy is reflected back to the ultrasound transducer. For best imaging results, the incident beam should be perpendicular to the tissue imaged. This obviously is not always possible.

Refraction

Waves that are transmitted across an interface undergo a change in direction, similar to the refraction of light. For example, when you look into a container of water and reach into the water to fetch an object that you see lying on the bottom, you are likely not to find it at first try, since the light rays from the object change direction when they go from water into air. The ultrasound beam undergoes similar distortion. The amount of refraction varies with the following factors:

- The difference in acoustic impedance between the two tissue types
- The angle of incidence; the farther from the perpendicular, the greater the refraction

Refraction affects image quality because of the loss of reflected energy and distortion of the image, which make it more difficult to establish tissue location.

Scattering

When the reflecting surface is uneven, less energy is returned. Scattering results in less accurate localization of the reflecting interface and of underlying structures (see Fig. 6-3).

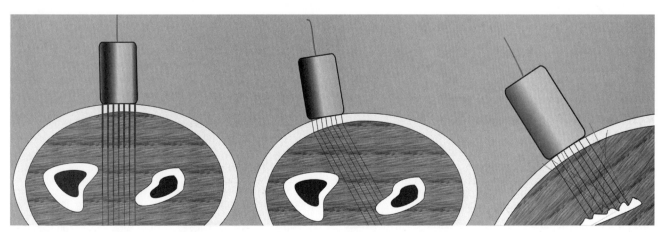

Figure 6-3 Absorption (left); refraction (middle), and reflection/scattering (right) of the ultrasound beam.

The Ultrasound Image

Energy reflected from the tissues back to the transducer is used for creating the image based on the piezoelectric effect.

Applying the Transducer

Ultrasound imaging is different from other imaging methods in several ways:

- The ultrasound transducer is applied directly to the skin, with an intervening layer of gel.
- The ultrasonographer can continuously monitor and change the imaging process during the examination.
- Musculoskeletal structures are often located by palpation before the application of the transducer and even through the transducer during application.
- The examiner can locate painful areas with palpation and perform musculoskeletal tests during the examination process.

Approaches to Scanning Various Tissues

The performance of diagnostic ultrasound may depend on the tissue being scanned:

- Ligaments are often superficial structures. They are best imaged using high-frequency transducers, because higher frequencies have less penetration and shorter focal lengths. The examination of ligaments can be supplemented by ligament stress tests during the ultrasound examination.
- Bursae are typically superficially located and are best imaged using high-frequency transducers. Care must be taken in how the transducer is applied; too firm a contact can displace the bursal fluid out of the field of view during the examination; but adequate distention of the bursa is prerequisite for being able to view it.
- Scanning of a muscle or a tendon may be supplemented by simultaneous manual testing of the muscle. A tear may not be visible until resistance is applied to the muscle or it is passively lengthened.

Information Used to Create the Image

The most important information used for image creation consists of the following:

- Amplitude of the reflected waves
- Timing of the reflected waves
- Transverse location of the reflected waves

Amplitude

It is important to keep in mind that in ultrasound imaging, unlike CT and MRI, tissues do not have "set" characteristic signal intensities. The pattern and intensity of reflection from the tissues depend on the nature of the tissue interface from which the signal originates and the angle at which the

sound waves strike the interface as well as on the type of tissue. Tissues or interfaces that reflect much energy are called hyperechoic, and tissues that reflect little energy are called hypoechoic. When there is no reflection, tissues may be referred to as anechoic. The waves reflected off hyperechoic tissues and interfaces between tissues that are dissimilar in density have high amplitude and produce bright images. The waves reflected off hypoechoic tissues have low amplitude and produce a dark image.

Timing

The distance from the transducer to the tissues, reflecting the signal, is determined by the time it takes the sound wave to reach the structure of interest and travel back to the transducer. Signals from the various depths return to the transducer at different times, allowing calculation of their distance from the transducer based on return times (Fig. 6-4).

Transverse Location

Across the transducer there are hundreds of individual crystals. The transverse location of an incoming signal (its location along the transducer's surface) is determined based on which crystal, on the long axis of the transducer, receives the signal.

Viewing the Ultrasound Image

The ultrasound monitor displays the intensity of the signals returned from the tissues in terms of different levels of brightness, depending on the echogenicity of the tissues and interfaces. As in CT and MRI, the image shows a slice of tissues. In ultrasound using a linear array transducer, this slice is oriented in the direction of the ultrasound beam and the field of view can be considered to be a direct continuation of the transducer—the width of the slice is the same as that of the

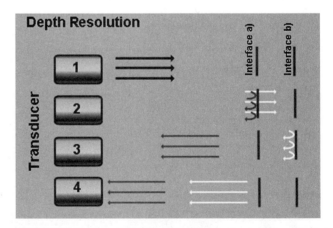

Figure 6-4 Depth resolution, based on return times of the reflected ultrasound. The time it takes the sound waves to arrive at the tissue interface, where it is reflected, and reflect back to the transducer, allows the determination of distance (depth resolution). Some of the ultrasound waves (gray arrows) are reflected from interface (a), whereas the remainder (white arrows) is reflected from interface (b). The former waves arrive back to the transducer earlier than the waves reflected off interface (b), indicating less depth.

long axis of the transducer. The width of this slice, however, can be increased in ultrasound units capable of providing an extended field of view. "Extended field of view" displays sequentially acquired frames on the monitor, not just the one that is currently being acquired, allowing structures that are longer than the long axis of the transducer to be displayed. This technique allows circumferential limb scanning, producing images that resemble the axial images of CT or MRI.

Scanning Planes: Nomenclature

The terminology used to describe the planes of view, for diagnostic ultrasound, is different from that used in CT and MRI. Whereas CT and MRI refer to the three orthogonal planes (although sometimes with modifications), the sonogram is described relative to the structures being examined. For example, when the long axis of the transducer is aligned with the long axis of a muscle, this is referred to as a longitudinal sonogram. A comparison of ultrasound scanning planes and orthogonal planes helps illuminate this difference:

- For a longitudinal sonogram of the long head of the biceps tendon, the transducer is applied along the tendon and the resulting image shows a sagittal slice of the tendon (Fig. 6-5).
- For a transverse sonogram of the same tendon, the transducer is applied across the tendon, resulting in an axial image of the tendon (Fig. 6-5).
- A longitudinal sonogram of the supraspinatus muscle results in an oblique coronal image.

Imaging Characteristics of Different Tissues

The different imaging characteristics of the tissues mainly relate to their echogenicity and the reflective characteristics of the interface the tissues form with adjacent tissues. For example, the cortex of a bone is echogenic, and so is a tendon; the signal from these structures will be bright. But if there is tissue superficial to the tendon that has very different reflective characteristics, the signal will be even brighter. The brightness of the signal is frequently described with reference to that of surrounding tissues (Table 6-1). What follows is a discussion of the ultrasound imaging characteristics:

- Ultrasound does not penetrate bone. Therefore, the bone–soft tissue interface returns a bright echo while no ultrasound is returned from subcortical bone, which is displayed thus as hypoechoic (Fig. 6-6).
- Tendons relative to muscle, are hyperechoic, and display a distinct pattern of parallel fibers in the longitudinal sonogram. In the transverse sonogram, the fibers have a dense, spotted appearance (Fig. 6-6).
- Ligaments are hyperechoic relative to muscle and display a distinct fiber pattern, more compact than that of tendons. Ligaments and tendons have anisotrophic properties, meaning that a slight alteration in the angle of the ultrasound probe may change the appearance of the tendon from hypo- to hyperechoic; this may help distinguish it from surrounding fat, which is uniformly hypoechoic.

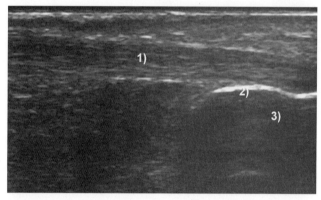

Figure 6-6 Longitudinal sonogram of the Achilles' tendon. (1) Achilles' tendon, (2) cortical bone of the calcaneus, (3) subcortical bone of the calcaneus. This longitudinal sonogram corresponds to a sagittal view, using the terminology of orthogonal planes of MRI and CT. Note the parallel fibers within the tendon.

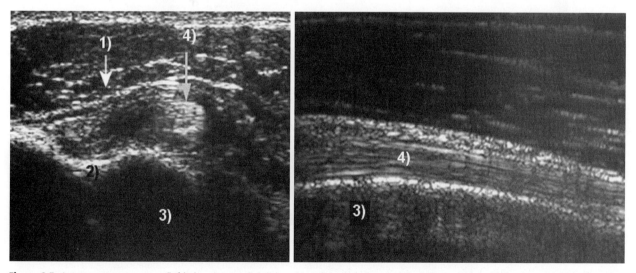

Figure 6-5 A transverse sonogram (left) showing medial dislocation of the long head of the biceps tendon. (1) Tendon of pectoralis major; (2) empty bicipital groove; (3) humerus (subcortical bone), (4) biceps tendon. A longitudinal normal sonogram (right) shows the tendon within the bicipital groove. *(Image courtesy of John Lin, MD.)*

- Muscles are hypoechoic relative to the adjacent fasciae or tendons (Fig. 6-7). Fibrous bands of fasciae and fibroadipose tissue within the substance of the muscle can be discerned in longitudinal sonogram as parallel hyperechoic bands with a slightly brighter signal. In the transverse sonogram, these fibrous bands appear as dots across the relatively hypoechoic substance of the muscle.

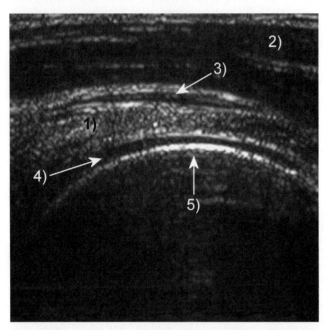

Figure 6-7 Longitudinal sonogram of the infraspinatus tendon (1). The overlying deltoid muscle is relatively hypoechoic, with faint striations (2); the subacromial bursa is displayed as a thin hypoechoic line (3); the articular cartilage (4) is also displayed as a thin hypoechoic line, separating the cortex of the humeral head (5) from the tendon.

- A bursa is a potential space that contains only minuscule amounts of fluid, so it is most often displayed as a hypoechoic line (no wider than 2 mm) between two more hyperechoic structures, for example, between tendon and bone or between tendon and muscle (Fig. 6-7).
- Hyaline cartilage is displayed as a hypoechoic layer next to hyperechoic cortical bone (Fig. 6-7).
- Fibrocartilage, which is found in articular surfaces of the temporomandibular joint and in the menisci of the knee, is hyperechoic and sometimes difficult to distinguish from cortical bone.
- Nerve tissue is hypoechoic relative to tendons; hyperechoic relative to muscle. It has a faint striated pattern in the longitudinal sonogram but a speckled appearance in the transverse sonogram.
- Cysts are anechoic (fluid) and are imaged as dark with enhancement of structures posterior to the cyst (Fig. 6-8).

Characteristic Abnormal Findings[3,4]

- Muscle strains involve some disruption of the fibrous bands; this differs according to the grade of the injury. Injuries are often associated with a hypoechoic hematoma. In a substantial or complete rupture, there is retraction of muscle fibers.
- Tendon pathology is most often associated with focal or diffuse thickening of the tendon and disruption of fiber pattern and mixed echogenicity (Fig. 6-9). Where there is associated inflammation of synovial sheath, this will appear as a hypoechoic layer in the longitudinal sonogram or as a hypoechoic ring around the circular tendon in the transverse sonogram. Tendon ruptures are seen as disruptions of the fibrous structure, initially filled with hypoechoic hematoma and fibrous debris. It may be necessary to put the tendon on mild stretch in order to verify a complete rupture. Frequently the stumps of the tendon

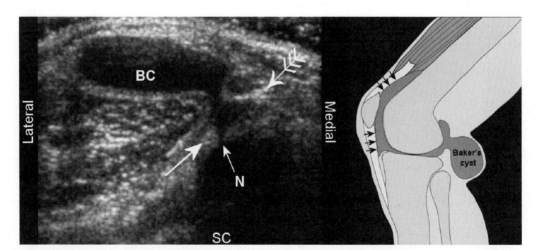

Figure 6-8 A transverse sonogram of the popliteal fossa, showing a Baker's cyst (BC). The cyst communicates with the synovial cavity (SC) of the knee joint posteromedially. This communication takes place via a narrow channel, called a "neck" (N), between the medial head of the gastrocnemius (arrow) and the semimembranosus (feathered arrow). The bursa fills during flexion owing to pressure on the anterior part of the capsule; but during extension, this fluid has difficulty escaping from the cyst, because tightening of the gastrocnemius and semimembranosus closes the channel. *(Source of ultrasound image: http://www.medcyclo.com by GE Healthcare.)*

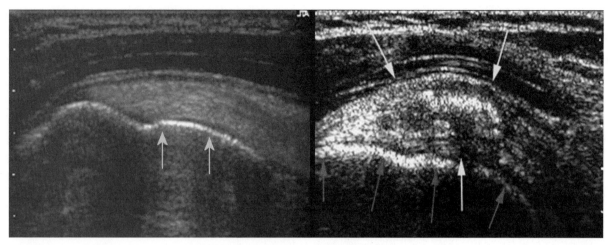

Figure 6-9 Longitudinal sonograms of normal (left) and degenerated (right) supraspinatus tendons. In the degenerated tendon, note the cortical outline (gray arrows), the increased thickness of the tendon (white arrows above), and the mixed echogenicity within the tendon. There is also a partial tear in the articular surface of the tendon (white arrow pointing upward). *(Image courtesy of John Lin, MD.)*

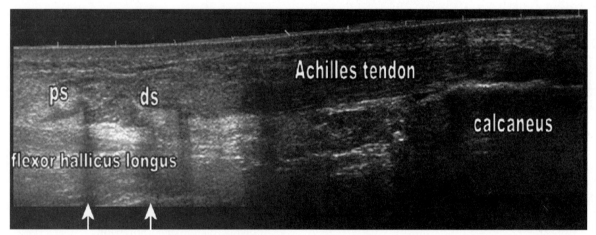

Figure 6-10 An extended field of view longitudinal sonogram of a rupture at the gastrocnemius–musculotendinosus junction. The torn proximal (ps) and distal (ds) stumps are curled up and cast acoustic shadows (arrows) on the underlying tissues. *(Source of image: http://www.medcyclo.com by GE Healthcare.)*

retract and bundle up; their ends then cast an acoustic shadow on the underlying tissues (Fig. 6-10).

- Bursitis is seen as a widening of the hypoechoic space. The fluid tends to pool at the lower end of the bursa in the dependent position or may accumulate where anatomic spaces allow. Thickening of the walls of the bursa, appearing as hyperechoic lines, is associated with chronic bursitis; normally the walls of the bursa are not visible.
- Ligament strains and partial tears are seen as a disruption of fiber patterns; strains may be associated with thickening and hypoechogenic thickening of the ligament.
- Where cartilage is accessible to ultrasound scanning, ultrasound can demonstrate beginning pathological changes, displayed as inhomogeneous thickening of the cartilage.
- Nerve compression, as in carpal tunnel syndrome, is seen as flattening of the nerve at the point of compression and swelling proximal to the compression.

- Cysts may contain thickened synovium, hemorrhage, septations, and debris from an associated joint space.

For a review of abnormal findings see Table 6-1.

The Quality of the Image

Lateral and Axial Resolution

Resolution in ultrasound imaging is discussed in terms of lateral resolution and axial resolution. Lateral resolution is the ability to differentiate between structures in the plane perpendicular to the ultrasound beam; it is best when employing smaller transducers and higher frequency. Axial resolution is the ability to differentiate between structures that lie one above the other in the longitudinal axis of the ultrasound beam. It is greater than lateral resolution and, like lateral resolution, improves with increasing ultrasound

TABLE 6-1 ● *Imaging Characteristics of Ultrasound*

Normal Tissue	
Cortical bone	Hyperechoic, smooth, continuous
Tendons and ligaments	Hyperechoic; distinct parallel fiber pattern
Muscle	Hypoechoic, with parallel fibrous hyperechoic bands
Bursae	Thin hypoechoic line
Hyaline cartilage	Hypoechoic layer next to hyperechoic cortex
Nerve	Hyperechoic, relative to muscle
Cysts	Anechoic
Disease/Disorders	
Fracture	Break in continuity, uneven surfaces
Tendon/ligament strains	Thickening, of mixed echogenicity (hypoechoic if inflammation or hematoma); disrupted fiber pattern
Tendon/ligament rupture	Disruption of structures, initially fills with hypoechoic hematoma, and separation of ends
Muscle strain	Disruption of fibrous bands; hypoechoic hematoma in early stages
Muscle rupture	Retraction of muscle stumps
Bursitis	Increased width of bursa. In later stages, hyperechoic thickening of bursal walls
Cartilage damage	Early changes display as inhomogeneous thickening; later irregularity and disruption
Nerve compression	Flattening; swelling proximal to compression
Distended/abnormal cyst	Increased volume, thickened walls; septations; debris

TABLE 6-2 ● *Advantages and Disadvantages of Ultrasound Relative to MRI*

General Advantages	
Low cost and portability	
No contraindications; orthopedic hardware not a problem	
Ability to visualize structures is not limited by orthogonal planes	
Continuous modification of imaging based on findings	
Palpation, stress, testing, and application of resistance while imaging	
Advantages Over MRI	
Muscles	Architecture; imaging while testing with resistance
Tendons	Fiber structure, degenerative changes, longitudinal tears
Ligaments	Fiber structure, ability to stress test while imaging
Cysts and bursae	Septations, debris not seen on MRI
Disadvantages	
Joints; intra-articular structures	Limited ability to show joint surfaces and intra-articular structures
Bones	Can show only cortical outline of bone
Scanning across lung fields	Ultrasound does not cross air–tissue interfaces

frequency. There are two main reasons for this improvement of resolution with increasing frequency:

- The signal is stronger because higher frequencies increase the amount of reflection at interfaces.
- Higher frequencies allow the visualization of smaller structures along the longitudinal axis, whereas lower frequencies are associated with longer waves, which may penetrate through the tissues of interest without returning a signal.

Clinical Uses of Ultrasound

Diagnostic ultrasound is rapidly gaining ground in the diagnosis of the soft tissues of the musculoskeletal system. A number of studies find its diagnostic sensitivity and specificity to be comparable to those of MRI.[5–6] Ultrasound is discussed here in comparison with MRI, because these two modalities represent the most sensitive methods for soft tissue diagnosis.

General Advantages[7]

The general advantages of ultrasound over MRI include the following (Table 6-2):

- Higher resolution
- Low cost and portability
- No known hazards; can be used to image soft tissues in the presence of orthopedic hardware
- Ready comparison with opposite side

Ability to follow a structure, like peripheral nerve, from beginning to end, regardless of orthogonal planes.

Another advantage of ultrasound is the ability to modify the imaging while it is being performed; palpating for the area of tenderness and performing various examination procedures during the imaging procedure. This decreases the risk of emphasizing clinically irrelevant findings. Furthermore, concurrent use of physical examination techniques may reveal lesions not visible in the resting position. Examples include the following:

- Placing the affected joint in a symptom-provoking position
- Using resisted contractions or passive muscle stretching
- Applying traction or compression
- Stress testing ligaments
- Palpating for tenderness and applying the probe accordingly

Imaging Characteristics

Muscles

For imaging of muscles, ultrasound is just as accurate as MRI and additionally provides intricate details of the muscle's internal architecture. Ultrasound is as accurate as MRI for measuring the cross-sectional area of muscles.[8]

Tendons

Ultrasound has the advantage over MRI that it can demonstrate the internal architecture of tendons. Ultrasound clearly shows the fibers within the tendon and thus can reveal pathology not easily diagnosed with MRI. Examples include the following:

- Degenerative changes, which frequently precede tendon ruptures
- Longitudinal tears within the tendon substance (Fig. 6-11)

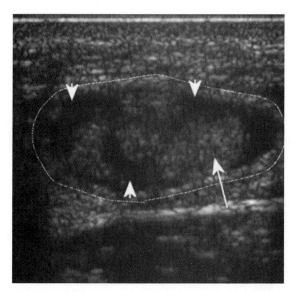

Figure 6-11 Transverse sonogram of the Achilles' tendon (dotted line). The long arrow points to normal tendon substance, while the arrowheads show longitudinal, fluid-filled interstitial tears, returning a low signal. *(Image courtesy of John Lin, MD.)*

Ligaments

Ultrasound imaging of ligaments rivals that of MRI, with the added advantage of a better display of fiber structure and the ability to perform stress tests during the examination process.

Nerves

Ultrasound can demonstrate inflammation of a nerve as well as changes in nerve diameter that indicate entrapment neuropathies.

Joints

Compared with MRI, ultrasound imaging is limited in its ability to show intra-articular structures, although the peripheral parts of the menisci can be visualized. However, ultrasound is valuable for the detection of joint effusion and in pediatrics, where other imaging methods are associated with health risks or are difficult to perform. Here ultrasound is primarily used for the evaluation of developmental dysplasias of the hip.

Cysts and Bursae

Ultrasound provides greater detail on cysts and bursae than does MRI. Frequently, what appears on MRI to be a simple fluid-filled bursa is found on ultrasound to contain septations, debris from an adjacent joint, or thickened synovial tissue.

Bone

Ultrasound can image only the cortical outline of bone and is therefore limited compared with CT and MRI. This, however, is valuable in the assessment of enthesopathy, which entails roughening of bone at the attachments of tendons or ligaments, frequently associated with degenerative or inflammatory changes (Fig. 6-12). Ultrasound can also be used to evaluate osteoporosis. The principles behind these measurements are different from those of radiographic methods, which measure bone mineral density based on absorption of radiation. Ultrasound evaluates the strength of bone based on attenuation and the speed of the ultrasound within the bone. This method can accurately predict the risk of osteoporotic fractures.[9]

What Are the Limitations of Ultrasound?

One of the main limitations of ultrasound is its limited field of view, caused by the limited size of the transducer (see Table 6-2). Other limitations include the following:

● Ultrasound is more operator-dependent than other imaging methods.
● Ultrasound does not penetrate bone, so structures deep to bone, such as intra-articular ligaments, are not visualized.

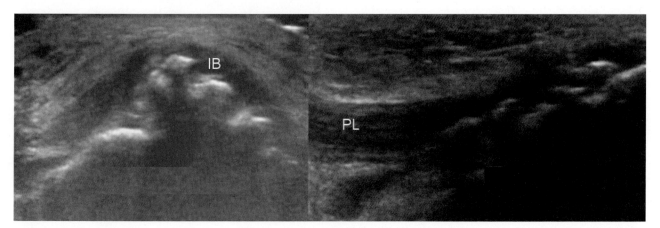

Figure 6-12 Transverse (left) and longitudinal (right) views of the tibial tuberosity in a person with Osgood–Schlatter disease. The cortical irregularity at the insertion of the patellar ligament (PL) on the tibial tuberosity is displayed as hyperechoic mounds. The superficial infrapatellar bursa (IB) is distended.

- Ultrasound waves do not cross air interfaces. This is problematic in attempting to image structures obscured by the lungs or by gas in the intestine.
- Obese patients are not imaged well. This limitation is caused both by loss of acoustic energy and by difficulty in obtaining the correct focal length.

Summary and Future Developments

Ultrasound rivals or surpasses MRI for musculoskeletal soft tissue diagnosis, although it is not as widely used. Its low cost, portability, safety of use, and possibilities for integration with the clinical examination are bound to lead to more widespread use among physical therapists.

Clinical Thinking Point

Real-Time Ultrasound Imaging—Biofeedback

Numerous studies have employed ultrasound in order to obtain real-time information about the role of the multifidus and transversus abdominis (TrA) muscles in stabilization of the lumbar spine.[10,11] The importance of the TrA for spinal stability was established partly through studies demonstrating that contraction of the transversus abdominis precedes movement of the extremities in healthy individuals[12] while this activity is decreased in individuals with low back pain. This difference in activation patterns, and other dysfunctions of the stabilizing musculature in individuals with low back pain, may help to explain the high recurrence rate of low back pain.[13] Findings related to normal and abnormal function of the TrA have been used in order to devise exercise regimes for stabilization employing low-level cocontraction of transversus abdominis and multifidus that have been successfully used in the treatment of nonspecific low back pain, spondylolisthesis, and instability of the sacroiliac joint.[14–15] Dynamic ultrasound imaging has played a key role in this development and is routinely used in physical therapy clinics in order to examine the activity of the stabilizing musculature and providing feedback to the patient about correct activation of the stabilizing musculature. Figures 6-13 and 6-14 demonstrate correct and incorrect activation of the TrA.

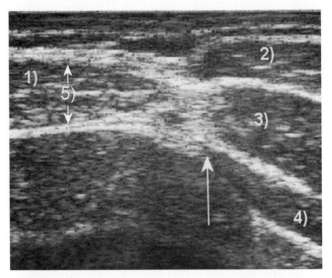

Figure 6-13 Transverse image of the abdominal muscles, showing correct activation of the transversus abdominis. Note that muscle is hypoechoic relative to the bright fibrous bands of tendons and aponeuroses. The structures displayed are the (1) rectus abdominis, (2) external oblique, (3) internal oblique, and (4) transversus abdominis. Note the fibrous sheaths separating these muscles, as well and the anterior and posterior rectus sheath (5). The muscles are dark relative to the fasciae on either side. Correct activation is evidenced by lateral movement of the medial attachments of the transversus abdominis (white arrow) and thickening of its muscle belly.

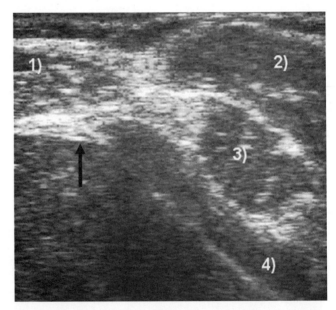

Figure 6-14 Incorrect activation of the transversus abdominis. Note the thickening of the rectus abdominis (1) as well as the external (2) and internal (3) obliques. Note the passive elongation of the transversus abdominis (4) and medial movement of the medial attachments (arrow).

Summary of Key Points

1. Ultrasound was the first imaging modility for accurate diagnosis of soft tissue.

2. Ultrasonography is real-time imaging that can be continuously modified based on the imaging findings.

3. The images are typically not referenced in terms of the orthogonal planes, but as longitudinal or transverse images of the the structure being scanned.

4. Both lateral and axial resolution improve with increasing frequency; higher frequency is better suited for viewing superficial structures.

5. In the tissues of the body, ultrasound is partly absorbed, reflected, and diffused (through refraction and scattering).

6. The images are based on the amplitude and timing of returned signals, and the transverse location of waves returned to the ultrasound transducer.

7. The amplitude of signals is highest from echogenic structures with smooth surfaces; interfaces between structures with highly different echogenicity are also strong reflectors.

8. Echogenic structures include cortical bone, tendons, and ligaments.

9. Hypoechoic structures include cysts, bursae, and fat.

10. The advantages of ultrasound include high resolution, low cost, safety of use, and the ability to modify the examination; the disadvantages include operator dependency and inability to scan intra-articular structures.

11. Ultrasound has greater resolution for the internal architecture of tendons, ligaments, and muscles than MRI does.

References

1. Woo, J: A Short History of the Development of Ultrasound in Obstetrics and Gynecology. Accessed October 4, 2008 at http://www.ob-ultrasound.net/history.html.

2. Brown, AK, Roberts, TE, O'Connor, PJ, et al: The development of an evidence-based educational framework to facilitate the training of competent rheumatologist ultrasonographers. Rheumatology (Oxford) 46:391, 2007.

3. Chew, K, Stevens, KJ, Wang, TG, et al: Introduction to diagnostic musculoskeletal ultrasound: Part 2. Examination of the lower limb. Am J Phys Med Rehabil 87:238, 2008.

4. Lew, HL, Chen, CP, Wang, TG, and Chew, KT: Introduction to musculoskeletal diagnostic ultrasound: Examination of the upper limb. Am J Phys Med Rehabil 86:310, 2007.

5. Beggs, I: Ultrasound of the shoulder and elbow. Orthop Clin North Am 37:277, 2006.

6. Warden, SJ, Kiss, ZS, Malara, FA, et al: Comparative accuracy of magnetic resonance imaging and ultrasonography in confirming clinically diagnosed patellar tendinopathy. Am J Sports Med 35:427, 2007.

7. Nazarian, LN: The top 10 reasons musculoskeletal sonography is an important complementary or alternative technique to MRI. AJR Am J Roentgenol 190:1621, 2008.

8. Hides, JA, Richardson, CA, and Jull, GA: Magnetic resonance imaging and ultrasonography of the lumbar multifidus muscle. Comparison of two different modalities. Spine 20:54, 1995.

9. Guessous, I, Cornuz, J, Ruffieux, C, et al: Osteoporotic fracture risk in elderly women: Estimation with quantitative heel US and clinical risk factors. Radiology 248:179, 2008.

10. Wilke, HJ, Wolf, S, Claes, LE, et al: Stability increase of the lumbar spine with different muscle groups: A biomechanics study. Spine 20:192, 1995.

11. Macintosh, JE, Bogduk, N, and Gracovetsky, S: The biomechanics of the thoracolumbar fascia. Clin Biom 2:78, 1987.

12. Hodges, PW, and Richardson, CA: Contraction of the abdominal muscles associated with movement of the lower limb. Phys Ther 77:132, 1997.

13. Hodges, PW, and Richardson, CA: Inefficient muscular stabilization of the lumbar spine associated with low back pain. A motor control evaluation of transversus abdominis. Spine 21:2640, 1996.

14. Richardson, CA, and Jull, GA: Muscle control–pain control. What exercises would you prescribe? Man Ther 1:2, 1995.

15. Richardson, CA, Snijders, CJ, Hides, JA, et al: The relation between the transversus abdominis muscles, sacroiliac joint mechanics, and low back pain. Spine 27:399, 2002.

SELF-TEST

Image A

This is a longitudinal (midline sagittal) ultrasound image of the posterior leg.

1. What are the structures labeled 1 through 8 in the image?

2. What are the imaging characteristics of ultrasound that help you identify them?

Image B

The image on the left is a longitudinal sonogram of the patellar ligament (1) and its insertion on the patella (cortical outline = 2). The middle image, also longitudinal, shows a partial tear of the quadriceps tendon. Note the cortical outline of the femur (3) and the infrapatellar fat pad (4). The image to the right is a transverse image across the upper patella.

3. What pathological changes are represented by *a*, *b*, and *c*?

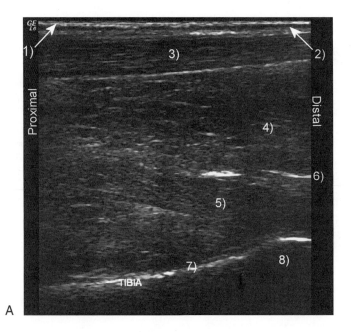

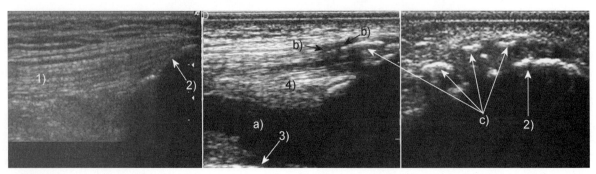

(Image courtesy of John Lin, MD.)

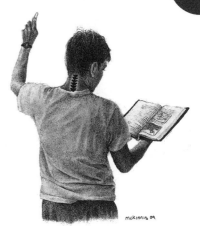

RADIOLOGIC EVALUATION OF THE CERVICAL SPINE

The cervical spine region is one of the most common areas of dysfunction treated by clinicians. Conditions resulting from acute trauma, degenerative disorders, and chronic postural strains can cause pain and debilitation that lead the patient to seek therapeutic or surgical intervention. Important to the clinical evaluation in any of these patient groups is an understanding of the underlying degenerative changes of the spine revealed on radiograph. The degree of severity of degeneration will affect the ability of the spine to withstand trauma, assume postural changes, and make functional gains in mobility and movement patterns.

In radiology, the cervical spine is one of the most frequently evaluated body segments. A busy emergency department frequently evaluates the cervical spine for direct trauma and also screens for indirect trauma if the patient has been in a severe fall or accident. The mobility of the cervical spine allows for protection of the neural contents but at the same time predisposes it to certain types of injury. If some trauma has occurred, the injury potential of this vulnerable area of the body should never be underestimated, even if the trauma is at a site in the body far from the neck. Clinicians should review the radiologist's consultation prior to initiating the evaluation of a patient who has suffered a cervical spine injury. Equally important, the clinician should never rely on the results of any diagnostic study alone. Physical evaluations, including ligamentous stability tests, are also important and should be performed on every patient who has sustained a cervical spine trauma. The determination of treatment is based on all components of the examination—the history, clinical evaluation, and laboratory tests as well as the radiologic findings.

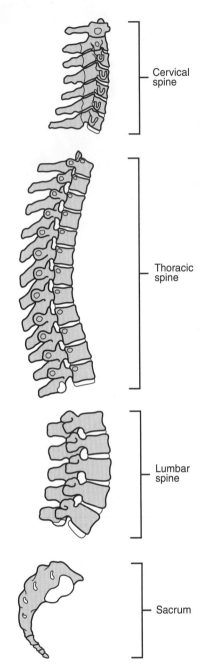

Figure 7-1 Divisions of the spinal column.

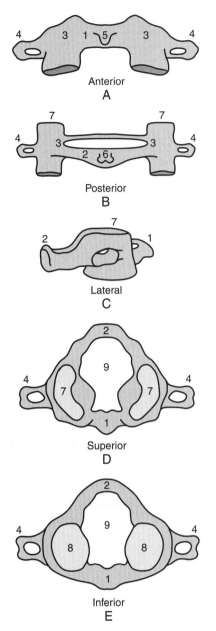

Figure 7-2 (A–E) Atlas (C1). 1 = anterior arch; 2 = posterior arch; 3 = lateral mass; 4 = transverse process; 5 = anterior tubercle; 6 = posterior tubercle; 7 = occipital condyles; 8 = inferior facets; 9 = vertebral foramen.

ⓡ Review of Anatomy[1–7]

Osseous Anatomy

The cervical spine (Fig. 7-1) consists of seven vertebrae positioned in a lordotic curve. The *atlas (C1)* (Fig. 7-2) and *axis (C2)* (Fig. 7-3) have unique characteristics. The remaining vertebrae, *C3* (Fig. 7-4) through *C7*, share common osseous features.

The *atlas,* so named for the mythical earth-supporting giant, supports the globe of the head. The atlas is composed of *anterior* and *posterior arches* united by *lateral masses* and forming a bony ring. Long, perforated *transverse processes* extend from the lateral masses and are easily palpated behind

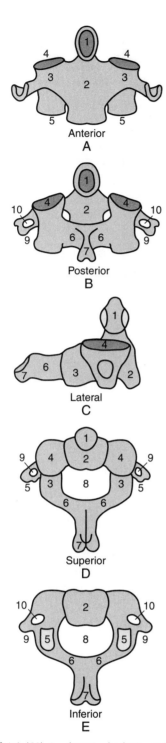

Figure 7-3 (A–E) Axis (C2). 1 = dens; 2 = body; 3 = pedicles; 4 = superior articulating processes; 5 = inferior articulating processes; 6 = laminae; 7 = bifid spinous process; 8 = vertebral foramen; 9 = transverse processes; 10 = transverse foramen.

the angles of the mandible. The anterior arch has a midline *anterior tubercle* on its outer surface and a midline *facet* on its inner surface for articulation with the superiorly projecting *odontoid process* or *dens* of C2. The posterior arch has a

midline *tubercle*, which is a rudimentary spinous process. The lateral masses support large, concave, medially inclined facets that articulate with the *occipital condyles*, forming the *atlanto-occipital (AO) joint*. The inferior facets lie in a relatively transverse plane and articulate with the superior facets of C2, forming the *atlantoaxial (AA) joint* (Figs. 7-5 and 7-6).

The *axis* is so named as it is the pivot on which the head rotates. The axis is composed of a small *body* with the distinctive *dens (odontoid process)* arising from the anterior portion. The dens has two articulating facets. The anterior surface of the dens articulates with the inner anterior arch of the atlas, and the posterior surface articulates with the *transverse ligament* of the atlas. Short, thick *pedicles* extend laterally from the body and provide support for the *superior and inferior articulating processes* and associated *facets*. The inferior articulating facets are offset posteriorly from the superior pair and lie in a plane common to the remainder of the cervical facet joints. *Transverse processes* are small and not bifid at this level. The *laminae* project medially and unite in a *bifid spinous process*.

C3 through C7 are each characterized by the presence of a *vertebral body*, stout *pedicles*, paired *superior and inferior articulating processes*, bifid *transverse processes*, and *laminae* uniting in *bifid spinous processes*. All of the cervical vertebrae have large *vertebral foramina* for passage of the *spinal cord*, *transverse foramina* for transmission of the *vertebral artery and vein*, and grooves on the superior surfaces of the transverse processes for transmission of the *spinal nerves*. *Intervertebral disks* are present beginning at the C2–C3 interspace. *Uncinate processes* project from the superolateral margins of the bodies articulating with adjacent bodies to form small *uncovertebral joints*, which offer some stability to the interposed disks (Fig. 7-7). The cervical *zygapophysial joints*, more commonly referred to as *facet joints*, are formed by the articulating processes of adjacent vertebrae. The expanse of bone that encompasses the superior and inferior articulating processes is referred to as the *articular pillar* and is distinct from the pedicle. The expanse of bone between the superior and inferior articulating processes is known as the *pars interarticularis*.

Ligamentous Anatomy

The primary ligaments of this region are reviewed to assist in the understanding of mechanisms of injury and the resultant instabilities. Ligaments are of a water density and so do not possess enough radiodensity to be specifically visualized on radiographs. However, ligaments can be assessed *indirectly* by assessing the articular relationships that intact ligaments provide. Loss of normal articular relationships implies a loss of ligamentous support. Ligaments can be *directly* visualized by magnetic resonance imaging (MRI) (Fig. 7-8).

The *cervicocranial ligaments* intricately support the articulating relationships between the occiput, atlas, and axis (Fig. 7-9). The principal ligamentous stabilizers are (1) the

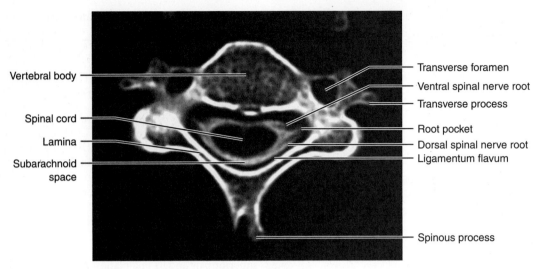

Figure 7-4 CT myelography, axial view, of a typical cervical vertebra.

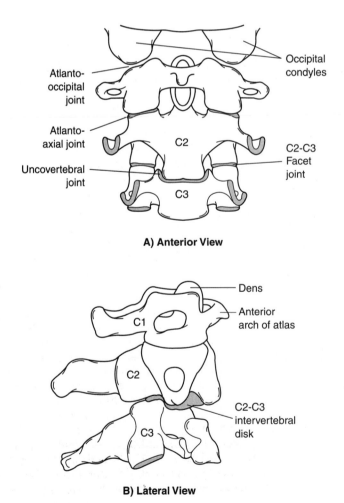

A) Anterior View

B) Lateral View

Figure 7-5 (A) Anterior and **(B)** lateral views of the craniovertebral and intervertebral joints.

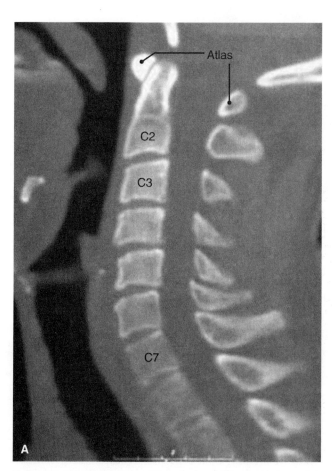

Figure 7-6 CT, three-dimensional reconstruction of the upper cervical spine.

alar ligaments, extending upward and outward from the superolateral surfaces of the dens to the occiput, providing a restraint against excessive rotation at the atlanto-occipital joint; (2) the *transverse ligament of the atlas,* extending horizontally across the dens and attached to the lateral masses of the atlas, securing the articulation between these two bones; (3) the *anterior* and *posterior atlanto-occipital ligaments,* extending from the superior margins of the atlas to the foramen magnum; and (4) *the tectorial membrane,* extending from the posterior body of the axis and attached to the anterior margins of the foramen magnum, providing support to the subcranial region.

The lower cervical vertebrae are supported posteriorly by the (1) *ligamentum nuchae,* stretching from the occipital crest to the spinous processes; (2) the *ligamenta flava,* joining the laminae of adjacent vertebrae; (3) the *interspinous ligaments,* joining adjacent spinous processes; and (4) the *posterior longitudinal ligament,* located within the vertebral canal and attached to the disks and posterior vertebral bodies. All of these ligaments assist in limiting forward flexion and rotation of the cervical spine. The *anterior longitudinal ligament* stretches from the occiput to the sacrum, attaching to the anterior disks and margins of the vertebral bodies and limiting backward bending.

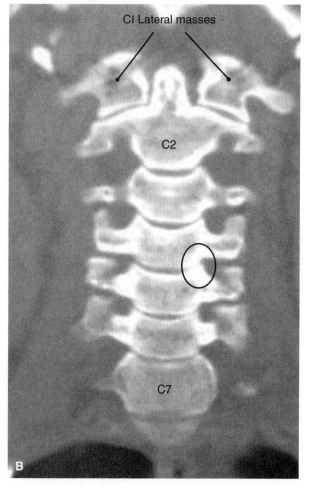

Figure 7-7 CT reformatted as **(A)** sagittal and **(B)** coronal views of the cervical spine. The first intervertebral disk space is at C2–C3. Uncinate processes articulate with adjacent bodies to form uncovertebral joints (oval).

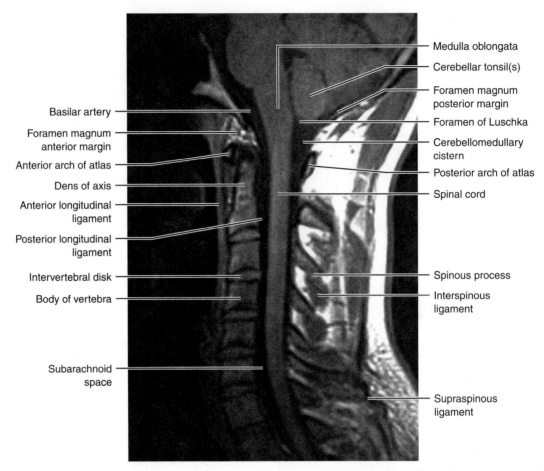

Basilar artery

Foramen magnum anterior margin

Anterior arch of atlas

Dens of axis

Anterior longitudinal ligament

Posterior longitudinal ligament

Intervertebral disk

Body of vertebra

Subarachnoid space

Medulla oblongata

Cerebellar tonsil(s)

Foramen magnum posterior margin

Foramen of Luschka

Cerebellomedullary cistern

Posterior arch of atlas

Spinal cord

Spinous process

Interspinous ligament

Supraspinous ligament

Figure 7-8 MRI, sagittal view of the cervical spine with ligaments and major structures labeled. *(Image courtesy of www.medcyclopedia.com.)*

Joint Mobility

The cervical spine possesses great mobility, allowing for a wide range of movements for the head. Combined motions at all cervical spine joints produce about 145 degrees of flexion and extension, 180 degrees of axial rotation, and 90 degrees of lateral flexion. The unique structural anatomy of the upper cervical joints produces unique functional mobility. The cervical joints below C2 are similar in their functional contributions to cervical mobility.

Approximately 10 to 15 degrees of both flexion and extension are possible at the atlanto-occipital joint. Less than 10 degrees of lateral flexion is possible to each side, and very minimal or no rotation occurs at this articulation.

The atlantoaxial joint is the most mobile segment of the cervical spine. Approximately 50 degrees of rotation is possible to each side, accounting for half of the rotation mobility present in the entire cervical spine. Less than 10 degrees of both flexion and extension takes place, and minimal or no lateral flexion exists.

All the cervical joints below C2 allow for flexion, extension, rotation, and lateral flexion. Distributed from C3 through C7 are approximately 40 degrees of flexion, 25 degrees of extension, 45 degrees of rotation to either side, and 50 degrees of lateral flexion to either side.

Growth and Development

The process of ossification of the vertebrae begins in the sixth week of fetal life. At birth at least three primary ossification centers are present at each vertebral level. (See the radiograph of an infant skeleton, Fig. 11-7.)

The anterior arch of the atlas is completely cartilaginous at birth (Fig. 7-10). Complete fusion of the synchondroses will unite the anterior arch by age 8 and the posterior arch by age 4. The odontoid process is formed by two vertically positioned ossification centers. The odontoid fuses inferiorly to the vertebral body between the ages of 3 and 6. The superior tip fuses by age 12 (Fig. 7-11).

The bodies of the axis and the lower vertebrae are ossified at birth. The neural arches and spinous processes fuse by the age of 2 or 3. The posterior spinal elements then fuse with vertebral bodies between the ages of 3 and 6. The vertebral bodies are wedge-shaped anteriorly until they take on a more squared-off shape by age 7. After age 8 the cervical spine has attained its gross adult form (Fig. 7-12).

Continued vertebral growth throughout childhood occurs via periosteal apposition, similar to the periosteal growth of long bones. At puberty, secondary centers of ossification develop in the superior and inferior endplates of the vertebral bodies. Secondary ossification centers also

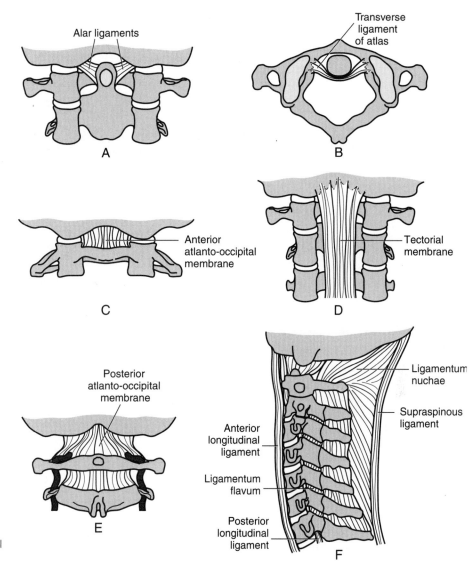

Figure 7-9 (A–F) Ligaments of the cervical spine.

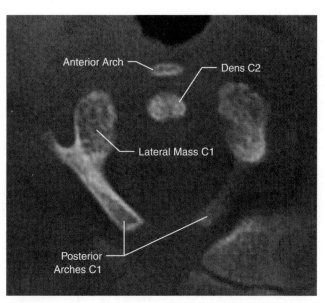

Figure 7-10 Axial CT of a 10-month-old child's atlas. Note that only ossification centers are visible. Much of the atlas is cartilaginous at this age.

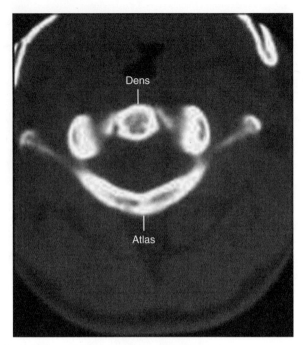

Figure 7-11 Axial CT of the atlas at skeletal maturity.

appear for the bifid spinous processes, transverse processes, and articular processes at this age. Each of these structures completes fusion by age 25.

The uncovertebral joints are not present in early life and appear to be the result of degenerative fibrotic changes associated with normal aging.

Postural Development

At birth the spinal column exhibits one long curve, which is convex posteriorly: the *primary curve* of the spine. As the baby learns to lift its head from prone lying, the *secondary curve of cervical lordosis* begins to develop (Fig. 7-13). The onset of walking develops the secondary curve of *lumbar lordosis*. These secondary curves continue to develop until the growth of the vertebral column matures postpuberty.

Postural changes in the spine throughout adult life appear to be influenced by multiple factors including genetics, health, occupation, and type of recreational activities. Degenerative conditions and disease processes often render characteristic alterations in spinal posture (Fig. 7-14). Trauma to the spine or any extremity may affect spinal posture as the body attempts compensatory strategies to lessen pain. The cervical spine appears to adapt with the additional goal of maintaining the eyes in a forward and horizontal orientation.

Routine Radiologic Evaluation[8–20]

Practice Guidelines for Spine Radiography in Children and Adults[8]

The American College of Radiology (ACR), the principal professional organization of radiologists in the United States, defines the following practice guidelines as an

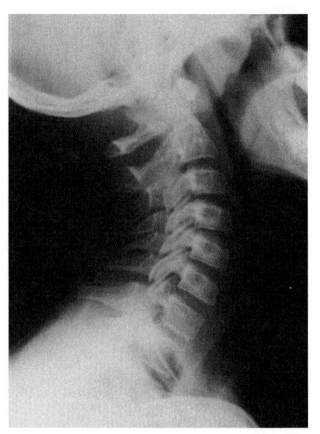

Figure 7-12 Normal radiographic appearance of the cervical spine of an 11-year-old female, lateral view. The vertebrae exhibit their gross adult form, although the anterior vertebral bodies still show some slight wedging. The tips of the spinous processes have just begun to fuse.

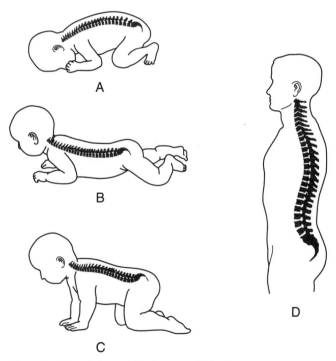

Figure 7-13 (A–D) Postural development of spinal curvatures progresses from the primary convex curve of the newborn **(A)** to the secondary concavities of the cervical and lumbar spines in the adult **(D)**.

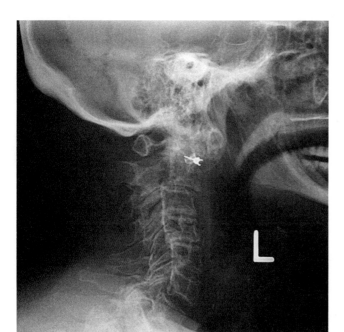

Figure 7-14 Lateral radiograph of a patient with advanced rheumatoid arthritis. The progression of the disease has caused an erosion of the odontoid process as well as a complete loss of the normal lordotic curve of the spine. Note the kyphosis at C2 to C4, resulting in an "S" shaped spine. The metal artifact is an earring. *(Image courtesy of John C. Hunter, MD, University of California, Davis School of Medicine.)*

educational tool to assist practitioners in providing appropriate radiologic care for patients.

Goals

The goal of cervical spine radiographic examination is to identify or exclude anatomic abnormalities or disease processes of the spine.

Indications

The indications for radiologic examination include but are not limited to trauma, shoulder or arm pain, occipital headache, limitation in motion, planned or prior surgery, evaluation of primary and secondary malignancies, arthritis, suspected congenital anomalies and syndromes associated with spinal abnormality, evaluation of spinal abnormality seen on other imaging studies, follow-up of known abnormality, and suspected spinal instability.

Basic Projections and Radiologic Observations

A complete examination includes the entire cervical spine from the craniocervical junction to the superior endplate of the first thoracic vertebra. Standard projections include *anteroposterior (AP)* and *lateral views*. An *open-mouth AP view* may be indicated, depending on clinical circumstances. A *swimmer's lateral* projection should be performed if necessary to assess the lower cervical segments and cervicothoracic junction.

In trauma cases with significant clinical suspicion of cervical spine fracture, *cross-table lateral, AP,* and *AP open-mouth* views should be obtained on the immobilized patient prior to moving the patient for further examination.

Additional projections may be needed in some clinical circumstances. Bilateral *oblique* projections can be obtained when assessment of the neural foramina is necessary. Flexion-extension lateral views can assess instability. *Articular (pillar) views* should be considered if a facet fracture is suspected on the initial examination.

In the pediatric population, *AP, AP open-mouth,* and *lateral* radiographs are sufficient for most clinical indications. Additional views are less often necessary than in adults but include the same views just discussed. Examination of pediatric patients at a high risk for instability (such as those with Down's syndrome) should include active *lateral flexion/extension views*.

Trauma at the Cervical Spine[4,31–33]

Diagnostic Imaging for Trauma of the Cervical Spine

Controversy exists regarding what is the most efficient imaging protocol for patients with acute trauma to the cervical spine. In the past it has been accepted that radiographs are obtained first. However, computed tomography (CT) has been found to be significantly more sensitive to detecting subtle injuries, and better at visualizing the craniovertebral and cervicothoracic junctions. Additionally, MRI is recommended for any patient with a neurological deficit for its ability to demonstrate the position of bony fragments as well as injury to the spinal cord, disk, and soft tissues in the same exam. Thus, radiographic examination is not necessary in patients with suspected *significant* injury, if these advanced modalities are available. Significant injury includes fracture, dislocation, or instability.

Two evidence-based guidelines have been established to help the clinican decide if a patient has the potential for a significant cervical spine injury and if radiographic examination *is* or *is not* necessary. The *Canadian C-Spine Rule (CCR)* and the *National Emergency X-Radiography Utilization Study (NEXUS)* identify similar clinical criteria. To summarize, patients who have sustained an acute trauma *should* have radiography if the mechanism of injury was dangerous (diving accident, fall from a height, motor vehicle accident), are older than 65 years of age, have paresthesias in the extremities, have midline tenderness over the spine, or are unable to rotate the neck 45 degrees to the left and right.

If the patient meets the clinical criteria of the CCR or NEXUS guidelines, current *ACR Appropriateness Guidelines for Suspected Spinal Trauma* recommend CT with sagittal and coronal reformatting or both CT and MRI as complementary studies to assess instability or myelopathy. See Chapter 18 for more on clinical decision rules and ACR Guidelines for variants of suspected spine trauma.

Routine Radiologic Evaluation of the Cervical Spine

Anteroposterior Open-Mouth

This view demonstrates the articulation of C1 and C2, the atlantoaxial joint. The patient is positioned with the mouth wide open to remove the superimposition of the density of the mandible from obscuring the upper cervical spine.

Radiologic Observations

The important observations are:

1. The atlas is positioned symmetrically on the axis. The widths of the lateral masses should be equal (*a, a* in Fig. 7-15). Asymmetry in the widths of the lateral masses suggests rotation of the atlas. The lateral mass with the wider dimension is the side with anterior rotation.
2. The lateral borders of the lateral masses of the atlas should not appear more lateral than the superior articular processes of C2 (*b, b* in Fig. 7-15). An "overhanging" of the atlas suggests fracture or dislocation. A mild degree of overhanging may be a normal variant in children.
3. The dens is positioned symmetrically between the lateral masses of the atlas, shown by equal dimensions of vertical space on either side of the dens (*c, c* in Fig. 7-15).
4. The bilateral joint spaces at the lateral atlantoaxial facet articulations are of equal height (*d, d* in Fig. 7-15).
5. The C2 spinous process is positioned in the midline (*e* in Fig. 7-15).
6. The dens is superimposed on both the anterior and posterior arches of the atlas. The borders of the arches image as lines that cross over the dens. These border images must be distinguished from fracture lines.

Any alterations in these landmarks may be indicators of ligamentous laxity or tear, fracture, or dislocation, relative to the atlanto-occipital and atlantoaxial articulations.

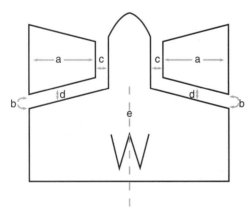

Figure 7-15 Radiographic spatial relationships at C1–C2.

Basic Projections

- **AP open-mouth**
- AP lower C-spine
- Lateral
- Right oblique
- Left oblique

Setting up the Radiograph

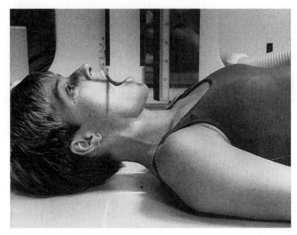

Figure 7-16 Patient position for AP open-mouth cervical spine radiograph.

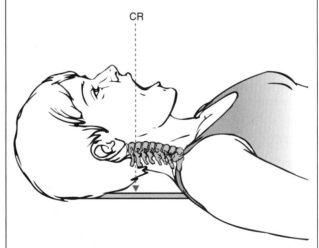

Figure 7-17 The central ray passes through the C1–C2 joint space.

What Can You See?

Look at the radiograph (Fig. 7-18) and try to identify the radiographic anatomy. Trace the outlines of structures using a marker and transparency sheet. Compare results with the book tracing (Fig. 7-19). Can you identify the following:

- Long curved line that is the base of the occiput
- Angle of the mandible
- Dens and body of C2
- Anterior arch of the atlas
- Posterior arch of the atlas
- Lateral atlantoaxial facet joints
- Transverse processes of the atlas
- Bodies and spinous processes of C2 through T1

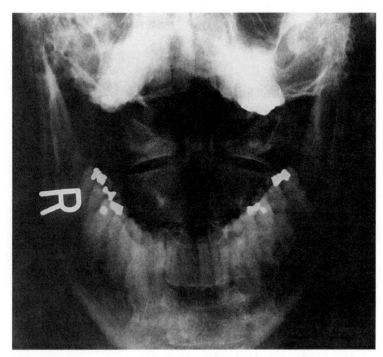

Figure 7-18 AP open-mouth cervical spine radiograph.

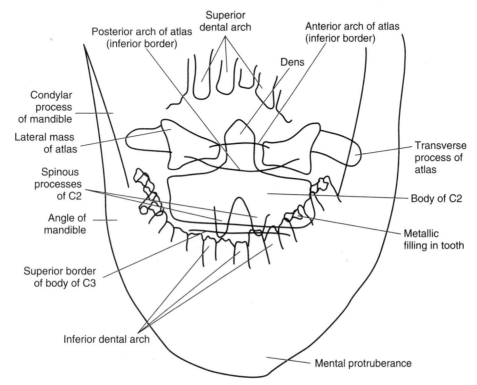

Figure 7-19 Tracing of AP open-mouth cervical spine radiograph.

Routine Radiologic Evaluation of the Cervical Spine

Anteroposterior Lower Cervical Spine

This view demonstrates the five lower cervical vertebrae, the upper thoracic vertebrae and associated ribs, medial thirds of the clavicles, and trachea. The superimposition of the mandible and skull will obscure the upper cervical vertebrae. In identifying the level of cervical vertebrae, remember that the joint C2–C3 possesses the first intervertebral disk and T1 possesses the first rib articulation.

Radiologic Observations

The important observations are:

1. The cervical and thoracic vertebral bodies are aligned in a relatively vertical column.
2. The spinous processes are positioned in the midline throughout the spine. The distance from the spinous process to the lateral borders of the vertebral body should be equal on either side of the spinous process (*a, a* in Fig. 7-20). Note normal irregularities in the shape of the processes.
3. The superimposition of the overlapping facet joints and articular pillars creates a radiographic illusion of one smoothly undulating column of bone on either side of the vertebral bodies, the "lateral column."
4. The transverse processes are mostly within the image of this lateral column. The superimposed densities of the lateral column make the transverse processes difficult to discern.
5. The pedicles are also somewhat superimposed by the lateral column image but can be identified by their radiodense oval-like cortical outline. Like that of the spinous processes, this image is analogous to the image created by the pipe radiographed end-on (see Fig. 1-12C).
6. The interpedicular distance between opposing paired pedicles is typically 30 mm in the cervical spine (*b* in Fig. 7-20).
7. The disk spaces are not evaluated in this frontal view. The sagittal plane of the lordosis and the angle of the

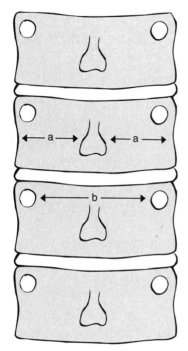

Figure 7-20 Radiographic spatial relationships of AP cervical spine.

Basic Projections

- AP open-mouth
- **AP lower C-spine**
- Lateral
- Right oblique
- Left oblique

Setting up the Radiograph

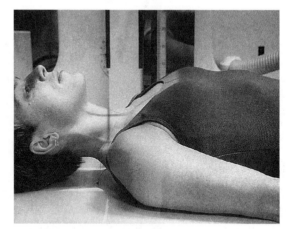

Figure 7-21 Patient positioning for AP lower cervical spine radiograph.

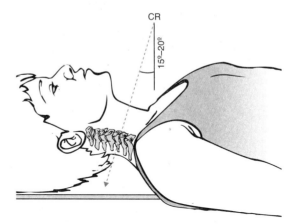

Figure 7-22 The central ray is angled 15 to 20 degrees cephalad, enters below the thyroid cartilage, and passes through the C5–C6 joint space.

central ray results in some distortion and prevents the true dimensions of the disk spaces from being visualized. The lateral view best demonstrates disk spaces.

8. Note the uncinate processes extending from the superior vertebral bodies and the formation of uncovertebral joints at some levels.
9. Note the radiolucent image of the air-filled trachea overlying the cervical spine at midline.
10. The clavicles are farthest from the film plate and thus are imaged with the greatest degree of size distortion in comparison to the other structures. Note the *magnification* of the radiographic image of the clavicles.

What Can You See?

Look at the radiograph (Fig. 7-23) and try to identify the radiographic anatomy. Trace the outlines of structures using a marker and transparency sheet. Compare results with the book tracing (Fig. 7-24). Can you identify the following:

- Vertebral bodies of C3 through T1 (note the presence of *uncinate processes* at some levels)

- Spinous processes of C3 through T1
- Large transverse process of T1
- First ribs and costotransverse joints
- Clavicles
- Air-filled trachea

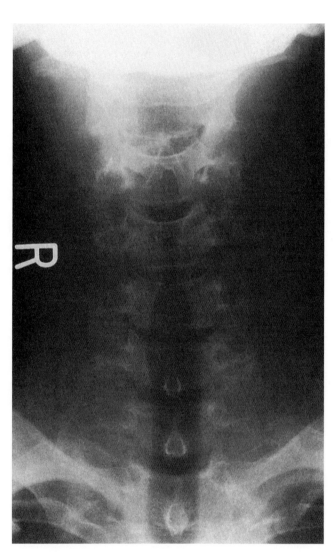

Figure 7-23 AP lower cervical spine radiograph.

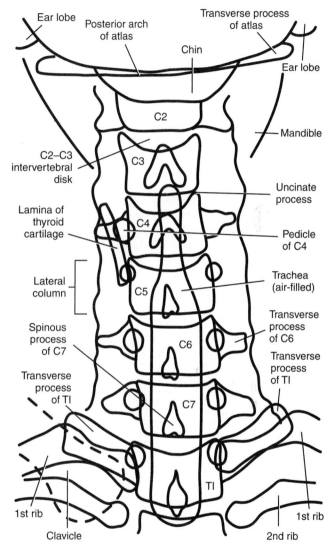

Figure 7-24 Tracing of AP lower cervical spine radiograph.

Routine Radiologic Evaluation of the Cervical Spine

Lateral

This view demonstrates the seven cervical vertebrae, intervertebral disk spaces, articular pillars and facet joints, spinous processes, and prevertebral soft tissues.

Radiologic Observations

The important observations are:

1. The alignment of the lateral cervical spine can be imagined as three roughly parallel lines (*a* in Fig. 7-25). In a normal spine, *the spatial relationship of these lines will remain constant whether the neck is positioned in neutral, flexion, or extension.* Disruption of this spatial relationship may be due to fracture, dislocation, or severe degenerative changes.

   - *Line 1:* The anterior borders of the vertebral bodies normally align in a lordotic curve. Osteophytes may project anteriorly and are thought to be traction spurs from tension at the attachment of the anterior longitudinal ligament or related to degenerative intervertebral disk changes. They are ignored in evaluating the *spatial* relationships of these lines.
   - *Line 2:* The posterior borders of the vertebral bodies normally follow the same curve as the anterior bodies. Osteophytes that project from this line encroach upon the spinal canal and intervertebral foramina and have the potential to compress the spinal cord or nerve roots.
   - *Line 3:* The spinolaminar line is the junction of the lamina at the spinous processes. This line represents the posterior extent of the central spinal canal. The spinal cord lies between lines 2 and 3.

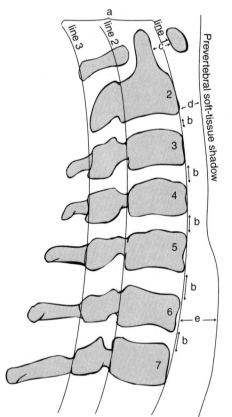

Figure 7-25 Radiographic spatial relationships in lateral view of the cervical spine.

172

Basic Projections

- AP open-mouth
- AP lower C-spine
- **Lateral**
- Right oblique
- Left oblique

Setting up the Radiograph

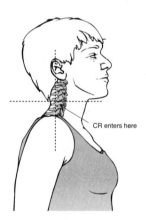

Figure 7-26 Patient position for lateral cervical spine radiograph.

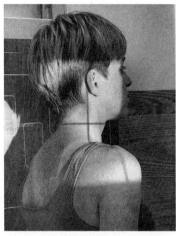

CR enters here

Figure 7-27 The central ray passes horizontally through the C4–C5 joint space.

2. The vertebral bodies are box-like in appearance with distinct, smoothly curved osseous margins. Note any osteophyte formation as described earlier.
3. The intervertebral disk spaces are well preserved in height at each level (*b* in Fig. 7-25).
4. The articular pillars and facet joints are superimposed as a pair at each level. The facet joints can be individually defined on the oblique views, but the lateral view is best for visualizing joint margins and joint spaces.
5. The bursa between the dens and its articulating facet on the atlas is represented by the dark radiolucent line anterior to the dens. This *atlantodental interface* or *predental space* is a

distance kept constant by the transverse ligament of the atlas during all neck ranges of motion (*c* in Fig. 7-25). Upper limits of this distance in adults is 2.5 mm. In younger children, the upper limits are 4.5 mm. See the lateral flexion–extension films for more information regarding this point.

6. The transverse processes are superimposed over the vertebral bodies.

7. The retropharyngeal space is the distance from the posterior pharyngeal wall to the anteroinferior aspect of C2 (*d* in Fig. 7-25). It normally measures 6 mm or less. Distention of the soft tissue shadow is often the result of hemorrhage or effusion and is a sign of trauma.

8. The retrotracheal space is the distance from the posterior wall of the trachea to the anteroinferior aspect of C6 (*e* in Fig. 7-25). It normally measures 22 mm in adults and 14 mm in children. A helpful way to remember these prevertebral soft tissue distances in adults is "6 at 2 and 22 at 6."

What Can You See?

Look at the radiograph (Fig. 7-28) and try to identify the radiographic anatomy. Trace the outlines of structures using a marker and transparency sheet. Compare results with the book tracing (Fig. 7-29). Can you identify the following:

- Arches of C1
- Dens
- Vertebral bodies of C2 through C7
- Articular pillars and lamina (note the facet joints formed by adjacent articular processes)
- Intervertebral disk spaces from C2–C3 through C6–C7
- Spinous processes (note the vertebra prominens of C7)
- Transverse processes
- Facet joint surfaces

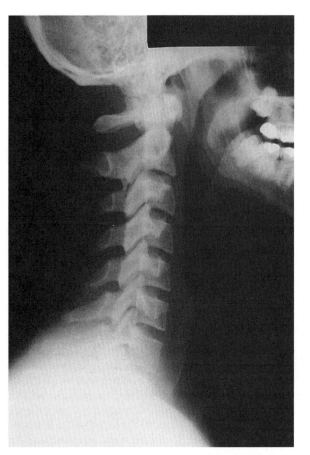

Figure 7-28 Lateral cervical spine radiograph.

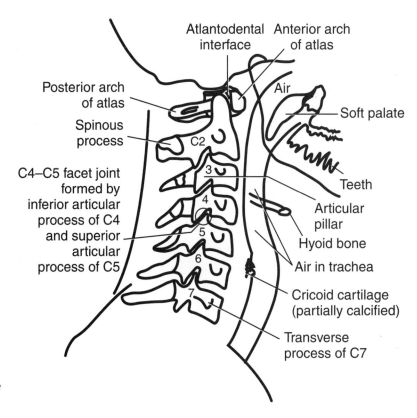

Figure 7-29 Tracing of lateral cervical spine radiograph.

Routine Radiologic Evaluation of the Cervical Spine

Right and Left Obliques

This view demonstrates the intervertebral foramina, uncovertebral joints, facet joints, and pedicles of the cervical vertebrae. Both right and left obliques are obtained so that each of these structures is viewed individually, as opposed to the lateral view, which superimposes the posterior vertebral elements.

Radiologic Observations

The important observations are:

1. The intervertebral foramina, through which the spinal nerves exit, are normally imaged as radiolucent ovals (*a* in Fig. 7-30). Narrowed, ragged margins of the ovals may indicate bony encroachment on the spinal nerves. The contralateral foramina are not seen. The intervertebral foramina are named by spinal segment (e.g., the C4–C5 foramen or the C5–C6 foramen).

2. In this view the head and body are in neutral alignment and rotated as a unit 45 degrees from the lateral view. The 45-degree rotation may be to either side of the lateral, depending on the preference of the facility. A left anterior oblique (LAO) projection (the patient's left anterior neck is closest to the film plate) will image the *open left intervertebral foramina,* and the right anterior oblique (RAO) will image the *open right intervertebral foramina.* Conversely, the left posterior oblique (LPO) projection (the patient's left posterior neck is closest to the film plate, as in Figure 7-31B) images the right intervertebral foramina, and the right posterior oblique (RPO), as in Figure 7-31A, images the left intervertebral foramina. See Chapter 1 for positioning diagrams. This distinction is rarely discussed in daily exchanges except by radiographic technicians. Referring to "the right oblique" means that the patient's right-side IV foramina are visible; it is not always critical to know whether the image was obtained as RAO or LPO.

Basic Projections

- AP open-mouth
- AP lower C-spine
- Lateral
- **Right and left obliques**

Setting up the Radiograph

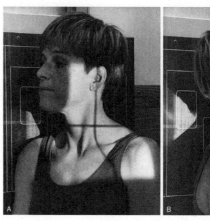

Figure 7-31 Patient position for **(A)** right posterior oblique and **(B)** left posterior oblique cervical spine radiograph.

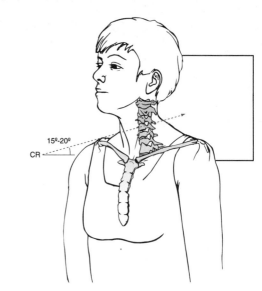

Figure 7-32 For the posterior oblique view, the central ray is angled 15 to 20 degrees cephalad, passing through C4.

3. The pedicles are viewed *en face* or parallel to the image receptor; minimal distortion is imposed. The contralateral pedicles are superimposed behind the vertebral bodies and image as tubes seen end-on.

4. The irregular shape of the laminae, becoming larger in descending vertebrae, is normal. They too image as a structure seen end-on.

What Can You See?

Look at the radiographs (Fig. 7-33) and try to identify the radiographic anatomy. Trace the outlines of structures using

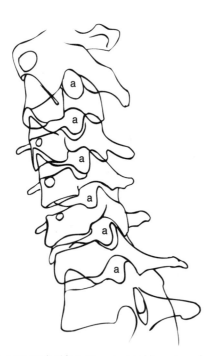

Figure 7-30 Intervertebral foramina seen on oblique view of cervical spine.

a marker and transparency sheet. Compare results with the book tracings (Fig. 7-34). Can you identify the following:

- Vertebral bodies
- Pedicle, lamina, and spinous process at each level

- Inferior and superior articulating processes of the facet joints
- Intervertebral foramina
- Contralateral pedicle
- Angle of the mandible
- Thoracic ribs

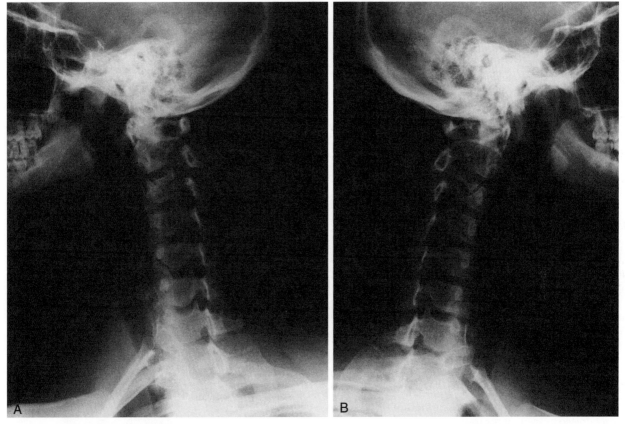

Figure 7-33 **(A)** Right posterior oblique cervical spine radiograph. **(B)** Left posterior oblique cervical spine radiograph.

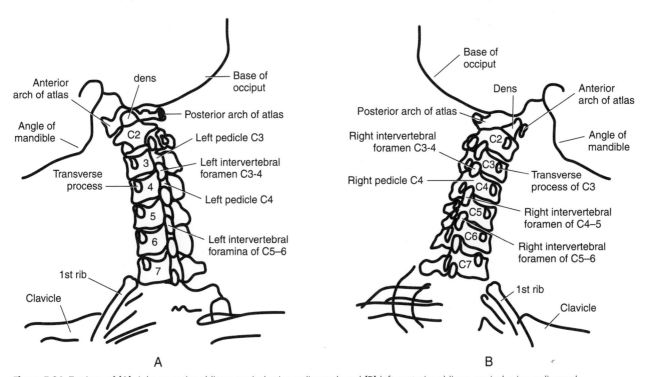

Figure 7-34 Tracings of **(A)** right posterior oblique cervical spine radiograph and **(B)** left posterior oblique cervical spine radiograph.

Optional Projections for Radiologic Evaluation of the Cervical Spine

Lateral Flexion and Extension Stress Views

These projections are not part of the routine radiographic examination of the cervical spine but are common optional projections. The purpose of these projections is to observe joint alignment while the supporting soft tissue structures are stressed by gross neck flexion or extension positions. Thus, these views are also referred to as *stress films* or *functional studies* because they examine the joints at the end ranges of voluntary flexion and extension. Joint instabilities that were not apparent on the routine lateral view may be effectively demonstrated here.

Radiologic Observations

The important observations are:

1. As noted on the routine lateral projection, the spatial relationship of the three parallel lines designating normal cervical spine alignment (see Fig. 7-25) will, under normal conditions, remain constant through any degree of flexion or extension. Note the preservation of this relationship on these normal films. Disruption of this spatial relationship may be due to fracture, dislocation, or severe degenerative changes.

2. The cortical outlines of the vertebral bodies, articular pillars, and spinous processes appear as on the routine lateral projection. The joint positions will change slightly on these views, however. In *flexion,* the anterior intervertebral disk spaces narrow and the posterior intervertebral spaces and interspinous spaces widen. In *extension,* the anterior intervertebral spaces widen and the posterior intervertebral spaces and interspinous spaces narrow.

3. The *atlantodental interface,* represented by the radiolucent line anterior to the articulating facet of the dens, is recognized as seen on the routine lateral view. The width of this space will, under normal conditions, remain constant in any degree of flexion or extension. An increase in this distance to more than 3 mm indicates C1–C2 subluxation. (See Fig. 2-38 for a radiographic example of an increased atlantodental interface, representing C1–C2 joint instability.)

Optional Projections

- **Lateral flexion and extension stress views**

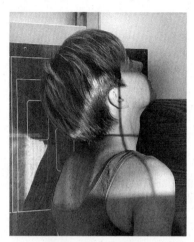
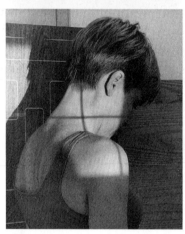

Figure 7-35 Patient position for lateral views of cervical spine in **(A)** extension and **(B)** flexion.

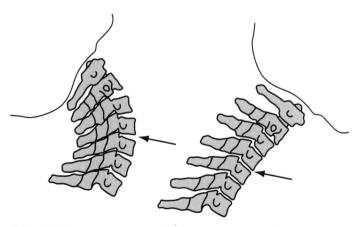

Figure 7-36 The central ray passes horizontally through C4–C5.

What Can You See?

Look at the radiographs (Fig. 7-37) and verify the relationships shown in the drawings (Fig. 7-38).

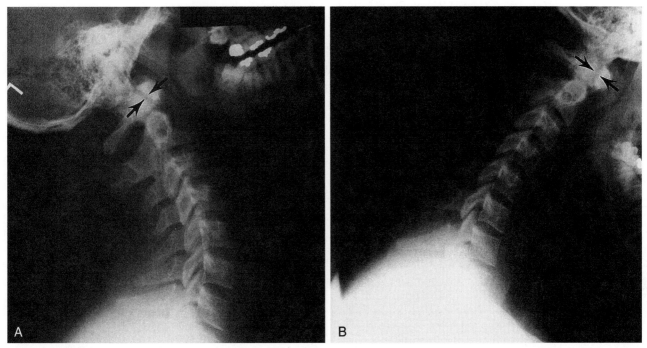

Figure 7-37 **(A)** Lateral extension and **(B)** flexion stress radiographs of the cervical spine. Arrows indicate the atlantodental interface, which has remained at a constant distance in either radiograph.

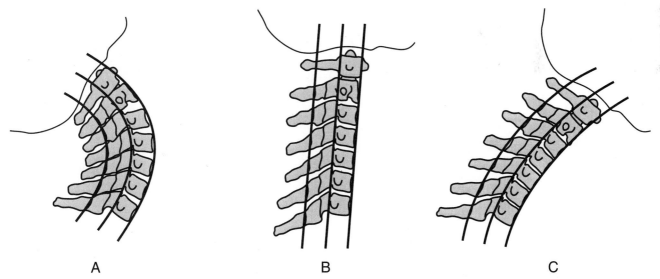

Figure 7-38 The lines of reference for vertebral alignment remain constant whether the neck is positioned **(A)** in extension, **(B)** neutrally, or **(C)** in flexion.

Cross-Table Lateral

The lateral view is the first radiograph made and evaluated if the patient has a history of trauma and is not being evaluated in a trauma center where advanced imaging is readily available. The significance of the lateral view is that normal cervical alignment is easily evaluated in the aforementioned series of parallel vertebral line images. Discontinuity or obvious step-offs in bony alignment may indicate the presence of fracture or dislocation. In severe trauma cases the cross-table lateral view, performed on a supine, immobilized patient, functions as a preliminary diagnostic screen. The majority of cervical spine injuries can be grossly identified on the lateral view.

Lateral Flexion and Extension Stress Views

The lateral flexion and extension stress views are performed to expose excessive segmental motion during functional movement. At times there is sufficient historical evidence or patient symptoms to support the presence of serious injury, but little radiographic evidence of such. Consider that conventional radiographs are static pictures that capture the joints only at one point in time. Instability may be present, but the joint position at that moment may not show it. Stress films give the joints more opportunity to reveal instability by imposing mechanical stress on them. A normal conventional radiograph on a patient who exhibits clinical signs or symptoms of joint instability (such as spinal cord compression signs) warrants further imaging studies.

Radiologic Signs of Cervical Spine Trauma

Evaluation of radiographs for significant signs of cervical trauma includes examination of the soft tissues, vertebral alignment, and joint characteristics (Table 7-1).

Abnormal soft tissue signs include (1) widened retropharyngeal or retrotracheal spaces, (2) displacement of the trachea or larynx, and (3) displacement of the prevertebral fat pad. Any of these signs suggest the presence of edema or hemorrhage, indicating associated pathology.

Abnormal vertebral alignment signs include (1) loss of the parallelism as outlined for the lateral view, indicating fracture, dislocation, or severe degenerative changes; (2) loss of lordosis, indicating muscle spasm in response to underlying injury; (3) acute kyphotic angulation with a widened interspinous space, indicating rupture of the posterior ligaments; and (4) rotation of a vertebral body, indicating unilateral facet dislocation, a hyperextension fracture, muscle spasm, or disk or capsular injury.

Abnormal joint signs are (1) widened atlantodental interface, indicating degeneration, stretching, or rupture of the transverse ligament; (2) widened interspinous process space (known as "fanning"), indicating rupture of interspinous and other posterior ligaments; (3) widened intervertebral disk space, indicating posterior ligament rupture; (4) narrowed intervertebral disk space, indicating rupture of disk and extrusion of nuclear material; and (5) loss of facet joint articulation, indicating dislocation.

Potential Injury to the Spinal Cord and Spinal Nerves

Stable Versus Unstable Injuries

Injuries to the cervical spine are first broadly classified as stable or unstable injuries, in reference to the immediate or subsequent potential risk to the spinal cord and spinal nerve roots. Stable injuries are protected from significant bone or joint displacement by intact posterior spinal ligaments. Examples of stable injuries are compression fractures, traumatic disk herniations, and unilateral facet dislocations. Unstable injuries may show significant displacement initially or have the potential to become displaced with movement. Examples of unstable injuries are fracture–dislocations and bilateral facet dislocations.

C1–C2 and C6–C7 are the most frequently injured levels in the cervical spine. Adults characteristically injure their lower cervical spine and children more frequently injure their upper cervical spine. Cervical spine fractures, overall, have a 40% incidence of associated neurological injury. Approximately two-thirds of all spinal cord injuries occur in the cervical spine.

SCIWORA Syndrome

The spinal cord can also be injured without fracture or dislocation. This is known as the *SCIWORA* syndrome, an acronym for *spinal cord injury without radiographic abnormalities*. It is predominant in children, due to the inherent elasticity in the pediatric spine. Causes include ligamentous injury and cartilaginous vertebral endplate fractures. Instability would be revealed on lateral flexion and extension views or with visualization of soft tissue

---

TABLE 7-1 ● Radiologic Signs of Cervical Trauma

Abnormal Soft Tissues
Widened retropharyngeal space (normally 2–5 mm at C2–C4)
Widened retrotracheal space (normally 18–22 mm in adults at C5–C7)
Displacement of prevertebral fat pad
Tracheal displacement
Laryngeal displacement

Abnormal Vertebral Alignment
Reversal of lordosis
Acute kyphotic angulation
Rotation of vertebrae
Widened intervertebral space
Step-offs in vertical alignment

Abnormal Joint Relationships
Widened atlantodental interspace
Widened interspinous space
Widened intervertebral disk space
Narrowed intervertebral disk space
Facet disarticulation

disruption via advanced imaging. In adults, acute disk prolapse and/or excessive buckling of the ligamentum flavum into a canal that is already compromised by posterior vertebral body osteophytes can result in a central cord syndrome.

Fractures

Mechanism of Injury

The mechanism of cervical spine injury is broadly classified as either being direct force, such as in a blow to the head, or indirect force, such as the rapid acceleration and deceleration of the body in a motor vehicle accident. Mechanisms of injury are further defined by the motion or position of the neck during the injury. The cervical spine will suffer injury when forced past the extreme end ranges of extension, flexion, lateral flexion, or rotation or when axially loaded by compression (as when the head strikes the windshield). A summary of the injuries that can happen as a result of these mechanisms is presented in Table 7-2.

Characteristics of Cervical Spine Fractures

Two fracture configurations are characteristically seen in the cervical spine: *avulsion fractures* and *compression or impaction fractures*. Avulsions occur as a bone fragment is pulled off by violent muscle contraction or, more commonly, by the passive resistance of a ligament applied against an oppositely directed force. For example, an avulsion of the C7 spinous process may occur as a result of forceful contraction of the rhomboids and trapezius or of the resistance of the supraspinous and interspinous ligaments during hyperflexion.

Compression or impaction fractures will result when adjacent vertebrae are forced together. For example, an axial compression force will cause a comminuted or "burst" fracture of the impacted vertebral body. A flexion force will compress the impacted vertebral body into an anterior wedge shape. An extension force will fracture and compress the articular pillars.

Descriptions of some common fractures specific to levels in the cervical spine follow.

Fractures of the Atlas (C1)

A common compression fracture at atlas is a posterior arch fracture, sustained during a hyperextension force that compresses the arch between the occipital condyles and posterior elements of axis. Another common compression fracture occurs through both the anterior and posterior arches of the atlas, called a burst fracture or Jefferson fracture. The mechanism of this fracture is axial compression that forces the occiput onto the atlas. Diving into shallow water head-first and motor vehicle accidents are the usual causative actions. Atlas fractures are rarely associated with neurological injury.

Imaging

Diagnosis of fractures at the atlas can be difficult on conventional radiographs. The AP open-mouth view may demonstrate a lateral shift in the lateral masses of C1 or a spreading out of the lateral masses. CT scans are definitive in diagnosis. However, if a horizontal fracture occurs across the anterior arch, it can be missed on an axial CT slice. Sagittal and coronal CT reformations are valuable to disclose these injuries. Post healing, lateral flexion and extension stress views assess stability.

Treatment

Generally, the patient is immobilized in halo traction for 6 to 8 weeks, followed by a cervical brace for 6 to 8 weeks. Less stable fractures require prolonged halo traction. Chronic instability or pain sometimes necessitates C1–C2 fusion. Rehabilitation to restore range of motion usually begins 4 months after injury.

Fractures of the Axis (C2): The Pedicles

A common compression fracture of the axis is the bilateral fracture of the pedicles, causing a dislocation of C2 on C3. This fracture–dislocation is called a traumatic spondylolisthesis and also a hangman's fracture, because it bears a pathological skeletal resemblance to the fatal characteristics of a judicial execution by hanging. The precipitating mechanism is hyperextension, as seen in motor vehicle accidents. These fractures are unstable.

Imaging

Lateral radiographs demonstrate this fracture well. CT can define compromise of the spinal canal and MRI is used to provide information on the spinal cord.

Treatment

Treatment is determined by the amount of displacement and stability present and may include rigid cervical orthosis, halo traction, or fusion of C2–C3. Rehabilitation after healing addresses restoration of mobility, strength, and function.

Fractures of the Axis: The Dens

Dens (odontoid process) fractures comprise about 20% of cervical spine fractures. They have a high association with other fractures of the cervical spine, and there is a 10% incidence of associated neurological involvement. Dens fractures are divided into type I, an avulsion of the tip caused by alar or apical ligament stress; type II, a fracture at the junction of the dens to the body, most common and most difficult to heal; and type III, a fracture deep below the junction, which heals readily. The mechanism for these fractures is usually a motor vehicle accident in younger adults and a simple fall in the elderly.

Imaging

Dens fractures can be difficult to visualize on the AP open-mouth view because the arches of the atlas, or the

TABLE 7-2 ● *Cervical Spine Injuries*

Structures Involved	Mechanism	Appearance	Stable +/–
Hyperflexion sprain: Disruption of superficial posterior ligaments and capsules with transient anterior subluxation of vertebral joints	Hyperflexion		+
Bilateral facet joint dislocation	Hyperflexion		–
Disruption of alar, apical, and transverse ligaments; possible C1–C2 dislocation; possible odontoid fracture	Hyperflexion		–
Avulsion fracture of spinous process, "clay shoveler's fracture"	Hyperflexion		+
Unilateral facet dislocation	Hyperflexion + rotation		+
Anterior vertebral body compression fracture; "wedge fracture"	Hyperflexion ± compression		+
Anterior inferior vertebral body fracture with posterior displacement of the rest of the vertebra; "flexion teardrop fracture"	Hyperflexion ± compression		±
Fracture-dislocation at C1–C2	Hyperflexion ± compression		–
Fracture-dislocation at any other vertebral segments C3–C7	Rotation		–
Unilateral facet dislocation	Rotation		+
Dislocation of C1 on C2	Rotation		–

TABLE 7-2 ● *Cervical Spine Injuries (continued)*

Structures Involved	Mechanism	Appearance	Stable +/−
Odontoid fracture	Rotation		±
Fracture of anterior and posterior arches of C1; "Jefferson fracture"	Axial compression		−
Comminuted fracture of vertebral body; "burst fracture"	Axial compression		±
Hyperextension sprain: disruption of anterior ligaments and soft tissues with transient posterior subluxation	Hyperextension		+
Anteroinferior vertebral body fractures	Hyperextension		±
Posteriorly displaced odontoid fractures	Hyperextension		−
Avulsion fracture of the anterior arch of C1	Hyperextension		+
Fracture of the posterior arch of C1	Hyperextension		+
Fracture of the pedicles of C2 with dislocation of the body of C2 on C3; "hangman's fracture"	Hyperextension		−
Fracture of the uncinate process	Lateral flexion		+
Avulsion fracture of transverse process	Lateral flexion		+

(continued)

TABLE 7-2 ● *Cervical Spine Injuries (continued)*

Structures Involved	Mechanism	Appearance	Stable +/−
Lateral compression fracture of vertebral body	Lateral flexion		+
Compression fracture of articular pillar	Lateral flexion		+

teeth, may be superimposed. Axial CT scans can miss dens fractures oriented in the horizontal plane, but coronal reconstructions demonstrate them well (Fig. 7-39). Some clinicians advocate the use of three-dimensional CT reconstruction as both a diagnostic aid and also as a surgical template.

Treatment

Treatment depends on type, stability, and whether other fractures of the cervical spine are present. Treatment can include rigid cervical orthosis, halo traction, screw fixation through the odontoid, or late fusion to achieve stability. Rehabilitation addresses neurological deficits, if present (which can range from Brown-Séquard syndrome to hemiparesis or quadriparesis) and general restoration of mobility, strength, and function.

Fractures of C3–C7

Fractures of the mid- and lower cervical vertebrae may occur at any site on the vertebral structure. Some of the more commonly seen fractures are:

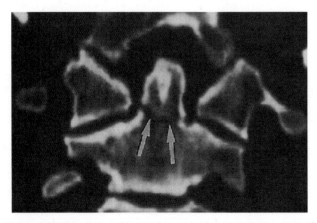

Figure 7-39 Type II dens fracture (arrows), located at the junction of the base to the body, is the most common and most difficult to heal. This is a CT image reformatted to the coronal plane.

- *Wedge fracture:* This fracture occurs when an interposed vertebra is compressed anteriorly by two adjacent vertebrae owing to hyperflexion forces. Two-thirds of these fractures in the cervical spine occur at C5, C6, or C7. This fracture is stable because ligamentous structures are at least partially intact (Fig. 7-40).
- *Burst fracture:* This fracture occurs when an intervertebral disk is axially compressed and the nucleus pulposus is driven through an adjacent vertebral endplate, causing a literal bursting apart of the vertebral body and resulting in comminution. This fracture may be stable or unstable, depending on the fracture configuration (Fig. 7-41).
- *Teardrop fracture:* This fracture occurs when a triangular fragment of bone is separated from the anteroinferior corner of the vertebral body because of either an avulsion force sustained during hyperextension or a compressive force sustained during hyperflexion. The flexion teardrop fracture is the most severe of the lower cervical fractures. The force necessary to cause this fracture is often associated with additional injury, such as intervertebral disk tearing, ligament rupture, and facet dislocation, rendering this a potentially unstable injury. The posterior displacement of the vertebral body can cause anterior cord compression, resulting in quadraplegia (Fig. 7-42).
- *Articular pillar fracture:* The articular pillar, the rhomboid structure composed of the superior and inferior articulating processes, is fractured by a compressive hyperextension force combined with a degree of lateral flexion. This fracture occurs most frequently at C6 and is usually a stable injury.
- *Clay shoveler's fracture:* This fracture is an avulsion fracture of the spinous process produced by hyperflexion forces or forceful muscular contraction of the trapezius and rhomboids often associated with the repetitive heavy labor of the upper extremities, as seen in shoveling. Occurring most frequently at C6, C7, and T1, this fracture is stable (see Fig. 7-40A).
- *Transverse process fracture:* This uncommon fracture, when present, usually occurs at the largest transverse process in the cervical spine, C7. This fracture usually results from lateral flexion forces causing an avulsion at the tip of the contralateral transverse process.

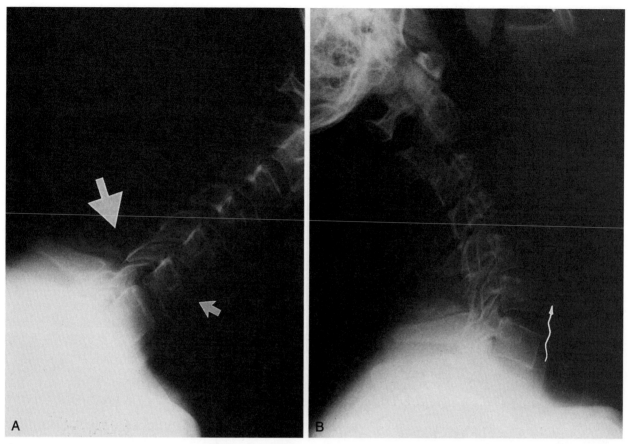

Figure 7-40 Lateral hyperflexion and hyperextension films of the cervical spine in a 38-year-old woman involved in a motor vehicle accident. **(A)** Note the avulsion fracture of the spinous process of C6 (large arrow). A compression fracture is present at the anterior superior corner of the vertebral body of C6 (small arrow). **(B)** Hyperextension film shows widening of the C6–C7 interspace (wavy arrow). The wide interspaces are signs of ligamentous disruption at that segment.

Imaging

Radiologic imaging consists of AP, AP open-mouth, and lateral views. If an instability is suspected and the patient is without neurological complaint, willing, cooperative, and fully conscious, flexion and extension stress views are obtained. CT with reconstructions may be obtained to characterize fracture patterns and assess the degree of spinal canal compromise. MRI may be used to delineate spinal cord, disk, and canal abnormalities further. Follow-up imaging studies are used to monitor the progress of healing as well as segmental stability.

Treatment

Initially, in the emergency setting, stable fractures are immobilized with a cervical orthosis, and unstable fractures are immobilized with tong traction to decompress the canal indirectly. After imaging studies are completed and the extent of injuries is defined, treatments vary depending on stability. Conservative treatment for stable fractures involves some kind of rigid orthosis (such as a Philadelphia collar, four-poster brace, other cervicothoracic brace, or halo traction). Operative treatments can achieve stabilization via interspinous wiring, bilateral plating, anterior plating, and bone grafts.

Dislocations

Dislocations in the spine are described by the direction that the superior vertebra of the segment moved. For example, an anterior dislocation of C2–C3 indicates that C2 displaced anteriorly on C3.

Dislocations Associated With Fractures

The most serious and life-threatening injuries to the cervical spine are fracture–dislocations (see Fig. 7-41). In the upper cervical spine, a fracture through the base of the dens combined with a ligament rupture will cause a fracture–dislocation of the atlantoaxial joint, C1–C2. The hangman's fracture of the axis, described earlier, is usually associated with anterior dislocation of C2 on C3. At any lower vertebral level, fractures of the posterior vertebral structures combined with tears of the posterior ligaments may cause a vertebral body to displace anteriorly, transecting or contusing the spinal cord.

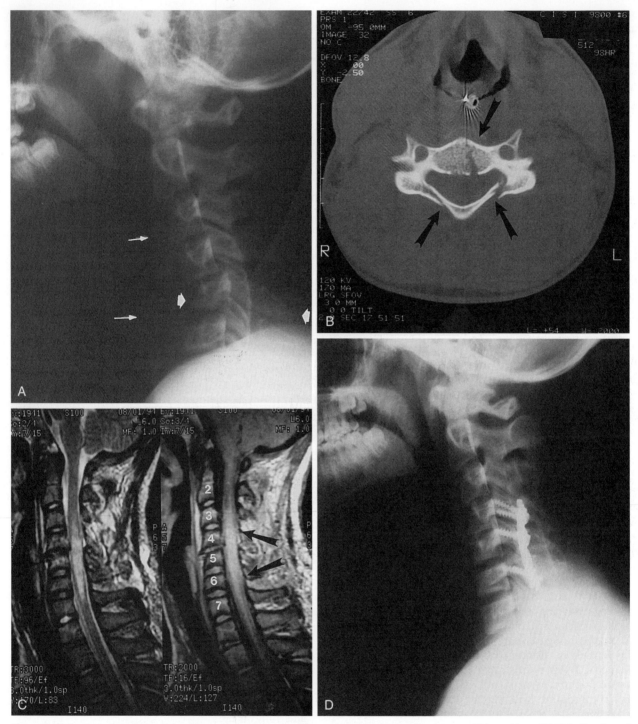

Figure 7-41 Fracture–dislocation of the fifth cervical vertebra in a 15-year-old boy who was in a motor vehicle accident. **(A)** Plain film, lateral view, shows the posterior displacement of the C5 vertebra (wide arrows). Small arrows point to the prevertebral shadow (normal soft tissue image of the anterior neck), which is displaced anteriorly because of edema. **(B)** CT axial view of C5 shows a burst fracture of the vertebral body and fractures of both laminae (arrows). **(C)** MRI, sagittal plane, reveals edema of the spinal cord from the level of C3 through C7 (arrows). **(D)** Plain film, lateral view, of internal fixation restoring vertebral alignment and stabilizing the spinal segments.

Dislocations Not Associated With Fractures

Dislocations not associated with fractures may be either complete or self-reducing and are in reference to the facet joints. In self-reducing dislocations, a force momentarily disengages the articulations, which then return to normal alignment once the force dissipates. These momentary dislocations are also referred to as transient dislocations or subluxations. It is critical to remember that transient joint injuries will not be revealed on radiographs; the joint has

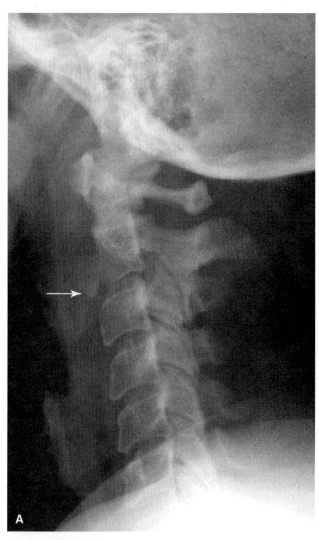
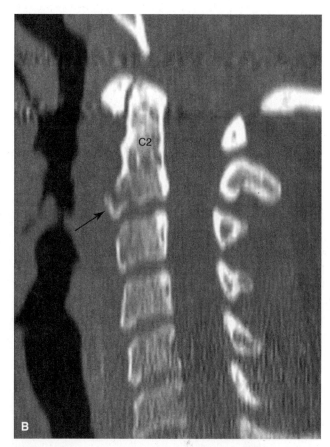

Figure 7-42 (A) Lateral radiograph of the cervical spine with a anteroinferior fracture of the body of C2 (arrow), known as a teardrop fracture. **(B)** Same patient, CT sagittal reformation, with white arrow pointing to triangular fragment on the body of C2. *(Image courtesy of John C. Hunter, MD, University of California, Davis School of Medicine.)*

returned to its normal position. Soft tissue signs may give clues to the severity of the prior insult. The absence of abnormal radiologic findings puts the responsibility on the clinician to exercise caution at all times in the evaluation maneuvers performed on any patient with a cervical spine injury.

Complete facet joint dislocation may occur *unilaterally* at a segment as a result of a flexion–rotation force or *bilaterally* as a result of a hyperflexion force. In either case, the inferior articulating process of the uppermost vertebra will come to lie in front of the superior articulating process of the subjacent vertebra, locking the joint out of normal articulation; hence the term *locked facets* (Fig. 7-43).

Unilateral facet dislocations tear one facet capsule and the posterior ligaments. In the absence of vertebral body

subluxation, unilateral facet dislocation is a stable injury. Frequently, however, there is a 25% anterior subluxation of the vertebral body (observed as a step-off at the anterior vertebral body line). These patients are at risk for nerve root injury or, rarely, Brown-Séquard–type spinal cord injury.

Bilateral facet dislocations are unstable injuries because of the extensive disruption of the posterior ligaments, the facet joint capsules, the annulus fibrosus, and sometimes the anterior longitudinal ligament. These dislocations are frequently associated with spinal cord injuries (Fig. 7-44).

C1–C2 Rotary Subluxation and Dislocation

Atlantoaxial rotary subluxation occurs when the forces of flexion or extension combine with rotation to cause one inferior facet of C1 to slip anterior to the superior facet of C2 and become fixed in this position. In some cases, it can occur spontaneously without a history of trauma. The patient presents with marked limitation of motion, especially

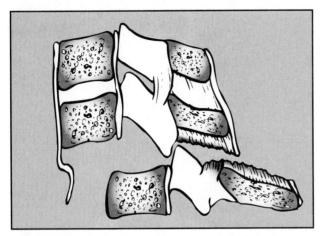

Figure 7-43 Schematic of bilateral cervical facet joint dislocation.

toward the subluxed side. In chronic cases, patients may present with torticollis.

Imaging AP open-mouth radiographs demonstrate asymmetry of the joint space between the dens and the lateral masses of the atlas. Lateral radiographs may demonstrate the inferior facet of C1 positioned anterior to the superior facet of C2.

Treatment Reduction involves traction techniques supplemented by active range-of-motion exercises to restore alignment. Immobilization with a cervical orthosis for several weeks follows reduction.

C3–C7 Dislocations

Imaging On the lateral view, dislocations of single facet joints may be difficult to see because of superimposition of the pair of facet joints. A clue to facet dislocation is in the alignment of the posterior vertebral body line; anterior displacement of the vertebral body is evident with facet dislocation. Unilateral facet dislocation can result in forward displacement up to 25% of the AP diameter of the disk

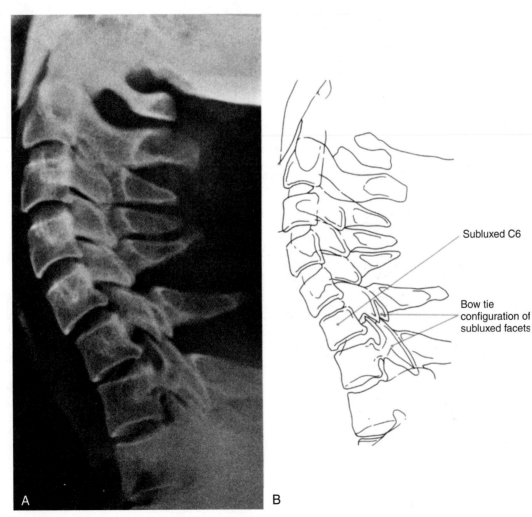

Subluxed C6

Bow tie configuration of subluxed facets

A   B

Figure 7-44 Bilateral facet joint dislocation at C6–C7.

space. Bilateral facet dislocation can result in at least 50% forward subluxation.

On the AP view, facet dislocation may result in a wide interspinous space at one level and an abnormally wide intervertebral disk space. Deviation in spinous process alignment may also be evident. Oblique radiographs are necessary to view the facet joints.

Treatment Reduction is achieved with traction techniques, either manual mobilization techniques or mechanical techniques via skull traction and applied weights. Some patients require several weeks of postreduction immobilization in a cervical orthosis because of rupture of the posterior ligament complex. Rare cases that cannot be reduced by closed methods or those that demonstrate persistent instablity on flexion and extension stress films may require open reduction and surgical fusion.

Cervical Spine Sprains

Cervical sprains are injuries to the ligaments of the spine. The terms *hyperflexion* and *hyperextension sprains* more accurately define the mechanism of injury, direction of force, and the ligaments susceptible to disruption. The layman's term *whiplash* is often substituted for these terms.

Hyperflexion Sprains

Hyperflexion sprains disrupt the posterior ligament complex. The posterior ligament complex includes all of the posterior ligaments and the facet joint capsules. With extreme force, injury to the posterior annulus fibrosus and posterior aspect of the intervertebral disk, transient facet dislocations, avulsion fractures of the spinous processes, and impaction fractures of the anterior vertebral bodies may occur (see Fig. 7-40). The magnitude of the force, direction, and degree of flexion determine the injury severity and number of structures compromised.

Imaging

Tears of the posterior ligaments allow the superior vertebra of a segment to rotate or translate anteriorly on its subjacent vertebra. That vertebral segment will no longer align in a normal lordotic curve and will instead show a *hyperkyphotic angulation* on the lateral radiograph (Fig. 7-45). Thus, the injured segment appears to be *flexed,* whereas the remainder of the spine is in relatively neutral alignment.

At times the posterior complex may be torn, but the lateral radiograph does not reveal any signs of joint instability. If there is a history of trauma and joint instability or hypermobility, or if either is clinically suspected or needs to be ruled out, lateral flexion and extension stress films should be obtained. These two films are then evaluated to identify joint hypermobility revealed by misalignment (excessive angulation or excessive glide) of the injured segment. Misalignment is judged by referencing the anatomic spatial relationship of the lines described on the routine neutral lateral film. Routine radiographs also screen for associated fractures.

Hyperextension Sprains

Hyperextension sprains result when the neck is forced past the end ranges of extension. Hyperextension injuries

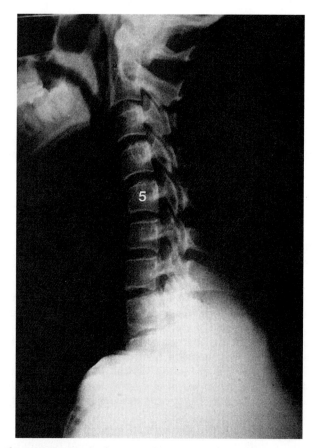

Figure 7-45 Hyperkyphotic angulation of a spinal segment. Lateral view of the cervical spine of a 40-year-old woman with complaints of chronic neck pain. The only history of injury was an incident 5 years earlier whereby the patient ran into a wall while playing racquetball. The most striking feature is the loss of cervical lordosis and the hyperkyphotic angulation of the C4–C5 and C5–C6 segments. Assuming that there were no professional errors in positioning the patient for this view, one possible assumption is that a ligamentous injury occurred at one or more segments in the past and adaptive shortening of the soft tissues has occurred over time. Lateral hyperflexion and hyperextension films would provide valuable information regarding the segmental mobility available.

may happen as an isolated injury, or as a rebound action of the head and neck following hyperflexion. Severe sprains disrupt the anterior ligaments and soft tissues, resulting in a transient posterior subluxation of the vertebral segment. Associated vertebral fractures can occur when increased magnitude of the extension force converts to a compressive force. Compression during hyperextension is due to the parallel pull of the neck flexor muscles on the spine while the vertebrae are already in bony approximation.

Imaging

The lateral view may demonstrate vertebral misalignment secondary to ligamentous or intervertebral disk disruption. Lateral flexion and extension stress views are obtained to evaluate joint stability (Fig. 7-46). Routine radiographs screen for associated fractures.

Treatment

The length of immobilization varies according to the severity of soft tissue disruption. Soft or rigid cervical orthoses are used to provide support and allow tissues time to heal. Pain management with medication and therapeutic modalities is helpful in the acute stages. Rehabilitation focuses on restoration of normal posture, joint arthrokinematics, active movement, and strength.

Intervertebral Disk Herniations

Acute Injury

Acute disk herniation that results in nerve root compression is uncommon in the cervical spine, owing to inherent anatomic protection. The anteriorly positioned nucleus pulposus, posteriorly reinforced annulus fibrosus, wide and double-layered posterior longitudinal ligament, and uncovertebral joints offer security to the disks that is lacking in the more commonly herniated lumbar intervertebral disks. Traumatic injury to the cervical spine may, however, cause a posterior or lateral disc herniation that results in neural compression. The patient seeks medical attention for radiating arm pain.

Intervertebral disks that herniate without causing neural compression are more common but are not as recognized; the patient does not suffer significant symptoms. Additionally, acute disk injuries may result in anterior herniations or intravertebral herniations, which also do not cause neural compression.

Imaging

Conventional radiographs are of little diagnostic value in the diagnosis of acute cervical disk herniation. Myelography, CT–myelography, and MRI are used, often in combination, to assist in determining treatment protocols or necessity for surgery (Fig. 7-47).

Chronic disk herniations result in degenerative changes that are visible on conventional radiographs (see the discussion of degenerative disk disease in the following section).

Treatment

Conservative treatment usually involves medications to decrease inflammation, such as nonsteroidal anti-inflammatory drugs or short-term steroids, pain management, and therapeutic modalities to relieve symptoms, such as cervical spine traction, joint mobilization, soft tissue techniques to reduce spasm, and therapeutic modalities.

Surgical treatment is considered when conservative treatment fails to improve symptoms over a length of time. Anterior cervical diskectomy, with or without fusion via preformed bone grafts and sometimes plating, has been the most common procedure of recent decades. Posterior approaches for microlaminectomy or microforaminotomy with diskectomy without fusion are more recent developments.

Degenerative Diseases of the Cervical Spine[12,25,32–38]

Degenerative changes can involve the cervical spine at multiple sites:

1. Degeneration of the intervertebral disks leads to the condition known as *degenerative disk disease (DDD)*.
2. Osteoarthritic changes at the synovial facet joints of the cervical spine lead to the condition known as *degenerative joint disease (DJD)* of the cervical spine.
3. Diminished normal dimensions of the intervertebral foramina secondary to degenerative changes in adjacent structures lead to the condition known as *foraminal encroachment*.
4. Osteophyte formation at joint margins leads to the condition known as *cervical spine spondylosis*.
5. Advanced spur formation from degeneration of the vertebral bodies and annulus fibrosus lead to the condition known as *spondylosis deformans*.
6. Flowing ossification along the anterior vertebral bodies and disk spaces is known as *diffuse idiopathic skeletal hyperostosis (DISH)*.

It is common practice, in both the literature and verbal exchanges, to use some of these terms interchangeably. The word *spondylosis*, for example, is frequently used as a general descriptor for any degenerative change in the vertebral segment. The most effective communication, however, avoids generalities and employs anatomically exact information.

Degenerative Disk Disease

Evidence of degenerative disk disease (DDD) is seen radiographically in most persons over age 60. Degenerative changes in the disk may include dehydration, nuclear herniation, annular protrusion, and fibrous replacement of the annulus. These degenerative changes within the disk cause an overall decrease in disk height. As the intervertebral space decreases, the vertebral endplates approximate. Uncovertebral joints experience excessive friction, which leads to osteophyte formation at the articulation site and eventually around the entire osseous margin of the endplates. DDD also presents with *Schmorl's nodes* (intravertebral herniation of nucleus pulposus through the vertebral endplate into the spongiosa of the vertebral body) and *vacuum phenomenon* (nitrogen gas from extracellular spaces accumulates in the degenerative dehydrated fissures of the disk).

Imaging

The radiographic hallmark of DDD is decreased height of the disk space as assessed on the lateral view (Fig. 7-48). Schmorl's nodes are identified as radiolucent focal defects in the vertebral endplates. Osteophytes at the uncovertebral joints and vertebral endplates can be seen on the lateral or AP view. The vacuum phenomenon presents as a horizontally oriented

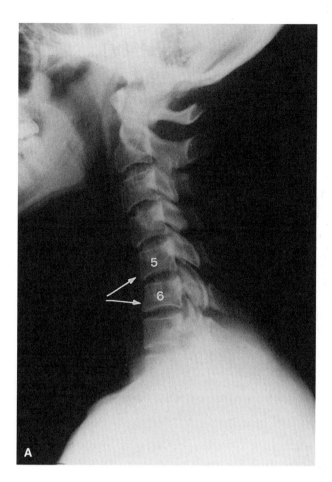

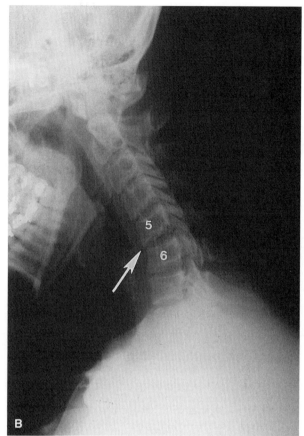

Flexion

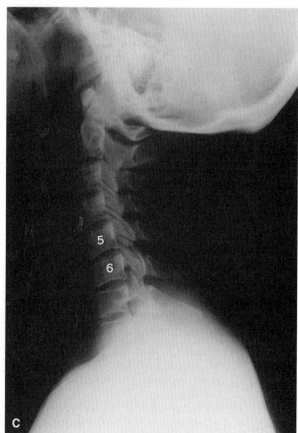

Extension

Figure 7-46 Cervical sprain. This 22-year-old woman sustained a hyper-flexion–hyperextension sprain to her cervical spine while driving in a demolition derby contest. **(A)** Plain film, lateral view, shows a loss of cervical lordosis and hyperkyphotic angulation at C5–C6. **(B)** Lateral flexion film shows slight anterior displacement of C5 on C6 (arrow) and widening of the C5–C6 interspinous space. **(C)** Extension film shows reluctance or inability of patient to hyperextend the neck and a persistent hyperkyphotic angulation of the C5–C6 segment. These findings suggest ligamentous disruption at the C5–C6 segment.

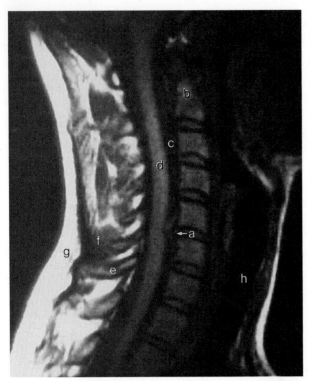

Figure 7-47 Sagittal MR image of the cervical spine. A posterior intervertebral disk herniation is present at C5–C6 (a). Other structures are the dens (b), cerebrospinal fluid (c), spinal cord (d), spinous process of C6 (e), muscle (f), skin and fat (g), and trachea (h).

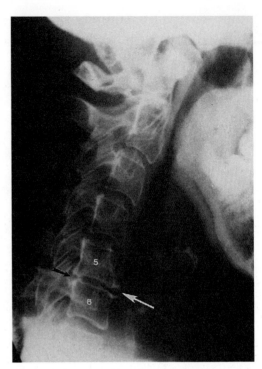

Figure 7-48 Degenerative disk disease of the cervical spine. On this lateral view decreased disk space is evident at C5–C6. Note the osteophyte formation both anteriorly (white arrow) and posteriorly (black arrow).

radiolucency within the disk space. Only in very advanced cases of DDD are all of these characteristics radiographically present.

Degenerative Joint Disease

Degenerative joint disease (DJD) of the cervical spine involves osteoarthritic changes of the facet joints. The facet joints are vulnerable to DJD because of the great mobility of the cervical spine, postural strains, and repetitive occupational or recreational actions that contribute to the abnormal tissue and joint biomechanics and biochemistry. As in degenerative joint disease elsewhere in the body, articular facets undergo articular cartilage thinning, subchondral bone sclerosis, eburnation, and development of osteophytes at joint margins. Cervical spine DJD may develop in isolation or concomitantly with degenerative disk disease. Indeed, one process often predisposes or accelerates the joint's development of the other process.

Imaging

The hallmarks of DJD—decreased joint space, subchondral sclerosis, and osteophytosis—are observed in the facet joints on either the lateral view or the oblique view (Fig. 7-49).

Foraminal Encroachment

Foraminal encroachment is the result of degenerative changes in adjacent structures, including DDD and DJD, that diminish the size of the intervertebral foramina. The spinal nerve root that exits through a structurally constricted foramen is susceptible to mechanical compression. The resultant radiating arm pain is what brings the patient to seek medical attention.

Imaging

The oblique views permit assessment of the intervertebral foramina. Encroachment can be seen as a narrowing of the radiolucent ovals that represent the foramina (Fig. 7-50). Be aware that only ossified degenerative changes are visible on the radiograph. Fibrotic thickening of the facet capsule, for instance, will not be evident, but it will contribute to constriction of the space the nerve has available through which to exit.

Cervical Spine Spondylosis

Cervical spine spondylosis is the formation of osteophytes in response to degenerative disk disease. Osteophyte formation has been shown to be most predominant at the points in the curvatures of the spine farthest from the center of gravity line, or at the apices of the concavities, as a result of greater segmental mobility. In the cervical spine these sites are at C4–C5 and C5–C6. Osteophyte formation may be the body's attempt to repair friction damage or to protect from friction

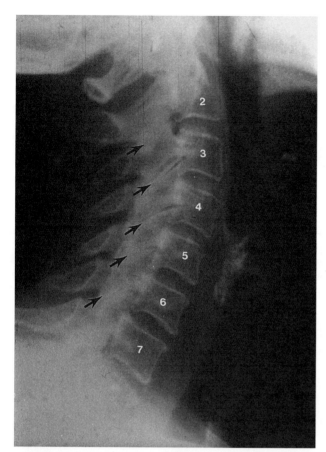

Figure 7-49 Degenerative joint disease of the cervical spine. On this lateral view of the cervical spine the black arrows indicate the facet joint spaces. Note the narrowing of the joint spaces and sclerosis of the articular surfaces at all levels. Note also that the disk spaces at all levels are well preserved and without degenerative changes. This is true degenerative joint disease of the cervical spine; that is, the facet joints show the classic hallmarks of osteoarthritis.

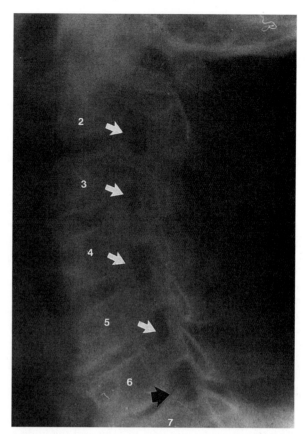

Figure 7-50 Foraminal encroachment is best demonstrated on the oblique view of the cervical spine. Arrows indicate the foramina. Note the foramen of C2–C3 not constricted by any osteophyte (spur) formation. The remaining foramina show varying amounts of encroachment. The most severely compromised level is C6–C7 (black arrows). Note the large osteophytes projecting from the posterior bodies of these two vertebrae.

damage, but osteophytes can become a source of friction themselves. Osteophyte protrusion from the vertebral endplates into the intervertebral foramina will narrow the passageway of the spinal nerves, contributing to foraminal encroachment.

Imaging

Osteophytes are visible on the AP, lateral, or oblique views as radiodense irregularities at vertebral joint margins.

Spondylosis Deformans

Spondylosis deformans is a degenerative condition characterized by anterior and lateral vertebral endplate osteophytosis that results from anterior or anterolateral disk herniation. Initiating factors in the development of this condition may be abnormalities in the peripheral fibers of the annulus that weaken the attachment of the disk to the endplate. In contrast to DDD, the intervertebral disk spaces are not decreased in height.

Imaging

The AP or lateral views will demonstrate the osteophytes, often clawlike in formation, cupping toward the intervertebral disk (see Fig. 11-53).

More than one vertebral segment is involved; however, this condition is to be differentiated from the characteristic multiple level involvement of DISH, discussed in the following subsection.

Diffuse Idiopathic Skeletal Hyperostosis

Diffuse ideopathich skeletal hyperostosis (DISH) is different from spondylosis deformans, although both involve extensive osteophytosis. DISH has an undefined etiology, although investigators have associated it with diabetes, growth hormone, vitamin A or retinoid derivatives, and metabolic syndromes. DISH appears to develop around age 40 and to increase with age; it appears more frequently in men. The most common sites of involvement are the middle to lower thoracic spine and upper lumbar spine as well as the lower cervical spine.

Clinical symptoms of DISH are mild pain and stiffness. Although uncommon, patients may develop dyspnea, dysphagia, aspiration pneumonia, myelopathies, peripheral nerve entrapment, or tendinitis.

Imaging

Assessed on the lateral view, three radiographic criteria define DISH and distinguish it from spondylosis deformans:

1. Flowing ossification along the anterolateral aspects of at least four contiguous vertebral bodies
2. Relative preservation of disk height and absence of radiographic evidence of DDD
3. Absence of facet joint DJD or sacroiliitis

A condition related to DISH is *ossification of the posterior longitudinal ligament (OPLL)*. OPLL may develop alone or in conjunction with DISH. Some studies show OPLL present in 50% of patients with DISH. The cervical spine is most commonly involved.

OPLL appears on the lateral view as a thin, linear calcification running parallel and posterior to the vertebral bodies. A radiolucent cleft may be sandwiched between the calcified ligament and the vertebral bodies.

Clinical Considerations of the Degenerative Spine

Significant for the clinician to appreciate is that all of these degenerative processes are slow to form and the body has time to adapt. However, the body may at some time reach limits in its ability to adapt. At this point, the cervical spine may become symptomatic to even minor trauma. The normal, nondegenerative spine has a margin of safety in its elastic capsules, resilient and flexible ligaments, hydrated and cushioning disks and cartilage, and wide-open foramina. The degenerative spine, in contrast, has lost its margin of safety and, in trauma, suffers greater dysfunction and requires longer time to heal. A review of the acute patient's radiographs, with special observation of the underlying chronic degenerative changes, is necessary to understand the patient's pain pattern and assist in developing a comprehensive treatment plan.

Degenerative changes cannot be reversed. However, the surrounding environment of the joints can be optimized to prevent or control pain and preserve functional range of motion. Rehabilitation can include (1) segmental mobilization techniques to restore joint mobility, (2) therapeutic exercise to balance muscle strength and flexibility to promote optimal posture, (3) patient education in occupational and leisure activity accommodations that decrease stressful postures or maladaptive behaviors, and (4) therapeutic modalities such as cervical traction, heat/cold, and ultrasound to provide relief of acute symptoms.

Cervical Arthroplasty: Total Disk Replacement

When conservative treatment fails and neural decompression is sought, the standard surgical treatment has been anterior cervical diskectomy and fusion. The immediate benefit of this procedure is neural decompression and relief of radicular symptoms. The long-term disadvantage is accelerated degenerative changes in the intervertebral segment *above* the fused level. As an alternative to fusion, *cervical arthroplasty* with a prosthetic total disk replacement that preserves intervertebral motion has been performed since the early 1990s in Europe, and over the past few years in the United States. Refinement of cervical arthroplasty in terms of materials and models continues, and although more long-term studies are needed, this procedure appears to have the potential to fundamentally change the field of spine surgery (Fig. 7-51).

Cervical Spine Anomalies[2,28]

Congenital or developmental anomalies of the spine appear with frequency at the transitional segments or junctions of the curvatures. The atlanto-occipital region and the lumbosacral region are common sites of anomalies. Spinal anomalies consist of one or more of the following in a structure:

1. Failure to develop
2. Arrested development
3. Development of accessory bones
4. Asymmetrical structural development

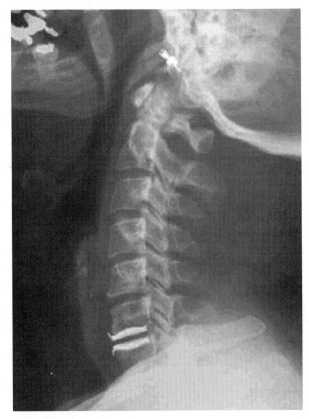

Figure 7-51 Cervical arthroplasty with placement of an artifical disc at C6–C7. One of two models currently approved by the Food and Drug Administration, this Bryan device consists of a polyethylene core between the two metal endplates. The core acts as a spacer and is shaped so that the endplates pivot in a way that imitates normal motion of the two vertebrae. There are small prongs on one side of each endplate. The prongs help anchor the endplate to the surface of the vertebral body.

Spinal anomalies may occur in isolation or in combination with other spinal, visceral, and soft tissue malformations.

Clinically significant in cervical spine anomalies, especially in the upper cervical region, is the potential for joint instability. Mobilization, manipulation, manual resistance, or traction applied without prior knowledge of the anomaly may result in neurological deficit, paralysis, or even death.

Although spinal anomalies are present in only a small portion of the general population, the potentially devastating effects of mishandling these patients warrants the clinician's attention to any spinal structural variant.

Examples of cervical anomalies, their clinical significance, radiographic features, and appearance are presented in Table 7-3. See Figures 7-52, 7-53 for radiographic examples.

TABLE 7-3 ● Cervical Spine Anomalies

Anomaly	Clinical Considerations	Radiographic Features	Appearance
Atlas			
Occipitalization of C1	No motion possible at AO joint. Excessive compensatory motion at subjacent joints with resultant degenerative joint changes.	Lateral film: see decreased or absent space between occiput and posterior arch.	
Agenesis of posterior arch of C1	Transverse ligament integrity may be compromised; possible AA instability.	Lateral film: absent posterior neural arch, enlarged anterior arch (from stress), enlarged C2 spinous process representing fusion of rudimentary posterior arch with spinous process.	
Absence of transverse ligament	AA joint instability; possible cord compression.	Lateral flexion film: required to determine AA stability.	
Axis			
Dens anomalies: Ossiculum terminale—failure of tip of dens to unite	Usually no clinical significance.	View dens anomalies on AP open-mouth films: cephalic portion of dens separate from peg, bounded by smooth osseous margins.	
Os odontoideum—failure of dens to unite with body of C2	Possible AA joint instability. Associated with Klippel–Feil and Morquio syndromes; present in 20% of Down's syndrome cases.	Dens separated from body by a radiolucent cleft. Lateral flexion film required to determine AA joint stability.	
Hypoplastic dens— abbreviated development	Possible AA instability.	Small, malformed dens. Lateral flexion film required to determine AA stability.	
Cervical Vertebrae			
Block vertebrae—two adjacent vertebrae fused at birth. Partial or complete fusion of bodies, facets, spinous processes	No motion at fused segment. Excessive compensatory motion at adjacent free joints with resultant degenerative changes Most common at C5–C6, C2–C3; associated with Klippel–Feil syndrome.	Lateral film: Small AP diameter of bodies with indented "waspwaist" fused intervertebral disk space. Facets fused in 50% of cases. Spinous processes may be fused or malformed.	
Sprengel's deformity— congenital elevation of scapula	Present in 25% of Klippel–Feil syndrome cases; frequently associated with scoliosis, block vertebrae, spina bifida occulta, hemivertebrae, and cervical ribs.	AP film: 30%–40% of cases have an omovertebral bone appearing as a bony bar projecting from the lamina of C7 to the vertebral border of the scapula.	

(continued)

TABLE 7-3 ● *Cervical Spine Anomalies (continued)*

Anomaly	Clinical Considerations	Radiographic Features	Appearance
Cervical Vertebrae			
Cervical ribs—extra bone projecting from and sometimes forming a joint with transverse process	Possible source of compression in thoracic outlet syndrome. Most common at C7, less often present at C6 and C5; often bilateral but usually asymmetric in size and shape.	AP film: rib projecting caudally from cervical transverse process. (Thoracic ribs project cephalically.) Joint may be formed at distal end of rib. When no joint is formed distally, there is sometimes a fibrous band anchoring the distal rib. A fibrous band would not appear on radiograph but could contribute to compression of the NV bundle.	
Spina bifida occulta—failure of laminae to unite and form a spinous process	Usually no clinical significance.	AP film: see a vertically oriented radiolucent cleft between the laminae. The spinous process will be absent or malformed at the involved level.	

AA, atlantoaxial joint; AO, atlantooccipital joint; NV, neurovascular.

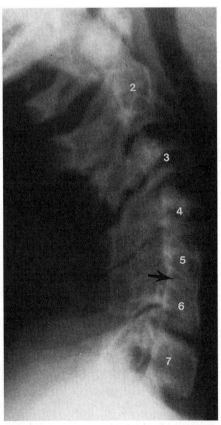

Figure 7-52 Multiple congenital deformities of the cervical spine and scapula in a 3-year-old boy. The left scapula is elevated (arrow points to the spine of the scapula). This condition is commonly known as Sprengel's deformity. The etiology is a failure of the scapula to descend to normal position from its high level in the early weeks of gestation. The cause of this failure is unknown. It is usually associated with other deformities as seen here. A group of deformities in the cervical spine, commonly known as Klippel–Feil syndrome, is present. Note failure of the laminae to unite at midline at some levels, and synostosis of much of the lower cervical spine into one bony mass. There is an omovertebral bar connecting the scapula to the cervical spine.

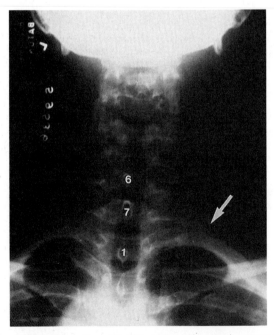

Figure 7-53 Cervical rib at C7. This congenital anomaly occurs most commonly at the seventh cervical vertebra. Cervical ribs are usually bilateral, and when this is the case, one rib is always higher and presents a more advanced stage of development than the other, as seen here. The left rib is larger and has formed an articulation with the first thoracic rib (arrow).

Summary of Key Points

Routine Radiologic Evaluation

1. The routine radiologic evaluation of the cervical spine includes five projections:
   - ➤ *AP open-mouth*—demonstrates the atlantoaxial joint
   - ➤ *AP lower cervical spine*—demonstrates the five lower cervical vertebrae
   - ➤ *Lateral*—demonstrates the normal alignment of all seven cervical vertebrae and paired facet joints
   - ➤ *Right and left obliques*—demonstrate single-side intervertebral foramina

2. Normal vertebral alignment is demonstrated on the lateral view by three approximately parallel line images:
   - ➤ The anterior borders of the vertebral bodies
   - ➤ The posterior borders of the vertebral bodies
   - ➤ The junctions of the laminae to the spinous processes (spinolaminar line)

   A discontinuity in the spatial relationships of these lines may indicate fracture or dislocation.

Trauma

3. A *trauma screen* is the series of radiographs and selected advanced imaging performed to screen and prioritize injuries in a trauma victim.

4. The *cross-table lateral* view screens for fracture or dislocation of the cervical spine.

5. Radiographic indicators of trauma include abnormal soft tissue images, abnormal vertebral alignment, and abnormal joint relationships.

6. Injuries to the cervical spine are broadly classified as *stable* or *unstable* injuries with regard to the immediate or subsequent threat to the spinal cord.

7. The role of MRI in spinal trauma is to aid in the characterization of soft tissue injury, neural element injury, and disk injury; thus it is mandatory in any trauma patient with a neurological deficit.

Fractures

8. *Avulsion fractures* and *compression fractures* are characteristic types of fractures seen in the cervical spine.

9. Fracture–dislocations are the most unstable injuries and as such are the most serious and life-threatening injuries in the cervical spine.

Dislocations

10. Isolated dislocations can ocurr unilaterally at a facet joint, secondary to a flexion–rotation force, or bilaterally at a pair of facet joints, secondary to a hyperflexion force.

11. Unilateral dislocations without anterior translation are stable injuries. Bilateral dislocation or unilateral dislocations with anterior translation are considered unstable injuries.

Other Injuries

12. Cervical sprains are injuries to the ligaments of the spine. *Hyperflexion sprains* injure the posterior ligaments and related soft tissues; *hyperextension sprains* injure the anterior ligaments and related soft tissues. The degree of severity of a sprain may range from minimal soft tissue involvement to ligamentous tearing with possible transient joint subluxations and compression fracture.

13. *Acute disk herniations* are not diagnosed by conventional radiography and require ancillary techniques such as myelography or MRI for diagnosis.

Degenerative Diseases

14. *Degenerative disk disease (DDD)* is demonstrated on the lateral view by decreased disk space height.

15. *Degenerative joint disease (DJD)* at the facet joints is demonstrated on the lateral view by decreased joint space, sclerosis, and osteophytes. DJD is seen radiographically in most persons over age 60.

16. *Foraminal encroachment* is the result of degenerative changes in adjacent structures that narrow the intervertebral canal; the potential exists for compression of the spinal nerve.

17. *Cervical spine spondylosis* is the spurring that forms at the vertebral endplates in response to DDD.

18. *Spondylosis deformans* is extensive osteophytosis at the anterior and anterolateral aspects of the vertebral bodies and annulus. Disk height is not decreased.

19. *Diffuse idiopathic skeletal hyperostosis (DISH)* presents as flowing ossification along the anterior aspects of at least four contiguous vetebrae with an absence of DDD or DJD. *Ossification of the posterior longitudinal ligament (OPLL)* is a separate entity but associated with DISH in as many as 50% of cases.

Anomalies

20. *Anomalies* represent failure of a structure to develop, arrested or asymmetrical development, or the development of accessory bones. They appear most frequently in the transitional vertebrae between regions of the spine.

21. Anomalies at the upper cervical segment, such as a diminutive dens, may have potential for instability and life-threatening consequences.

Please refer to the text's enclosed CD-ROM for the American College of Radiology's current Musculoskeletal Appropriateness Criteria for the following topics: *Chronic Neck Pain and Suspected Spine Trauma.*

CASE STUDIES

CASE STUDY 1

Cervical Spine Instability? Positive!

The patient is a 45-year-old woman referred to physical therapy by her family practice physician for management of neck pain following a motor vehicle accident.

History of Trauma

While returning by car from vacation in a neighboring state, the patient, who was in the passenger seat, was involved in a motor vehicle accident. Her vehicle rolled twice and came to rest in a ditch after the driver fell asleep at the wheel. The patient, restrained by a seat belt, was trapped in the vehicle for 30 minutes until rescue personnel arrived on the scene. She was immediately transported to the emergency room of a local hospital and evaluated by an emergency room physician. Her primary complaint at the time was of neck pain. She was also bleeding from the head as a result of superficial scalp lacerations.

Initial Imaging

In the emergency room, conventional radiographs were ordered, including AP, lateral (Fig. 7-54), and open-mouth views. The radiologist's report noted no abnormalities other than decreased cervical lordosis, presumably attributable to cervical paraspinal muscle spasm.

Intervention

The patient was treated for the scalp lacerations, given pain medications, and released from the hospital. The next day, she returned home and followed up by phone with her family practice physician. She saw the physician in his office 2 days later, at which time he recommended physical therapy for management of her neck pain, to be initiated 2 weeks after the date of the accident.

Physical Therapy Examination

Patient Complaint

At the patient's initial physical therapy appointment, she complained of continued neck pain and diffuse tingling in both hands, which had developed over the past week. She had not discussed the tingling with her physician and did not have a follow-up appointment scheduled for another week. She had not noticed any symptoms of dizziness, nausea, weakness in the extremities, or gait disturbances.

Physical Examination

The physical therapist did not have access to the patient's initial radiographs but did read the radiologist's report. The therapist examined the patient carefully with a limited number of tests. Her posture was still characterized by decreased cervical lordosis. Cervical active range of motion movements increased the patient's bilateral tingling in both flexion and extension. At this point the therapist ended the examination, contacted the patient's family practice physician, and voiced concerns about possible cervical instability. The therapist and physician agreed that further investigation with imaging was warranted.

Additional Imaging

Another series of cervical spine conventional radiographs and an MRI were ordered. The lateral radiograph (Fig. 7-55) revealed anterolisthesis of C6 on C7, and the sagittal MR image (Fig. 7-56) confirmed the forward slippage and showed encroachment into the spinal canal with moderate spinal cord compression.

Outcome

The patient was immediately referred to an orthopedic spine surgeon. The surgeon scheduled the patient for spinal fusion surgery to stabilize the C6–C7 motion segment. The case is summarized in Figure 7-57.

Discussion

Although the physical therapist in this example did not have first contact with the patient following the initial trauma, the therapist was the first professional to examine the patient *after the development of new symptoms.* In this sense, the therapist did assume a primary care role. The therapist was astute in recognizing a potentially dangerous situation. Bilateral numbness and tingling symptoms following cervical spine trauma are "red flags" signifying potential threat to the integrity of the spinal cord and requiring referral to another practitioner.

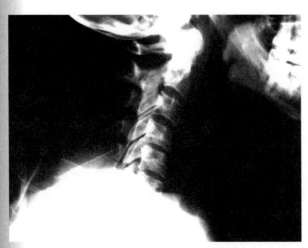

Figure 7-54 Lateral cervical spine, no abnormal findings.

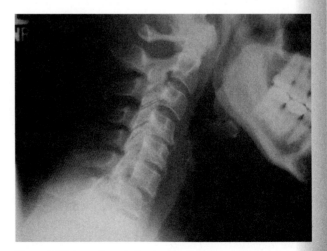

Figure 7-55 Lateral cervical spine demonstrating anterolisthesis of C6 on C7.

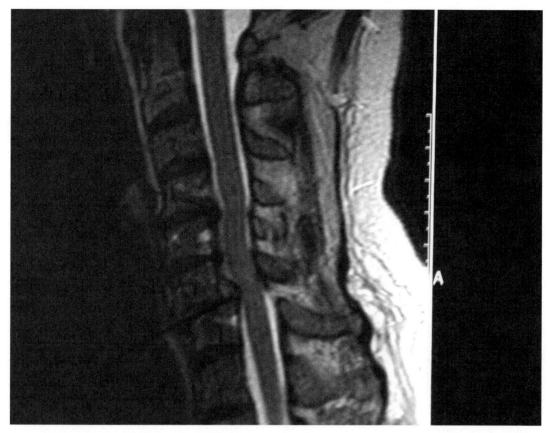

Figure 7-56 Sagittal MRI demonstrating C6 anterolisthesis, spinal canal encroachment, and moderate spinal cord compression.

Why Did Initial Radiographs Read Normal?

First, it is not unusual for an unstable joint to appear normal on static radiographs. At the moment the initial radiographs were made, the unstable joint may have simply been in normal alignment. It follows that if a joint is unstable, it has the capacity to move. Postural splinting and muscle spasm may have assisted in maintaining temporary joint position. Subluxation occurred later as a consequence of many factors; mechanical forces and pain medication that reduced protective spasm are the most obvious.

Second, perhaps the instability was present at the time of the initial radiograph—but it was not diagnosed because not all seven vertebrae are visualized! Look at Figure 7-54 again. C7 is not visible! The patient may have had her shoulders elevated because of guarding or spasm; superimposition of the shoulders obscured C7. Inadequate visualization of all seven vertebrae is one of the most common reasons for missed cervical spine injuries.

CRITICAL THINKING POINT

Even when the radiologic reports do not identify an abnormality, this does not mean that no abnormalities exist. The radiologist reports only on what is found on the radiograph. Neither the radiologist nor the family practice physician had the patient in front of them 2 weeks later. The therapist has the responsibility to complete a thorough history, recognize the potential consequences from the mechanism of injury, be aware of the clinical signs and symptoms of serious cervical spine injury, and exercise the appropriate caution in the initial evaluation. In this case, the therapist might have caused irreparable damage to the spinal cord if evaluation or treatment had been too vigorous. The therapist's knowledge of imaging, its limitations and capabilities, permitted effective communication with the referring physician and the ability to make recommendations about appropriate follow-up imaging studies.

CASE STUDY 2

Cervical Spine Instability? Negative!

The patient, a 37-year-old man, was referred to physical therapy by his primary care physician for management of neck pain following a motor vehicle accident.

History of Trauma

The patient was returning home from work during rush hour traffic. He had to stop suddenly in response to the quickly slowing vehicles ahead of him. The car behind him struck his vehicle, causing his neck to snap backward and then forward when his car hit the vehicle ahead of him. He immediately experienced pain in the anterior and posterior neck. He was taken by ambulance to the emergency room and examined by an emergency room physician.

Initial Imaging

Conventional radiographs of the cervical spine were ordered, including AP, lateral and open-mouth views. The radiologist's report noted no evidence of cervical spine fracture or joint instability.

Intervention

Experiencing no other symptoms beside neck pain, the patient was given a soft cervical collar for comfort and released from the emergency room with a prescription for pain medications and instructions

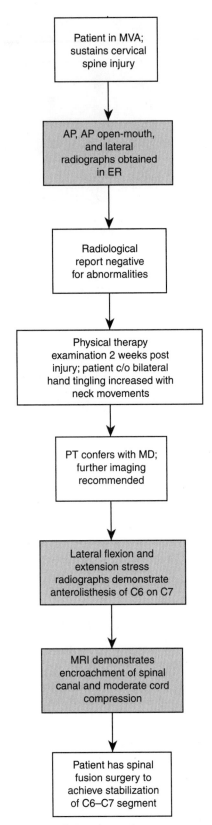

Figure 7-57 Case Study 1, pathway of events.

to follow up with his primary care physician. The next day the patient saw his physician, who also looked at the emergency room radiographs. The physician recommended that the patient continue with the collar and pain medication as necessary and return in

2 weeks. At that appointment, 2 weeks later, the patient reported continued neck pain and also intermittent tingling in the right thumb. The physician discontinued the soft collar and referred the patient to physical therapy, to begin in 2 more weeks.

Physical Therapy Examination

Patient Complaint

At the initial physical therapy appointment, 4 weeks after injury, the patient's chief complaint was posterior neck pain, especially on the right, and right thumb tingling, which was increasing in frequency. He did not report any other symptoms.

Physical Examination

The therapist was able to look at copies of the patient's radiographs from the emergency room and read the radiologist's report. Upon examination of cervical active range of motion, extension and rotation to the right resulted in an increase in right thumb tingling. Cervical compression also increased the tingling, whereas manual distraction decreased it. The therapist was concerned about dysfunction at the C5–C6 vertebral segment. The therapist communicated with the physician and requested follow-up radiographs to confirm stability of the cervical spine and to determine whether manual interventions would be safe.

Additional Imaging

Lateral flexion and extension stress radiographs were performed (Figs. 7-58 and 7-59). The radiographs were normal, showing no excessive anterior translation at the C5–C6 levels with cervical movements.

Outcome

The therapist initiated treatment with manual cervical traction and soft tissue mobilization. The patient's tingling symptoms resolved, and neck pain gradually diminished over the next 3 weeks. The case is summarized in Figure 7-60.

Discussion

In contrast to the patient in Case Study 1, this patient did not report the spinal cord compression "red flag" of bilateral upper extremity symptoms. His new neurological symptoms were unilateral and isolated to the thumb. Therefore spinal cord compression due to cervical spine instability was unlikely.

CRITICAL THINKING POINTS

The clinical lack of evidence for cervical instability did not warrant flexion/extension stress radiographs. The unilateral symptoms and clinical signs narrowed the diagnostic possibilites considerably. A unilateral encroachment at the intervertebral foramina would be a more common cause of the clinical presentation. An oblique-view conventional radiograph would allow observation of the foramina, but only bony encroachment would be visible on the radiograph. It is unlikely, however, that a 37-year-old with no prior history of radiating symptoms has a degenerative intervertebral foramen. An oblique view, in his case, would also read normal; the soft tissues responsible for his symptoms would not be visible.

This case illustrates:

1. The good intentions of the physical therapist to be cautious in the treatment of a patient with cervical trauma

2. A physician–physical therapist working relationship that includes consultation and recommendation to each other regarding the patient

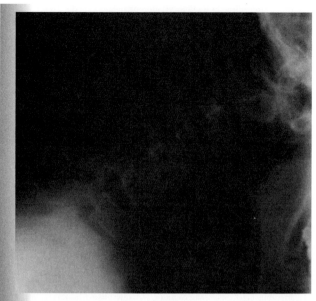

Figure 7-58 Lateral flexion radiograph of the cervical spine. No abnormalities noted.

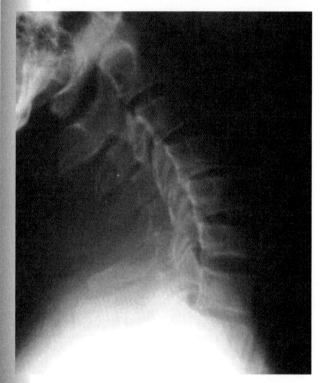

Figure 7-59 Lateral extension radiograph of the cervical spine. No abnormalities noted.

3. The performance of unnecessary imaging

4. Absence of consultation with the radiologist; if the radiologist had been aware of the clinical symptoms at 4 weeks after injury via a discussion with the therapist or physician, different recommendations might have been made (such as to allow a trial of conservative treatment prior to further imaging)

_____
Case studies adapted by J. Bradley Barr, PT, DPT, OCS.

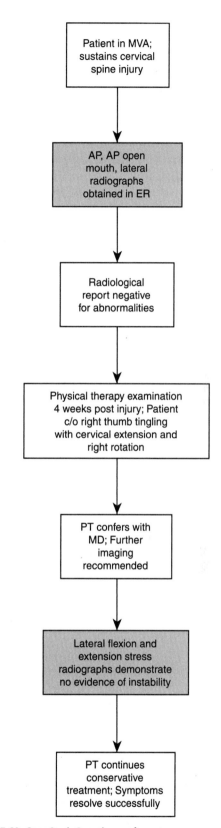

Patient in MVA; sustains cervical spine injury

↓

AP, AP open mouth, lateral radiographs obtained in ER

↓

Radiological report negative for abnormalities

↓

Physical therapy examination 4 weeks post injury; Patient c/o right thumb tingling with cervical extension and right rotation

↓

PT confers with MD; Further imaging recommended

↓

Lateral flexion and extension stress radiographs demonstrate no evidence of instability

↓

PT continues conservative treatment; Symptoms resolve successfully

Figure 7-60 Case Study 2, pathway of events.

References

1. Netter, FH: Atlas of Human Anatomy, ed. 4. WB Saunders, Philadelphia, 2006.
2. Yochum, TR, and Rowe, LJ: Essentials of Skeletal Radiology, ed. 3. Williams & Wilkins, Baltimore, 2004.
3. Nordin, M, and Frankel, VH: Basic Biomechanics of the Musculoskeletal System, ed. 3. Lippincott Williams & Wilkins, Philadelphia, 2001.
4. Whiting, W, and Zernicke, R: Biomechanics of Musculoskeletal Injury, ed. 2. Human Kinetics, Champaign, IL, 2008.
5. Gehweiler, JA, et al: The Radiology of Vertebral Trauma. WB Saunders, Philadelphia, 1980.
6. Meschan, I: An Atlas of Normal Radiographic Anatomy. WB Saunders, Philadelphia, 1960.
7. Weber, EC, Vilensky, JA, and Carmichael, SW: Netter's Concise Radiologic Anatomy. WB Saunders, Philadelphia, 2008.
8. American College of Radiology: Practice Guideline for the Performance of Spine Radiography in Children and Adults. 2007 (Res. 39). Accessed May 18, 2008 at http://www.acr.org.
9. Bontrager, KL: Textbook of Radiographic Positioning and Related Anatomy, ed. 6. Mosby, St. Louis, MO, 2005.
10. Chew, FS: Skeletal Radiology: The Bare Bones, ed. 2. Williams & Wilkins, Baltimore, 1997.
11. Fischer, HW: Radiographic Anatomy: A Working Atlas. McGraw-Hill, New York, 1988.
12. Greenspan, A: Orthopedic Radiology: A Practical Approach, ed. 4. Lippincott, Williams & Wilkins, Philadelphia, 2004.
13. Harris, JH, and Edeiken-Monroe, B: Radiology of Acute Cervical Spine Trauma. Williams & Wilkins, Baltimore, 1987.
14. Helms, CA: Radiology of Acute Cervical Spine Trauma. WB Saunders, Philadelphia, 1989.
15. Whitley, A: Clark's Positioning in Radiography, ed. 12. Oxford University Press, New York, 2005.
16. Frank, E, Smith, B, and Long, B: Merrill's Atlas of Radiographic Positions and Radiologic Procedures, ed. 11. Elsevier Health Sciences, Philadelphia, 2007.
17. Grey, ML, and Ailinani, JM: CT and MRI Pathology: A Pocket Atlas. McGraw-Hill Medical, New York, 2003.
18. Kelley, LL, and Peterson, CM: Sectional Anatomy for Imaging Professionals, ed. 2. Mosby, St. Louis, MO, 2007.
19. Lazo, DL: Fundamentals of Sectional Anatomy: An Imaging Approach. Thomson Delmar Learning, Clifton Park, NY, 2005.
20. Weber, EC, Vilensky, JA, and Carmichael, SW: Netter's Concise Radiologic Anatomy. WB Saunders, Philadelphia, 2008.
21. American College of Radiology: Appropriateness Criteria. Clinical Condition: Suspected Spine Trauma. Available at http://www.acr.org/Secondary MainMenuCategories/quality_safety/app_criteria/pdf/ExpertPanelonMus culoskeletalImaging/SuspectedCervicalSpineTraumaDoc22.aspx.
22. Steil, I, et al: The Canadian C-Spine Rule versus the NEXUS Low Risk Criteria in Patients with Trauma. N Engl J Med 349:2510, 2003.
23. Berquist, TH: Imaging of Orthopedic Trauma, ed. 2. Raven Press, New York, 1989.
24. Bucholz, RW, Heckman, J, and Court-Brown, C (eds): Rockwood and Green's Fractures in Adults, ed. 6. Lippincott Williams & Wilkins, Philadelphia, 2005.
25. McCort, JJ, and Mindelzun, RE: Trauma Radiology. Churchill Livingston, New York, 1990.
26. Drafke, MW, and Nakayama, H: Trauma and Mobile Radiography, ed. 2, FA Davis, Philadelphia, 2001.
27. Koval KJ, and Zuckerman, JD: Handbook of Fractures, ed. 3, Lippincott Williams & Wilkins, Philadelphia, 2006.
28. Hodler, J, von Schulthess, GK, and Zollikofer, CL: Musculoskeletal Diseases: Diagnostic Imaging and Interventional Techniques. Springer-Verlag Italia, Milan, Italy, 2005.
29. Bernstein, J: Musculoskeletal Medicine. American Academy of Orthopaedic Surgeons, Rosemont, IL, 2003.
30. IP, D: Orthopedic Traumatology: A Resident's Guide. Springer, Berlin, Germany, 2006.
31. McConnell, J, Eyres, R, and Nightingale, J: Interpreting Trauma Radiographs. Blackwell, Oxford, UK, 2005.
32. Salter, RB: Textbook of Disorders and Injuries of the Musculoskeletal System, ed. 2. Williams & Wilkins, Baltimore, 1983, p 227.
33. Brashear, HR, and Raney, RB: Shand's Handbook of Orthopaedic Surgery, ed. 10. Mosby, St. Louis, MO, 1986, p 340.
34. Daffner, RH: Clinical Radiology: The Essentials, ed. 3. Williams & Wilkins, Baltimore, 2007.
35. Marchiori, DM: Clinical Imaging with Skeletal, Chest, and Abdomen Pattern Differentials, ed. 2, Mosby, St. Louis, MO, 2004.
36. Chi, JH, et al: General considerationsfor cervical arthroplasty with technique for ProDisc-C. Neurosurg Clin North Am 16(4):609, 2005.
37. Sekhon, LH, and Ball, JR: Artificial cervical disc replacement: principles, types, and techniques. Neurol India 53(4):445, 2005.
38. Eroken, WE: Radiology 101: The Basics and Fundamentals of Imaging. Lippincott Williams & Wilkins, Baltimore, 1998.

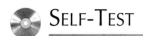 SELF-TEST

Radiographs A and B belong to the same patient.

Radiograph A

1. Identify the projection.

2. Are any abnormalities present in the structure of the vertebral bodies?

3. Which disk spaces appear narrowed?

4. What signs of degenerative disk disease do you see?

Radiograph B

5. Identify the projection.

6. What anatomic feature is best assessed on this view?

Radiographs C and D belong to the same patient.

Radiograph C

7. Identify the projection.

8. What signs of degenerative disk disease do you see? At what levels?

Radiograph D

9. Identify the projection.

10. What nerve root is susceptible to compression?

Comparing both patients

11. Considering the degenerative changes in the joints, which patient probably has the greater degree of *restricted range of motion* in the cervical spine?

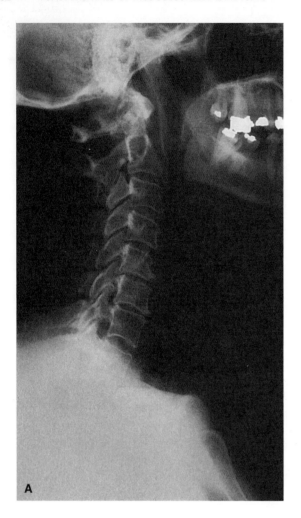

A

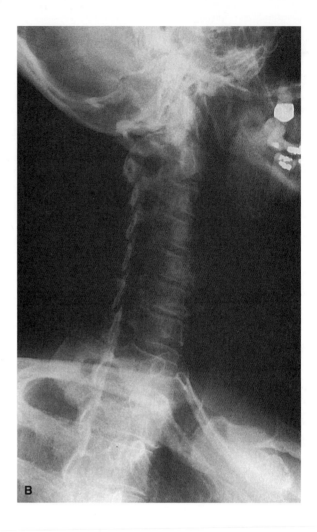

B

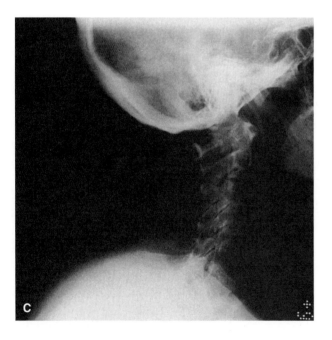

C

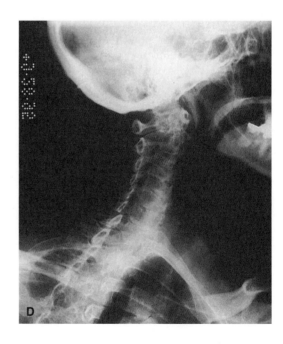

D

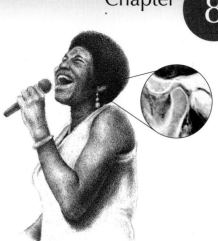

Chapter 8

RADIOLOGIC EVALUATION OF THE TEMPOROMANDIBULAR JOINT

Hilmir Agustsson, MHSc, DPT, MTC, CFC

Historical Perspective

Treatment of the temporomandibular joint (TMJ) was first described in Egyptian papyri 4,000 years ago and the technique currently used for reducing TMJ dislocation was developed by the ancient Greeks.[1] However, the construct of TMJ disorders was first introduced in the 1930s, when James Costen, an otolaryngologist, put forth the theory that pain in the muscles of mastication, facial pains, headaches, ringing in the ears, and numerous other symptoms originated in the TMJ. Disorders of the TMJ were presumed to be caused by dental malalignment, occlusal disharmonies, and missing teeth—the implication being that TMJ disorders were dental problems, best treated with structural corrections. This view survived for half a century; but in the last 30 years, the discussion of TMJ-related problems has taken a very different turn. Occlusal factors have been all but abandoned as a major cause of

symptoms and current treatment guidelines generally do not recommend invasive interventions and structural changes.[2]

Causes of TMJ Disorders

TMJ disorders have been attributed to a variety of causes, but in recent years the focus has shifted away from the TMJ as the sole cause of the symptoms previously attributed to this joint. Structures outside the TMJ, including the joints and muscles of the cervical spine, are now recognized as common sources of symptoms. An example of the changing emphasis is a decreasing concern with diseases and dysfunctions. The discussion is shifting away from presumed mechanical or structural problems toward a focus on symptoms; consequently, symptoms associated with TMJ disorders are now most commonly referred to simply in terms of craniofacial pain or orofacial pain.[3]

Review of Anatomy

The TMJ is a compound synovial joint between the mandible and the cranium. This joint is considered a part of a larger functional unit, the craniomandibular system, encompassing the TMJ, the cranium, and the cervical spine.

Osseous Anatomy

The osseous components of the TMJ consist of two surfaces, covered with fibrocartilage, and an interposed articular disk. The osseous components are (1) the anterior part of the mandibular fossa of the temporal bone, and the articular eminence anterior to it, and (2) the condyle of the mandible (Fig. 8-1). The anatomy of the joint is described here in the sagittal, coronal, and axial planes:

- *Sagittal plane:* The temporal articular surface covers the anterior slope of the fossa and the articular eminence; the mandibular (condylar) cartilage primarily covers the anterosuperior condyle. Note that both these osseous surfaces are convex; the disk makes up their lack of congruence (see Fig. 8-1).
- *Coronal plane:* The mandibular fossa, concave in the coronal plane, articulates with the medial side of the convex condyle only (Fig. 8-2).
- *Axial (horizontal) plane:* The mediolateral dimension of the condyle is greater than the anteroposterior dimension, giving the condyle an elliptical shape (Fig. 8-3).

The long axis of the condyle is directed posteriorly and medially by about 15 to 30 degrees from the coronal plane, whereas the temporal surface is directed anteriorly and laterally; forming an acute angle of about 40 degrees between the two.

Articular Disk

The fibrocartilaginous articular disk is an oval-shaped structure that is interposed between the osseous components of the joint. The disk is biconcave in the sagittal plane, so each surface of the disk forms a convex-on-concave joint with the corresponding convex osseous surface. This arrangement improves the congruency of the articular surfaces and contributes to the stability of the TMJ.

The disk, unlike the meniscus of the knee, is not perforated. It has a thin central portion and thicker anterior and posterior bands; acting as wedges within the joint, which stabilize the concave intermediate zone on the convex condyle. The posterior band of the disk, furthermore, maintains the vertical "articular height," preventing the condyle from ascending into the apex of the mandibular fossa. The posterior band is partly vascularized and innervated.

Ligamentous Anatomy

The ligaments of the TMJ play a secondary role in the stabilization of the joint; the main role is played by co-ordiated action of the musculature.

Articular Capsule

The articular capsule is attached superiorly to the circumference of the mandibular fossa and distally around the neck of the condyle of the mandible. The capsule is attached to the periphery of the disk, dividing the joint into

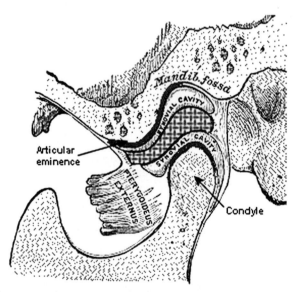

Figure 8-1 Sagittal section of the left TMJ. *(Adapted from Gray, 1918. [Gray, H: Anatomy of the Human Body, ed. 20. Lea & Febiger, Philadelphia, 1918. Accessed November 7, 2003 at http://www.bartleby.com/br/107.html.])*

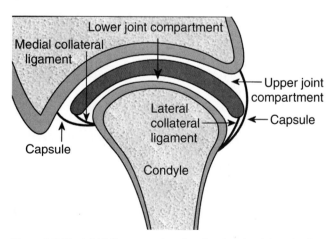

Figure 8-2 The left TMJ: a coronal section showing the disk and collateral ligaments; demonstrating the concave-on-convex nature of the joint in this plane.

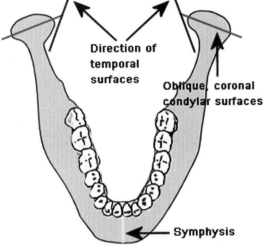

Figure 8-3 Axial view of the mandible demonstrating the orientation of articular surfaces and the symphysis of the mandible.

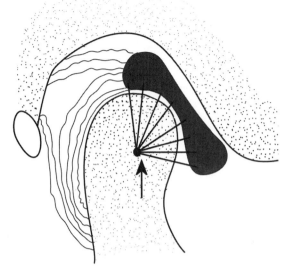

Figure 8-5 Lateral collateral ligament, stabilizing the disk on top of the condyle.

two compartments: (1) a smaller lower compartment, the condyle and the inferior surface of the disk, and (2) a larger upper compartment, consisting of the temporal surfaces and the superior surface of the disk.

Lateral and Medial Ligaments

Medially and laterally, there are ligaments that (1) guide the movement of the joint, (2) control the position the articular disk, and (3) limit excessive opening.

1. The temporomandibular ligament restricts downward and backward movement of the mandible and guides the forward motion of the condyle during the opening movement (Fig. 8-4).
2. The medial and lateral collateral ligaments stabilize the disk on the top of the condyle (Fig. 8-5).
3. The sphenomandibular and stylomandibular ligaments, medial to the joint, limit excessive opening (Fig. 8-6).

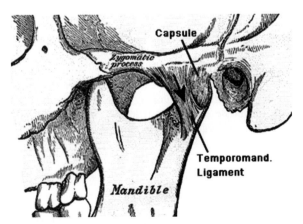

Figure 8-4 The temporomandibular ligament. *(Adapted from Gray, 1918.)*

Posterior Ligaments

The posterior ligamentous structures are often collectively referred to as the bilaminar zone (Fig. 8-7). These structures consist of superior and inferior ligamentous strata enveloping the highly vascular and innervated retrodiskal tissue, the volume of which changes during forward and backward translation of the condyle. The posterior ligaments restrict forward movement of the disk during opening, and its lower part assists in pulling the disk posteriorly during the closing movement.

Biomechanics of the TMJ

Because of the activities of speaking, swallowing, chewing (mastication), and facial expression, the TMJ moves almost continuously. These movements are discussed in terms of osteokinematic movements (the gross movements of the mandible) and arthrokinematic movements (the motions of the joint surfaces relative to each other).

Osteokinematics

The osteokinematic movements consist of opening/closing, protrusion/retrusion, and lateral excursion. Note the following:

● The normal range of motion for opening at the TMJ is equal to or greater than 40 mm as measured between the central incisors.
● Combined range of motion for protrusion and retrusion is 10 mm.
● The range of lateral excursion is 10 mm to each side.
● The ranges of opening and of lateral excursion are interrelated; 10 mm of active lateral excursion to either side is necessary for full opening.

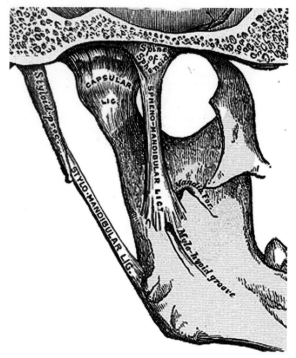

Figure 8-6 The stylomandibular and sphenomandibular ligaments. *(Adapted from Gray, 1918.)*

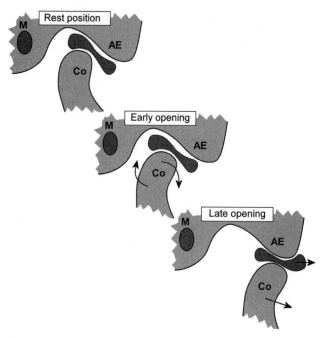

Figure 8-8 The movements of the TMJ in opening. M = extenal auditory meatus, Co = condyle, AE = articular eminence. Note the rotation of the condyle during early opening and the predominant translation during late opening as well as the changing configuration of the disk during movement.

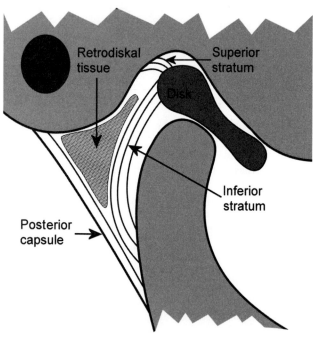

Figure 8-7 The bilaminar zone and retrodiscal tissue. The inferior stratum pulls the disk back as the mandible rotates posteriorly during closing.

Arthrokinematics

Imaging has greatly contributed to our understanding of the arthrokinematics of the TMJ, allowing us to visualize normal and abnormal motion. Magnetic resonance imaging (MRI),

and arthrography before that, offers visualization of the movements of the articular surfaces and the disk at various phases of opening and closing.

Opening and closing involve the same events in opposite order. The arthrokinematics of opening involve (1) rotation and (2) translation (Fig. 8-8).

1. Rotation of the condyle takes place in the lower joint compartment during the early phase of opening.
2. Anterior translation of the condyle takes place in the upper joint compartment during the latter half of opening.

Rotation and translation each contribute approximately half of the opening movement. Because of the anterolateral direction of the temporal articular surfaces, the condyles also translate laterally during opening, necessitating a symphysis anteriorly in the mandible around which the posterior widening of the mandible takes place (see Fig. 8-3). Note that the two TMJs are interdependent; if motion at one joint is restricted, the other joint will compensate, resulting in deflection of the mandible to the restricted side during opening of the mouth owing to the increased anterior translation on the nonrestricted side. During translation, the disk moves with the condyle down the articular eminence toward its apex because of its condylar attachment by the collateral ligaments and capsule (Fig. 8-8).

Growth and Development

The face and skull grow rapidly during the first 6 years of life, during which time the dimensions of the face, including the mandible, grow more rapidly than those of the skull. The ramus of the mandible grows in length and assumes a more vertical orientation with maturity, resulting in a decrease in the angle between the ramus and the body of the mandible from 140 degrees in early childhood to 110 degrees in adulthood.

The facial structures undergo continuous remodeling throughout life, and the shape of the mandible and maxilla as well as dental equilibrium affect the function of the TMJ. However, the function of the craniomandibular system also affects the development of dentofacial structures. Examples of this can be seen in cases of muscle weakness and forward head posture, which commonly leads to anterior open bite, lengthening of the lower part of the face, and increased mandibular angle. The impact of abnormal posture and muscle tone is clearly demonstrated in patients with severe neurological involvement, who often develop marked facial and dental malformation.

Imaging in the Evaluation of the TMJ

The imaging modalities used to evaluate the TMJ include conventional radiography, tomography, computed tomography (CT), ultrasound, and MRI. Selection of imaging studies is based on a number of considerations, including availability, applicability for the proposed diagnosis, cost, and radiation exposure.[4]

A thorough examination of the patient plays a central role. Although imaging accurately demonstrates structural changes and associated movement abnormalities, there is low correlation between imaging findings and the patient's symptoms. Up to one-third of asymptomatic individuals may have disk displacement and, conversely, a normal position of the disk may be found in up to 23% of symptomatic patients.[5]

Conventional Radiographs

Conventional radiographs are of limited use for imaging the TMJ, partly because of difficulties in getting an unobstructed view of the articular surfaces. Conventional radiography is most commonly used to evaluate arthritides, fractures, or disease processes. The transcranial radiograph is the basic examination, but lateral cephalometry and cervical radiographs may be used to aid in clinical decision making.

(Continued on page 210)

Routine Radiologic Evaluation of the TMJ

Transcranial View (Lateral Oblique Transcranial)

The transcranial view represents a lateral oblique projection of the TMJ.[6] The side of the patient's face is against the image receptor, and the TMJ closest to the image receptor is visualized. The central ray enters from a superior and oblique direction, which is parallel to the long axis of the condyle (Fig. 8-9). The transcranial view provides a gross view of the osseous structures of the TMJ as well as the condyle, articular eminence, and mandibular fossa.

Radiologic Observations

The important observations are:

1. The shape of the articular eminence, which determines the path of condylar translation during opening and lateral excursion.
2. The shape and size of the condyle.
3. The position of the condyle within the fossa. A vertical line drawn from the apex of the mandibular fossa should intersect a point midway between the poles of the condyle.
4. The position of the petrous line (normally the petrous line should intersect the condyle).
5. The long horizontal axis of the condyle, which comes into view because of the inferiorly directed x-rays, displaying the lateral (inferiorly) and medial (superiorly) poles of the condyle.
6. The joint height. In some cases two transcranial radiographs may be made; one with the mouth fully closed and one with the mouth fully open. The difference in joint height on the two images is noted; if the joint space increases on full opening and decreases in the closed position, this could indicate disk displacement.

Note that the transcranial view is limited to the lateral aspect of the joint; the middle and medial aspects of the joint are less clearly visualized because of superimposition of the condyle and the petrous part of the temporal bone.

What Can You See?

Look at the radiograph (Fig. 8-10) and identify the radiographic anatomy. Trace the outline of the structures, using a marker and a transparent sheet. Then compare your tracing with the tracing in Figure 8-11. Can you identify the following:

- External auditory meatus
- Petrous line
- Lateral and medial poles of the condyle
- Neck of the condyle
- Articular eminence
- Mandibular fossa

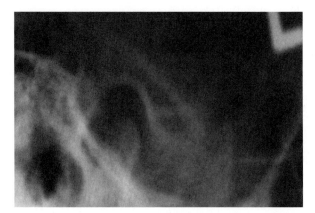

Figure 8-10 Conventional transcranial radiograph of the left TMJ. The radiograph is made in the rest position of the mandible. *(Courtesy of M. Rocabado.)*

Setting up the Radiograph

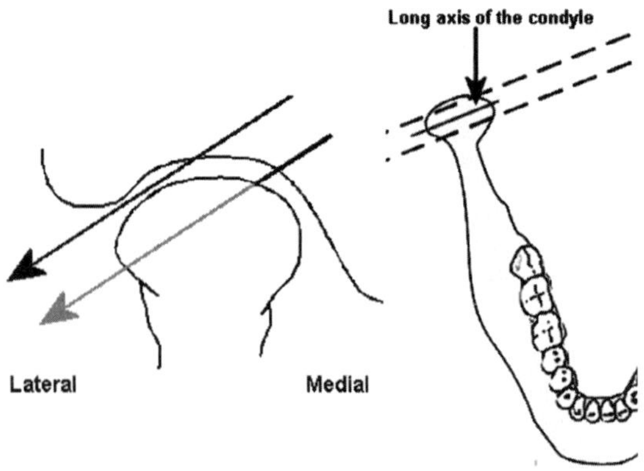

Long axis of the condyle

Lateral   Medial

Figure 8-9 Direction of x-rays for transcranial radiography for the right TMJ. The film plate is placed against the lateral aspect of the TMJ and the x-rays are aligned with the long axis of the condyle (anteriorly by 15 to 30 degrees) and directed down by about 25 degrees.

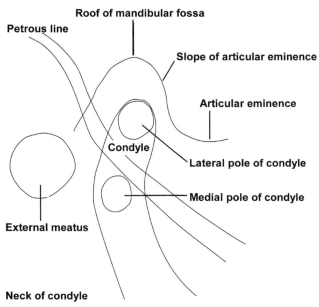

Roof of mandibular fossa
Petrous line
Slope of articular eminence
Articular eminence
Condyle
Lateral pole of condyle
Medial pole of condyle
External meatus
Neck of condyle

Figure 8-11 Tracing of the conventional transcranial radiograph.

Cephalometry: Lateral Radiographs

Lateral cephalometry is a method of measuring the dimensions of the head. It is used by orthodontists in planning and monitoring treatment. Cephalometric images (Fig. 8-12) are also of interest to clinicians who treat patients with TMJ problems. The cephalographs display the craniovertebral relationship and cervical alignment and help guide treatment of the subcranial region, which exerts influence on the movements of the TMJ and can be the source of craniofacial pain.

Radiologic Observations

The radiologic evaluation for the lateral view of the cervical spine is described in Chapter 7. Additional observations for cephalographs, important in the assessment of craniofacial pain and TMJ disorders, are:

1. The odontoid plane, found by drawing a line from the anterior inferior angle of the C2 vertebral body through the tip of the odontoid process (dens).
2. The sagittal plane inclination of the head; a line from the posterior hard palate to the base of the occiput (McGregor's line) should be horizontal.
3. Posterior osseous spaces in the subcranial area; note whether the spaces between the occiput and C1 and between C1 and C2 are open (each space should be at least 6 mm).
4. The degree of lordosis of the cervical spine, quickly assessed by drawing a line along the posterior vertebral bodies, from C2 to C7.
5. The position of the hyoid bone, which is related to the position of the tongue and the resting position of the mandible because of the attachment of the genioglossus (tongue) to the hyoid bone.
6. The angle of the mandible; long-standing muscular weakness increases this angle.
7. The size and the shape of the ramus of the mandible.
8. The height of the coronoid process relative to the condyle; if the condyle is lower than the coronoid process, this could indicate severe condylar degenerative changes.

The alignment of the head relative to the cervical spine is described in terms of the craniovertebral angle. This angle can be measured as the angle where McGregor's line and the odontoid plane intersect posteriorly. Normal values for the craniovertebral angle are between 96 and 106 degrees.

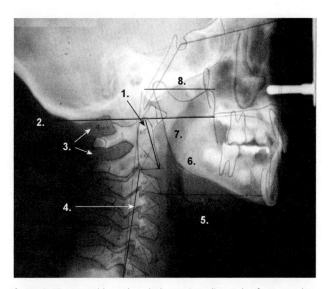

Figure 8-12 Normal lateral cephalometric radiograph of a young boy: (1) odontoid plane; (2) McGregor's line; (3) posterior subcranial spaces; (4) line connecting posterior vertebral borders of C2 and C7; (5) hyoid bone; (6) angle of mandible; (7) ramus of mandible; (8) line demonstrating the height of the coronoid processes relative to the condyle. Note that the lines across the vertebral bodies are for the purpose of locating their centers. *(Image courtesy of M. Rocabado.)*

Other Projections

The submentovertex view represents an axial view of the TMJ. The central ray enters the head under the chin, near the symphysis of the mandible, and exits at the vertex, where the image receptor is placed. This view demonstrates the alignment and shape of the condyles in the axial plane and is useful for demonstrating condylar asymmetry (Fig. 8-13). Furthermore, submentovertex radiographs may be made prior to transcranial radiography to help align the central ray with the long axis of the condyle and to plan conventional tomography—an approach called axially corrected tomography.

A panoramic radiograph allows a view of the both TMJs, mandible, and teeth in one image. It is routinely used in dentistry and can be used to be used for the initial radiographic examination of the TMJ. However, it is of limited value in the diagnosis of TMJ disorders owing to the superimposition of other structures and shape distortion.

Conventional Tomography

Conventional tomography of the TMJ is capable of showing sagittal slices as thin as 1 mm through mediolateral dimensions of the TMJ (Fig. 8-14), thus complementing conventional transcranial radiography, which can show only the lateral aspect of the joint. It is performed with the patient in the upright seated position by moving the x-ray source and the image receptor in opposite directions around the focal point of interest: the TMJ. Typically the tomogram is made in a parasagittal plane, at right angles to the long axis of the condyle. This method is now less frequently used, since CT is offers superior spatial resolution. However, for diagnosing joint erosions and osteophytes, the value of conventional axially corrected tomography has been found to equal CT.[7]

Computed Tomography

CT provides accurate tomography of the osseous structures of the TMJ, relatively free of blurring or superimposition of different tissues (Fig. 8-15). Modern scanners are increasingly able to display soft tissue structures as well. CT

of the TMJ is performed in the axial plane, although it is possible to create images in any of the orthogonal planes when data are acquired using volumetric spiral scanning. Volumetric scanning also offers the possibility of three-dimensional presentations, a technique that is likely to have significant impact on orthodontics and maxillofacial surgery as well as the treatment of TMJ disorders.[8] Scanning of the TMJ typically produces 12 to 15 slices 1 to 3 mm thick, but cone beam CT offers submillimeter slices. Scanning covers the area from above the roof of the mandibular fossa and down to the maxillary teeth.

Clinical Application

CT clearly demonstrates the morphology of the osseous structures of the TMJ, although it does not equal MRI for demonstrating soft tissues. Its advantages, compared with MRI, include thinner slices, better spacial resolution, shorter imaging times, and lower cost. The main disadvantage is the fairly high radiation dose, although the use of cone beam CT may decrease this. CT excels in the evaluation of complex fractures,

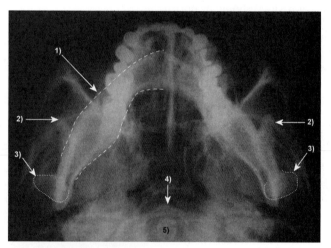

Figure 8-13 Submentovertex view of the mandibles and cranium: (1) mandible, (2) coronoid processes, (3) condyles, (4) anterior arch of atlas, and (5) dens.

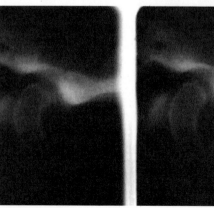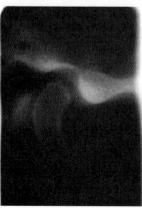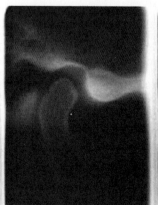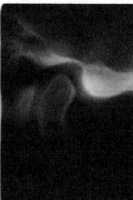

Figure 8-14 Conventional tomogram of the right TMJ, showing the changing osseous outlines of the joint from the medial to the lateral aspect of the joint. Note the deepening of the articular fossa as the cuts are made progressively more laterally. *(Image courtesy of M. Rocabado.)*

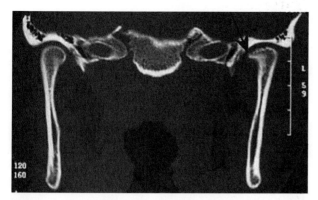

Figure 8-15 This CT image, reconstructed in the coronal plane, shows an osteophyte on the anteromedial aspect of the left condyle (arrow). Note the flattening of the left condylar head. *(Image courtesy of M. Rocabado.)*

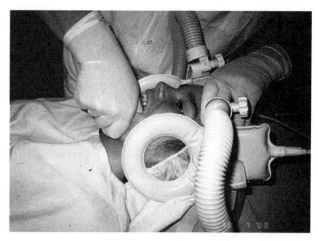

Figure 8-16 MRI. Simultaneous scanning of both TMJs. The clinician positions the joint in the desired degree of opening before scanning. *(Image courtesy of M. Rocabado.)*

ankylosis, and bone pathology and has greater sensitivity and specificity for detecting joint erosions and osteophytes than does MRI.[7] Although CT can demonstrate the disk, it is less accurate than MRI for displaying disk displacement because of the small difference in density between the disk and the surrounding soft tissue.

Viewing CT Images

Axial images are viewed from below and sagittal images are viewed from the left toward the right for both joints. Three-dimensional images are viewed on the computer screen, where they can be rotated to be viewed from any angle.

Magnetic Resonance Imaging

MRI is the imaging modality of choice for visualizing the soft tissues surrounding the TMJ and the articular disk. In the 1990s, it replaced arthrography as the preferred method for evaluating disorders of the articular disk, although arthrography may still be the best method for identifying disk perforations. MRI accurately images the position of the disk and changes in its morphology. Disadvantages of MRI relative to CT include long imaging times, high cost, and thick slices.

Method and Scanning Planes

MRI can acquire high-definition images of both TMJs simultaneously, using specialized surface receiver coils about 7.5 mm in diameter. The slice thickness is typically 3 to 4 mm. With a field of view of 10 to 12 cm and a matrix of 256 by 256, the pixel size is approximately 0.5 mm[9] (Fig. 8-16). The scanning planes include the axial plane (Fig. 8-17), the oblique sagittal plane—which is perpendicular to the long axis of the condyle, and the oblique coronal plane along the long axis of the condyle (Fig. 8-18). Scanning times are kept as brief as possible in order to minimize the need for swallowing, which causes a motion artifact.

Viewing the TMJ

Viewing MR images of the TMJ can be difficult; structures in this area are very small relative to slice thickness, and slight variations in the alignment of the scanning plane can alter

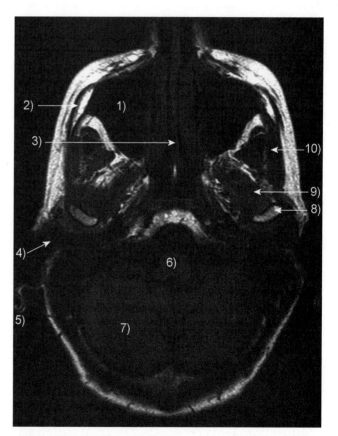

Figure 8-17 Axial T1 MRI at the level of the mandibular condyles, showing (1) maxillary sinuses, (2) zygomatic arch, (3) nasal septum, (4) external auditory meatus, (5) ear, (6) medulla, (7) cerbellum, (8) condyle, (9) lateral pterygoid, and (10) masseter. *(Source of image: http://www.medcyclo.com by GE Healthcare.)*

the appearance of the structures displayed. It is therefore important to focus on identifying the main points of reference: the articular eminence, external auditory meatus, and condyle. The challenge of sectional anatomy in CT and MRI is that structures of interest are typically not seen in their entirety and can be appreciated only if consecutive slices are

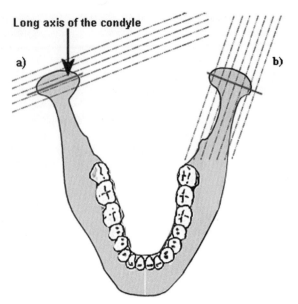

Figure 8-18 MRI scanning planes for the TMJ: (a) oblique coronal plane, aligned with the long axis of the condyle; (b) oblique sagittal plane, perpendicular to the long axis of the condyle.

viewed. Thus one should not be too concerned if structures in a particular slice look unfamiliar; they may become recognizable in an adjacent slice (Figs. 8-19, 8-20, and 8-21).

Findings on MRI

As in other joints, the strength of MRI lies in imaging changes in soft tissues and bone marrow, while it does not equal the ability of CT to demonstrate changes in cortical bone. Some changes seen on MRI can be diagnostics in themselves, such as altered position of the articular disk, while other changes, such as bone marrow edema and effusion, may be pathognomonic for several disease entities.

- Changes in bone marrow, referred to as bone edema or bone bruise, are important in the diagnosis of avascular necrosis (AVN) and osteoarthritis (OA), both of which are preceded by a period of inflammatory reaction in bone. Although imaging findings and patient symptoms may not correlate well, bone bruise correlates highly with pain from the TMJ.[10]
- Effusion, defined as an increase in joint fluid, is rarely found in asymptomatic individuals. It is associated disk displacement, early OA, and trauma; it is the hallmark of rheumatoid arthritis (RA). MRI can distiguish distention of the capsule due to synovial proliferation, as seen in RA, from simple effusion.[11] Sometimes intravenous gadolinium is employed for the purpose of diagnosis of synovial proliferation; the synovium shows increased signal intensity following gadolinium administration, which the joint fluid does not.

TMJ Movements on MRI

MRI allows clear visualization of changes in the position of the condyle and of the position and shape of the disk at different points in the range of motion. This is not accomplished by true dynamic imaging but by sequentially imaging the TMJ during different degrees of opening. Figure 8-22 shows

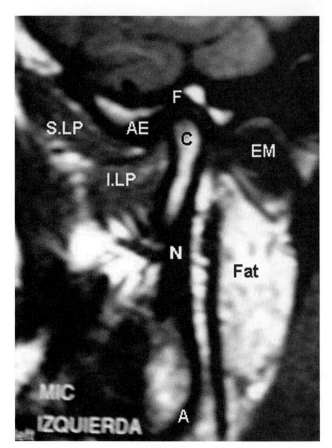

Figure 8-19 Sagittal T1 MR image of the left TMJ in full occlusion. Here the following structures can be identified: articular fossa (F), articular eminence (AE), superior and inferior heads of the lateral pterygoid (S.LP and I.LP), external auditory meatus (EM), neck of the condyle (N), and angle of the mandible (A). The disk forms a thin, low-signal line above the condyle, still not as dark as the cortex of the condyle, but the outlines of the disk are not clearly seen. Note that the condyle is seen both as cortical bone (dark) and bone marrow (white). Further down the neck of the condyle, however, only cortical bone is visible. *(Image courtesy of M. Rocabado.)*

sagittal images of the left TMJ at various degrees of opening, starting with full occlusion, and Figure 8-23 shows coronal slices of the joint lateral excursion to the opposites sides.

Ultrasound

During the last few years, ultrasound has increasingly been used for the diagnosis of disk displacement, providing a portable, low-cost alternative to MRI. It can show, in real time, the position of the disk and condyle throughout the range of the opening movement and has recently been used to demonstrate differences in condylar motion of patients with different types of occlusion.[12] The sensitivity and specificity of this method have been found to be good compared with MRI, although the absence of a classification system for sonography of the TMJ makes a comparison between MRI and ultrasound difficult. Ultrasound yields almost perfect sensitivity and specificity for the detection of degenerative changes and effusion of the TMJ.[13] However, as discussed in Chapter 6, ultrasound is a dynamic imaging method; it is highly susceptible to factors such as transducer pressure, orientation, and angulation, all of which creates difficulties in viewing and reproducing images.

Pathological Conditions of the TMJ

Osteoarthritis

OA is a common condition of the TMJ. However, there is limited correlation between radiographic findings of OA on one hand and symptoms and signs on the other. Furthermore, signs and symptoms do not seem to increase concurrent with progression of degenerative changes; indeed long-term studies show that symptoms of osteoarthritis of the TMJ tend to decrease with time.[14] However, in spite of favorable symptomatic outcomes, degenerative changes can lead to functional changes, malocclusion, and facial asymmetry.

OA, most commonly results from disk displacement; it is rarely seen in the presence of normally positioned disks.[15] Displaced disks with extensive degenerative changes are frequently seen in children and adolescents, and 20% of

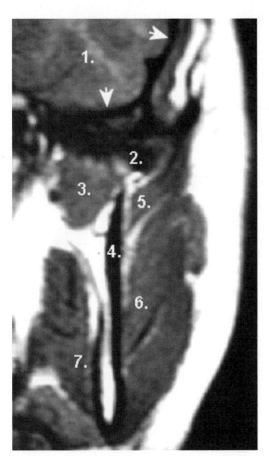

Figure 8-20 Coronal T1 image. The slice is made just anterior to the condyle itself, so there is no condyle to be seen. The temporal bone is marked by arrowheads. Other structures: (1) brain, (2) articular disk, (3) lateral pterygoid, (4) anterior border of the ramus of the mandible, (5) deep portion of the masseter, (6) superficial portion of the masseter, (7) medial pterygoid. *(Image courtesy of M. Rocabado.)*

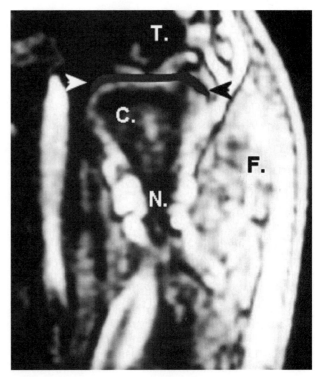

Figure 8-21 Coronal T1 image in full occlusion. This slice is made posterior to the one in Fig. 8-20. The neck of the condyle (N) is visible below the condyle (C). Subcutaneous fat (F) is bright, and the temporal bone (T) is black. Arrowheads mark the outline of the disk, which has here been enhanced. *(Image courtesy of M. Rocabado.)*

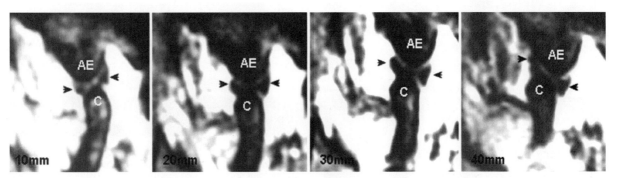

Figure 8-22 Sagittal MRIs showing the TMJ at various degrees of opening. Arrowheads indicate the articular disk. The condyle (C) and the articular eminence (AE) are marked. This series demonstrates hypermobility of the disk-condyle complex, but no instability of the disk. This is in spite of the excessive translatory motion (hypermobility) of the condyle; at 20 mm of opening, the disk is already on the top of the eminence, and at 30 and 40 mm of opening, the disk and the condyle move beyond the articular eminence. Note that fat appears bright, while the osseous structures and the disk are dark. *(Image courtesy of M. Rocabado.)*

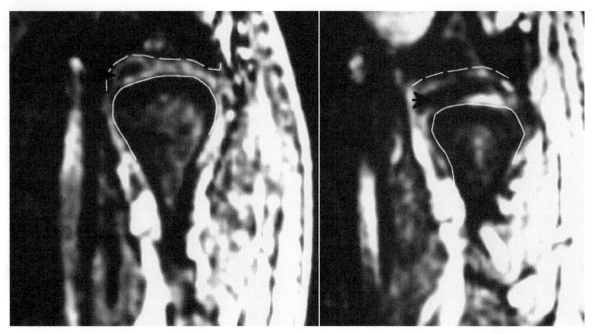

Figure 8-23 Image on the left: Coronal MR image of left TMJ during full *left* lateral excursion. An arrowhead marks the disk. Note that left lateral excursion involves anterior translation of the right condyle, while the left condyle functions more or less as a pivot. The condyle is marked by a solid outline; the eminence, with a dotted line. The image shows good condyle-disk relationship. Note that increased lateral joint pressure can be expected where the condyle abuts against the lateral region of the fossa. Image on the right: Coronal MR image of left TMJ during full *right* lateral excursion. Now the disk is clearly visible between the osseous surfaces. At full translation the joint space has opened up and the lateral pole of the condyle translated laterally. *(Image courtesy of M. Rocabado.)*

patients already have OA at the time of initial consult for disk disorders (Fig. 8-24).

Clinical Presentation and Treatment

Signs and symptoms of osteoarthritis include pain in the TMJ, pain in the ear, restricted motion, and crepitus on movement.[16] Although degenerative changes cannot be reversed, the signs and symptoms can be treated effectively by exercise, mobilization, relaxation, and postural correction.[17]

Radiologic Findings

Radiologic findings of osteoarthritis at the TMJ include the following:

1. Decreased joint space between the condyle and the articular eminence
2. Subchondral sclerosis
3. Flattening of the condyle, eminence, or both
4. Irregular joint surfaces
5. Osteophytes, typically close to the anterior attachments of the capsule, presenting as a "beak" on the anterior condyle (see Figs. 8-24 and 8-25)
6. Subchondral cysts, representing intrusion of synovial fluid into subchondral bone

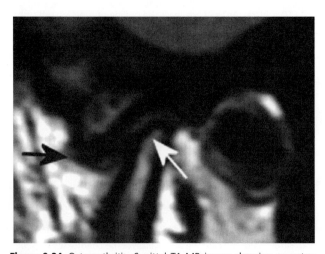

Figure 8-24 Osteoarthritis. Sagittal T1 MR image showing an osteophyte and severe flattening of the condylar head (white arrow) of the condyle in a 17-year-old girl with a permanent disk displacement (black arrow). *(Image courtesy of M. Rocabado.)*

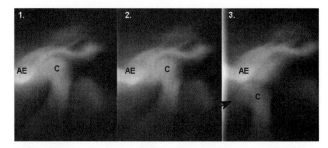

Figure 8-25 Conventional tomography demonstrating degenerative changes. Both in full occlusion (1 and 2) and in opening (3), a decrease in the joint spaces can be observed. There is subchondral sclerosis, in particular of the articular eminence (AE). The eminence is eroded, and the head of the condyle (C) flattened. When the patient attempts full opening (3), a decrease in translatory movement can be noted. Note the typical beak-shaped osteophyte anteriorly on the condyle. *(Image courtesy of M. Rocabado.)*

Rheumatoid Arthritis

Approximately half the patients diagnosed with RA demonstrate changes in the TMJ, although typically other joints are involved first. TMJ involvement tends to be bilateral.

Clinical Presentation and Treatment

RA is characterized by pain localized to the TMJ, swelling, crepitus, and limited motion.[18] It typically results in occlusal changes as a result of destruction of the joint. Treatment is focused on decreasing the inflammation with anti-inflammatory medications as well as rest, education, and splint therapy aimed at stabilizing the joint and decreasing joint loads.

Imaging Findings

Characteristic changes of RA of the TMJ include the following:

1. Decreased joint space
2. Subchondral cysts
3. Rapid resorption of the condylar head[19]
4. Anterior open bite with molar contact due to condylar changes
5. Soft tissue edema and joint effusion, seen on T2 MRI; synovial proliferation, best seen on gadolinium-enhanced images

Disk Displacement

Disk displacement represents the loss of the normal disk-condyle relationship, most commonly displacement of the disk medial and anterior to the condyle. This condition, which most often has an onset in the fourth decade, is the most common structural abnormality of the TMJ. It is three to five times more common in women than in men. Changes associated with disk displacement may include condylar bone marrow edema, hyperplasia of the posterior ligament, and fibrosis of the lateral pterygoid muscle, which may form an area of decreased signal intensity parallel to the disk ("double disk sign").

Etiology

The causes of disk displacement are rarely known. Excessive opening or prolonged stretch, as associated with lengthy dental procedures, may be contributing factors. Disk displacement has been associated with TMJ hypermobility, characterized as excessive translation of the condyle during opening. Other predisposing factors include stretched collateral ligaments and loss of elasticity of the posterior ligaments, which may allow the disk to displace anteriorly to the condyle.

One possible complication of disk displacement is AVN of the condyle, resulting from backward and upward displacement of the condyle, which causes compression of the bilaminar zone containing the collateral blood supply to the condyle.

Clinical Presentation

Disk displacement, and the subsequent soft tissue and osseous changes, can be seen as a progressive disorder with identifiable stages.[19] The first signs of disk displacement are clicking in the joint and disturbance of smooth movement. Motion may be severely restricted and painful in the early stages of permanent displacement, but later movement may return to almost normal.

Classification

Disk displacements are commonly classified into reducible and nonreducible types (permanent displacements). In reducible disk displacements, the disk returns to its normal position on top of the condyle during the opening movement but displaces each time the condyle moves back during the closing movement. Nonreducible displacements are characterized by a disk that remains displaced and deformed in front of the condyle throughout the opening movement (Fig. 8-26). Although the disk most commonly displaces anterior to the condyle, it is now believed that coronal plane displacement, resulting from weakening of one of the collateral ligaments, precedes anterior displacement.[20]

Grading Displacements

For grading purposes, the superior and anterior aspects of the condyle are divided into four segments, and disk displacement is graded based on the position of the posterior edge of the disk relative to these segments (see Fig. 8-26). In joints with reducible disk displacement, the disk is located anterior to the condyle when the mouth is closed but reduces to again be positioned on the top of the condyle at some degree of opening. When the disk is displaced for any length of time, it becomes deformed, often assuming a biconvex shape, which makes reduction of the disk more difficult.

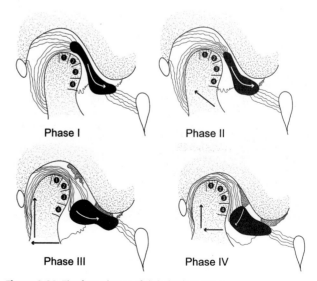

Figure 8-26 The four phases of disk displacement.

Radiologic Findings

No definitive diagnostic conclusions regarding the position of the disk can be made based on conventional radiographs or tomograms. However, loss of joint height between the condyle and the roof of the mandibular fossa could indicate disk displacement, which allows the condyle to migrate up and backward (Fig. 8-27). If the joint height increases once the condyle reaches the eminence during forward translation, it is likely that the disk will be reducible.

MRI of Disk Displacements

MRI is the definitive imaging modality for evaluating disk displacement. It can be used to evaluate the direction and phase of displacement as well as morphologic changes of the disk. The main difficulty in visualizing the disk lies in its low signal intensity, which often makes it difficult to differentiate from the adjacent cortical bone of the condyle and the articular eminence.

Anterior displacement of the disk is usually easy to identify. However, a disk that appears to be sitting on top of the condyle in the sagittal image may actually be displaced sideways when examined in the coronal view, indicating failure of one of the collateral ligaments. In the case of sideways disk displacement, the condyle may also be abnormally positioned; in such cases the disk tends to subluxate in the opposite direction to the condyle (Fig. 8-28).

Treatment of Disk Displacement

With signs of impending displacement, preventive measures are critical. These include postural correction and restoration of normal joint surface relationships through exercises. In the case of a reducible disk displacement, longitudinal traction or lateral excursion to the opposite side is frequently used to reduce displaced disks (Fig. 8-29). This treatment is followed up by measures aimed at stabilizing the disk in this position, such as exercises and splint therapy.

Retrusion With Occlusive Force in the Treatment of Disk Displacement

Following disk reduction during protrusion (note that this is easier than reduction with opening, which has a tendency to push the disk forward), contraction of the muscles of mastication can serve to stabilize the disk on the condyle while the condyles translate posteriorly to the fully occluded position. The disk now follows the condyle, because the contractile force keeps the condyle seated in the concavity of the disk (Fig. 8-30). Lasting success for this treatment depends on the patient's ability to perform functional movements without losing the correct disk–condyle relationship.

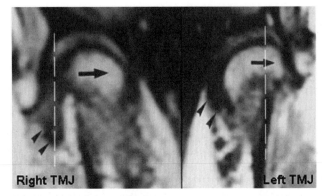

Figure 8-28 Bilateral disk displacements, with condylar subluxation in direction opposite to the disk displacements. The arrowheads show the outlines of the displaced disks. The dashed lines demonstrate the condylar displacement relative to the temporal bone. *(Image courtesy of M. Rocabado.)*

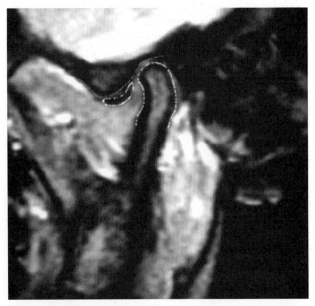

Figure 8-27 Disk displacement in full occlusion. This MR image shows the left TMJ of a 14-year-old girl with anterior disk displacement. The disk is sitting on the eminence, whereas the condyle has migrated superiorly and is positioned deep within the fossa. *(Image courtesy of M. Rocabado.)*

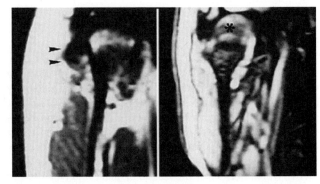

Figure 8-29 Reduction of a laterally displaced disk. In these coronal MR images showing the right TMJ, the lateral disk displacement is evident in the image to the left (arrowheads). The image on the right shows reduction of disk (asterisk) accomplished with lateral excursion to the left. This presumably results from the distraction accompanying lateral excursion to the opposite side. *(Image courtesy of M. Rocabado.)*

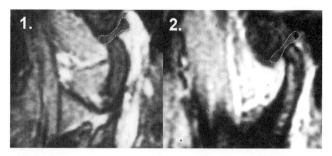

Figure 8-30 Disk reduction, using on occlusal force. These sagittal MR images show the right TMJ of a patient with a disk that displaced during the closing movement. Once the disk has been reduced with full protrusion of the mandible (1), the patient bites on a hyperbole. The occlusal force, which stabilizes the disk on top of the condyle, is maintained during retrusion. The condyle can now translate back without displacing posteriorly out of the concavity of the disk (2). The normal articular height has been restored (+). *(Image courtesy of M. Rocabado.)*

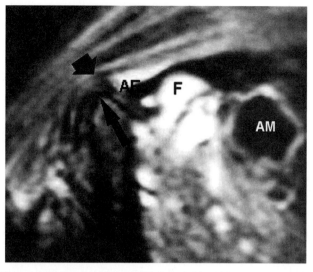

Figure 8-31 Hypermobility resulting in impingement on temporalis tendon. This MR image demonstrates excessive translation of the condyle (long arrow) beyond the articular eminence (AE). The translation causes considerable deformation of the temporalis tendon (short arrow). *(Image courtesy of M. Rocabado.)*

Other Disorders and Findings

TMJ Hypermobility

Hypermobility of the TMJ presents mechanical problems and results in an increased load on muscles and soft tissues surrounding the joint, such as the anterior capsule and the posterior aspect of the temporalis tendon (Fig. 8-31). Hypermobility of the TMJ has been linked to an increased incidence of OA and is thought to contribute to disk displacement.[21]

Disk Adhesion

Conversely, the disk may be hypomobile; stuck on the articular eminence. The biomechanical consequences of this condition vary according to where the disk is 'stuck.' If it is stuck in the resting position, the condyle displaces out of the concavity of the disk when the joint moves beyond mid–range of motion; if it is stuck further along the eminence, the disk–condyle articulation reduces with full opening. The MRI diagnosis is made not by visualizing an adhesion, but on account of lack of disk motion.

Fractures

Fractures of the mandible or condyle most frequently result from sports participation or manual blows. If the teeth are in contact during the blow, this may help to diffuse the impact. Fractures can involve the condylar neck, the upper part of the ramus, or the body of the mandible (Fig. 8-32). Fractures are usually adequately demonstrated with conventional radiography, although CT may be used for complex fractures.

The type of displacement associated with fractures depends in part on the forces acting on the fragments. In the case of a condylar neck fracture, the lateral pterygoid may externally rotate the fragment and displace it anterior to the ramus. In the case of a coronoid process fracture, the fragment may be displaced upward.[22]

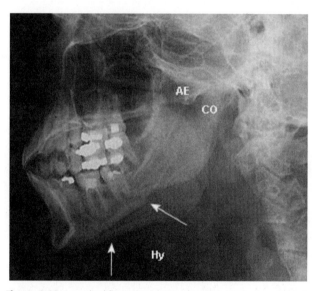

Figure 8-32 Lateral oblique projection showing bilateral mandibular fracture (arrows). *(Image courtesy of Amilcare Gentili, MD, http://www.gentili.net/)*

Craniomandibular Anomalies

The craniomandibular region can be affected by various congenital or acquired anomalies. The bones may be asymmetrical, and this can affect the function of the TMJ, just as changes in function can lead to asymmetry. Clinicians working in the field of craniofacial pain are particularly interested in facial asymmetry, which is found more commonly in patients diagnosed with TMJ disorders and unilateral headaches than in asymptomatic individuals.[23] Facial asymmetry is frequently caused by degenerative and pathological changes in the condyles. Craniomandibular anomalies are most often assessed and measured clinically and with cephalometry.

One anomaly that can affect TMJ function is Eagle syndrome, an elongation of the styloid process, or ossification of the stylohyoid ligament, first described by American otorhinolaryngologist Watt Weems Eagle in 1937.[24] This ossification can cause facial pain, tracheal pain, and dysphagia and present a mechanical impediment to cervical and TMJ motions (Fig. 8-33).

The TMJ and the Cervical Spine

Imaging of the cervical spine may be included in the assessment of TMJ disorders for the following reasons:

- Pain associated with TMJ disorders is usually in the sensory distribution of the trigeminal nerve and the C2, C3, and C4 dermatomes; thus the cervical spine is a plausible source of pain.
- The position of the subcranial joints can influence the biomechanics of the TMJ.[25]

Although discussion of the biomechanics of the cervical spine is beyond the scope of this chapter, keep in mind that the subcranial spine is responsible for up to half of all cervical spine rotation. Loss of subcranial mobility leads to increased demands on the midcervical spine and possibly results in cervical hypermobility (Fig. 8-34). If the cervical spine is not properly aligned, compensation may take place in the subcranial spine for the purpose of achieving a position where the eyes are level and facing forward. For example, if the midcervical spine is rotated and laterally flexed to the right, the following subcranial compensation takes place:

1. The C0–C1 joint must be extended and laterally flexed to the left, in order to keep the eyes level.
2. The C1–C2 joint must rotate to the left, in order to keep the eyes facing forward.

Positional Faults of the Cervical Spine

The term *positional fault* is frequently used by clinicians who specialize in treating the spine to describe an asymmetrical position of a vertebra. In the context of craniofacial pain, extension of the subcranial joints, accompanied by a loss of cervical lordosis, is the most common positional fault. These postural changes can be triggered by changes in mandibular position, often due to changes in breathing patterns.[26]

Cervical Position in the Sagittal Plane

The sagittal alignment of the cervical spine is intricately linked with the position of the subcranial joints and affects

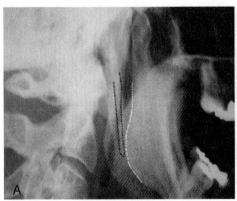
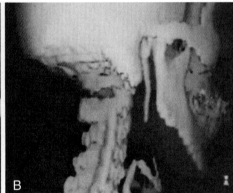

Figure 8-33 Eagle syndrome resulting in limited opening of the mouth. The image on the left is a lateral radiograph of the upper cervical spine and mandible, made during full opening. Note that the head is slightly rotated to the left, with the result that the right mandible (white dotted line) appears to be anterior to the left mandible. The elongated right styloid process is outlined in gray. The image on the right is a three-dimensional reformatted CT image, demonstrating the extensive ossification of the stylohyoid ligament and its relationship to the mandible. *(Image courtesy of M. Rocabado.)*

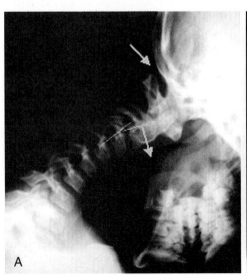
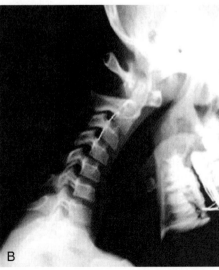

Figure 8-34 Loss of C0–C1 flexion in a 9-year-old boy. The radiograph to the left shows full cervical flexion. The posterior arch of the C1 vertebra, however, does not move relative to the occiput, so the C0–C1 posterior interspace is reduced, while the C1–C2 space is increased. The major compensation, however, takes place at the C2–C3 level. Here excessive angulation, due to hypermobility, can be seen; note the lines drawn along the posterior vertebral borders of C2 and C3. The right radiograph is made following treatment aimed at mobilizing C0–C1, resulting in normalized relationships. *(Image courtesy of M. Rocabado.)*

the position of the mandible, but it is also associated with clinical problems, such as the following:

- Increased TMJ muscle activity
- Increased muscle tension in the subcranial area
- Compression of soft tissue structures in the posterior subcranial spaces (Fig. 8-35)
- Loss of cervical lordosis

Loss of Cervical Lordosis

The chain of events associated with extension of the sub-cranial spine (decreased craniovertebral angle) and loss of cervical lordosis can be summarized as follows:

1. The head is brought level (McGregor's line horizontal), even if the subcranial spine is extended.
2. This produces flexion of the C2 vertebra.
3. The retroverted inferior endplate of the vertebral body of C2 now produces flexion of the C2–C3 joint, resulting in a flexed position of the C3 vertebra.
4. The mid-cervical lordosis is flattened or reversed, with a forward head position (see Fig. 8-35).

The problems associated with loss of cervical lordosis include the following:

1. A shift of load from the lower cervical to the midcervical and subcranial spine
2. Premature osteoarthritic changes of the facet joints[27]
3. Increased incidence of headaches, which can be due to:
   a. Increased activity of the muscles of mastication
   b. Static tension of the subcranial muscles
   c. Compression of the C1 and C2 nerves
   d. Compression of the vertebral artery
   e. Loss of shock absorption in the cervical spine

Note that subcranial spaces can be decreased both between C1 and the occiput (see Figs. 8-34 and 8-35) and between C1 and C2 (Fig. 8-36).

Positional Faults in the Coronal Plane

Positional faults in the coronal plane can lead to an altered pattern of movement of the TMJ. For example, lateral flexion to the left may be associated with hypermobility of the right TMJ. Subcranial asymmetries may also result in compression of neural structures. These positional faults, best seen on the anterioposterior (AP) open-mouth view (Fig. 8-37) and better described in Chapter 7, most often involve rotation at the C1–C2 joint (Fig. 8-38).

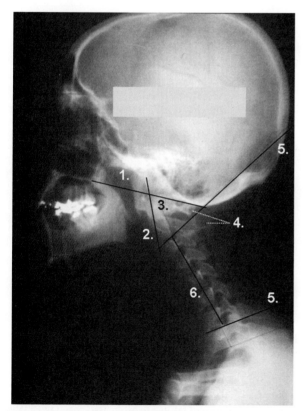

Figure 8-35 Forward head posture resulting in severe disturbances of cervical alignment. Note the following: (1) McGregor's line is directed 12 degrees anterosuperiorly instead of beieng horizontal; (2) the odontoid plane is directed anteriorly by 10 degrees instead of posteriorly by 6 to 16 degrees; (3) the craniocervical angle is decreased, measuring only 68 degrees; (4) there is a loss of the posterior subcranial space as the spinous process of C2 is up against the occiput, with the posterior arch of C1 barely visible; (5) the lordosis is reversed, as seen by the fact that lines drawn from the inferior aspects of the vertebral bodies of T1 and C2 diverges posteriorly instead of converging, producing 20 degrees of kyphosis instead of the normal 35 degrees of lordosis; (6) the posterior borders of the vertebral bodies of C4 through C6 all fall behind the C2–C7 line. *(Image courtesy of M. Rocabado.)*

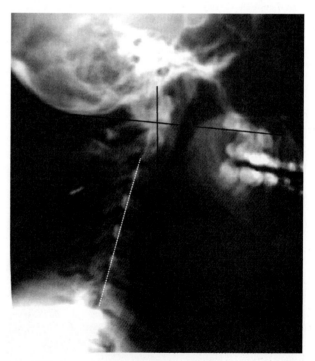

Figure 8-36 A young girl with an extended position at the C1–C2 joint. The space between the occiput and the posterior arch of C1 is normal, but the C1–C2 space is decreased. The inferior vertebral endplate of C2 is directed posteriorly, resulting in a cervical kyphosis. The craniovertebral angle, however, is normal, possibly owing to the fact that the head is held in flexion (downward-sloping McGregor's line). This compensation may not last: The odontoid plane is vertical, so once the eyes are brought level, the craniovertebral angle will be close to 90 degrees, which by definition is too small. Note that the C2–C7 line intersects all the intervening vertebrae. *(Image courtesy of M. Rocabado.)*

C1–C2 Rotational Fault

In the case of a C1–C2 rotational fault, an open-mouth radiograph may show the following:

- Decreased joint space between the inferior facet of the lateral mass of C1 and the upper facet of C2
- Apparent increased distance between the lateral mass of C1 and the dens on the side to which C1 is rotated (see Fig. 8-38); the reasons for this are explained in Figure 8-39.

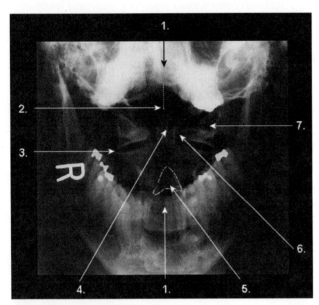

Figure 8-37 Points of interest in the AP open-mouth view. Note the following: (1) position of the central incisors; (2) intervestibular line; (3) congruity and alignment of the C1–C2 facets; (4) position of the dens relative to other midline structures; (5) C2 spinous process; (6) distance between the dens and the lateral masses of the atlas; (7) size and symmetry of the lateral masses of the atlas.

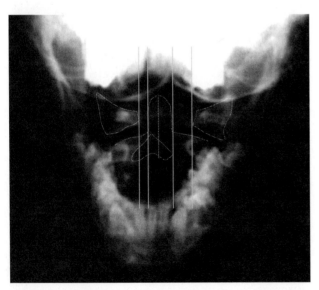

Figure 8-38 Left rotation and lateral translation of C1. The atlanto-odontoid space on the left is increased. Note that the facet joint space on the left is decreased, as the lateral mass of C1 has descended with the posterior glide accompanying the rotation. Notice in this image that the spinous process of C2 is positioned just to the right (left in the image) of a vertical line drawn through the tip of the dens. That position indicates left C2 rotation. *(Image courtesy of M. Rocabado.)*

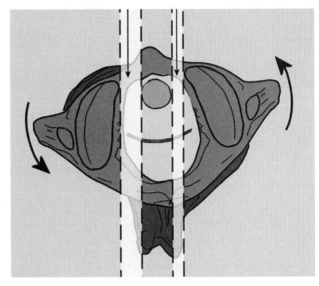

Figure 8-39 Left rotation of the C1–C2 joint. The left lateral mass moves away from the midline, opening up the apparent space on that side, but the right lateral mass closes down the right atlanto-odontoid space as seen on the AP projection.

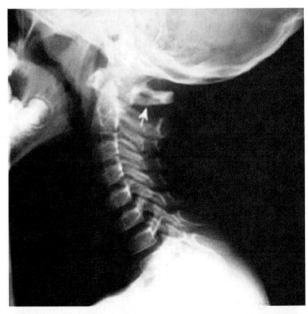

Figure 8-40 Rotation and lateral flexion of C1. Because both the left and right posterior arches of C1 can be seen on lateral view at slightly different heights, C1 is in a position of rotation and lateral flexion.

Note that rotational faults are often associated with lateral flexion, and this fault may show up on a lateral radiograph as a double image of the posterior arch of C1 (Fig. 8-40).

Acknowledgment

I would like to acknowledge the contribution of Professor Mariano Rocabado, who for over 30 years has been a leader in the field of physical therapy for the TMJ. He has graciously allowed the use of his unique collection of imaging studies for this chapter.

Summary of Key Points

Radiographic Evaluation

1. The routine radiographic evaluation related to the TMJ may consist of:
   - ➤ Transcranial view, providing a gross view of the osseous structures of the lateral part of the TMJ
   - ➤ Lateral cephalometry

Advanced Imaging

2. CT provides accurate tomography of the osseous structures of the TMJ, relatively free of superimposition.

3. MRI best demonstrates intra-articular structures and can demonstrate the shape of the disk and its position at various points of the range of motion.

4. Ultrasound offers a portable, low-cost alternative to MRI for the diagnosis of disk displacement and effusion.

Arthritides at the TMJ

5. The radiologic findings of OA include decreased joint space, subchondral sclerosis, osteophytosis, and flattening and irregularity of the joint surfaces of the condyle and articular eminence.

6. The radiologic findings of RA include decreased joint space, subchondral cysts, and resorption of the condylar head. MRI will demonstrate soft tissue edema and joint effusion.

Disk Displacements

7. Disk displacements are classified as reducing or nonreducing displacements or graded according to position of the disk relative to the condyle.

8. Radiological findings include decreased joint height. MRI, CT, or ultrasound will demonstrate the disk displaced in front of condyle and reducing at various degrees of opening or demonstrate a sideways displacement.

Other Disorders

9. TMJ hypermobility is excessive translation of the condyle during opening. It is demonstrated on conventional radiographs or MRI.

10. Fractures are most often associated with manual blows and impacts sustained in sports. Fractures frequently involve the condylar neck and are best demonstrated by conventional radiography.

TMJ and the Cervical Spine

11. Imaging of the cervical spine may be included in the assessment of TMJ disorders because the position of the subcranial joints can influence the biomechanics of the TMJ and may be the cause of referred craniofacial pain.

12. The radiologic evaluation of the cervical spine includes these additional observations:
   - ➤ *Lateral radiograph:* craniovertebral angle and loss of cervical lordosis
   - ➤ *AP open-mouth view:* positional faults in the coronal plane

---

CASE STUDY

Cervical Influence on TMJ Pain

History

Janet is a 31-year-old woman who works in a collection agency. She was involved in a rear-end collision 5 weeks ago. She immediately experienced pain in the right upper cervical area and upper trapezius as well as pain over the right side of the right mandible and painful clicking in the TMJ. At a follow-up visit, 2 weeks later, her cervical pain had subsided but there was still pain over the right TMJ. Her physician explained the symptoms as a whiplash injury to the TMJ and recommended that she visit her dentist. After a careful examination, her dentist referred her to physical therapy.

Imaging Findings

No imaging studies were performed at the emergency room, but the dentist had made transcranial radiographs. These revealed an elevated position of the right TMJ condyle as compared to the left.

Physical Therapy Examination

Complaints

Janet complained of unilateral right-sided headaches and pain in the right jaw that increased over the day. There was clicking in the right TMJ at midrange of opening and again during closing. Janet said her work involved almost continuous use of the computer, often while cradling the telephone receiver between her right shoulder and the ear. She said the computer monitor was located to the left of her keyboard.

Physical Examination

Janet demonstrated forward head posture, with visible hypertrophy of the right masseter. Active opening was accompanied by a deviation to the right that corrected, with an audible click, toward the end of range of motion. Terminal opening was limited and accompanied by pain over the right TMJ. Lateral excursion to the right was within normal limits, but left lateral excursion had only 50% of normal range of motion. Palpation revealed tenderness anterior to the right TMJ condyle. The subcranial spaces were decreased, and there was tenderness superior and medial to the C1 transverse process on the right. Active trigger points were found in the right superior oblique, sternocleidomastoid, and masseter muscles, with pain radiating to the TMJ.

Treatment

Treatment focused on the following:
- Education about workplace ergonomics and posture
- Soft tissue manipulation for the right masseter, sternomastoid, and subcranial muscles

- Cervical distraction
- Light, repetitive exercises for jaw opening
- Resisted opening exercise
- Distraction to right TMJ

Outcome

After 2 weeks and six visits, Janet reported that she was free of headaches and there was no pain on opening. The opening movement, while it was of normal range of motion, was still associated with some deviation to the right. The range of motion for left lateral excursion of the mandible was within normal limits. In spite of good resolution of signs and symptoms, further treatment was planned in order to stabilize the disk over the condyle.

Discussion

Although Janet most likely had a reducible disk displacement, which in itself is a cause for concern, her symptoms are probably related to her working conditions. Referred pain from the superior oblique and sternocleidomastoid is a likely explanation for her pain. As a result of her working conditions, both muscles are overworked in a shortened position. The masseter is obviously a source of pain as well as limitation of movement. It is, however, unlikely that the TMJ was injured during the rear-end collision, although it is likely that the injury triggered her symptoms. How can that be?

During rear-end collisions, the sternocleidomastoid muscle undergoes eccentric lengthening as it attempts to stop the backward movement of the head, and is activated before other cervical muscles.[28] This could result in injury, which in turn could produce referred pain. Her asymmetrical working positions perpetuated this injury.

CRITICAL THINKING POINT

The presumed mechanism of the TMJ whiplash injury is a forced opening of the mandible as it gets "left behind" during hyperextension. This has not been substantiated. Indeed, it has been found that sudden extension of the neck results in reflex activity of the masseter and temporalis muscles, with closing of the mouth and subsequent elevation of the mandible into full occlusion.[29] The infrahyoid and suprahyoid muscles are now in a position of mechanical advantage to resist extension of the head provided that the masseter and temporalis adequately fix the mandible. The synergy of these muscles is well known.[30]

This model could explain injury to the anterior cervical muscles and the elevator muscles of the TMJ as well as pain and changes in function, including displacement of the articular disk. It follows that soft tissue work in this area and improvements in posture could go a long way toward alleviating signs and symptoms in an individual without prior TMJ disorder.

References

1. Molin, C: From bite to mind: TMD–A personal and literature review. Int J Prosthodont 12:279, 1999.
2. Okeson, JP (ed): Orofacial Pain: Guidelines for Assessment, Diagnosis, and Management. Quintessence, Chicago, 1996.
3. Greene, CS: The etiology of temporomandibular disorders: Implications for treatment. J Orofac Pain 15:93, 2001.
4. Brooks, SL, Brand, JW, Gibbs, SJ, et al: Imaging of the temporomandibular joint: A position paper of the American Academy of Oral and Maxillofacial Radiology. Oral Surg Oral Med Oral Pathol Oral Radiol Endod 83:609, 1997.
5. Katzberg, RW, Westesson, PL, Tallents, RH, and Drake, CM: Anatomic disorders of the temporomandibular joint disc in asymptomatic subjects. J Oral Maxillofac Surg 54:147, 1996.
6. Tucker, TN: Head position for transcranial temporomandibular joint radiographs. J Prosthet Dent 52:426, 1984.
7. Hussain, AM, Packota, G, Major, PW, and Flores-Mir, C: Role of different imaging modalities in assessment of temporomandibular joint erosions and osteophytes: A systematic review. Dentomaxillofac Radiol 37:63, 2008.
8. Periago, DR, Scarfe, WC, Moshiri, M, et al: Linear accuracy and reliability of cone beam CT derived 3-dimensional images constructed using an orthodontic volumetric rendering program. Angle Orthod 78:387, 2008.
9. Vilanova, JC, Barceló, J, Puig, J, et al: Diagnostic imaging: magnetic resonance imaging, computed tomography, and ultrasound. Semin Ultrasound CT MR 28:184, 2007.
10. Sano, T, Otonari-Yamamoto, M, Otonari, T, and Yajima, A: Osseous abnormalities related to the temporomandibular joint. Semin Ultrasound CT MR 28:213, 2007.
11. Tomas, X, Pomes, J, Berenguer, J, et al: Temporomandibular joint soft-tissue pathology, II: Nondisc abnormalities. Semin Ultrasound CT MR 28:205, 2007.
12. Landes, CA, and Sader, R: Sonographic evaluation of the ranges of condylar translation and of temporomandibular joint space as well as first comparison with symptomatic joints. J Craniomaxillofac Surg 35:374, 2007.
13. Jank, S, Emshoff, R, Norer, B, et al: Diagnostic quality of dynamic high-resolution ultrasonography of the TMJ–A pilot study. Int J Oral Maxillofac Surg 34:132, 2005.
14. de Leeuw, R, Boering, G, Stegenga, B, and de Bont, LG: Symptoms of temporomandibular joint osteoarthrosis and internal derangement 30 years after non-surgical treatment. Cranio 13:81, 1995.
15. Westesson, PL: Magnetic resonance imaging of the temporomandibular joint. In Pertes, RA, and Gross, SG (eds): Clinical Management of Temporomandibular Disorders and Orofacial Pain. Quintessence, Chicago, 1995, pp 175–196.
16. Lobbezoo-Scholte, AM, Lobbezoo, F, Steenks, MH, et al: Diagnostic subgroups of craniomandibular disorders. Part II: Symptom profiles. J Orofac Pain 9:37, 1995.
17. Nicolakis, P, Burak, EC, Kollmitzer, J, et al: An investigation of the effectiveness of exercise and manual therapy in treating symptoms of TMJ osteoarthritis. Cranio 19:26, 2001.
18. Pertes, RA, and Gross, SG: Disorders of the temporomandibular joint. In Pertes, RA, Gross, SG (eds): Clinical Management of Temporomandibular Disorders and Orofacial Pain. Quintessence, Chicago, 1995, pp 69–89.
19. Bayar, N, Kara, SA, Keles, I, et al: Temporomandibular joint involvement in rheumatoid arthritis: A radiological and clinical study. Cranio 20:105, 2002.
20. Nebbe, B, and Major, PW: Prevalence of TMJ disc displacement in a pre-orthodontic adolescent sample. Angle Orthod 70:454, 2000.
21. Dijkstra, PU, de Bont, LG, de Leeuw, R, et al: Temporomandibular joint osteoarthrosis and temporomandibular joint hypermobility. Cranio 11:268, 1993.
22. Cohen HV, and Pertes, RA: Congenital, developmental and acquired disorders of the temporomandibular joint. In Pertes, RA, and Gross, SG (eds): Clinical Management of Temporomandibular Disorders and Orofacial Pain. Quintessence, Chicago, 1995, pp 109–121.
23. Schokker, RP, Hansson, TL, Ansink, BJ, and Habets, LL: Craniomandibular asymmetry in headache patients. J Craniomandib Disord 4:205, 1994.
24. Murtagh, RD, Caracciolo, JT, and Fernandez, G: CT findings associated with Eagle syndrome. AJNR Am J Neuroradiol 22:1401, 2001.
25. Zafar, H: Integrated jaw and neck function in man. Studies of mandibular and head-neck movements during jaw opening-closing tasks. Swed Dent J Suppl 143:1, 2000.
26. Solow, B, Siersbaek-Nielsen, S, and Greve, E: Airway adequacy, head posture, and craniofacial morphology. Am J Orthod 86:214, 1984.
27. Harrison, DE, Harrison, DD, Janik, TJ, et al: Comparison of axial and flexural stresses in lordosis and three buckled configurations of the cervical spine. Clin Biomech (Bristol, Avon) 16:276, 2001.
28. Brault, JR, Siegmund, GP, and Wheeler, JB: Cervical muscle response during whiplash: Evidence of a lengthening muscle contraction. Clin Biomech (Bristol, Avon) 15:426, 2000.
29. Christensen, LV, and McKay, DC: Reflex jaw motions and jaw stiffness pertaining to whiplash injury of the neck. Cranio 15:242, 1997.
30. Porterfield, JA, and DeRosa, C: Mechanical Neck Pain: Perspectives in Functional Anatomy. WB Saunders, Philadelphia, 1995.

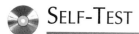

SELF-TEST

Image A

This is a transcranial radiograph of the TMJ.

1. What are the structures labeled *a* through *e* in the image?

2. How is the position of the condyle in Figure 1 different from that in Figure 2?

Image B

This is an open-mouth AP radiograph of the upper cervical spine.

3. Is the atlas rotated? To which side?

4. Is the axis rotated? To which side?

5. Is the atlas side-bent?

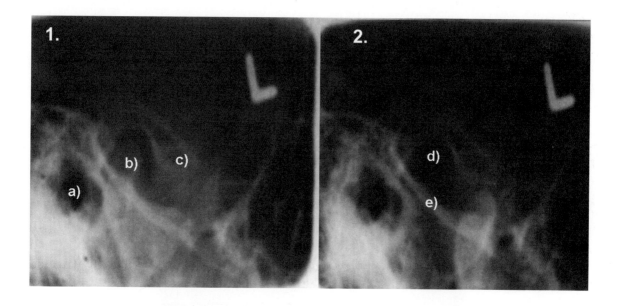

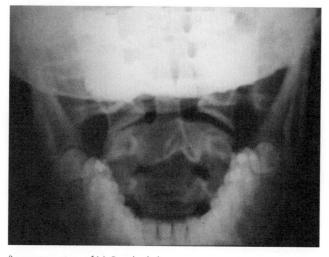

(Images courtesy of M. Rocabado.)

RADIOLOGIC EVALUATION OF THE THORACIC SPINE, STERNUM, AND RIBS

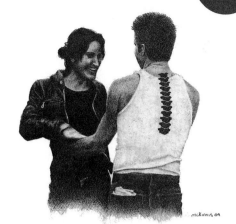

The differences in the regional characteristics of the thoracic spine result in a variety of developmental and postural deformities, fracture types, and joint dysfunctions. The cervicothoracic and thoracolumbar transitional regions are prone to specific mechanical problems, because these areas represent the junctions between the flexible cervical and lumbar spines with the less flexible thoracic spine.

Radiographically, almost all features of the thoracic spine are accountable on the anteroposterior (AP) and lateral views. The sternum and ribs are assessed on their own separate radiographic evaluations. They are included in this chapter as associated articulations often involved in injury, disease, and developmental abnormalities related to the thoracic spine.

Review of Anatomy[1–6]

Osseous Anatomy

Thorax

The bones of the thorax include the 12 thoracic vertebrae, 24 ribs, and the sternum. The thorax forms a protective cage to house the heart, lungs, and upper abdominal viscera.

The articulations of the thorax allow for flexibility to accommodate the actions of respiration and trunk mobility. Additionally, the thorax provides stability for movements of the neck and upper extremities.

Thoracic Vertebrae

Thoracic vertebrae are positioned in a convex posterior (kyphotic) curve spanning from 20 to 40 degrees of arc in the sagittal plane (Fig. 9-1). Mild lateral curves are commonly noted and are believed to be related to hand dominance. The upper thoracic vertebrae, T1–T4, exhibit some of the characteristics of cervical vertebrae, while the lower thoracic vertebrae, T9–T12, exhibit some of the characteristics of lumbar vertebrae. These transitional vertebrae are often referred to as components of the cervicothoracic and thoracolumbar regions, respectively. The vertebrae considered to be typical thoracic vertebrae are T5–T8.

Thoracic vertebrae have shield-shaped *vertebral bodies;* paired *superior and inferior costal demifacets* on the posterolateral surfaces of the bodies; round *vertebral foramina* and stout *pedicles;* short, thick *laminae* that partially overlap adjacent laminae in a shingle effect; long and downwardly inclined *spinous processes;* and long and posterolaterally inclined *transverse processes* with *costal facets* at the tips (Figs. 9-2 and 9-3). The paired *superior and inferior articular processes* form *zygapophysial joints (facet joints)* with adjacent vertebrae. Typical thoracic facet joints are oriented vertically in the frontal plane, although the upper thoracic facets gradually approach the angled frontal cervical facet orientation and the lower thoracic facets gradually approach the sagittal lumbar facet orientation. Twelve pairs of *spinal nerves* exit the *intervertebral foramina* formed by coadjacent pedicles.

Ribs

Ribs are semicircular flat bones that are continuous anteriorly with hyaline costal cartilage (Fig. 9-4). Anteriorly the first rib attaches to the sternal manubrium, the second rib to the sternal angle, and the third through sixth ribs to the sternal body. The remaining ribs attach in turn to each other, forming the costal margin. The exceptions are the 11th and 12th ribs, the "floating" ribs, which are unattached anteriorly. Posteriorly the ribs attach to the thoracic spine via the synovial costovertebral joints. Each rib head forms a costocentral joint with two adjacent vertebral bodies and the interposed intervertebral disk. Each rib tubercle forms a costotransverse joint with a transverse process. The exceptions are the first rib, which forms a costocentral joint with only one vertebral body, and the 11th and 12th ribs, which also form costocentral joints with only one vertebral body and do not articulate with the transverse processes.

Sternum

The sternum consists of a body joined superiorly via the sternal angle to the manubrium and joined inferiorly to the xiphoid process. These joints allow some movement to occur in the sternum but will generally fuse into a rigid unit after middle age.

Ligamentous Anatomy

Thoracic Vertebral Joints

The thoracic spine is supported anteriorly by the anterior longitudinal ligament attaching to the anterior margins of the vertebral bodies and intervertebral disks, increasing in

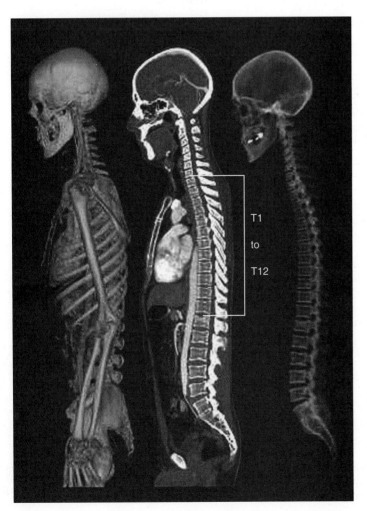

Figure 9-1 Contrast-enhanced CT study of the body, obtained in one exam in less than 17 seconds. On the left is a three-dimensional reformatted image display showing the skeleton and organs. In the middle is a two-dimensional sagittal reformatted image displayed in a *mediastinal window,* meaning that both contrast-enhanced soft tissues and bone are displayed. On the right is an image that looks like a conventional radiograph but is a sagittal reformation of the osseous spine. *(Image courtesy of Toshiba Medical Systems, Europe.)*

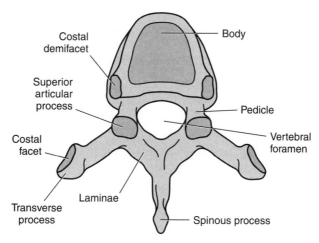

Figure 9-2 Typical thoracic vertebra, superior view.

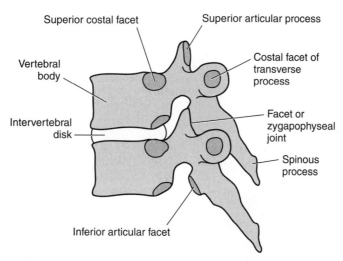

Figure 9-3 Typical thoracic vertebrae, lateral view.

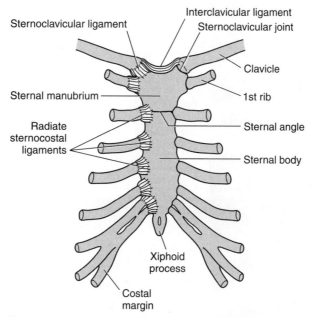

Figure 9-4 The attachment of the ribs to the sternum forms the anterior portion of the thoracic cage.

width as it extends downward from the atlas to the sacrum. Posteriorly the thoracic spine is supported by the posterior ligament complex (Fig. 9-5). The posterior ligament complex consists of the following:

1. *Posterior longitudinal ligament,* attaching to the posterior margins of the vertebral bodies and intervertebral disks and decreasing in width as it descends from the axis to the sacrum
2. *Ligamenta flava,* joining adjacent laminae

3. *Supraspinous* and *interspinous ligaments,* joining adjacent spinous processes
4. *Intertransverse ligaments,* joining adjacent transverse processes
5. *Articular capsules,* supporting the facet joints

Sternoclavicular Joint

The sternoclavicular joint is the synovial articulation between the manubrium of the sternum and the proximal

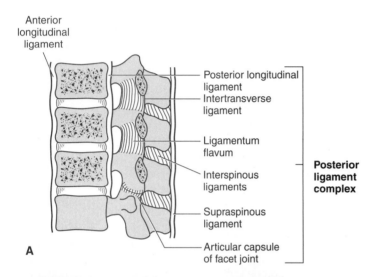

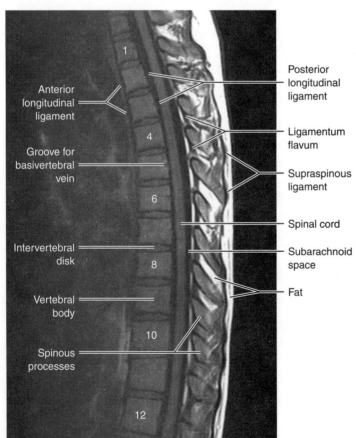

Figure 9-5 Ligaments of the thoracic spine. **(A)** Drawing is a cutaway through the vertebral body and lamina. **(B)** Sagittal T1-weighted MRI. The ligaments of the spine are possible to see on this slice. *(Image courtesy of http://www.medcyclopaedia.com by GE Healthcare.)*

end of the clavicle. A fibrocartilaginous disk, or meniscus, is interposed between the articulating surfaces. This disk facilitates anteroposterior and superoinferior gliding of the joint, as well as rotation of the clavicle. The principal stabilizing structure is the costoclavicular ligament.

Rib Joints

The ribs are attached to both the vertebral bodies and the vertebral transverse processes (Figs. 9-6 and 9-7). The costocentral joints, between the ribs and the vertebral bodies, are supported by the following:

1. *Articular capsules*
2. *Intra-articular ligaments,* blending with the fibers of the intervertebral disk
3. *Radiate or stellate ligaments* extending from the rib heads to the vertebral bodies and interposed disks

The costotransverse joints, between the ribs and the transverse processes, are supported by the following:

1. *Articular capsules*
2. *Middle costotransverse ligaments,* attaching the rib necks to the transverse processes
3. *Superior costotransverse ligaments,* attaching the rib necks to the transverse processes of the vertebrae above
4. *Lateral costotransverse ligaments,* extending from the tips of the transverse processes to the nonarticular portion of the rib tubercle

Anteriorly the ribs are joined to the sternum via radiate *sternocostal ligaments* (see Fig. 9-4).

Joint Mobility

The mobility of the thoracic vertebral segments allows for flexion, extension, lateral flexion, and rotation of the trunk to occur. The associated articulations of the bony thorax

additionally play a role in orienting and restricting trunk motion. Thus the thoracic spine, rib cage, and sternum are considered as a unit during movement, as these related articulations not only limit each other but adapt in response to movement produced by each other.

Trunk flexion, extension, and lateral flexion each incur approximately 20 to 45 degrees of motion in the thoracic spine. Trunk rotation incurs approximately 35 to 50 degrees of rotation within the thoracic spine. The elasticity of the ribs and their articulations allows for adaptive increases or decreases in the intercostal spaces and the costovertebral, sternocostal, and chondrocostal angles as the spine moves.

Growth and Development

Ossification of the Thoracic Vertebrae

Ossification of the thoracic vertebrae begins in the sixth week of fetal life. At birth the bodies of the vertebrae are ossified, and at least three ossification centers are present at each vertebral level to continue development of the body and posterior structures (see the radiograph of newborn skeleton in Fig. 11-7). Fusion of the neural arches to the spinous processes occurs by age 2 or 3, and these posterior elements fuse to the vertebral body by ages 3 to 6. At puberty, secondary centers of ossification appear at the vertebral endplates and the spinous, transverse, and articular processes. These structures complete ossification by age 25.

Radiographic Appearance of Neonate Spine

At birth the shape of the thoracic and lumbar bodies is rounded. Radiographically the superior and inferior aspects of the vertebral bodies show dense calcification, appearing as clearly defined white margins with relatively darker, more radiolucent bodies. Occasionally the opposite will be seen, and the centrum of the bodies will appear densely calcified, causing a "bone-within-bone" radiographic image. The

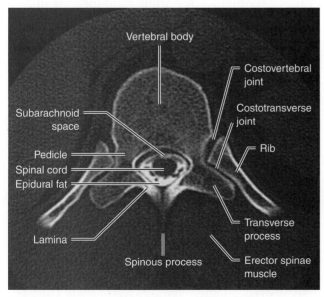

Figure 9-6 Attachment of ribs to thoracic vertebra via costocentral and costotransverse joints as seen on a CT myelographic image. *(Image courtesy of http://www.medcyclopaedia.com by GE Healthcare.)*

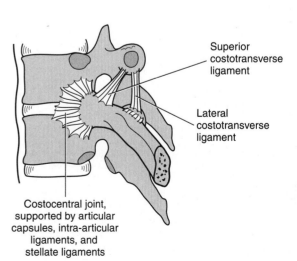

Figure 9-7 Attachment of ribs to thoracic vertebrae via costocentral and costotransverse joints, lateral view.

middle anterior aspects of the vertebral bodies will also show indentations, which are grooves for vertebral veins (Fig. 9-8). Single or double grooves may also be seen on the posterior aspects of the vertebral bodies, and these may persist into adulthood.

Vertebral Ring Apophyses

At approximately age 6, vertebral ring apophyses appear on the anterolateral superior and inferior surfaces of the middle and lower thoracic and upper lumbar vertebrae (Fig. 9-9). Less often, the cervical and upper thoracic vertebrae share in this development. Radiographically these apophyses appear as thin rims of bone slightly separated from the vertebral body. Ossification of the apophyses to the bodies is most

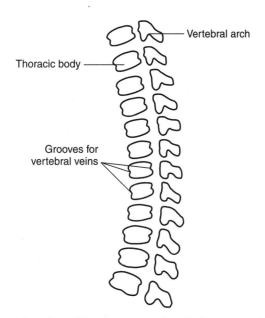

Figure 9-8 Radiographic appearance of ossified structures in the newborn thoracic spine.

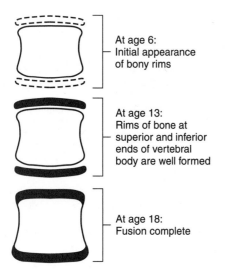

Figure 9-9 Radiographic appearance of vertebral ring apophyses.

pronounced at age 13, and fusion is usually complete by age 18. These apophyses are outside of the true epiphyseal plates and do not contribute to vertebral growth. The significance of these structures is as a radiographic indicator of skeletal age. Determination of the time frame available for effectively bracing and correcting a scoliotic curve, for example, is largely predicated on this reliable sign of skeletal maturity.

Thoracic Spine Kyphosis

The normal thoracic kyphosis increases with postural maturity from approximately 20 degrees in childhood to approximately 30 to 40 degrees in adulthood.

Excessive kyphosis can result from numerous and highly variable conditions such as the degenerative changes associated with osteoporosis, genetic predisposition, postural habits, congenital anomalies, paralysis, tuberculosis, arthritis, ankylosing spondylitis, vertebral epiphysitis (Scheuermann's disease), Paget's disease, osteomalacia, or rickets.[8-10]

Ossification of the Sternum and Ribs

Ossification of the sternum and ribs begins in the eighth to ninth week of fetal life. At birth the sternum is largely cartilaginous, with vertically positioned ossification centers at each sternebra. Fusion of the sternebrae into the sternal body takes place after puberty. At birth the xiphoid process is cartilaginous; its ossification center does not appear until 3 years of age. The xiphoid process remains cartilaginous into young adulthood.

The chondrocostal extensions of the ribs gradually undergo ossification throughout late adulthood, progressively limiting flexibility of the rib cage and in turn limiting flexibility of the thoracic spine.

Routine Radiologic Evaluation[8-17]

Practice Guidelines for Spine Radiography in Children and Adults[8]

The American College of Radiology (ACR), the principal professional organization of radiologists in the United States, defines the following practice guidelines as an educational tool to assist practitioners in providing appropriate radiologic care for patients.

Goals

The goal of thoracic spine radiographic examination is to identify or exclude anatomic abnormalities or disease processes of the spine.

The sternum is examined to assess fracture, inflammatory processes, or other pathology. The sternoclavicular joint is examined to assess joint separation or other pathology of the joint.

Indications

The indications for radiologic examination include but are not limited to trauma, pain radiating around the chest wall, limitation in motion, planned or prior surgery, evaluation of primary and secondary malignancies, arthritis, osteoporosis, compression fractures, evaluation of kyphosis and scoliosis, suspected congenital anomalies and syndromes associated with spinal abnormality, evaluation of spinal abnormality seen on other imaging studies, follow-up of known abnormality, and suspected spinal instability.[14]

Basic Projections and Radiologic Observations

Recommended Thoracic Spine Projections

Routine projections include *anteroposterior (AP)* and *lateral* views. Lower cervical or upper lumbar anatomy should be visualized to ensure accurate numbering of thoracic levels.

Additional evaluation may be needed in some circumstances and may include some or all of the following:

- *Swimmer's lateral view* of the upper thoracic region: This is a lateral view with the patient's arm placed overhead, to remove superimposition of the shoulder from obscuring the lower cervical and upper thoracic vertebrae.
- *Oblique views:* These demonstrate facet joints. This view is not included in the routine projections, because the thoracic facet joints are rarely involved in pathology.
- *Thoracolumbar* or other *coned* views: A coned view is a close-up view of a designated area. *Cone* refers to the circular aperture attachment on the x-ray tube, which limits the exposure field.

Recommended Sternum Projections

The sternum is almost impossible to see on an anteroposterior projection because of the superimposition of the denser thoracic spine. Therefore, a frontal view of the sternum is obtained by rotating the body just enough to bring the sternum out of the shadow of the spine. A posterior oblique projection, with the patient in a right anterior oblique (RAO) position, is most commonly used, as this will project the sternum over the homogeneous density of the heart, providing contrast.

If the sternoclavicular joints are the area of interest, the patient position and projection is the same, but the central ray passes through the joint area. The RAO position will image the right sternoclavicular joint; a left anterior oblique (LAO) position will image the left sternoclavicular joint.

The lateral view of the sternum is easily visualized, because the sternum is the most anterior structure in the thorax and there is a minimum superimposition of overlying tissue.

Recommended Rib Projections

The great expanse of bone, multiplanar curves, and superimposition of the muscular diaphragm necessitates the radiographic evaluation of the rib cage to be done in sections. The entire rib cage is not often radiographed in an evaluation. Rather, the clinical history and symptoms define a region of interest, and only those sections are radiographed.

Rib sections include the anterior ribs, the posterior ribs, and the axillary ribs. These sections are further divided into their right or left sides. These sections are again divided into the upper ribs, 1 to 9, which can be visualized above the density of the diaphragm, and the lower ribs, 8 to 12, which can be imaged with altered exposure below the level of the diaphragm.

Rib sections are radiographed with either AP or posteroanterior (PA) projection for the posterior or anterior ribs, and oblique projections for the axillary ribs. A PA chest film is often included in a trauma rib series to rule out possible pneumothorax or hemothorax. See Chapter 10.

Trauma at the Thoracic Spine[16,18–36]

The thoracic spine is most commonly injured because of flexion forces. The vertebrae most commonly injured are the transitional vertebrae of the cervicothoracic and thoracolumbar regions. These regions are predisposed to injury because they are the junctions between the relatively immobile thoracic spine and the more flexible cervical and lumbar spines.

The incidence of acute injury is highest in the thoracolumbar vertebrae. The 12th thoracic and first lumbar vertebrae are most frequently involved and less often the 11th thoracic and second lumbar vertebrae. Compression fractures and fracture–dislocations commonly occur in this region. Neurological injury complicates 15% to 20% of fractures at the thoracolumbar level.

Diagnostic Imaging for Trauma of the Thoracic Spine

Imaging of the thoracic and lumbar spine after blunt trauma (high energy injury mechanisms such as motor vehicle accidents) has changed in recent years due to the availability of high speed computed tomography (CT) in trauma centers and emergency departments. Patients with serious injuries are often assessed with *thorax–abdomen–pelvis body (TAP)* CT scans. The data from these scans can be reformatted to evaluate the spine without further cost or radiation exposure and without additional time required to perform separate radiographic studies.

The literature supports the superiority of CT over radiographs in the detection of spinal fractures. Some factors that account for this is that noncontiguous spinal injuries are often multiple (as many as 25%); thus identification of a spinal fracture at one level may imply a need to survey the remainder of the spine. Also, thoracolumbar injuries are often multiple and known to be frequently missed in patients with multiple other injuries, especially patients with significant *distracting* injuries. Distracting injuries are defined as acute injuries requiring immediate attention, such as long bone fractures or visceral injuries requiring surgery. Again, the utility of CT scan to acquire all data in one exam is unsurpassed.

Children age 14 or older are usually treated as adults, as their spines are fully developed. Recommendations for patients 16 years of age or younger are to initially evaluate the thoracic and lumbar spine with AP and lateral radiographs

Routine Radiologic Evaluation of the Thoracic Spine

Anteroposterior

This view demonstrates the thoracic vertebral bodies; the intervertebral disk spaces; alignment of the pedicles, spinous processes, transverse processes, and articular processes; and the costovertebral joints and posterior ribs.

Radiologic Observations[11,15–21]

The important observations are:

1. The alignment of the vertebral bodies forms an approximately vertical column with well-preserved intervertebral disk spaces.
2. Rotation in the thoracic column is identified by the rotation of a pedicle image toward the midline or of the spinous process away from midline. Mild rotation is not an abnormal finding; it can be a result of positioning inaccuracy or related to postural patterns.
3. The pedicles are spaced equidistantly from the midline spinous processes. The width between opposing paired pedicles, *the interpedicular distance,* is normally 20 mm in the thoracic spine (*a* in Fig. 9-10). The interpedicular distance represents the transverse diameter of the spinal canal. Compromise of this space is a threat to the spinal cord. Significant misalignment may be an indication of fracture–dislocation.
4. Intervals between each spinous process, from the vertebra above to the vertebra below, are compared for consistency

Basic Projections

- **AP thoracic spine**
- Lateral thoracic spine

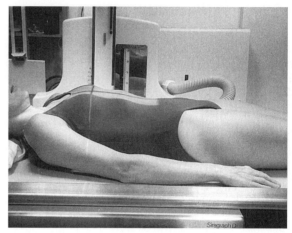

Setting up the Radiograph

Figure 9-11 Patient position for an AP projection of the thoracic spine.

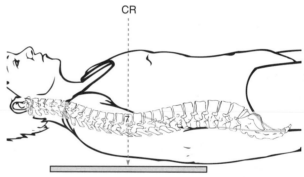

Figure 9-12 The central ray is perpendicular to the image receptor and passes through the ninth thoracic vertebra.

(*b* in Fig. 9-10). An increased interval at one level may indicate a torn posterior ligament complex.
5. The articular processes cast a butterfly-shaped shadow over the vertebral body. Although the plane of the facet joints is not visible, the alignment of the articular processes is evident. Misalignment is an indication of fracture–dislocation or subluxation.
6. The costocentral and costotransverse joints are visible, although they are normally superimposed at many vertebrae.
7. The ribs normally form smooth, curving margins.

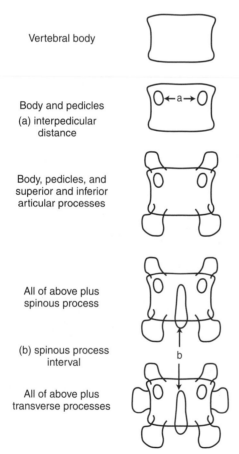

Vertebral body

Body and pedicles
(a) interpedicular distance

Body, pedicles, and superior and inferior articular processes

All of above plus spinous process

(b) spinous process interval

All of above plus transverse processes

Figure 9-10 Schematic to distinguish vertebral structures on an AP radiograph. *(Adapted from Squires and Novelline,[22] p. 169.)*

What Can You See?

Look at the radiograph (Fig. 9-13) and try to identify the radiographic anatomy. Trace the outlines of structures using a marker and transparency sheet. Compare results with the book tracing (Fig. 9-14). Can you identify the following:

- Thoracic vertebral bodies
- Spinous processes
- Pedicles
- Transverse processes (note the size distortion of the transverse processes of T8–T10 owing to slight rotation of the bodies)
- Superior and inferior articular processes
- Ribs and their vertebral articulations

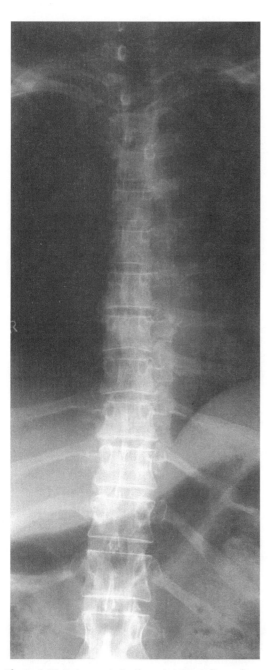

Figure 9-13 Anteroposterior thoracic spine radiograph.

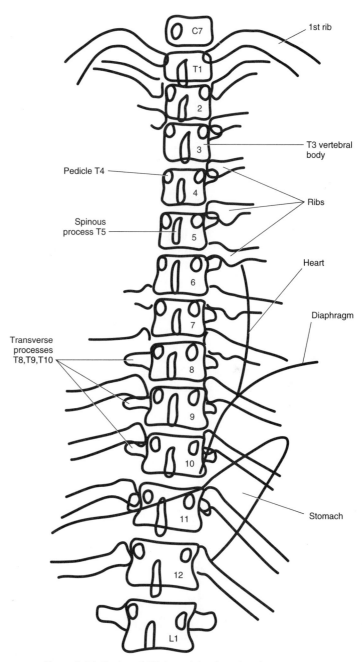

Figure 9-14 Tracing of AP view of the thoracic spine.

Routine Radiologic Evaluation of the Thoracic Spine

Lateral

This view demonstrates the thoracic vertebral bodies, intervertebral disk spaces, and intervertebral foramina. The uppermost two or three thoracic vertebrae are not well visualized because of superimposition of the shoulder. If these vertebrae are of special interest, a *swimmer's lateral* projection is done with the arm positioned overhead to remove the obstruction of the shoulder.

Radiologic Observations

The important observations on the lateral view are:

1. As observed in the cervical spine, normal alignment of the thoracic vertebrae is similarly verified by identifying three roughly parallel lines (Fig. 9-15).

   - *Line 1:* the *anterior vertebral body line,* representing the connected anterior borders of the vertebral bodies, forms a smooth, continuous curve.
   - *Line 2:* the *posterior vertebral body line,* representing the connected posterior borders of the vertebral bodies, forms a continuous curve parallel to line 1.
   - *Line 3:* the *spinolaminar line,* representing the junctions of the laminae at the spinous processes, forms a continuous curve parallel to lines 2 and 3. Because of overlapping laminae and long, downwardly inclined spinous processes, the spinolaminar line in the thoracic region exhibits a shingle effect.

   The spatial relationship of these three lines will normally remain constant during any amount of thoracic flexion or extension. Disruptions in these parallel lines may indicate fracture or dislocation. Remember that the spinal canal lies between lines 2 and 3, and compromise of this space seriously threatens the integrity of the spinal cord. In the presence of a fracture or dislocation, this space may show an increase or decrease in diameter, relative to adjacent levels.

2. The vertebral bodies are box-like in appearance with distinct, smoothly curved osseous margins.

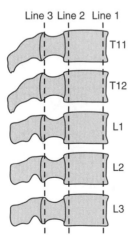

Figure 9-15 Normal alignment of thoracic vertebrae on the lateral view is verified by identifying three approximately parallel lines. Line 1 = anterior vertebral body line; line 2 = posterior vertebral body line; line 3 = spinolaminar line. This spatial relationship will normally hold true in any degree of flexion or extension.

Basic Projections

- AP thoracic spine
- **Lateral thoracic spine**

Setting up the Radiograph

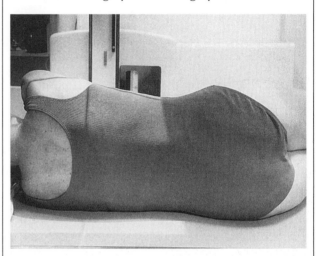

Figure 9-16 Patient position for a lateral thoracic spine projection.

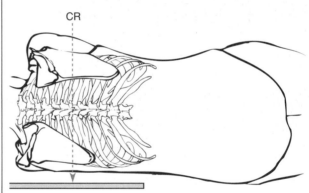

Figure 9-17 The central ray is perpendicular to the image receptor and passes through the ninth thoracic vertebra.

3. The intervertebral foramina, through which the spinal nerves exit, are normally imaged as radiolucent ovals. Narrowed, ragged margins of the ovals indicate bony encroachment upon the spinal nerves or the spinal canal.
4. The intervertebral disk spaces normally exhibit well-preserved joint space. Note any osteophyte formation at the joint margins, indicating degenerative changes.
5. The pedicles are superimposed as a pair at each level.
6. The axillary portions of the ribs overlay the thoracic spine but are easily projected through, because they are less dense than the vertebrae. The posterior rib cage is projected tangentially and images as a dense border posterior to the vertebrae.
7. Zygapophyseal (facet) joint articulations are partially seen at some levels.
8. The soft tissue density representing the diaphragm may be seen as a shadow superimposed over the lower thoracic vertebrae.

What Can You See?

Look at the radiograph (Fig. 9-18) and try to identify the radiographic anatomy. Trace the outlines of structures using a marker and transparency sheet. Compare results with the book tracing (Fig. 9-19). Can you identify the following:

- Vertebral bodies
- Pedicles, laminae, and spinous processes

- Intervertebral foramina
- Facet joints that are visible
- Axillary portion of the ribs
- Diaphragm

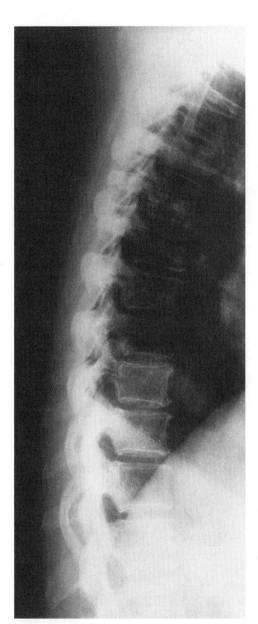

Figure 9-18 Lateral thoracic spine radiograph.

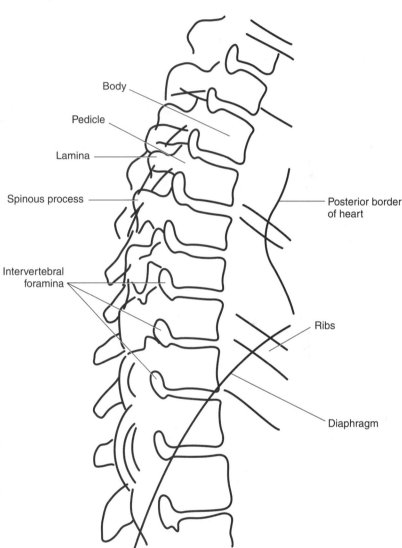

Figure 9-19 Tracing of lateral view of the thoracic spine.

Routine Radiologic Evaluation of the Sternum

Posterior Oblique

This view projects the sternum over the homogeneous density of the heart, allowing for contrast to delineate the image of the sternum. Some distortion of the sternum occurs because of the obliquity of the projection.

If the sternoclavicular joints are the area of interest, the central ray will pass through the joint area. The RAO position will image the right sternoclavicular joint; an LAO position will image the left sternoclavicular joint.

Radiologic Observations

The important observations are:

1. Many densities are superimposed over the image of the sternum. These include the radiodensities of anterior and posterior ribs, as well as the radiolucencies of the lungs and trachea.
2. A gross look at the manubrium and the sternal body is seen, with some distortion owing to the obliquity of the position and projection.
3. Articulation between the manubrium and sternal body is seen at the radiolucent sternal angle. Another articulation is seen at the junction of the sternal body to xiphoid process.
4. Joint articulations include the sternoclavicular joints and the sternocostal joints. Note the first rib articulation to the manubrium is immediately inferior to the clavicular articulation.

Basic Projections

- **Posterior oblique (in RAO position)**
- Lateral

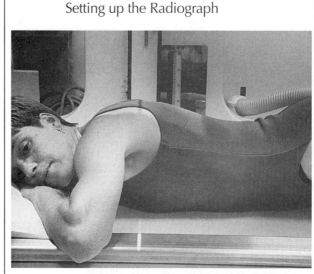

Setting up the Radiograph

Figure 9-21 Patient position for RAO projection of the sternum.

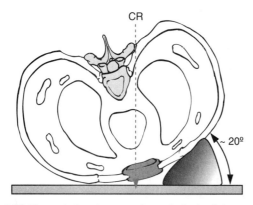

Figure 9-20 The central ray is centered over the body of the sternum. If the sternoclavicular joints are the area of interest, the positioning is the same but the central ray passes through the joint area.

What Can You See?

Look at the radiograph (Fig. 9-22) and try to identify the radiographic anatomy. Trace the outlines of structures using a marker and transparency sheet. Can you identify the following:

- Manubrium
- Body of the sternum
- Sternoclavicular joints
- Sternal angle
- Xiphoid process
- Costoclavicular joints

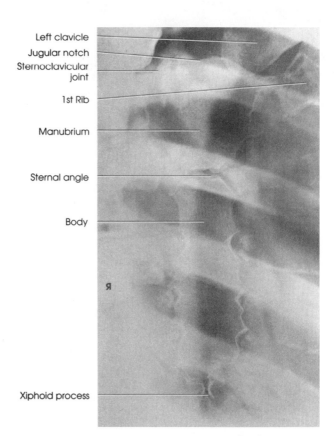

Left clavicle
Jugular notch
Sternoclavicular joint
1st Rib
Manubrium
Sternal angle
Body
Xiphoid process

Figure 9-22 PA oblique projection sternum, RAO position. *(Reprinted with permission from Merrill's Atlas of Radiographic Positions and Radiologic Procedures ed. 10. Mosby, St. Louis, MO, 2003, p. 501.)*

Routine Radiologic Evaluation of the Sternum

Lateral

This view of the sternum is easily visualized since the sternum is the most anterior structure in the thorax and there is a minimum superimposition of overlying tissue.

Radiologic Observations

The important observations are:

1. This lateral view of the thorax allows a gross look at the sternum from the manubrium to the xiphoid process.
2. Sternoclavicular and sternocostal joints are not seen as these structures lie tangent to the beam.

Basic Projections

- Posterior oblique (RAO position)
- **Lateral**

What Can You See?

Look at the radiograph (Fig. 9-24) and try to identify the radiographic anatomy. Trace the outlines of structures using a marker and transparency sheet. Compare results with the book tracing (Fig. 9-25). Can you see the following:

- Manubrium
- Body of the sternum
- Xiphoid process

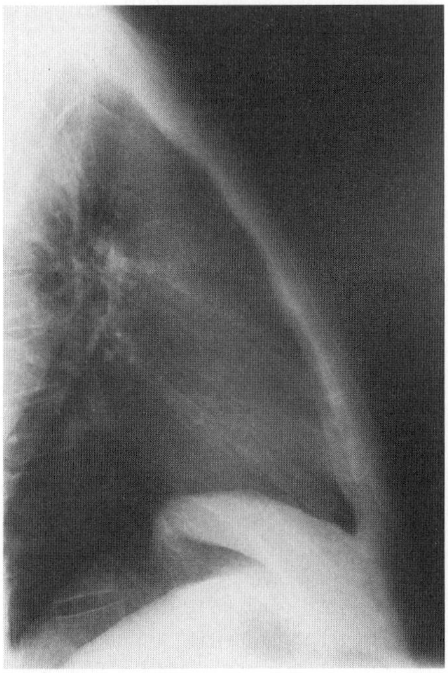

Setting up the Radiograph

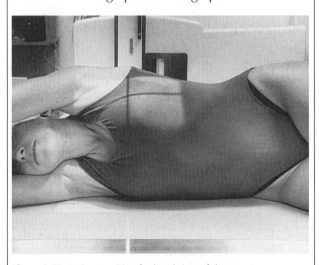

Figure 9-23 Patient position for latral view of the sternum.

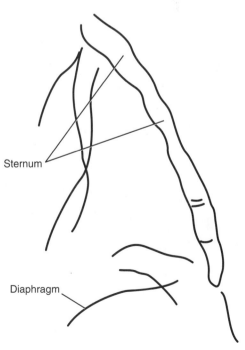

Figure 9-24 Lateral sternum radiograph.

Sternum

Diaphragm

Figure 9-25 Tracing of lateral view of the sternum.

Routine Radiologic Evaluation of the Ribs

Anteroposterior or Posteroanterior

The AP projection (Fig. 9-26) demonstrates the posterior ribs (shown here), as the posterior ribs are closest to the image receptor. A PA projection (with patient in a prone position) would be used to demonstrate the anterior ribs, which would then be closest to the image receptor.

Radiologic Observations

The important observations are:

1. The rib cage is radiographed in sections to best image one region, determined by clinical presentation. To overcome the difficulty of looking at multiple rib superimposition, try to identify that specific section that is being radiographed and use anatomic landmarks to organize your perception of which ribs are which.
2. In this AP projection, both anterior and posterior ribs are visible. The posterior ribs, however, are best defined due to minimal magnification, and can be seen attaching to the thoracic vertebrae. (On a PA projection of the anterior ribs, you would look for their attachment to the sternum, which is more difficult to see due to their cartilaginous density.)
3. Note that in the above-diaphragm radiograph images (Fig. 9-27), the ribs are superimposed over the radiolucent air-filled lungs and the radiodensity of the heart. The patient is instructed to take a deep breath to depress the diaphragm, which allows visualization of more ribs.
4. The below-diaphragm radiograph images (Fig. 9-28) the ribs superimposed over the radiodensites of the diaphragm and abdominal organs. The exposure is made at the end of full expiration, which elevates the diaphram and abdominal viscera, providing a more homogenous soft tissue density to view the ribs on.

Setting up the Radiograph

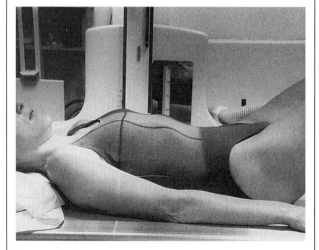

Figure 9-26 Patient position for anteroposterior projection of the right posterior ribs, above diaphragm.

Basic Projections

- **AP** or PA
- Anterior oblique (AO) or posterior oblique (PO)

What Can You See?

Look at the both radiographs of the posterior ribs. Can you identify the following:

- Thoracic vertebrae
- Costovertebral joints
- Soft tissues: diaphragm, heart
- Ribs 1 to 10 above diaphragm, ribs 8 to 12 below diaphragm

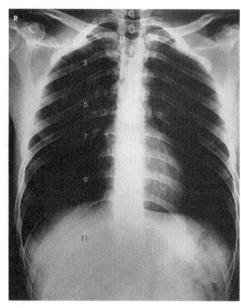

Figure 9-27 AP projection of posterior ribs (numbered) above diaphragm. *(Reprinted with permission from Merrill's Atlas of Radiographic Positions and Radiologic Procedures, ed. 10. Mosby, St. Louis, MO, 2003, p. 521.)*

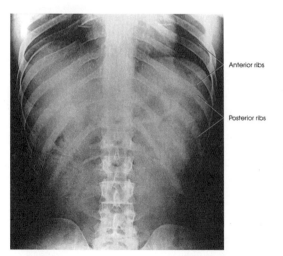

Anterior ribs

Posterior ribs

Figure 9-28 AP projection of the posterior ribs, below diaphragm. *(Reprinted with permission from Merrill's Atlas of Radiographic Positions and Radiologic Procedures, ed. 10. Mosby, St. Louis, MO, 2003, p. 521.)*

Routine Radiologic Evaluation of the Ribs

Anterior Oblique (AO) or Posterior Oblique (PO)

Oblique rib projections demonstrate the axillary ribs. The *projection* may be either AO or PO with the patient in either an AO or PO *position*. Shown here is an *anterior oblique projection* with the patient in a *right posterior oblique (RPO) position*.

Radiologic Observation

With the patient in an oblique position, the central ray is directed at the posterolateral rib cage, avoiding superimposition of the sternum and spine (Fig. 9-29).

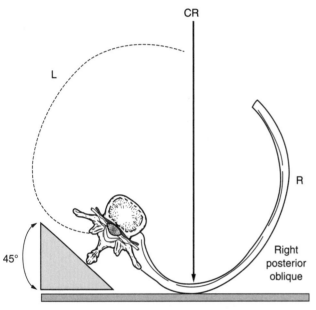

Figure 9-29 Patient position for posterior oblique projection of the right posterolateral axillary ribs, above diaphragm.

Basic Projections

- AP or PA
- AO or **PO**

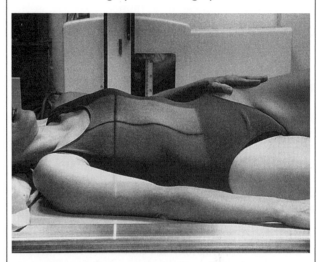

Setting up the Radiograph

Figure 9-30 AP oblique projection, RPO position. The central ray passes through the right posterolateral ribs, which are closest to the image receptor.

What Can You See?

Look at the AP radiograph (Fig. 9-31). Can you see the following:

- At least 8 ribs above diaphragm
- Soft tissues: the magnified heart, border of the diaphragm

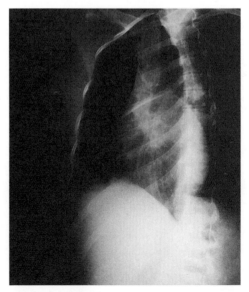

Figure 9-31 Anterior oblique radiograph of right posterolateral axillary ribs, above diaphragm.

unless they have already had a thorax–abdomen–pelvis CT scan. Considerations regarding radiation exposure in this age group are paramount; subsequent CT scanning as a supplement to radiographs should be used very selectively for complex problem solving only.

Magnetic resonance imaging (MRI) is the primary modality to evaluate the degree of neural compromise, cord edema, cord contusion, epidural hematoma, nerve root involvement, or ligamentous disruption. However, isolated ligamentous injury in the absence of fracture is rare in the thoracolumbar spine (unlike the cervical spine). MRI is not indicated if the CT scan is normal.

The Three-Column Concept of Spinal Stability

Viewing the thoracolumbar spine as three linear columns is a well-established concept developed to determine the stability of various vertebral injuries (Fig. 9-32). The *anterior column* consists of the anterior longitudinal ligament and the anterior two-thirds of the vertebral body and annulus fibrosus. The *middle column* consists of the posterior third of the body and annulus and the posterior longitudinal ligament. The *posterior column* consists of the posterior ligament complex and the vertebral arch structures.

Fractures involving only one column are considered stable injuries, and fractures involving all three columns are considered unstable injuries. Involvement of two columns may or may not be stable, depending on the degree of injury. Thoracolumbar stability usually follows the middle column; if it is intact, the injury is usually stable.

One- or Two-Column Injuries

A frequent type of thoracic spine injury involving only one column is a compression fracture to the anterior column. When greater force is imposed, this one-column injury can

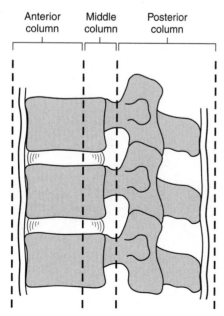

Figure 9-32 The three-column concept in viewing the thoracolumbar spine aids in determining the stability of various vertebral injuries.

become a two-column injury as the posterior column ligaments become damaged.

Anterior Vertebral Body Compression Fractures

Anterior compression fractures of the vertebral bodies are the most common spinal injury detectable on radiographs in all age groups. Over age 60, compression fractures comprise the majority of all vertebral injuries.

Mechanism of Injury

Flexion forces account for approximately 90% of compression fractures; lateral bending forces account for the remaining 10%. In younger adults, motor vehicle accidents or falls from great heights, are the precipitating events. When a person lands on his or her feet from a great height, the force that results in a hindfoot fracture can travel up the kinetic chain and also cause a fracture in the thoracolumbar vertebrae (see Fig. 11-38). In older adults, preexisting osteoporosis is a significant factor in vertebral body collapse, often with minimal imposed forces. The frequency of anterior compression fractures seen in the thoracic and thoracolumbar spines is the result of multiple factors:

- The vertebral bodies are composed of compressible, spongy cancellous bone, whereas the vertebral arches are composed of less compressible, dense cortical bone.
- An axial compressive force applied through the spinal column will result in a collapse of the anterior vertebral structures with relative sparing of the posterior structures.
- An axial force is often converted into a flexion force. A flexion force itself will load the anterior vertebral bodies first, and these areas will collapse when their weight-bearing threshold has been reached.
- The normal thoracic kyphosis predisposes the thoracic spine toward flexion.
- External factors, such as falls on the buttocks, items falling from above onto the back, or the sitting position in motor vehicles, place the spine in flexion at or prior to sustaining a compressive force.
- Additionally, humans move reflexively into flexion as a protective response; thus anticipated trauma is often sustained in a position of truncal flexion.

Characteristics

Anterior compression fractures deform the anterior vertebral body while the posterior body, vertebral arches, and posterior ligaments remain intact (Fig. 9-33). The loss of anterior vertebral body height may range in severity from barely perceptible to complete collapse with comminution.

Anterior compression fractures are considered stable fractures because only the anterior column is involved. However, if the force incurred exceeds the force that collapsed the anterior body, a distractive disruption of the posterior bony structures and ligaments can occur (Fig. 9-34). In such an instance, more than one column is involved and stability is questionable.

Differences Between Upper and Lower Thoracic Spine

The intervertebral disk is commonly injured in association with compression fractures. The different thickness of the

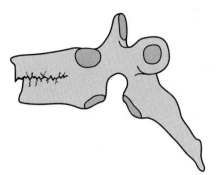

Figure 9-33 Anterior vertebral body compression fracture.

disks in the upper versus the lower thoracic spine alters the nature of both the injury to the disk and the deformity sustained by the vertebral bodies.

In the upper thoracic spine, disks are thinner and less shock-absorbing, so forces are readily transmitted to the vertebral body. The collapse of the body thus results in a true wedge-shaped deformity. In the lower thoracic and lumbar spine, disks are thicker and better shock absorbers, so forces are dispersed more readily to the disk itself and the vertebral endplates encasing it. The result is a greater occurrence of associated anterior or intervertebral disk herniations and vertebral endplate fractures and less of a vertebral body wedge deformity in this region (Fig. 9-35).

Additionally, the thickness of the disks in the lower thoracic spine also allows for greater distance between the vertebral bodies, and, in turn, greater facet joint translation is possible. A flexion force thus has the potential to translate into an anterior shearing force, tearing the outermost annular fibers that attach to the vertebral endplates (Sharpey's fibers) or avulsing the bony rims of the endplates (Fig. 9-36).

Anterior Compression Fractures in Older Adults

Compression fractures increase in incidence with age, in part as a result of degenerative changes in the vertebrae and intervertebral disks. Demineralization of bone renders the vertebrae less elastic, more brittle, and prone to fracture;

dehydration of the nucleus pulposus renders the disks less resilient to compression. These decreases in shock-absorbing qualities increase the degree of trauma suffered at the vertebrae (Fig. 9-37).

Radiologic Assessment

Radiographically, compression fractures will reflect the mechanical changes described earlier. The radiographic signs of compression fracture include the following:

1. *The step defect:* The anterior cortex of the vertebral body is the first structure to undergo strain and will suffer the greatest stress. The superior endplate is often displaced anteriorly, causing a buckling or step-off of the normally smooth concave anterior margin. This sign is best seen on the lateral view and is sometimes the only radiographic clue to a subtle compression fracture.
2. *The wedge deformity:* The collapse of the anterior vertebral body creates a triangular or trapezoidal body, apparent on the lateral view. This may result in increased kyphosis. Lateral wedging may also occur, resulting in a scoliosis, apparent on the AP view. It is estimated that at least a 30% loss of vertebral body height is required for the wedge deformity to be present on radiograph.
3. *Linear zone of impaction (white band of condensation):* A linear band of increased density is apparent beneath the involved endplate. Acutely, this represents the enmeshed trabeculae of the compression fracture. Later, this same appearance represents callus formation in the healing fracture. It is best seen on the lateral view.
4. *Displaced endplates:* The anterior shearing of the intervertebral disk may avulse the bony rim of an endplate or displace it anteriorly. The appearance on the lateral view will be a greater AP diameter of the vertebral body at the involved endplate.
5. *Loss of intervertebral disk height:* The intact disk is inferred from the well-preserved potential space between the vertebrae and the proper alignment of the vertebrae. Herniation of the disk will cause a decrease in the potential space and possibly a misalignment of adjacent vertebrae.

Figure 9-34 (A) Anterior vertebral body compression fracture with wedge deformity and intact posterior ligament complex. Involvement of only one column means this is a stable injury. **(B)** Anterior vertebral body compression fracture with torn posterior ligament complex. Two columns involved means this injury has the potential to be unstable.

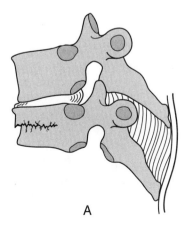

A

Stable

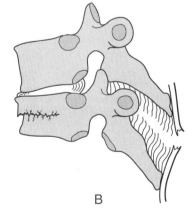

B

+/- Stable

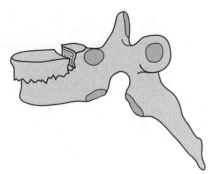

Figure 9-35 Anterior vertebral body compression fracture resulting in disruption of vertebral endplate.

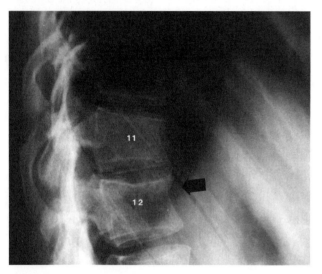

Figure 9-36 Traumatic compression fracture of the 11th and 12th thoracic vertebrae. This 40-year-old woman was operating a weed-whacker on a grassy slope when she slipped, sustaining these fractures as she landed on her buttocks. As is characteristic of compression fractures in the lower thoracic vertebrae, the flexion force has damaged the vertebral endplates by converting into anterior shear force, in addition to causing a compressive deformity.

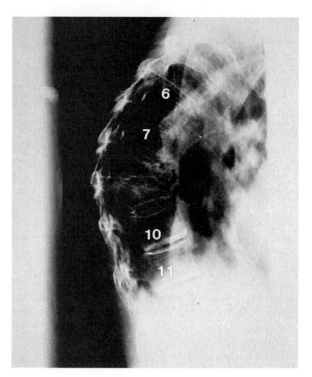

Figure 9-37 Multiple compression fractures secondary to osteoporosis in a 95-year-old woman. Note the collapse of T8 and T9. The severity of the deformity coincides with the severity of the postural thoracic kyphosis, as evident on this lateral view. Note the linear zone of impaction in both vertebral bodies, representing the enmeshed trabeculae of the compressed fracture fragments.

6. *Paraspinal edema:* Paraspinal soft tissue edemas or hematomas, often associated with compression fractures, are best seen on the AP view as increased areas of density adjacent to either side of the spine.
7. *Abdominal ileus:* Disturbance to the visceral autonomic nerves or ganglia may occur with paraspinal soft tissue trauma. The result will be excessive amounts of gas in the small or large bowel, best seen on the AP view. The significance of this sign is that it is an indicator of severe underlying trauma and the likelihood of fracture is great.

Determining the Age of a Compression Fracture

The age of a compression fracture is determined radiographically by the presence or absence of the foregoing radiographic signs (Table 9-1). The acute compression fracture will exhibit most of the indicators, although the less severe cases will not involve the soft tissue signs. The step defect and the linear zone of impaction are the most reliable signs of a recent or healing fracture that is less than 2 months old.

These two radiographic signs will disappear when union is complete, usually by 3 months postinjury. Bone scans may be helpful if the age of a compression fracture is in question because active healing will be evident. Bone scans are not precise, however, because they may stay positive for as long as 2 years postinjury.

Healing

Vertebral body fractures heal by both endosteal and periosteal callus formation. Union occurs in 3 to 6 months. Delayed union may be due to extensive disk herniation into the fracture site, interrupted nutrient vessels, or general poor health and advanced age. The anterior height of the vertebral body rarely returns to normal, and the wedge deformity persists after healing. Excessive cortical thickening at the anterior vertebral margin and excessive callus formation, even extending to the anterior longitudinal ligament, are not uncommon and may persist for years. Mildly damaged disks may revascularize and function normally. Severely torn disks may calcify and form a bony ankylosis at that segment.

TABLE 9-1 ● *Age Determination of Compression Fracture*

	New (Less than 2 months postfracture)	Old
Step defect	+	−
Wedge deformity	+	+
Linear zone of impaction	+	−

Treatment

Nonoperative treatment is the standard of care for vertebral compression fractures.

Anterior compression fractures are acutely painful; the most severe symptoms resolve in 10 to 14 days. Hospitalization is often required for a short stay to control pain and fit the patient for a thoracolumbar spinal orthosis (TLSO). In younger adults, bracing the trunk in extension relieves pain by unloading the anterior vertebral bodies from significant weight bearing. This allows immediate return to ambulation and activity as tolerated. Bracing continues for 4 to 6 weeks. Rehabilitation initially involves management of the TLSO, isometric back muscle strengthening, and ambulatory devices as needed.

Bracing is usually not effective, appropriate, or possible in the elderly because of pre-existing kyphotic deformities, loss of spinal extension mobility, or intolerance to confinement of the thorax. Rehabilitation involves pain-reducing modalities, ambulatory devices, interventions to promote ambulation and prevent generalized debility, measures to reduce the risk of falls, strengthening as tolerated, and instruction in postural adaptations to control pain during exacerbating movements (such as transfers from sitting to standing).

Two- or Three-Column Injuries

The majority of two- or three-column injuries in the thoracic spine are the results of high-energy hyperflexion forces. The injury patterns that result involve combinations of fracture and dislocation.

Fracture–Dislocation Injuries

Mechanism of Injury

Sixty-five percent of thoracolumbar fractures occur as a result of motor vehicle accidents and falls from great heights. The remaining injuries are caused by athletic participation or acts of violence. Hyperflexion forces in combination with rotary, shear, compressive, or distractive tension forces produce characteristic patterns of injury (Fig. 9-38). A summary of some fracture–dislocation injuries commonly seen in the thoracic and thoracolumbar spines is provided in Table 9-2.

Characteristics

Fractures and dislocations of the middle and posterior columns have the potential to be unstable injuries. The risk factors of these injuries involve the migration of a fracture fragment into the spinal canal or a compromise of the available space for the spinal cord in the canal.

Fractures combined with dislocations are common injury patterns in the thoracic spine. Pure dislocations of the facet joints in the thoracic spine are rare, because of the greater structural stability of these joints in comparison to the more mobile and dislocatable cervical facet joints. To dislocate a thoracic facet joint would require great force, and fractures are more likely to happen prior to a dislocation. Likewise, isolated fractures of the posterior column are also rare. To fracture the dense cortical bone of the vertebral arch would

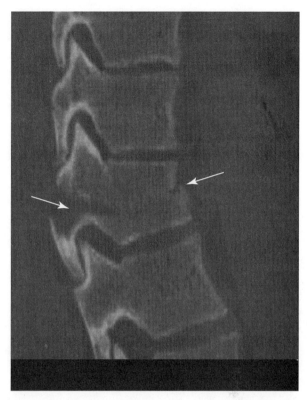

Figure 9-38 "Seatbelt" or "chance" fracture. This three-column injury is caused by hyperflexion over a fixed horizontal restraint, such as a seatbelt. The arrows indicate the horizontal split of the entire vertebra, including the vertebral body, pedicles, and laminae. *(Image courtesy of Nick Oldnall, http://www.xray2000.co.uk.)*

require great force; thus associated fractures and ligamentous damage are likely.

An exception to the rarity of isolated posterior column fractures is an avulsion fracture of the spinous process, commonly seen in the cervicothoracic region. This fracture is well known by the eponym "clay shoveler's fracture." The first thoracic vertebra, followed by the seventh cervical vertebra, followed by the second thoracic vertebra, is most frequently involved in this type of injury.

Radiologic Assessment

In the presence of a fracture and/or fracture–dislocation injury pattern, the lateral view allows assessment of the vertebrae using the three-column concept (see Table 9-2). A fracture and/or dislocation may demonstrate any of the following:

- Disruption of the three parallel lines that reference vertebral alignment, indicating translation or dislocation
- Hyperkyphotic angulation of a spinal segment, representing a torn posterior ligament complex
- Increased intervertebral joint space, representing rupture of the disk
- Decreased intervertebral joint space, representing herniation of nuclear material
- Osseous deformity, representing fracture or soft tissue disruption

TABLE 9-2 ● *Fracture–Dislocation Patterns in Thoracolumbar Space*

Mechanism	Injury	Appearance
A. Hyperflexion	Ant. Col: Vertebral body compression fracture Mid. Col: Tear of posterior longitudinal ligament (PLL) Post. Col: Tear of posterior ligament complex (PLC), dislocation of facet joints	
B. Hyperflexion plus rotation	Ant. Col: Vertebral endplate fracture, disk rupture Mid. Col: Tear of PLL Post. Col: Tear of PLC; dislocation or fracture at facet joints	
C. Hyperflexion plus shear: "traumatic spondylolisthesis"	Ant. Col: Shear fracture through vertebral body or disk Mid. Col: Body fracture and PLL tear Post. Col: Fracture of pedicles and PLC tear	
D. Hyperflexion over fixed horizontal restraint; "seatbelt injury"	Ant. Col: Horizontal body fracture Mid. Col: Horizontal body fracture Post. Col: Fissuring of laminae, pedicles, and transverse processes	
E. Hyperextension	Ant. Col: Rupture of anterior longitudinal ligament and intervertebral disk Mid. Col: Compression of posterior disk Post. Col: Compression fracture of vertebral arches or dislocation of facet joints	

The AP view may demonstrate any of the following:

- Alteration in the interpedicular distance
- Alteration in the spinous process intervals
- Paraspinal edema
- Abdominal ileus

Treatment

Treatment of unstable fractures does not always require surgical fixation. Some unstable compression fractures or burst fractures may respond well to hyperextension casting if sagittal alignment is restored. Molded jackets, TLSOs, and braces provide various degrees of immobilization in the different regions of the thoracic spine; the choice of external fixation is predicated on this.

Operative treatment is required for any injury that is accompanied by a neurological deficit or is at high risk for instability that may later result in neurological deficit. If a thoracic injury is accompanied by rib fractures at the same level, the index of suspicion for instability is higher.

Fractures of the Bony Thorax

Rib Fractures

Mechanism of Injury

Rib fracture is the most common thoracic injury, highly associated with all types of traumatic injury. Ribs are usually fractured by direct blows. In frail patients, severe coughing may fracture the lower ribs. Elderly survivors of cardiopulmonary resuscitation commonly sustain left side rib fractures. Occasionally, fractures can be seen as a result of overuse stresses in certain sports such as rowing, golf, and pitching in baseball. First rib fractures in infants are virtually diagnostic of abuse, and rib fractures in children under age 3 are highly predictive of abuse when other causes are excluded based on the clinical exam and history.

Characteristics

Clinically, rib fractures announce themselves by history, localized tenderness, and pain on deep inspiration. Ribs are seldom dislocated, because of the stability provided by the intercostal muscles.

Manual compression of the rib cage in an AP direction will flare the rib cage and reproduce painful symptoms.

Complications of rib fractures include puncturing of the pleura, causing a hemothorax; puncturing of the lung, causing a pneumothorax; or contusion to the underlying lung. The principal goal in evaluating rib fractures is to detect complications. In the absence of complications, the goal is pain relief.

Radiologic Assessment

Radiographically, rib fractures can be difficult to assess because of the numerous planes of the ribs (Fig. 9-39). Nondisplaced rib fractures are typically seen as a vertical or oblique fracture line with an offset of the cortical margin of the rib. The surrounding soft tissue density of the associated hematoma is often a reliable clue to a nearby fracture. Rib fractures are often easier to detect on follow-up radiographs. The callus formation of a healing rib fracture, seen 10 to 14 days postinjury, is sometimes the first noticeable radiographic indication that a fracture has indeed occurred. Cough-induced rib fractures are often delayed in diagnosis because the reason for the coughing fit is usually a pathology that directs initial medical attention, such as pneumonia.

Stress fractures related to sports are often misdiagnosed clinically as intercostal muscle strains. They are theorized to result from rapid, forceful contraction of the serratus anterior and external oblique muscles in rowers and of the serratus, latissimus dorsi, and abdominal muscles in golfers. Because stress fractures are difficult to diagnose on conventional radiographs in any bone, rib stress fractures may require a bone scan or CT scan to diagnosis. Ultrasonography is far superior to radiographs in detecting fractures but has the limitations of being time-consuming and making it difficult to assess retroscapular or and infraclavicular rib areas.

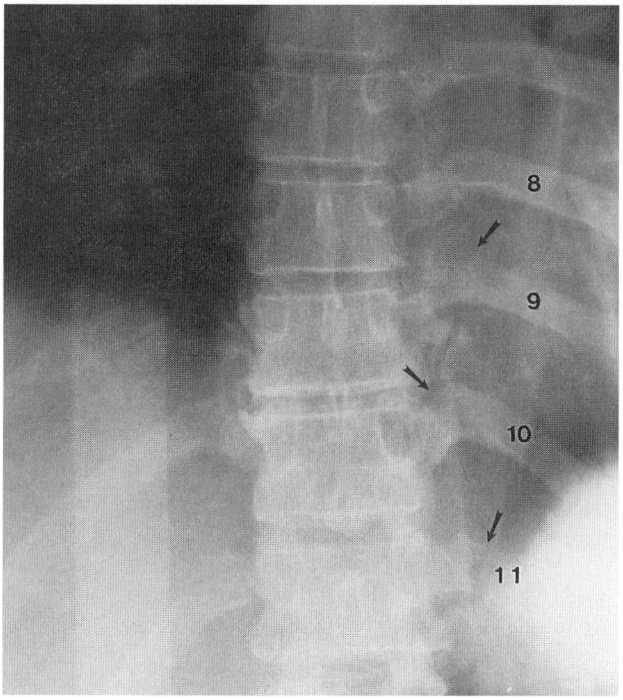

Healing

Ribs are well vascularized, and fractures occurring in them heal readily despite the continued movement of respiration. Most rib fractures heal, with rest, in 4 to 6 weeks. Nonunions or malunions of rib fractures are extremely uncommon and rarely cause symptoms if they do occur.

Treatment

Patients with uncomplicated rib fractures are treated conservatively with analgesics and a mildly compressive support, such as taping or a rib belt. Patients with three or more rib fractures are usually hospitalized on account of the increased risk of complications.

Sternum Fractures

Fractures of the sternum are caused by blunt-force trauma and are relatively uncommon. Fractures of the xiphoid process, however, are common because of its exposed position and brittleness after ossification.

Note that for surgical intervention, the sternum is cut vertically to gain access to the heart and lungs and is fixated with wire reduction postoperatively.

Abnormal Conditions

Osteoporosis[16,37–55]

Osteoporosis is a major public health threat for half of Americans over age 55. One in two women and one in four men will have an osteoporosis-related fracture in their remaining lifetimes. Vertebral compression fractures are among the earliest and most common of these osteoporotic fractures. With early radiographic identification, radiologists can help initiate early treatment intervention and minimize subsequent risk of fracture.

Clinical Presentation

Vertebral compression fractures are commonly associated with chronic back pain, limited spine mobility, and social isolation. Existence of one previous vertebral fracture increases the risk for subsequent vertebral fractures at multiple levels fivefold and hip fractures threefold. Resultant increases in the kyphosis of the thoracic spine are usually quite pronounced and deforming (see Fig. 9-37). Functional abilities are compromised as the spine and thorax lose flexibility. Ambulation is often impaired because of pain, compromised heart and lung volume, and the stressful compensatory cervical hyperextension required to bring the eyes to horizontal.

Figure 9-39 Multiple rib fractures are indicated by the black arrows to the left-side ribs 10 and 11. See Figures 11-38 and 14-50 for more fractures sustained by this patient in a fall.

Radiologic Assessment

Generalized osteoporosis, anywhere in the skeleton, demonstrates the classic radiologic hallmarks of increased radiolucency, cortical thinning, and trabecular changes. Osteoporosis in the spine demonstrates these same hallmarks and some others specific to the structure of the vertebrae:

- *Increased radiolucency of vertebrae.* Increased radiolucency is first evidenced at the cancellous vertebral bodies. This results in the "empty box" appearance of the vertebral body.
- *Thinning of cortical margins.* Thinning of the cortices is first noted at vertebral body margins, especially at the endplates, where the cortical outline is normally relatively thick. The cortical margins of the vertebral arches also become thinned.
- *Alterations in trabecular patterns.* Trabecular changes within the vertebral bodies often leave distinct vertical striations.
- *Wedge deformity.* The structurally weakened vertebral bodies often collapse under flexion or axial compressive forces. In severe osteoporosis, these vertebral compression fractures may be due to relatively minor or normal everyday forces. The preponderance toward fracture is directly related to the severity of the osteoporosis.
- *Other deformities of the vertebral body.* Chronic microfractures produce the *biconcave* appearance of a vertebral body without significant alteration of the anterior or posterior vertebral margins. This configuration results from structural weakness and expansile pressures of the disk. A single traumatic event results in *vertebra plana,* a flat-appearing vertebra. A summary of the various configurations of vertebral body collapse is presented in Figure 9-40.
- *Endplate deformities.* Smooth indentations are seen in the endplates centrally, in the region of the nucleus pulposus. Sclerosis along the endplates is most common in the thoracic and lumbar spines.
- *Schmorl's nodes.* Focal intrusion of nuclear material into the vertebral body through the structurally weakened endplates results in these radiolucent "nodes."

Unfortunately many vertebral fractures are missed, owing in part to a lack of standardization in radiologic interpretation, use of terminology that is nonspecific and does not adequately alert the referring clinican to the presence of vertebral fractures, and mild or moderate fractures not reported when the patient is asymptomatic. The radiologic report does not use the term *osteoporosis* as a descriptor; that term is the clinical diagnosis. *Diffuse demineralization* or *osteopenia* describes the radiolucency of bone. Osteoporotic bone is described on radiographs by the presence of pathologic changes in the cortex and trabeculae, new or old compression fractures, and structural deformities as related to the foregoing characteristics.

DEXA

Other imaging studies play an important role in the assessment of osteoporosis. The *dual energy x-ray absorptiometry test (DEXA scan)* is the most widely used method of measuring bone mineral density. Although quantitative CT (QCT) can directly measure bone density, DEXA is less expensive, exposes the patient to less radiation, and is more accurate at measuring subtle changes in bone density over time or in response to pharmacolgical therapy. DEXA is not interpreted visually, but modified radiographs of the thoracolumbar spine and nondominant hip are analyzed digitally. The patient is given two scores. A "T" score compares the patient's bone mineral density with that of a young, healthy person, and a "Z" score compares it with that of an age-matched healthy person. Pharmacological treatment is recommended based on parameters from these scores.

Treatment

Treatment options for osteoporotic vertebral fractures is focused primarily on pain reduction. Palliative care and analgesic medications are critical to promote activity and prevent complications of prolonged bed rest. Bracing, discussed in the prior section on anterior compression fractures, is not

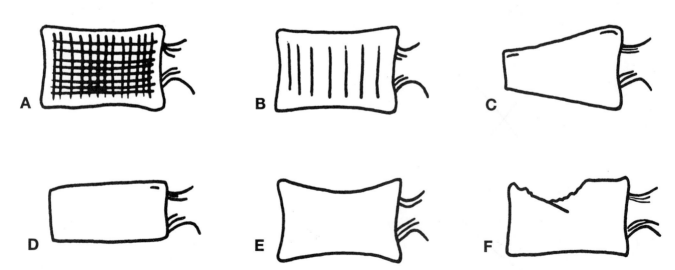

Figure 9-40 Osteoporosis: vertebral body configurations. **(A)** Normal. **(B)** Normal shape, with pencil-thin cortices. **(C)** Wedge shape due to anterior loss of height. **(D)** Vertebra plana with both anterior and posterior collapse. **(E)** Biconcave ("fish" vertebra) as a result of gradual endplate depression. **(F)** Angular endplate depressions from acute fractures.

effective in the elderly patient. Antiresorptive medications and bone forming hormones are often prescribed to slow or reverse bone loss.

Percutaneous vertebroplasty or balloon kyphoplasty are similar interventional techniques used to provide pain relief in select cases of vertebral compression fractures (Fig. 9-41). The procedures consist of an injection of a polymethyl methacrylate cement into the affected vertebral body via fluoroscopic guidance. In kyphoplasty, a balloon is inflated in the vertebral body first to create a premolded cavity for the cement. This has been shown to restore vertebral height to a greater degree and minimize cement leakage. These procedures are contraindicated in cases of complete vertebral collapse, as is seen in advanced cases of osteoporosis, as the cement will leak out.

Rehabilitation is valuable in the early stages of osteoporosis for improvement of posture via strengthening and flexibility exercises and improvement of general conditioning via weight-bearing activities and ambulation. In the later stages of osteoporosis, which are characterized by progressive vertebral fractures and spinal deformity, rehabilitation is

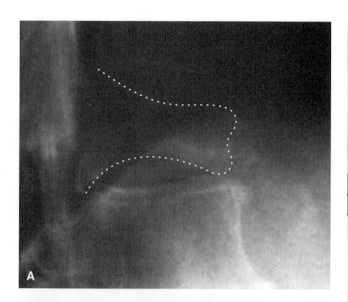

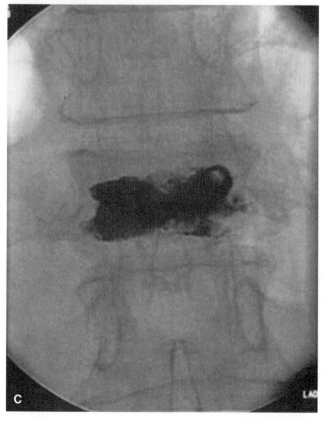

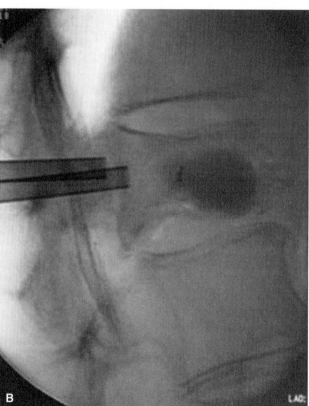

Figure 9-41 (A) Lateral view of the thoracic spine. Note the wedge-shaped collapse of the vertebral body. **(B)** Lateral fluoroscopic image with transpedicular trocars and balloon inflation in the vertebral body. **(C)** AP fluoroscopy of completed vertebroplasty with bone cement in place. The vertebral height is restored. *(Image courtesy of Harry Herkowitz, MD, William Beaumont Hospital, Royal Oak, MI.)*

important in providing adaptive modifications to preserve functional independence in activities of daily living and ambulation.

Scoliosis[16,56–68]

Scoliosis is a lateral deviation of the spine from the midsagittal plane combined with rotational deformities of the vertebrae and ribs. Pathological changes due to compressive forces on the concave side of a curvature include narrowed disk spaces, wedge-shaped vertebral bodies, shorter and thinner pedicles and laminae, and narrowed intervertebral foraminal and spinal canal spaces. Pathological changes on the convex side of a curvature include widened rib spaces and a posteriorly positioned rib cage, resulting in the deforming "rib hump" (Fig. 9-42).

Prevalence

The frequency of scoliosis is dependent on the degree of curvature. In adults, studies have shown that curves over 5 degrees appear in approximately 5% of the population, curves over 10 degrees appear in 2% to 4% of the population, and curves over 25 degrees occur in 1.5 per 1,000 individuals in the United States.[7] The greater the curve, the higher the female predilection. In children, 3 to 5 out of 1,000 will develop scoliotic curves large enough to warrant treatment.[29]

Classification

Scoliosis is broadly classified into structural and nonstructural scoliosis. Nonstructural scoliosis is characterized by a curvature that retains flexibility and will reverse or straighten on lateral flexion toward the convex side.

Nonstructural scoliosis can result from postural adaptations, nerve root irritation, inflammation, or leg length inequality.

Structural scoliosis is characterized by an inflexible curvature that remains unchanged during lateral flexion to the convex side. More than 50 pathological conditions are associated with structural scoliosis. However, approximately 80% of structural scoliosis cases are termed *idiopathic scoliosis* because the etiology remains unknown.

Idiopathic Scoliosis

Three types of idiopathic scoliosis are:

- *Infantile idiopathic scoliosis* appears before age 3 and may include neurological involvement. Many cases resolve spontaneously, although some progress to severe deformity.
- *Juvenile idiopathic scoliosis* appears between ages 3 and 10, more often in girls, and presents a high risk for progression.
- *Adolescent idiopathic scoliosis (AIS)* appears between age 10 and skeletal maturity at a 7:1 female:male ratio. The condition may become apparent at puberty or during a growth spurt. Skeletal maturity usually arrests the progressive development of a curve and also halts the effectiveness of treatment. Surgical treatment may be required if nonoperative treatment fails to halt curve progression.

Curve Patterns

Four distinct patterns of curvature are common (Fig. 9-43). Curves are named by the side of the convexity and are in reference to the patient's right and left sides.

1. *Right thoracic curve.* The most frequently seen curve is the right convex thoracic curve. This major curve extends from T4–T6 to T11–L1. Often, secondary or minor curves are seen above and below the major curve. These are compensatory and initially nonstructural curves that aid in balancing the spine and keeping the eyes oriented to the horizontal. Secondary curves may also be present in any of the following curve patterns.
2. *Right thoracolumbar curve.* This major curve is longer, extending from T4–T6 to L2–L4. It can appear to either side, but right is most common.
3. *Left lumbar curve.* This curve extends from T11 or T12 to L5. It also can appear to either side, but left is most common.
4. *Left lumbar, right thoracic curve.* This *double major curve* consists of two structural curves of equal prominence. This pattern may be the end result of what began as a major thoracic curve with a compensatory secondary lumbar curve, but progressed into two structural curves.

Radiologic Assessment

Radiographs are the most definitive and diagnostic modality in the management of the patient with scoliosis. Radiographs serve the following purposes:

1. To determine or rule out the various etiologies of the scoliosis
2. To evaluate the curvature size, site, and flexibility
3. To assess the skeletal maturity or bone age
4. To monitor the curvature progression or regression

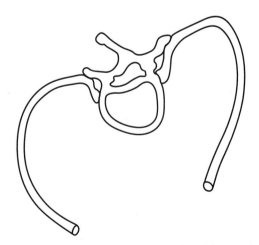

Figure 9-42 Rotational deformity of thoracic vertebrae and ribs in scoliosis, superior view.

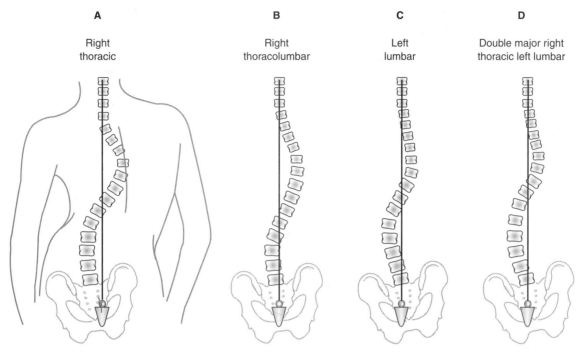

A Right thoracic

B Right thoracolumbar

C Left lumbar

D Double major right thoracic left lumbar

Figure 9-43 Four common curve patterns seen in scoliosis. This schematic represents the patient's spine from the perspective of a *clinical* (not radiographic) examination; that is, the viewer is looking at the patient's back. The curves are also named according to this perspective.

All of the foregoing influence the choice of treatment plan, modifications of the treatment plan, and the determination of when to discontinue treatment.

The diagnosis and management of scoliosis requires a high number of radiographs and thus repeated exposure to radiation at a young age. The risk-to-benefit ratio is of critical importance in management.

Diagnostic Radiographic Series

The radiographic series to diagnose and evaluate scoliosis consists of the following projections:

1. Erect AP
2. Erect lateral
3. Erect AP lateral flexion views of the spinal column
4. PA left hand

The erect AP lateral flexion views are taken at the end ranges of side bending right and side bending left. This will expose the flexibility or rigidity of a curve. Flexible nonstructural curves will reverse or straighten upon side bend to the convexity. Rigid, structural curves will not be altered during side bending (Fig. 9-44).

Additional lateral radiographs may be necessary to evaluate associated curves that may be present in the sagittal plane, such as a kyphosis or lordosis. A term such as *kyphoscoliosis* designates curves present in both the coronal and sagittal planes.

Figure 9-44 Schematic of AP side-bending radiographs done to evaluate the amount of flexibility present in a double major spinal curve. Side bending left shows a correction or reversal of the lumbar curvature, indicating a flexible, nonstructural curve in the lumbar spine. Side bending right, on the other hand, shows no correction of the thoracic curvature, indicating a rigid structural curve in the thoracic spine.

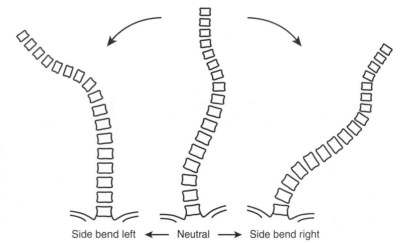

Side bend left ← Neutral → Side bend right

In addition to the spinal films, a radiograph of the left hand and wrist is made. This film is compared to standardized films in the Greulich and Pyle *Atlas*[28] to provide an accurate assessment of *skeletal age.* Skeletal age refers to the physiological stage of skeletal maturity and differs from chronological age, as discussed in Chapter 3.

Radiographic Indicators of Skeletal Maturity

Two other indicators of skeletal maturity are seen on the spine radiographs. Fusion of the vertebral ring apophyses closely parallels the end stages of skeletal maturity (see Fig. 9-9). Also, fusion of the iliac crest apophysis to the ilium appears at the end of skeletal maturity.

Risser's Sign of Skeletal Maturity The process of skeletal maturity as reflected in the radiographic appearance of the apophyses of the iliac crests is referred to as Risser's sign.

The apophyses first appear at the anterior superior iliac spines and progress over a year's time posteromedially to the posterior superior iliac spines. Fusion is completed in an additional 2- to 3-year period (Fig. 9-45).

The formation of the apophyses is graded in quarters relative to the excursion of the apophysis over the extent of the crest. This progression is assigned a Risser's value from 1+ to 5+:

- 1+ indicates an excursion of the apophysis over 25% of the crest.
- 2+ means 50% of the crest is "capped."
- 3+ is 75% capped.

- 4+ is 100% capped.
- 5+ indicates osseous fusion is complete.

Skeletal spinal maturity is thought to be complete when a 5+ Risser's sign is present *and* the vertebral ring apophyses complete fusion. Progression of a scoliotic curve is strongly inhibited after this point. Bracing is gradually weaned, because significant further corrective treatment is also inhibited.

Cobb Method of Measurement

The Cobb method is a widely accepted radiographic measurement of scoliotic curves. This method gives a value for curvature in the frontal plane, based on the AP radiograph (Figs. 9-46 and 9-47). The Cobb method is performed as follows:

1. Identify the uppermost involved vertebra of the curve that tilts significantly toward the concavity, and draw a line along its superior endplate.
2. Identify the lowermost involved vertebra of the curve that tilts significantly toward the concavity and draw a line along its inferior endplate.
3. Draw perpendicular lines through those two lines and measure the resulting intersecting angle. This angle represents the value assigned to the scoliotic curve.

Pedicle Method of Measurement

The pedicle method of measurement provides a value for the amount of axial rotation that has occurred in combination with the lateral curve.

This method of measuring rotation is done by identifying how far the convex-side pedicle has rotated toward midline (Fig. 9-48). The values of this grading system range from 0 to 4+:

- 0 indicates normal position.
- 1+ indicates the pedicle has moved a third of the way toward midline from its normal position.
- 2+ indicates the pedicle has moved two-thirds of the way.

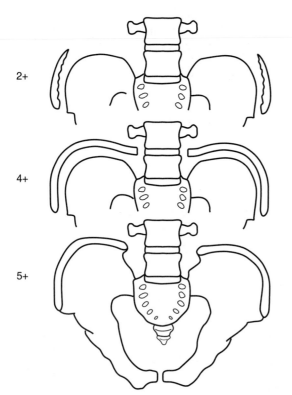

Figure 9-45 Radiographic appearance of the apophyses at the iliac crests at different stages of skeletal maturity. Referred to as Risser's sign, formation of the apophyses is graded by the percentage of bone covering the crests. Complete fusion is graded as 5+.

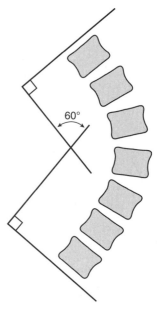

Figure 9-46 The Cobb method of measuring spinal curvatures on the AP radiograph.

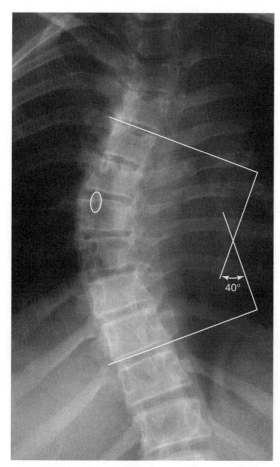

Figure 9-47 AP radiograph thoracic spine. Cobb method measures a 40-degree curve in the sagittal plane. Rotation is given a value by the pedicle method. As the spinous process rotated toward the convexity of the curve, one pedicle has "disappeared" and the outlined pedicle is seen in the 2+ position.

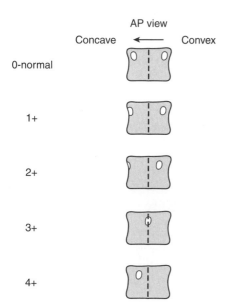

Figure 9-48 The pedicle method of measuring vertebral rotation in scoliosis.

- 3+ indicates that the pedicle is in the midline of the image of the vertebral body.
- 4+ indicates that the pedicle has rotated beyond midline.

Treatment

Treatment choices in adolescent idiopathic scoliosis are determined by a complex equation that factors in the patient's skeletal age, curve magnitude, curve location, and potential for curve progression. Thoracic curves are at a higher risk for progression than thoracolumbar or lumbar curves. Patients with curves of significant magnitude prior to onset of their adolescent growth spurt are at high risk for curve progression.

General treatment guidelines fall into three groups:

- *For patients with curves of minimal magnitude:* No active treatment but close observation for months or years to determine whether a curve is progressing
- *For patients with curves between 20 and 40 degrees:* Spinal bracing combined with exercise for several months or years until skeletal maturity is reached
- *For patients with curves over 50 degrees:* Surgical fixation

Bracing is most effective in children who have significant growth remaining. The primary goal of bracing is to stop progression of the curve. Any correction of a curve is considered a bonus.

The standard surgical procedure most often used to correct adolescent idiopathic scoliosis is a posterior spinal fusion with paravertebral rods and bone grafts. Recent advancements include minimally invasive thoracoscopic surgery, and also fusionless surgery utilizing convex anterior vertebral body stapling (Fig. 9-49). The goals of surgery are to prevent curve progression and to diminish spinal deformity. If the curve is more than 50 degrees at skeletal maturity, the natural history of idiopathic scoliosis during adulthood is one of continued progression.

Tuberculous Osteomyelitis (Pott's Disease)[16,38,69–82]

Tuberculous osteomyelitis, or bone tuberculosis, is always secondary to a tuberculous lesion elsewhere in the body. It is one of the oldest demonstrated diseases of humankind, documented in ancient mummies of Egypt and Peru. The terms *tuberculous osteomyelitis of the spine* and *tuberculous spondylitis* both refer to the eponym *Pott's disease,* so called after Percivall Pott, who presented its classic description in 1779. In developing countries spinal tuberculosis affects mostly children; adult infection is more common in North America and Europe, where the overall incidence is lower.

Clinical Presentation

Back pain is the earliest and most common symptom, with nerve root or spinal cord compression occurring in 50% of cases. Pain is usually localized and most common in the thoracic spine. A focal kyphosis is seen at the level of vertebral collapse. Standing and ambulating increase pain. Systemic

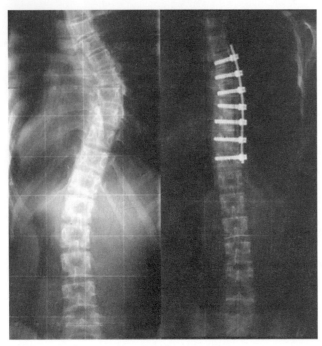

Figure 9-49 Pre- and postoperative AP radiographs of the thoracic spine. This minimally invasive thoracoscopic "keyhole" surgery is performed under fluoroscopic guidance. The hardware extends from T5 to T11. *(Image courtesy of Hee-Kit Wong, MD, University Spine Centre, National University Hospital, Singapore.)*

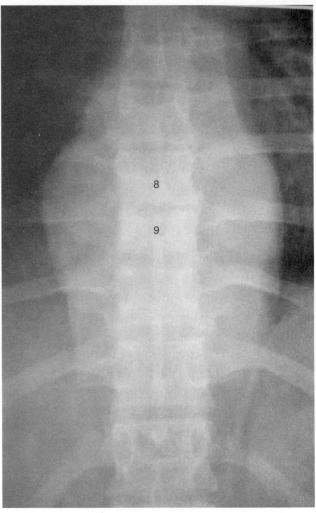

Figure 9-50 AP radiograph of a patient with tuberculous osteomyelitis shows osseous destruction of T8 with a paraspinal tuberculosis abscess. Note loss of vertebral body height, sclerosis of the vertebral endplates, and diminished disk spaces. *(Image courtesy of Laughlin Dawes, MD.)*

manifestations such as weight loss, fever, and fatigue are usually present.

As the infection progresses, a paravertebral abscess spans several vertebrae, with infection spreading up and down the spine under the anterior and posterior longitudinal ligaments.

Lower thoracic vertebrae are the usual sites (40% to 50%), followed by upper lumbar vertebrae (35% to 45%).

Radiologic Assessment

Conventional radiography demonstrates the characteristic *osteolysis*, or slowly progressive bone destruction with reactive sclerosis. This usually occurs in the anterior aspect of the vertebral body adjacent to the subchondral plate. Progressive destruction leads to collapse of the anterior vertebral bodies and associated increase in thoracic kyphosis. Most often more than one vertebra is involved; necrotic degeneration prevents reactive new bone formation and renders segments of bone avascular, producing tuberculous sequestra, especially in the thoracic region.

In contrast to pyogenic infections, the disk space may be spared. Paravertebral shadows suggest abcess formation (Fig. 9-50).

MRI is the diagnostic study of choice after radiographs. MRI demonstrates the relative sparing of the disk space, destruction of the vertebral bodies, extension of disease into the soft tissues, and reveals neural compression (Fig. 9-51).

A definitive diagnosis is made with needle biopsy via CT or MRI guidance.

Treatment

Early disease can be managed with multidrug therapy. Surgical intervention is necessary in advanced cases to prevent neurological deficits and spinal deformities.

Scheuermann's Disease[38,83–91]

Scheuermann's disease is a relatively common condition of adolescent boys and girls in which backache and thoracic kyphosis are manifestations of osteochondrosis of secondary centers of ossification in the spine. The eponym stems from Holger Scheuermann, a Danish radiologist of the early to mid 1900s.

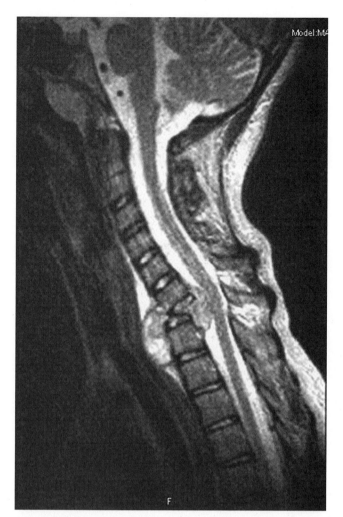

Figure 9-51 Tuberculous osteomyelitis of the first thoracic vertebra. Sagittal view, T2-weighted MRI findings include a complete destruction of the body of T1, sparing of the disks above and below T1, a large anterior subligamentous abscess, and extension of the mass posteriorly, resulting in neural compression. An incidental finding is the not uncommon congenital fusion of C2 to C3. Note the absence of an intervertebral disk at this level.

Clinical Presentation

This disorder most frequently affects the lower thoracic and upper lumbar spine, resulting in a thoracic kyphosis as well as a 50% occurrence of scoliosis. It is one of two conditions believed to mimic vertebral fractures in the thoracic spine, the other being physiological wedging. Some researchers categorize occurrence in the lumbar spine to be a subtype of Scheuermann's disease, usually found during late adolescence in male patients who are involved in heavy lifting tasks.

Scheuermann's disease has been implicated in secondary occurrence of thoracic outlet syndrome, specifically brachial plexopathy. The kyphosis of the spine increases the slope of the first ribs by rotating the scapulae, clavicles, and subclavius muscles. This increases tension on the anterior scalene muscles and neurovascular bundles. Raising the arms overhead from the sides (abduction with external rotation) also rotates the clavicles and subclavius muscles, which diminishes venous return. Complaints of migraine headache and thoracic outlet syndrome symptoms then result.

Etiology

The etiology of Scheuermann's disease is not currently known, although multiple minor injuries to the epiphyses and persistent anterior vascular grooves in the vertebral bodies have been incriminated.

The pathogenesis is also poorly understood. A consistent finding in the involved vertebral bodies is Schmorl's node, which is a herniation of an intervertebral disk through the anterior portion of the epiphyseal plate into the body of the vertebra. This results in less disk material between the vertebral bodies with narrowing of the disk space. It has been theorized that this disturbance may interfere with epiphyseal plate growth either directly or indirectly, causing irregular ossification in the anterior portion of the vertebral epiphysis. Continued deficient growth anteriorly with normal growth posteriorly produces the hallmark wedge-shaped vertebral body.

Radiologic Assessment

Current diagnostic criteria mandates at least three contiguous vertebrae to be involved with at least 5 degrees of anterior wedging of each affected vertebra and a thoracic kyphosis of greater than 40 degrees.

Conventional radiographs of the lateral thoracic spine show irregular ossification in the anterior portion of the epiphyses of at least three adjoining vertebrae, as well as indentations through their epiphyseal plates at the site of the Schmorl's nodes. The superior and inferior endplates appear undulating and show surrounding sclerosis. The intervertebral disk spaces are uniformly narrow, and the vertebral bodies are wedge-shaped.

MRI is used to demonstrate associated findings such as Schmorl's nodes and disk herniation (Fig. 9-52). Both MRI and magnetic resonance angiography (MRA) can be used to evaluate perfusion of the brachial plexus.

DEXA measures mineral density in the spine. Children with Scheuermann's disease may receive evaluation for bone mineral density with this procedure. One study found that 36% of the children with Scheuermann's disease who were evaluated were found to have osteopenia, theorized to be due to decreased physical activity secondary to back pain.

Treatment

Treatment is dependent upon the magnitude of the kyphotic deformity, pain complaints, and patient maturity. If the patient is skeletally immature, bracing may be indicated. Exercises to strengthen spinal extensor muscles and postural retraining are important. Spinal instrumentation and fusion are recommended for patients whose symptoms or deformities cannot be managed conservatively.

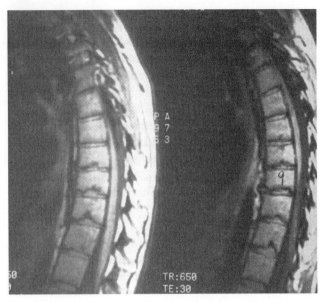

Figure 9-52 Scheuermann's disease, MRI findings. Note Schmorl's nodes at multiple levels and anterior disk protrusion at T9–10. *(Reprinted with permission from Marchiori,[36] p. 416, fig. 10-26.)*

Thoracic, Rib, and Sternal Anomalies[2,16,37,38]

Anomalies are related to a structure's (1) failure to develop, (2) arrested development, or (3) development of accessory bones.

Vertebral anomalies may occur in isolation or in combination with other spinal, visceral, or soft tissue malformations. The prevalence of vertebral anomalies is highest at the junctions of the spinal curvatures. The thoracolumbar junction is often the site of vertebral anomalies.

Rib and anterior chest anomalies are not uncommon and are usually clinically insignificant.

Examples of anomalies of the thoracic spine and thorax, their clinical significance, radiographic features, and appearances are presented in Table 9-3. See Figures 9-53 and 9-54 for radiographic examples of anomalies.

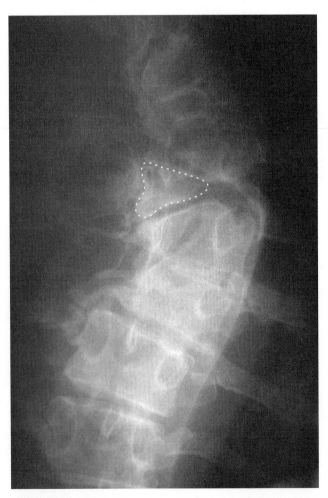

Figure 9-53 Congenital thoracic hemivertebrae, resulting in scoliotic deformity. The triangular vertebral body is outlined. *(Image courtesy of Nick Oldnall, http://www.xray2000.co.uk.)*

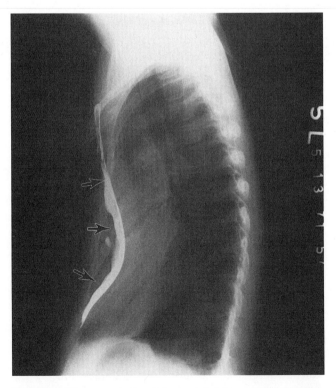

Figure 9-54 Pectus excavatum. This congenital anomaly of a posteriorly positioned sternum is demonstrated on this lateral film of a 9-year-old girl.

TABLE 9-3 ● Anomalies of the Vertebrae, Ribs, and Sternum

Anomaly	Clinical Considerations	Radiographic Features	Appearance
Block Vertebrae: Two adjacent vertebrae fused at birth. Partial or complete fusion of bodies, facets, spinous processes may be present.	No motion at fused segment. Excessive compensatory motion at adjacent freely moving joints with resultant accelerated degenerative changes. Common in both the thoracic and lumbar spines.	*Lateral film:* Small AP diameter of bodies with indented "wasp-waist" appearance of the fused intervertebral disk space. Facets fused in half the cases. Spinous processes may be fused or malformed.	
Butterfly Vertebrae: The endplates are indented toward the center of the body and filled with continuous disk material from adjacent superior and inferior disk spaces.	Usually clinically insignificant. The divided body halves are approximately symmetrical and maintain axial alignment of the vertebrae. Common in both the thoracic and lumbar spines.	*AP film:* The lucency of the invaginating disk material creates the appearance of the vertebral body as a pair of butterfly wings.	
Hemivertebrae: Failure of one half of the vertebral body to grow.	Often associated with other vertebral anomalies. In isolation a hemivertebra will become the apex of a structural scoliosis. Common in lower thoracic and upper lumbar spines.	*AP film:* The involved vertebral body presents a triangular appearance. Adjacent disk spaces are of normal height but adjacent vertebral endplates may be deformed, slightly altering the shape of the bodies.	
Schmorl's nodes: Weakening of the cartilaginous endplates that permit herniation of disk material through the plates and into the vertebral body.	Associated with developmental weakness of the endplates, trauma, or various pathologic conditions that weaken bone, such as osteoporosis, Paget's disease, DJD, sickle cell anemia, Scheuermann's disease, and malignancies. Common in thoracic and lumbar spines.	*Lateral film:* Protrusions of disk material into the body create cavities that eventually ossify. These cavities then radiograph as distinct squared-off sclerotic nodes. More nodes may be present but not seen on radiograph if the cavities have not ossified yet.	
Rudimentary 12th rib: Arrested development of the 12th pair of ribs.	Clinically insignificant.	*AP film:* Small irregularly shaped stubs of bone are present instead of well-formed ribs.	
Lumbar Ribs: Accessory ribs seen most often at L1. These ribs may have all the characteristics of a thoracic pair of ribs or may present only as rudimentary stubs of bone.	Clinically insignificant. Important in the differential diagnosis of transverse process fractures of the lumbar spine.	*AP film:* Note either well-developed thoracic-like rib pairs present at L1, or small irregularly shaped stubs of bone that are distinct from the transverse processes.	
Erb's anomaly: Diminished size or incomplete fusion of one or both first ribs.	Clinically insignificant.	*AP or PA film:* Note malformation of first ribs. May see congenital synostosis of the first rib to the second rib.	
Rib foramen: Formation of an opening within the shaft of the rib.	Clinically insignificant.	*AP or PA film:* Note radiolucent oval within the shaft of the rib.	
Luschka's bifurcated rib: A split at the anterior end of an upper rib.	Clinically insignificant. To be differentiated from a cavity within the lung.	*AP or PA film:* Note bifurcation of rib creating radiolucent area.	
Congenital synostosis: Developmental fusion of adjacent ribs.	Clinically insignificant.	*AP or PA film:* Note fusion of adjacent ribs.	

Chest Anomalies

Anomaly	Clinical Considerations	Radiographic Features	Appearance
Pectus excavatum: Congenital condition in which the sternum is abnormally depressed. Commonly termed "funnel chest."	Severe cases may compromise functioning of the heart and lungs and require surgical intervention.	*Lateral film:* Note posterior position of sternum.	
Pectus carinatum: Congenital abnormal prominence of the sternum. Commonly termed "pigeon breast."	Severe cases increase the AP diameter of the thorax enough to impair coughing and restrict the volume of ventilation. Surgery may be warranted to place the sternum in a more normal position via resection of the costal cartilages.	*Lateral film:* Note anterior position of sternum.	

Summary of Key Points

Routine Radiologic Evaluation

1. The routine radiographic evaluation of the thoracic spine includes two projections:
   - ➤ *Anteroposterior:* Demonstrates all 12 vertebrae.
   - ➤ *Lateral:* Demonstrates all vertebrae except the upper two or three, which are obscured by the shoulder; a swimmer's lateral, which positions the arm overhead, may be done for the purpose of evaluating these upper vertebrae.

2. The routine radiographic evaluation of the sternum includes two projections:
   - ➤ *Posterior oblique:* Demonstrates the sternum without superimposition of the spine.
   - ➤ *Lateral:* Demonstrates the entire sternum in profile.

3. The routine radiographic evaluation of the ribs includes at least two projections and is specific to the section of ribs indicated by clinical examination. Rib sections are further divided into above-diaphragm ribs (T1–T9) and below-diaphragm ribs (T8–T12).
   - ➤ *AP or PA:* Demonstrates the posterior or anterior ribs.
   - ➤ *AO or PO:* Demonstrates the axillary ribs.
   - ➤ *PA chest:* Screens for complications due to rib fracture, such as hemothorax or pneumothorax.

Trauma at the Thoracic Spine

4. Normal vertebral alignment is demonstrated on the lateral view by three approximately parallel line images representing the borders of the anterior vertebral bodies, the borders of the posterior vertebral bodies, and the spinolaminar junctions. Discontinuity in the spatial relationships of these lines may indicate fracture or dislocation.

5. In all age groups, anterior compression fractures of the vertebral bodies are the most common spinal injuries detectable on radiographs. Radiographic signs of anterior vertebral body compression fractures can include the step defect, wedge deformity, linear zone of impaction, displaced endplates, loss of intervertebral disk height, paraspinal edema, and abdominal ileus.

6. Fracture–dislocation injuries in the thoracolumbar spine are the result of high-energy hyperflexion forces usually sustained in motor vehicle accidents or falls from great heights. Two or three columns are involved, and the potential for instability exists. Neurological involvement is associated in 15% to 20% of thoracolumbar fractures.

Rib Fractures

7. Rib fractures can be difficult to identify on initial radiographs. Follow-up radiographs are often more diagnostic because of the presence of callus at the fracture site or the subsequent displacement of the fracture fragments due to the movement of respiration.

Osteoporosis

8. Radiographic characteristics of osteoporotic compression fractures can include increased radiolucency of the vertebrae, thinning of cortical margins, alterations in trabecular patterns, wedge deformity, biconcave deformity, vertebra plana deformity, endplate deformities, and Schmorl's nodes.

9. Treatment is limited; percutaneous vertebroplasty is appropriate in some cases. Pain reduction is the primary focus and includes palliative modalities and analgesic medications. Rehabilitation is important in preserving functional independence and ambulation.

Scoliosis

10. Radiography is critical in the management of scoliosis to determine etiology, demonstrate structural versus nonstructural curves, assess skeletal maturity, and monitor the effects of treatment.

11. The *Cobb method* of radiographic measurement gives a value to the deviation of the spine from the midsagittal plane. The *pedicle method* of radiographic measurement gives a value to the axial rotation of the curve.

12. Radiographic indicators of skeletal maturity include (1) comparative radiographs of the left hand and wrist to the general population as presented in the Greulich and Pyle *Atlas,* (2) the stage of ossification of the vertebral ring apophyses to the vertebral bodies, and (3) Risser's sign, a staging of the appearance and fusion of the iliac apophyses to the ilia.

Tuberculous Osteomyelitis

13. Tuberculous osteomyelitis (Pott's disease) is always secondary to a tuberculous lesion elsewhere in the body. Conventional radiography identifies lytic destruction of vertebral body. MRI is valuable in detecting spinal cord compression. MRI is also used to evaluate disk space infection and demonstrate the extension of disease into soft tissues.

Scheuermann's Disease

14. Scheuermann's disease is a relatively common condition of adolescence. Backache and thoracic kyphosis are manifestations of osteochondrosis of secondary centers of ossification in the spine.

15. Conventional radiographs of the lateral thoracic spine show irregular ossification in the anterior portion of the epiphyses of at least three adjoining vertebrae as well as indentations through their epiphyseal plates at the site of disk herniations (Schmorl's nodes). MRI demonstrates the disk herniations directly.

 Please refer to the text's enclosed CD-ROM for the American College of Radiology's current Musculoskeletal Appropriateness Criteria for the following topics: *Osteoporosis and Bone Mineral Density, Suspected Spine Trauma.*

CASE STUDY

Thoracolumbar Scoliosis

The patient, an 11-year-old girl, is referred to physical therapy by her pediatric orthopedist for management of thoracolumbar scoliosis.

History

The patient was referred to her family physician after a scoliotic curve was discovered during a routine school scoliosis screening. The family physician advised the family that she should be followed by a pediatric orthopedist.

Initial Imaging

The orthopedist ordered whole-spine conventional radiographs (Fig. 9-55) to define the location and magnitude of the scoliosis and assess skeletal maturity. Utilizing the Cobb method, it was determined that the patient had a left thoracic curve of 7 degrees extending from T7 to T11, and a right thoracolumbar curve of 8 degrees extending from T11 to L4. The iliac apophyses were graded with a Risser's sign grade of 4+.

Intervention

The orthopedist decided that bracing was not necessary initially. The scoliotic curve was mild and well below the threshold typical for effective brace management. However, since the patient had significant skeletal growth remaining, the curves had the potential to progress. The orthopedist therefore recommended repeat radiographs every 3 months over the next year to monitor the progression of the curve. The patient was also referred to physical therapy for a stretching and strengthening regimen.

Physical Therapy Examination

Patient Complaint

The patient reported only occasional, mild back pain. She stated that she did not feel limited in any of her normal activities, including participation in soccer and cheerleading, as a result of her back pain. She voiced some concern about the possibility of eventually needing to wear a brace.

Physical Examination

The physical therapist could observe the patient's scoliotic curves in both standing and forward flexion. Neither curve reversed with lateral flexion, consistent with the diagnosis of structural idiopathic scoliosis. The therapist read the orthopedist's report and viewed the patient's whole-spine radiographs. With this information, the therapist designed a home exercise program specific to the scoliosis. The patient was instructed in stretches for the paraspinal musculature on the concave sides of the curves as well as in general trunk-strengthening activities. The therapist saw the patient every week initially to monitor her progress with the home program.

Additional Imaging

Whole-spine conventional radiographs were obtained at 3-month intervals by the pediatric orthopedist. Slow progression of the curves was noted. One year after the inital radiographs were made, the left thoracic curve was measured at 18 degrees and the right thoracolumbar curve at 18 degrees (Fig. 9-56). At this point, the Risser's sign grade was 5+.

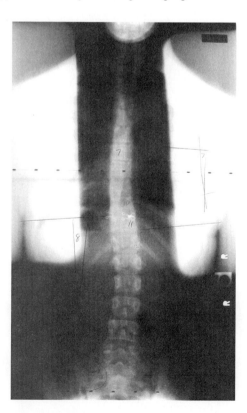

Figure 9-55 AP radiograph of the spine. The patient is an 11-year-old girl. Risser's sign is 4+.

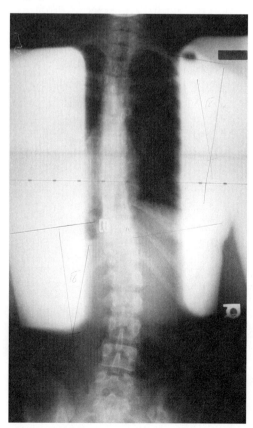

Figure 9-56 AP radiograph of the spine. The patient is now 12 years old. Risser's sign is 5+.

Outcome

At age 12 the patient was close to skeletal maturity, as evidenced by the fusion of the iliac apophyses and vertebral ring apophyses. She was 160 cm (5 ft 3in.) tall, close to her estimated adult height, at this time. The orthopedist felt that her spinal curves were unlikely to progress much further and therefore recommended continued monitoring at 6-month intervals over the next 2 years, also continuing follow-up with the physical therapist. After 2 years had passed, no evidence of progression was noted.

Discussion

This case is an example of appropriate management of adolescent idiopathic structural scoliosis in a patient with mild curvatures. The associated rib hump, detected on forward bending during a school scoliosis screening, was the instigating factor in the initiation of medical intervention. The patient was managed by radiographic interval monitoring and physical therapy until skeletal maturity was complete.

CRITICAL THINKING POINT

Treatment choices in adolescent idiopathic scoliosis can be complex. Factored into decisions are the patient's skeletal age, curve magnitude, curve location, and potential for curve progression. Thoracic curves are known to have a higher risk for progression than thoracolumbar or lumbar curves. In making the series of treatment decisions shown in Figure 9-57, the orthopedist balanced this patient's rate of progression, evidenced by radiographs, against the remaining projected time frame for her skeletal maturity.

Case study adapted by J. Bradley Barr, PT, DPT, OCS.

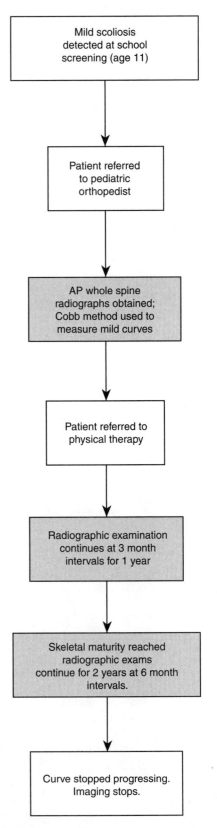

Figure 9-57 Pathway of case study events. Imaging is highlighted.

References

Anatomy

1. Netter, FH: Atlas of Human Anatomy, ed. 4. WB Saunders, Philadelphia, 2006.
2. Yochum, TR, and Rowe, LJ: Essentials of Skeletal Radiology, ed. 3. Williams & Wilkins, Baltimore, 2004.
3. Nordin, M, and Frankel, VH: Basic Biomechanics of the Musculoskeletal System, ed. 3. Lippincott Williams & Wilkins, Philadelphia, 2001.
4. Whiting, W, and Zernicke, R: Biomechanics of Musculoskeletal Injury, ed. 2. Human Kinetics, Champaign, IL, 2008.
5. Gehweiler, JA, et al: The Radiology of Vertebral Trauma. WB Saunders, Philadelphia, 1980.
6. Meschan, I: An Atlas of Normal Radiographic Anatomy. WB Saunders, Philadelphia, 1960.
7. Weber, EC, Vilensky, JA, and Carmichael, SW: Netter's Concise Radiologic Anatomy. WB Saunders, Philadelphia, 2008.

Routine Exam

8. American College of Radiology: Practice Guideline for the Performance of Spine Radiography in Children and Adults. 2007 (Res. 39). Accessed May 18, 2008 at http://www.acr.org.
9. Frank, E, Smith, B, and Long, B: Merrill's Atlas of Radiographic Positions and Radiologic Procedures, ed. 11. Elsevier Health Sciences, Philadelphia, 2007.
10. Bontrager, KL: Textbook of Radiographic Positioning and Related Anatomy, ed. 6. Mosby, St. Louis, MO, 2005.
11. Chew, FS: Skeletal Radiology: The Bare Bones, ed. 2. Williams & Wilkins, 1997.
12. Fischer, HW: Radiographic Anatomy: A Working Atlas. McGraw-Hill, New York, 1988.
13. Wicke, L: Atlas of Radiologic Anatomy, ed. 5. Lea & Febiger, Malvern, PA, 1994.
14. Weir, J, and Abrahams, P: An Atlas of Radiological Anatomy. Yearbook Medical, Chicago, 1978.
15. Squires, LF, and Novelline, RA: Fundamentals of Radiology, ed. 4. Harvard University Press, Cambridge, MA, 1988.
16. Greenspan, A: Orthopedic Radiology: A Practical Approach, ed. 4. Lippincott Williams & Wilkins, Philadelphia, 2004.
17. Krell, L (ed): Clark's Positioning in Radiology, Vol. 1, ed. 10. Yearbook Medical, Chicago, 1989.

Trauma

18. Denis, F: The three-column spine and its significance in the classification of acute thoracolumbar spinal injuries. Spine 8:817, 1983.
19. American College of Radiology: Appropriateness Criteria. Clinical Condition: Suspected Spine Trauma. Available at http://www.acr.org/Secondary MainMenuCategories/quality_safety/app_criteria/pdf/ExpertPanelonMus culoskeletalImaging/SuspectedCervicalSpineTraumaDoc22.aspx.
20. El-Khoury, GY: New trends in imaging of thoraco-lumbar spine trauma. Virtual Hospital, University of Iowa, Iowa City, 2003. Accessed November 5, 2003 at http://www.vh.org/adult/provider/radiology/thoracolumbarspine trauma/.
21. Kelley, LL, and Peterson, CM: Sectional Anatomy for Imaging Professional, ed. 2. Mosby, St. Louis, MO, 2007.
22. Lazo, DL: Fundamentals of Sectional Anatomy: An Imaging Approach. Thomson Delmar Learning, Clifton Park, NY, 2005.
23. Ip, D: Orthopedic Traumatology: A Resident's Guide. Springer, New York, 2006.
24. McConnell, J, Eyres, R, and Nightingale, J: Interpreting Trauma Radiographs. Blackwell, Malden, MA, 2005.
25. Bernstein, MR, Mirvis, SE, and Shanmuganathan, K: Chance-type fractures of the thoracolumbar spine: Imaging analysis in 53 patients. Am J Roentgenol 187:859, 2006.
26. Levi, AD, et al: Neurologic deterioration secondary to unrecognized spinal instability following trauma-A multicenter study. Spine 31(4):451, 2006.
27. Sava, J, et al: Thoracolumbar fracture in blunt trauma: Is clinical exam enough for awake patients? J Trauma 61(1):168, 2006.
28. Dai, LY, et al: Thoracolumbar fractures in patients with multiple injuries: Diagnosis and treatment-A review of 147 cases. J Trauma 56(2):348, 2004.
29. Diaz, JJ, et al: Practice management guidelines for the screening of thoracolumbar spine fracture. J Trauma 63(3):709, 2007.
30. Berry, GE, et al: Are plain radiographs of the spine necessary during evaluation after blunt trauma? Accuracy of screening torso computed tomography in thoracic/lumbar spine fracture diagnosis. J Trauma 59(6):1410, 2005.

31. Berquist, TH: Imaging of Orthopedic Trauma, ed. 2. Raven Press, New York, 1989.
32. Bucholz, RW, Heckman, J, and Court-Brown, C (eds): Rockwood and Green's Fractures in Adults, ed. 6. Lippincott Williams & Wilkins, Philadelphia, 2005.
33. McCort, JJ, and Mindelzun, RE: Trauma Radiology. Churchill Livingstone, New York, 1990.
34. Drafke, MW, and Nakayama, H: Trauma and Mobile Radiography, ed. 2. FA Davis, Philadelphia, 2001.
35. Koval, KJ, and Zuckerman, JD: Handbook of Fractures, ed. 3. Lippincott Williams & Wilkins, Philadelphia, 2006.
36. Eiff, M, et al: Fracture Management for Primary Care. WB Saunders, Philadelphia, 2003.

Abnormal Conditions

37. Daffner, RH: Clinical Radiology: The Essentials, ed. 3. Williams & Wilkins, Baltimore, 2007.
38. Marchiori, DM: Clinical Imaging with Skeletal, Chest, and Abdomen Pattern Differentials, ed. 2. Mosby, St. Louis, MO, 2004.

Osteoporosis

39. Lenchik, L, Rogers, L, Delmas, P, and Genant, H: Diagnosis of osteoporotic vertebral fractures: Importance of recognition and description by radiologists. Am J Roentgenol 183:949, 2004.
40. Ferrar, L, Jiang, G, Adams, J, and Eastell, R: Identification of vertebral fractures: An update. Osteoporos Int 16:717, 2005.
41. D'Costa, H, et al: Pitfalls in the clinical diagnosis of vertebral fractures: A case series in which posterior midline tenderness was absent. Emerg Med J 22(5):330, 2005.
42. Burton, AW, and Hamis, B: Kyphoplasty and vertebroplasty. Curr Pain Headache Rep 12(1):22, 2008.
43. Barbero, S et al: Percutaneous vertebroplasty: The follow-up. Radiol Med (Torino). 113(1):101, 2008.
44. Sun, G: Percutaneous kyphoplasty with double or single balloon in treatment of osteoporotic vertebral body compression fracture: A clinically controlled study. Zhonghua Yi Xue Za Zhi 88(3):149, 2008.
45. Schofer, MD, et al: Balloon kyphoplasty for recent vertebral fractures in the elderly. Orthopade 37(5):462, 2008.
46. Taylor, RS, et al: Balloon kyphoplasty and vertebroplasty for vertebral compression fractures: A comparative systemic review of efficacy and safety. Spine 31(23):2747, 2006.
47. Braunstein, V: Long-term reaction to bone cement in osteoporotic bone: New bone formation in vertebral bodies after vertebroplasty. J Anat 212(5):697, 2008.
48. He, SC, et al: Repeat vertebroplasty for unrelieved pain at previously treated vertebral levels with osteoporotic vertebral compression fractures. Spine 33(6):640, 2008.
49. Heffernan, EJ, et al: The current status of percutaneous vertebroplasty in Canada. Can J Assoc Radiol J 59(2):77, 2008.
50. Caudana, R, et al: CT-guided percutaneous vertebroplasty: Personal experience in the treatment of osteoporotic fractures and dorsolumbar metastases. Radiol Med (Torino) 113(1):114, 2008.
51. Pappou, IP, et al: Osteoporotic vertebral fractures and collapse with intravertebral vacuum sign (Kummel's disease). Orthopedics 31(1):61, 2008.
52. Baroncelli, GI: Quantitative ultrasound methods to assess bone mineral status in children: Technical characteristics, performance, and clinical application. Pediatr Res 63(3):220, 2008.
53. Freedman, BA, Potter, BK, Nesti, LJ, et al: Osteoporosis and vertebral compression fractures—Continued missed opportunities. Spine 8(5):756, 2008.
54. McCloskey, EV: Vertebral fracture assesment with desiometer predicts future fractures in elderly women unselected for osteoporosis. J Bone Miner Res 23(10):1561, 2008.
55. Qin, YX, et al: Longitudinal assessment of human bone quality using scanning confocal quantitative ultrasound. J Acoustic Soc Am 123(5):3638, 2008.

Scoliosis

56. Keim, HA: Clinical Symposia: Scoliosis, Vol 30, No 1. Ciba-Geigy Corporation, Summit, NJ, 1978.
57. Dawson, EG: Scoliosis in children: A complex disorder. Spine Universe, 2008. Accessed June 14, 2008 at http://www.spineuniverse.com.
58. Greulich, WW, and Pyle, SI: Radiographic Atlas of Skeletal Development of the Hand and Wrist, ed. 2. Stanford University Press, Stanford, CA, 1999.
59. Gilsanz, V, and Ratib, O: Hand Bone Age: A Digital Atlas of Skeletal Maturity. Springer, New York, 2004.

60. Hodler, J, Schulthess, GK, and Zollikofer, CL: Musculoskeletal Diseases: Diagnostic Imaging and Interventional Techniques. Springer-Verlag Italia, Milan, 2005.

61. Wong, HK, et al: Results of thoracoscopic instrumented fusion versus conventional posterior instrumented fusion in adolescent idiopathis scoliosis undergoing selective thoracic fusion. Spine 29(18):2031, 2004.

62. Zhang, J, Lou, E, Le, LH, et al: Automatic Cobb measurement of scoliosis based on fuzzy Hoough transform with vertebral shape prior. J Digital Imaging May 31, 2008. (Epub ahead of print).

63. Hedequist, DJ: Surgical treatment of congenital scoliosis. Orthop Clin North Am 38(4):497, 2007.

64. Guille, JT, et al: Fusionless treatment of scoliosis. Orthop Clin North Am 38(4):541, 2007.

65. Bernstein, RM, and Cozen, H: Evaluation of back pain in children and adolescents. Am Fam Physician 76(11):1669, 2007.

66. Qui, Y, et al: Radiological presentations in relation to curve severity in scoliosis associated with syringomyelia. J Pediatr Orthop 28(1):128, 2008.

67. Metz, LN, and Burch, S: Computer assisted surgical planning and image-guided surgical navigation in refractory adult scoliosis surgery: Case report and review of the literature. Spine 33(9):E287, 2008.

68. Kotwicki, T: Evaluation of scoliosis today: Examination, x-rays and beyond. Disabil Rehabil 30(10):742, 2008.

Tuberculous Spondylitis

69. Hidalgo, JA, and Alangaden, G: Pott disease (tuberculous spondylitis). Referenced article of eMedicine, 2006. Available at http://www.emedicine.com/med/topic1902.htm.

70. Sharif, HS, et al: Role of CT and MR imaging in the management of tuberculous spondylitis. Radiol Clin North Am 33:787, 1995.

71. Mitusova, GM, et al: Computed tomography in the diagnosis of tuberculous spondylitis complicated by neurological disorders. Probl Tuberk Bolezn Legk (6):13, 2003.

72. Hoffman, EB, et al: Imaging in children with spinal tuberculosis. A comparison of radiography, computed tomography and magnetic resonance imaging. J Bone Joint Surg Br 75(2):233, 1993.

73. Grover, SB, et al: Congenital spine tuberculosis: Early diagnosis by imaging studies. Am J Perinatol 20(3):147, 2003.

74. Marchiori, D: Clinical Imaging. Mosby, St. Louis, MO, 1999.

75. Beers, MH, and Berkow, R (eds): The Merck Manual of Diagnosis and Therapy, ed. 17. Merck Research Laboratories, Whitehouse Station, NJ, 1999, p 2414.

76. Bernstein, J: Musculoskeletal Medicine. American Academy of Orthopaedic Surgeons, Rosement, IL, 2003.

77. Medcyclopaedia: Tuberculous spondylitis. 2008. Available at http://www.medcyclopaedia.com/library/topics/volume_vii/t/tuberculous_spondylitis.

78. McLain, RF, and Isada, C: Spinal tuberculosis deserves a place on the radar screen. Cleve Clin J Med 71(7):537, 2004.

79. Fennira, H, et al: Vertebral tuberculosis revealed by thoracic manifestations. A study of five cases. Tunis Med 84(12):811, 2006.

80. Kotil, K, et al: Medical management of Pott disease in the thoracic and lumbar spine: A prospective clinical study. J Neurosurg Spine 6(3):222, 2007.

81. Danchaivijitr, N, et al: Diagnostic accuracy of MR imaging in tuberculous spondylitis. J Med Assoc Thai 90(8):1581, 2007.

82. du Plessis, J: Unusual forms of spinal tuberculosis. Childs Nerv Syst 24(4):453, 2008.

Scheuermann's Disease

83. Medcyclopaedia: Scheuermann's disease. 2008. Available at http://www.medcyclopaedia.com.

84. Scheuermann's disease. Scoliosis Research Society, 2008. Available online at: http://www.srs.org/professionals/resources/scheuermanns_kyphosis.pdf.

85. Collins, JD, et al: Scheuermann's disease as a model displaying the mechanism of venous obstruction in thoracic outlet syndrome and migraine patients: MRI and MRA. J Natl Med Assoc 95(4):298, 2003.

86. Popko, J, et al: Assessment of bone density in children with Scheuermann's disease. Rocz Akad Med Bialymst 42(1):245, 1997.

87. Weiss, HR, et al: The practical use of surface topography: following up patients with Scheuermann's disease. Pediatr Rehabil 6(1):39, 2003.

88. Summers, BN, et al: The radiological reporting of lumbar Scheuermann's disease: An unnecessary source of confusion amongst clinicians and patients. Br J Radiol 81(965):383, 2008.

89. Lowe, TG: Scheuermann's kyphosis. Neurosug Clin North Am 18(2):305, 2007.

90. Lowe, TG, and Line, BG: Evidence based medicine: Analysis of Scheuermann's kyphosis. Spine 32(19 Suppl):S115, 2007.

91. Kapetanos, GA, et al: Thoracic cord compression caused by disk herniation in Scheuermann's disease: A case report and review of the literature. Eur Spine J 15(Suppl 5):553, 2006.

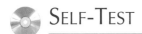

SELF-TEST

Radiograph A

1. What *section of ribs* is this film evaluating? Identify AP or PA, right or left, above or below diaphragm.

2. Give the radiographic or anatomic rationale for how you determined each part of the answer in question 1.

Radiograph B

3. Identify this *projection.*

4. How many *thoracic vertebrae* are visible? How many *lumbar vertebrae* are visible?

5. Note the *scoliosis.* Name the *curvature pattern.*

6. What can or cannot be said about the *lumbar spine* in regard to the scoliosis?

7. What *additional projections* would be helpful in determining whether the scoliosis is structural or nonstructural?

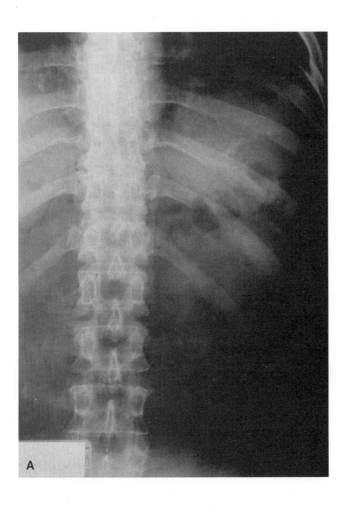

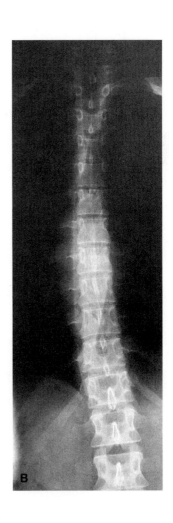

Chapter 10

THE CHEST RADIOGRAPH AND CARDIOPULMONARY IMAGING

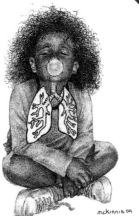

mckinnis 09

Where Does Cardiopulmonary Imaging Begin?

The evaluation of the cardiopulmonary system begins with *conventional radiography.* In the clinic, the radiograph of the heart and lungs is commonly referred to as the *chest radiograph, chest film,* or *chest x-ray.*

The chest radiograph has always been and continues to be a mainstay of basic health care. The chest radiograph is a quick, inexpensive, and noninvasive tool for screening and diagnosis. Many pathologies are adequately diagnosed and treated based on the chest radiograph itself. The chest radiograph also yields valuable information on the adjacent structures of the thyroid gland, gastrointestinal tract, and bony thorax. Additionally, metastatic disease from the skeleton and viscera often manifests in the lung. For these reasons, the chest radiograph has long been known as the "mirror of health or disease."

However, the chest radiograph has limitations. Modern cardiopulmonary imaging still *begins* with the static image of the chest radiograph but may extend to encompass images of organ motion, blood flow, ventilation, perfusion, even the molecular mechanisms of disease processes. Today, any physiological function can be observed noninvasively with the tools of advanced imaging.

Radiographic Anatomy[1-11]

A brief review of anatomy specific to viewing the chest radiograph follows.

Bony Thorax

First, it is a good idea to review the anteroposterior (AP) and lateral views of the thoracic spine in Chapter 9. Note a major difference between the thoracic spine radiograph and the chest radiograph is in *exposure technique.* Skeletal films are made in *high contrast* to see cortical margins. The chest radiograph is made in *low contrast* to see the soft tissues (see Fig. 1-22). Thus what you see of the bony thorax on a chest radiograph is incidental, but still useful. The bones help identify soft tissue anatomy and the location of lesions. For example, a lesion is reported to be located "at the seventh intercostal space." This is accepted to mean between the seventh and eighth posterior ribs.

A second major difference is the thoracic spine radiograph is made as an AP projection, thus details of the spine are easily seen because the vertebrae are closest to the image receptor. The chest radiograph is made as a posteroanterior (PA) projection (see Fig. 1-16). The sternum (now closest to the image receptor) and spine are superimposed and difficult to separate.

Ribs

A typical chest radiograph will show six anterior ribs and ten posterior ribs. How is it possible to tell them apart? The crosshatched image produced by the rib cage is very confusing for any beginner to decipher. Start by focusing on the posterior ribs. The posterior ribs are easiest to identify for two reasons: (1) they are furthest from the image receptor and so are magnified the largest and (2) they can be traced back to the vertebrae (Fig. 10-1). The anterior ribs become radiolucent—thus invisible!—at the anterior *costal cartilages*.

Respiratory Organs

The respiratory organs include the *larynx, trachea, bronchi,* and *lungs* (Fig. 10-2).

The larynx is at the level of C5, and is continuous with the trachea at C6. The trachea lies anterior to the esophagus, and is slightly shifted to the right of midline because of the arching of the aorta beside it. The trachea extends to the level of T4 or T5, where it bifurcates at the *carina* into the two primary bronchi.

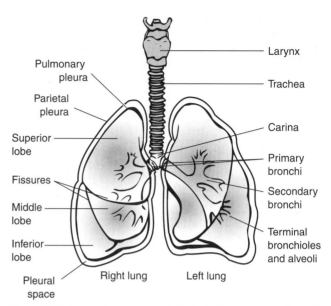

Figure 10-2 The respiratory organs include the larynx, trachea, bronchi, and lungs.

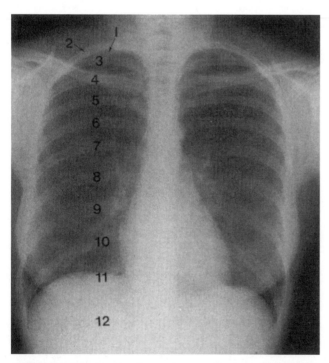

Figure 10-1 The posterior ribs can be traced back to the vertebrae. Usually 10 pairs of posterior ribs are visible on a normal inspiratory effort. (*Reprinted with permission from Textbook of Radiographic Positioning and Related Anatomy, ed. 3. 1993, Mosby, St. Louis, MO, fig. 2-30, p. 58.*)

On the posteroanterior (PA) radiograph, the air-filled trachea and primary bronchi form an inverted radiolucent "Y" over the heart.

The primary bronchi slant inferiorly into the lungs. The right primary bronchus is wider and more vertically inclined than the left, hence food, and foreign objects are more likely to lodge here. The right bronchus divides into three *secondary bronchi,* each entering one of the three lobes of the right lung. The left primary bronchus divides into two secondary bronchi which enter the two lobes of the left lung. (Fig. 10-3). All the secondary bronchi subdivide into *bronchioles* and terminate in *alveoli,* the air sacs where oxygen and carbon dioxide are exchanged with the blood. Note that normally, none of the airway vessels within the lungs are evident on the radiograph, because the vessel walls are thin and the vessels are filled with air. However, airway vessels can become visible if the alveoli around them fill up with fluid. The fluid then outlines the vessels. This is known as the *air bronchogram sign.* It is a nonspecific sign, however, as the fluid may be due to accumulation of infection (pneumonia), blood (hemorrhage), or serous fluid (pulmonary edema).

Each lung is contained in a double-walled sac called the *pleura.* The outer layer lines the chest wall and diaphragm and is called the *parietal pleura.* The inner layer covers the surface of the lungs and dips into the fissures between the lobes, and is called the *pulmonary* or *visceral pleura.* The potential space between the double-walled pleura is the *pleural cavity.* Normally the lungs abut the inner rib cage and the pleura are invisible between them. The pleura become radiographically visible if the pleural cavity is widened by fluid or a mass which will push the lung away from the rib cage.

Silhouette Sign

The *silhouette sign* is the loss of a normal interface between air and soft tissue. This usually refers to the interface between the heart and the lungs, or the interface between the diaphragm

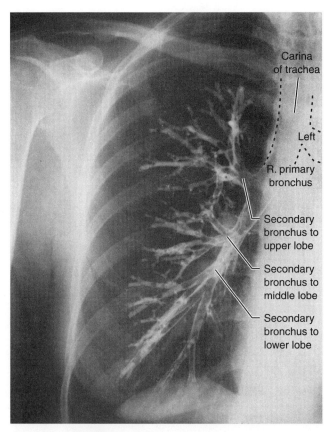

Figure 10-3 The bronchogram provides a great image of the divisions of the bronchial "tree." This test, rarely used today, involved the administration of a radiopaque contrast through a tracheal catheter. The dispersion of the contrast is seen out to the terminal bronchioles.

and lungs. The value of this sign is that it can localize a lesion to a specific lobe of the lung. How? Remember that radiographically, *there is no border between two similar densities.* So if a water density process such as *pneumonia* is in a lobe near the heart, the border between that lobe and the heart will be obliterated—and the heart will lose its silhouette. The following are commonly obliterated borders and their associated lung lobes (Fig. 10-4):

● Loss of border of superior mediastinum = lesion at the upper lobes
● Loss of border of right heart = lesion at right middle lobe
● Loss of border of left heart = lesion at left upper lobe or lingula
● Loss of border of right hemidiaphragm = lesion at right lower lobe
● Loss of border of left hemidiaphragm = lesion at left lower lobe

The Heart

The four-chambered heart and its great vessels are enclosed in a double-walled sac called the *pericardial sac.* Between the visceral and parietal layers is the *pericardial cavity,* which contains fluid that helps to reduce friction between the beating heart and the surrounding structures.

The great vessels are the *inferior* and *superior vena cava,* returning deoxygenated blood from the lower and upper body; the large *pulmonary arteries and veins,* exchanging

blood from the lungs; and the *aorta,* carrying oxygenated blood out to all parts of the body. The aorta can be divided into three parts: the *ascending aorta,* arising out of the heart; the *arch of the aorta;* and the *descending aorta,* which passes through the diaphragm, where it becomes the *abdominal aorta* (Fig. 10-5).

Cardiothoracic Ratio

The *cardiothoracic ratio* is a radiographic estimate of heart size. In adults, the widest width of the heart should *be less than half* the width of the chest at the level of the diaphragm. Disease processes that enlarge the heart include

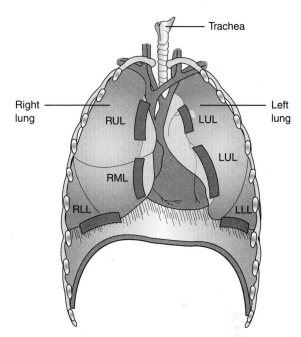

Figure 10-4 The *silhouette sign.* Consolidations can be localized to a lobe by observing which heart or diaphragm border has lost its silhouette. RUL = right upper lobe, RML = right middle lobe, RLL = right lower lobe, LUL = left upper lobe, LLL = left lower lobe.

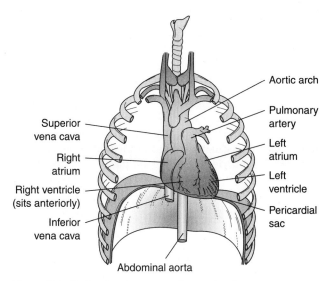

Figure 10-5 The heart and great vessels, anterior view.

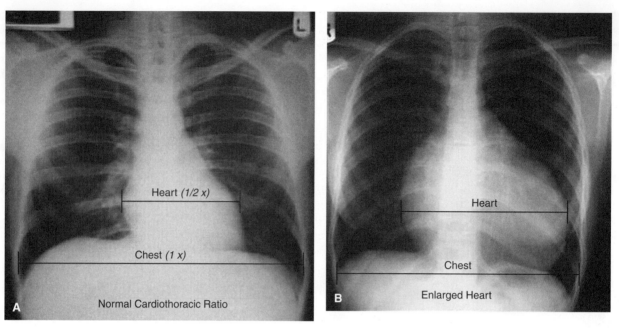

Figure 10-6 (A) Normal cardiothoracic ratio. The heart is less than half the width of the chest. **(B)** Abnormal cardiothoracic ratio. The heart is enlarged.

cardiomyopathy, congestive heart failure, or incompetent valves (Fig. 10-6).

Note that limitations exist with the cardiothoracic ratio estimate. A normal heart can *appear* enlarged for a variety of reasons: the projection is AP, the image is made at expiration not inspiration, the diaphragm is pushed up high from pregnancy or abdominal distention, or pericardial effusion is present and the surrounding fluid enlarges the entire cardiac image.

The Mediastinum

The *mediastinum* is the space between the lungs, bounded anteriorly by the sternum and posteriorly by the spine (Fig. 10-7). The mediastinum contains the bundled soft tissue structures of the heart, vessels, trachea, and esophagus sandwiched between the two inflated lungs. With the exception of the air-filled trachea and primary bronchi, *all of these structures have a similar radiodensity and merge into one homogenous shadow superimposed upon the spine.* Thus, on a PA chest radiograph, these structures cannot be separated from one another. Only the lateral borders of the bundle, outlined by the air-filled lungs, can be identified. The right mediastinal border is mostly composed of the superior vena cava and the right atrium. The left mediastinal border has three major "bumps": the aortic arch, the left atrial appendage (a muscular pouch connected to the left atrium), and the left ventricle. This is a good place for the novice to start. However, with practice, it is possible to see nine vascular structures as a series of intersecting arcs (Fig. 10-8).

Mediastinal Shift

A *mediastinal shift* means the soft tissue bundle is abnormally displaced to one side or the other. A shift may be permanent, as from a lung excision, or temporary, owing to any condition

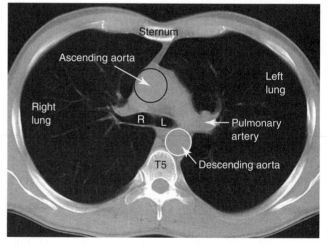

Figure 10-7 Axial CT scan with anatomy of the mediastinum labeled. R and L refer to the right and left primary bronchi.

that changes the volume in one hemithorax. The entire mediastinum may shift, or just a section of it. Examples of conditions that can cause a shift include *pleural effusion* (fluid in the pleural cavity), *pneumothorax* (air in the pleural cavity), or *atelectasis* (collapse of a lobe).

Mediastinal Masses

Many pathologies present on radiograph as a *mediastinal mass.* A comparison of the PA and lateral radiographs can localize the mass to a region of the mediastinum, such as the anterior mediastinum (in front of the heart), or posterior mediastinum (behind the heart), or superior mediastinum (from the neck to T4). Some common masses are:

- Anterior mediastinal masses; for example, goiter, thymoma, teratoma, lymphoma

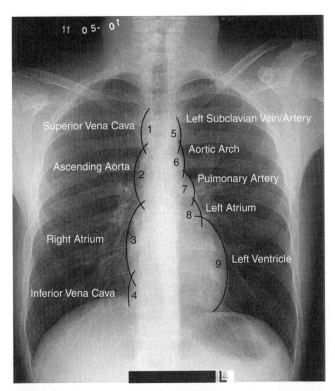

Figure 10-8 The "bumps" on the lateral borders of the homogenous density of the mediastinum can be identified as specific vascular structures: (1) superior vena cava, (2) ascending aorta, (3) right atrium, (4) inferior vena cava, (5) left subclavian vein and artery, (6) aortic arch, (7) pulmonary artery, (8) left atrium, (9) left ventricle.

- Middle mediastinal masses; for example, esophageal or bronchial carcinomas
- Posterior mediastinal masses; for example, aortic aneurysms, neurogenic masses

The Hilum

The *hilum* or "lung root" is where the bronchi, arteries, veins, and nerves enter and exit the lungs. On the radiograph, the hilum appears as a tangle of vessels on either side of the heart. These vessels are visible only because of the blood they contain. The hilum on the left side is partly obscured by the heart and also is higher than the hilum on the right because of the higher takeoff of the left pulmonary artery, which hooks up over the left primary bronchus.

The basic radiologic observation of the hilum is whether the vessels are of normal size or enlarged. Any obstruction to the return of oxygenated blood from the lung to the left side of the heart will enlarge the vessels. Examples include acute heart failure after myocardial infarct or chronic rheumatic heart disease with mitral valve stenosis. Nonvascular reasons for enlargement include enlarged lymph nodes responding to inflammatory lung disease or primary tumors.

The Diaphragm

The *diaphragm* is a thin, curved sheet of muscle that separates the abdominal cavity from the thoracic cavity. It is possible to see the *dome* of the diaphragm because it borders

on the air-filled lungs. Note that the large white density on the chest radiograph commonly referred to as "the diaphragm" is not actually the diaphragm but rather the *sum of the combined densities* of the liver, spleen, stomach, posterior lungs, and the part of the diaphragm tangential to the x-ray beam (Fig. 10-9). Above the level of the dome of the diaphragm, the sum of all densities is dominated by the air-filled lungs and appears black.

The dome of the diaphragm is normally seen (on inspiration) at the 10th rib intercostal space. Abnormal elevation of the diaphragm is due to excessive fluid in the peritoneal space, as seen with ascites or cirrhosis of the liver. Normal elevation is expected in late pregnancy or from "splinting" after recent abdominal surgery. Conversely, the diaphragm is abnormally flattened in any conditions that increase the volume of the lung, such as emphysema, large pleural effusions, or neoplastic masses within the lung (Fig. 10-10).

Hemidiaphragms

Another common radiographic phrase is the left or right *hemidiaphragm.* Although this is not anatomically correct, it is convenient for radiographic description, as the two halves of the diaphragm often respond independently to unilateral disease, either in the chest above or in the abdomen below.

Normally the highest point of each hemidiaphragm is in the middle third of each hemithorax. Note that the right hemidiaphragm is higher because of the presence of the liver and that the left hemidiaphragm contains the stomach, often with a radiolucent air bubble seen in the fundus. With hiatal hernia, the fundus may slip up through the esophageal hiatus, and this added density will be seen in the mediastinum.

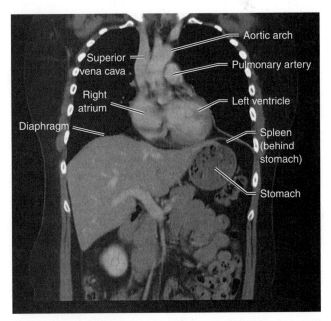

Figure 10-9 Coronal reformatting of a CT scan of the chest and abdomen. Note the position of structures superimposed in the radiographic "diaphragm."

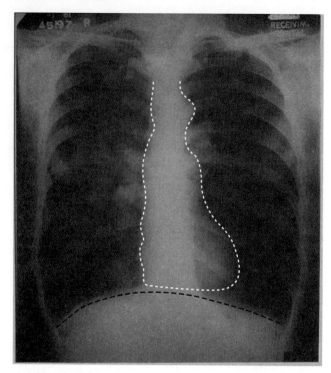

Figure 10-10 PA radiograph showing an abnormally flattened diaphragm as well as a narrowed mediastinum, elongated lung fields, and a heart that appears to "swing" suspended over the diaphragm. These are classic characteristics in a patient with advanced chronic obstructive pulmonary disease.

It is normal to see gastric air or bowel gas below the hemidiaphragms. It is *not* normal to see air outside the bowel in the *peritoneal cavity* of the abdomen. *Intraperitoneal air* or *free air* signifies that the bowel has been perforated, as from peptic ulcer disease, diverticulitis, or colon cancer. Free air is easiest to see in the right hemidiaphragm as it is interposed between the liver and diaphragm. Remember, with the patient in the upright position, air will rise superiorly. Note that free air is a normal finding for about 10 days after any abdominal surgery that exposes the peritoneal cavity to air.

Costophrenic Angles

The base of each lung is cupped convexly over each hemidiaphragm, and the parietal pleura reflects deep into a recess between the diaphragm and chest wall. This recess is the *costophrenic sulcus,* a circular ditch, if you will, where pleural fluid can gravitate. On the PA radiograph, the lateral parts of the sulcus, the *costophrenic angles,* are normally seen as sharply pointed, downward indentations between each hemidiaphragm and the adjacent chest wall.

If a pleural effusion is present, fluid will flow by gravity into the sulcus. The first 100 mm will fill up the deeper posterior sulcus and be evident only on the lateral radiograph. Additional fluid accumulation will fill the lateral sulci and then be evident on the PA radiograph as the costophrenic angles accumulate fluid. This can push the lung upward, resulting in blunting or blurring of the costophrenic angle image.

Routine Radiologic Evaluation[1–12]

Practice Guidelines for the Performance of Pediatric and Adult Chest Radiography[12]

The American College of Radiology (ACR), the principal professional organization of radiologists in the United States, defines the following practice guidelines as an educational tool to assist practitioners in providing appropriate radiological care for patients.

Goals

The goal of the chest radiographic exam is to help establish the presence, absence, or etiology of disease processes that involve the thorax or to follow their course.

Indications

The indications for chest radiography include but are not limited to evaluation of signs and symptoms potentially related to the respiratory, cardiovascular, and upper gastrointestinal systems. It is also indicated for the evaluation of extrathoracic disease that secondarily involves the chest; for follow-up of known thoracic disease processes; for monitoring of patients with life-support devices; or for surveillance studies as required by public law (as in screening for tuberculosis or occupational lung exposures).

Basic Projections and Radiologic Observations

A routine chest examination includes an erect *PA* and an erect left *lateral* projection made during full *inspiration.* The PA projection puts the heart and lungs closest to the image receptor and results in less distortion due to magnification. The less desirable AP projection is used only for patients who are too ill or unable to stand (see Fig. 1-25). The lateral projection is made in a left lateral position, since this places the heart closest to the image receptor.

The lateral view is important to localize the position of lesions seen on the PA view and to assess areas hidden on the PA view owing to superimposition of the midline structures. Note, however, that at times only a single PA or AP view is appropriate, as in pediatrics or with frail patients who are unable to lift their arms for the lateral view. Also, because the lateral view incurs more radiation exposure and less useful clinical information, some believe that it should always be a second-level decision based on findings obtained from the PA view.

Inspiration and Expiration

Inspiration increases the volume of the chest in three dimensions. The vertical expansion occurs via contraction of the diaphragm. A full inspiration in a healthy adult will expose at least 10 pairs of ribs on the radiograph. It is possible to see the ribs because the diaphragm has moved inferiorly; remember that this will also lengthen the heart and lungs as they are pulled downward with the diaphragm (Fig. 10-11).

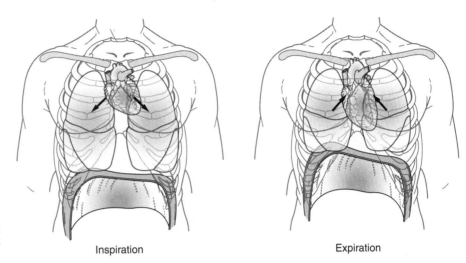

Figure 10-11 Comparison of movement of the diaphragm on inspiration versus expiration.

Inspiration   Expiration

Expiration decreases the volume of the chest via elastic recoil of the lungs combined with the weight of the thoracic walls. *Comparison radiographs* labeled "inspiration" and "expiration" are indicated in some situations to identify a small pneumothorax (air in the pleural cavity); the presence of a foreign body; lack of normal movement in the diaphragm; or to distinguish between an opacity in the rib or in the lung.

Viewing Conventions

Chest radiographs are viewed with the patient's image facing the examiner, so the patient's heart is on the viewer's right-hand side. It does not matter whether the radiograph was made as a PA or AP projection. Likewise it does not matter if a left or right lateral projection was made—lateral radiographs are viewed and presented in publications with the spine to the viewer's right-hand side.

Reading the Chest Radiograph

It is an understatement to say that there are many methods of "reading" a chest radiograph. Consider that prior to the common availability of advanced imaging, a wealth of diagnostic information was gleaned solely from the simple chest radiograph. Subtle changes in vessel size, lung field densities, heart contours, and so on provided enough diagnostic clues to fill entire textbooks for over half a century! The radiologic observations that follow are intended to be at a fundamental level; thus the approach is anatomic. An ABC checklist is presented in Table 10-1.

TABLE 10-1 ● *ABC Checklist for the Chest Radiograph*

A	Airways	Are the trachea and bronchi midline and patent?
B	Bones	Are fractures, osteolytic, or osteoblastic lesions present?
C	Cardiac contours	Normal cardiothoracic ratio? Normal lateral contours?
D	Diaphragm	Right higher than left? Dome-shaped or flattened? Presence of free air?
E	Effusion	Are the costophrenic angles sharp? Is the pleural cavity invisible or made evident by pathology?
F	Fields of the lungs	Any masses, infiltrates, silhouette, or air bronchogram signs?
G	Gastric bubble	Located in the stomach, on the left?
H	Hilum	Are vessels enlarged? Increased vascularity evident in branches?
I	Inspiration	Possible to count 10 posterior ribs?
J	Jazz, All that	Any lines, tubes, implants, prosthetic valves, foreign objects?

(Continued on page 274)

Routine Radiologic Evaluation of the Chest

Posteroanterior Chest

This view demonstrates the lung fields from the apices down to the costophrenic angles, the air-filled trachea, the heart, the great vessels, and the bony thorax.

Radiologic Observations

Body Position

1. Even a small amount of patient rotation can cause great distortion. Assess for rotation of the trunk by comparing the sternoclavicular joins to midline distance and the rib cage margin to midline distance. These should be equal bilaterally. The sternum should be midline, superimposed over the thoracic spine. Kyphosis or scoliosis may cause asymmetry.

Bony Thorax

2. Assess the scapulae, the visible portions of the humeri, the clavicles, and the ribs for bilateral symmetry in size, shape, and contour.
3. Assess bone density. Look for any erosions, osteolytic or osteoblastic lesions, fractures, or calcifications.
4. Look "through" the mediastinum to the thoracic spine and observe vertebral body height, disk spaces, and the integrity of the cortical margins of the vertebrae.
5. Count the posterior ribs in pairs from top to bottom. Usually 10 pairs are visible in a healthy adult.

Soft Tissues

6. Look for the overall amount of muscle and fat soft tissues in the supraclavicular regions, axillae, along the lateral chest walls, and the breast tissue. Observe any obvious masses, calcifications, or the absence of a breast due to mastectomy.

Basic Projections

- **PA**
- Left lateral

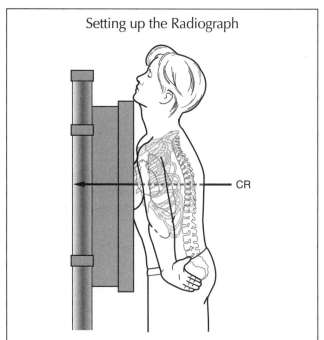

Setting up the Radiograph

Figure 10-12 Patient position for a PA radiograph. To remove unnecessary superimposition, the chin is elevated, the backs of the hands are placed on the hips to rotate the scapula forward, and the shoulders are depressed to move the clavicles below the lung apices. The exposure is made at the end of the second full inspiration to ensure maximum expansion of the lungs. The central ray passes through the seventh thoracic vertebra.

TABLE 10-2 ● *Medical Devices Seen on the Chest Radiograph*

Device	Position	Purpose
Nasogastric (NG) tube	From nose to stomach	To keep stomach empty of acids, bile, blood; also used to give medications and feedings in unconscious patient
Endotracheal tube	From mouth to above carina	To connect patient to a ventilator
Tracheostomy tube	Below cricoid cartilage to above carina	Long-term access for mechanical ventilation or pulmonary toilet
Intravenous central lines	Superior or inferior vena cava, subclavian, internal jugular, or right atrium	Has multiple lumens to deliver medications, chemotherapy, or total parenteral nutrition
Swan–Ganz catheter	From subclavian or internal jugular vein to the heart	To measure fluid balance, various pressures, core temperature, and cardiac output
Cardiac leads	Three or more electrodes placed around the chest surface	To monitor heartbeat and arrhythmias
Chest tubes	Midaxillary line between fourth and fifth ribs	To drain pleural effusions or pneumothorax
Pacemaker	Below left clavicle with leads that extend into the heart	To regulate heart rhythm, most often used for bradycardia
Defibrillator	Below left clavicle with leads that extend into the heart	To restore heart to normal rhythm via electric shocks
Prosthetic valves	Within the heart	To replace diseased valves; to replicate valve function to prevent heart failure

The Mediastinum

7. Look at the overall size and shape of the mediastinum. The trachea should be midline.
8. Check for lines, drains, tubes, electrical leads, implanted devices, and artificial valves (see Table 10-2).
9. Are any obvious masses or calcifications present?
10. Is a *mediastinal shift* present? Is the entire mediastinum shifted or just a section of it?

The Heart

11. Two-thirds of the heart is to the left of midline, one-third is to the right.
12. *Estimate* the heart's size with the *cardiothoracic ratio*. In adults, the width of the heart should be 50% or less of the width of the chest at the level of the diaphragm.
13. Identify the contours of the heart. Follow the right heart border up from the diaphragm to the hilum. This is the edge of the right atrium. From the hilum upward, the edge is formed by the superior vena cava.
14. Next, follow the left heart border up from the diaphragm to the lower left hilum. This border is the edge of the left ventricle. At the hilum there is a slight concavity representing the left atrial appendage. (This concavity is lost when the left atrium is enlarged, leading to a straightening or even a convexity of the left heart border.) Above the left atrial appendage at the level of the hilum is the pulmonary artery, and above this is the arch of the aorta.

The Lungs

15. Compare the overall size of each lung field. The lungs are aerated and should be equally radiolucent. Scan for any abnormally radiolucent or radiodense areas. Does an *air bronchogram sign* exist? If so, in what lobe?
16. Compare the right and left hila, remembering these vessels are visible because they are filled with blood. The key observation is whether they are of normal caliber or enlarged.
17. Are the borders between the lungs and heart and between the lungs and diaphragm clearly visible, or does a *silhouette sign* exist? If so, which lobe is involved?
18. Follow the pleural surface around each lung periphery. Is the pleural space abnormally wide? Note any calcifications or evidence of air or fluid in the pleural cavity.

The Diaphragm

19. Normally the diaphragm is at the level of the 10th pair of posterior ribs. Is the diaphragm abnormally elevated or abnormally flattened?
20. The costophrenic angles should be sharp and downwardly inclined. Note any abnormal blunting due to pleural effusion.
21. Look below the domes of the diaphragm for normal amounts of gastric or bowel gas and their locations. The gastric bubble should be seen in the stomach under the dome of the left hemidiaphragm. Scan the soft tissues of the abdomen for abnormal calcifications, masses, or free peritoneal air.

What Can You See?

Look at the radiograph (Fig. 10-13) and tracing (Fig. 10-14). Identify the following:

- Right mediastinal borders: superior vena cava, right atrium
- Left mediastinal borders: aortic arch, left atrial appendage, left ventricle
- Lung fields from apices to costophrenic angles
- Dome of the diaphragm
- Trachea, carina, primary bronchi

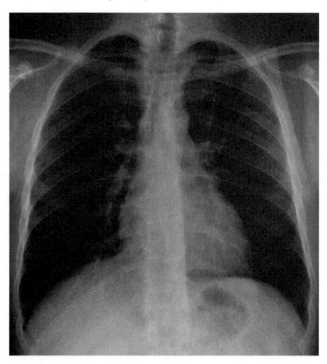

Figure 10-13 Normal PA chest radiograph.

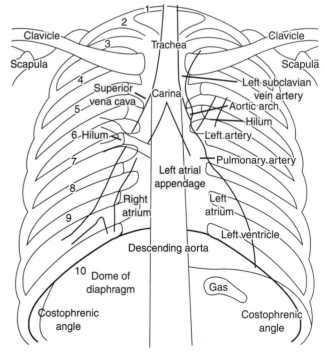

Figure 10-14 Tracing of normal PA chest radiograph.

Routine Radiologic Evaluation of the Chest

Lateral Chest

This view demonstrates the lung fields from the apices down to the costophrenic angles, from the sternum anteriorly to the posterior ribs and thorax posteriorly. Structures best seen are the heart, aorta, posterior tracheal wall and posterior esophageal wall, and left lung *(a right lateral projection would demonstrate the right lung best)*.

Radiologic Observations

Body Position

1. Determine whether the patient is rotated by looking at the profile of the sternum.

Bony Thorax

2. Check the overall alignment of the thoracic spine, noting vertebral body height and disk spaces. Assess the integrity of the cortical margins of the vertebral structures.
3. Assess bone density. Look for any erosions, osteolytic or osteoblastic lesions, fractures, or calcifications.
4. The right and left axillary ribs are superimposed. Note if the anterior cartilages are calcified.

Soft Tissues

5. Look for the overall amount of soft tissues and the breast tissue. Observe any obvious masses, calcifications, or the absence of a breast due to mastectomy.

Basic Projections

- PA
- **Left lateral**

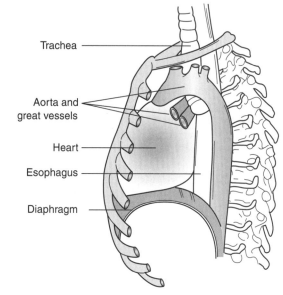

Figure 10-16 Anatomy of the heart, lateral aspect.

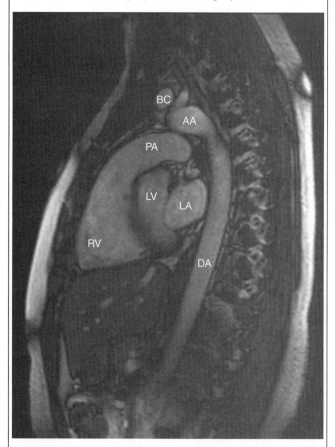

Setting up the Radiograph

Figure 10-17 Sagittal MRI. BC = brachiocephalic trunk, AA = ascending aorta, DA = descending aorta, PA = pulmonary artery, RV = right ventricle, LV = left ventricle, LA = left atrium.

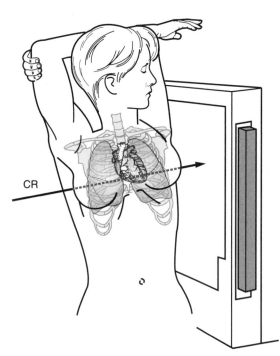

Figure 10-15 Patient position for a lateral chest radiograph. The arms are overhead to remove superimposition. The exposure is made at the end of the second full inspiration to ensure maximum expansion of the lungs. The central ray passes through the seventh thoracic vertebra.

The Mediastinum

6. The areas anterior, superior, and posterior to the mediastinum are normally radiolucent because they are filled with aerated lung.
7. Check for lines, drains, tubes, electrical leads, a pacemaker, or prosthetic valves.
8. Are any obvious masses or calcifications present?

The Heart

9. The anterior border of the heart is the right ventricle. The posterior border is composed of the left atrium superiorly and the left ventricle inferiorly.
10. The trachea and aorta may be visible posterior to the heart (Figs. 10-15 and 10-16).

The Lungs

11. Assess the anterior and posterior lung fields. Look for any abnormal radiolucency or density. Does an *air bronchogram sign* exist? If so, in which lobe?
12. The right and left hila are superimposed on the lateral view and it is difficult to identify abnormalities here.
13. Are the borders between the lungs and heart and between the lungs and diaphragm clearly visible, or does a *silhouette sign* exist? If so, which lobe is involved?
14. Follow the pleural surface around each lung periphery and posterior sternal margin. Is the pleural space abnormally wide? Note any calcifications, fluid, or air in the pleural cavity.
15. Normally the posterior costophrenic angle is sharp and downwardly inclined. Note any abnormal blunting due to pleural effusion.

The Diaphragm

16. Is the diaphragm abnormally elevated or abnormally flattened?
17. The hemidiaphragms can be distinguished by remembering that the heart "sits" on the left hemidiaphragm. The right hemidiaphragm is higher than the left.
18. Look at the abdomen for normal amounts and locations of gastric or bowel gas. Note any abnormal calcifications, masses, or free peritoneal air.

What Can You See?

Look at the radiograph (Fig. 10-18) and tracing (Fig. 10-19). Identify the following:

- Anterior mediastinal border: right ventricle
- Posterior mediastinal borders: left atrium, left ventricle
- Anterior and posterior lung fields
- Right and left hemidiaphragms
- Posterior costophrenic angle

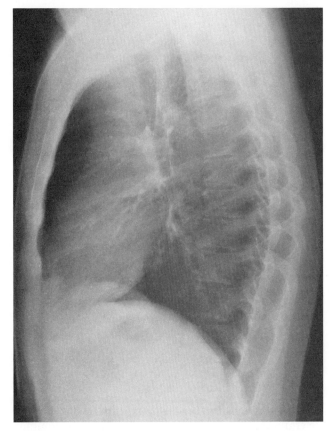

Figure 10-18 Normal lateral radiograph.

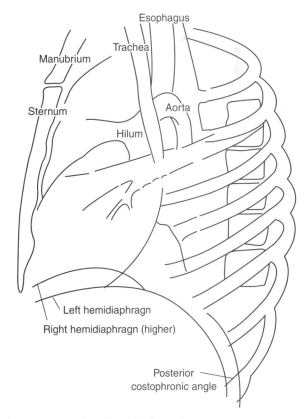

Figure 10-19 Tracing of lateral radiograph.

Pathology[5–11,21–35]

Imaging Choices in Cardiopulmonary Assessment

ACR Appropriateness Criteria[21–35] are established for an extensive scope of cardiopulmonary pathologies. These criteria, based on reviews of research literature, rank the usefulness of an imaging modality to diagnose a suspected pathology with respect to time/cost/benefit/risk/specificity factors. Interestingly, the century-old technology of the chest radiography ranks *first* in the diagnostic investigation for virtually every suspected cardiopulmonary pathology. See Table 10-3 for an example of appropriateness criteria for the clinical condition of *shortness of breath—suspected cardiac origin*.

The chest radiograph begins each imaging investigation for the following reasons:

- The radiographic findings will separate cardiac from pulmonary disease.
- The radiographic findings may define the pathology sufficiently to initiate treatment.
- The radiographic findings may *exclude* the possibility of some differential diagnoses, narrow the diagnostic choices, and thus direct the subsequent advanced imaging evaluation.

Advanced imaging can help to refine a diagnosis or determine treatment or surgical options. The most common imaging modalities used in cardiopulmonary assessment today include ultrasound in the form of echocardiography and Doppler studies, nuclear medicine studies for the evaluation of myocardial or pulmonary perfusion, computed tomography (CT) angiography, magnetic resonance (MR) angiography, as well as standard CT and MR imaging

(MRI). A brief review of these modalities follows later in the chapter.

Diagnostic Categories

A common method of assessing pathology on the chest radiograph is to divide the most obvious abnormalities into the following categories:

- Lung field is *abnormally white.*
- Lung field is *abnormally black.*
- Mediastinum is *abnormally wide.*
- Heart is *abnormally shaped.*

Although this sounds simplistic, it is useful because most pathologies in the chest will have a predominant alteration in either water densities or air densities. Although a discussion on the pathologies themselves is outside the scope of this chapter, the following section notes the radiographic characteristics of some common pathologies in each category and highlights some advanced imaging.

The Lung Field Is Abnormally White

Pneumonia

Pneumonia is a general term representing dozens of *pulmonary infections* arising from diverse etiologies. Pneumonia may involve any lobe or an entire lung; it may be unilateral or bilateral. As the body releases white blood cells to combat the infection, fluids fill up around and within the alveoli and bronchi. It is this fluid buildup that produces the characteristic *infiltrate* or *consolidation* on the chest radiograph (Fig. 10-20). Treatment for pneumonia is based on the causative microorganism and its known antibiotic

TABLE 10-3 ● *American College of Radiology ACR Appropriateness Criteria[27]*

Radiologic Procedure	Rating	Comments	RRL*
X-ray chest	9	For evaluation of pulmonary vascularity and edema.	Min
US echocardiography transthoracic	8		None
NUC myocardial perfusion scan	7		High
NUC Tc-99m ventriculography	6		Med
INV arteriography coronary	6		Med
INV left ventriculography	6		Med
CT heart function and morphology with contrast	5	Multidetector with maximal temporal and spatial resolution. For detection of coronary artery disease.	High
CT chest	5	For evaluation of pulmonary vascularity and edema.	Med
US echocardiography transesophageal	5		None
MRI heart function andmorphology with or without contrast	4		None
US peripheral venous	3	Only if DVT or PE suspected.	None
NUC Tc-99m V/Q scan lung	3	Only if PE suspected.	Med
INV arteriography pulmonary	2	Only if PE suspected.	High

Rating Scale: 1 = Least appropriate, 9 = Most appropriate
*Relative Radiation Level

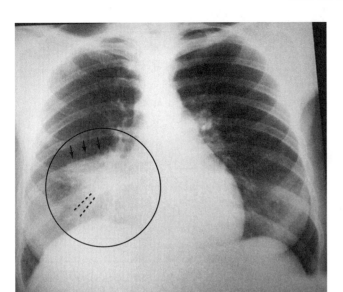

Figure 10-20 This 25-year-old female patient's PA chest x-ray shows evidence of right-middle-lobe consolidation. There is an opacity in the right mid-to-lower zone medially, which silhouettes the right heart border (circled). The opacity has a straight upper border suggesting margination along the horizontal fissure (arrows). Air bronchograms are present (dotted lines outline a vessel). There is little evidence of volume loss. The lateral film confirmed right middle lobe consolidation. *(Image courtesy of Laughlin Dawes, MD.)*

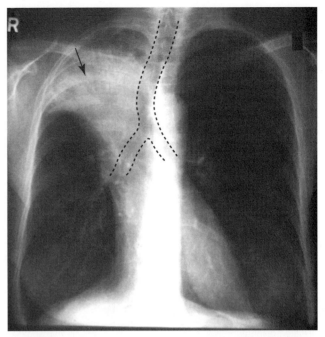

Figure 10-21 Atelectasis of the right upper lobe (arrow). The collapsed lobe is white due to deflation of the alveoli. The entire mediastinum has been pulled to the collapsed side. The trachea is no longer midline but curved to the right (dotted lines). Bronchocarcinoma is a frequent cause of obstruction resulting in this pattern of collapse.

sensitivity. However, a specific cause for pneumonia is identified in only 50% of patients.

Radiographic findings of pneumonia include the following:

- A water density *consolidation* in one or more lobes
- A *silhouette* sign if the consolidation is in a lobe that borders the heart or diaphragm
- Air *bronchogram* signs due to fluid accumulation around the terminal airway vessels

Atelectasis

Atelectasis is volume loss of a portion of the lung. It may be acute or chronic and can range from a complete collapse of an entire lung or, more commonly, involve one segment (Figs. 10-21 and 10-22). Atelectasis is not a disease itself but results from one of three causes: *obstruction* in the bronchi (foreign object, mucous plug, neoplasms), *compression* (pleural effusion, enlarged heart), or *traction* (scarring, fibrosis, adhesions). Treatment depends on the cause of the collapse. Atelectasis is a common postoperative complication due to poor inspiratory effort related to pain medications or location of the surgical incision. Secretion retention in the peripheral airways is the cause of the obstructed airflow. This atelectasis responds well to physical therapy emphasizing postural drainage and manual techniques to the area of focal pathology, along with deep breathing, coughing, and ambulation.

Radiographic findings of atelectasis include the following:

- Increased whiteness of the collapsed lobe because it is no longer filled with air.
- Lobes adjacent to the collapsed lobe may appear hyperinflated (darker) to compensate.
- The mediastinum will shift *toward* the collapsed lobe due to that lobe's loss of volume.
- The hemidiaphragm will elevate on the affected side.

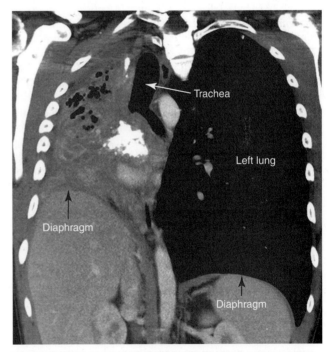

Figure 10-22 Coronal CT of the thorax demonstrating collapse of the entire right lung. The mediastinum is completely shifted to the right and the trachea can be seen pulled to the right. The right hemidiaphragm is elevated owing to loss of volume in the right hemithorax.

Pleural Effusion

Pleural effusion is excess fluid in the pleural cavity produced by an underlying pathology, such as infection, heart failure, liver failure, malignancies, pulmonary emboli, tuberculosis,

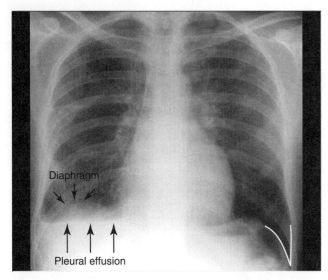

Figure 10-23 Pleural effusion. A flat density is present on the right side, characteristic of an effusion (straight arrows). The dome of the diaphragm can be seen above it (curved arrows). The effusion may also be concave; this shape helps to differentiate an effusion from an elevated diaphragm. Note the loss of a normal costophrenic angle as compared with the normal angle on the left (white outline). *(Image courtesy of www.med.yale.edu.)*

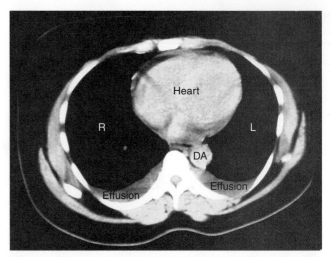

Figure 10-24 Axial CT at the level of the lower lobes. Because the patient is supine, the fluid has accumulated under the influence of gravity into the posterior pleural cavity at midline. DA refers to the descending aorta. *(Image courtesy of http://www.umdnj.edu.)*

and trauma. Four types of fluids can accumulate in the pleural space: (1) serous fluid *(hydrothorax)*; (2) blood *(hemothorax)*; (3) chyle *(chylothorax)*; and (4) pus *(pyothorax or empyema)*. The lung fields appear white because of the superimposition of the added water density in the pleural space (Fig. 10-23).

Once the effusion is diagnosed on the radiograph, the cause is determined by analyzing the fluid composition. The fluid is obtained through *thoracentesis*—a needle inserted into the pleural space at a posterior intercostal space withdraws a sample of fluid. A *thoracostomy* or *chest tube* may be inserted to drain large or recurrent effusions. CT imaging may be performed to help identify the etiology. Remember, because a patient is supine for a CT scan, fluid will accumulate under the influence of gravity in the *posterior* chest wall pleural cavity (Fig. 10-24).

Radiographic findings of pleural effusion include the following:

- *Blunting* of the normally sharp *costophrenic angles,* as the fluid accumulates by gravity in the *costophrenic sulcus.* However, at least 300 mL of fluid must be present before it is detectable on upright radiographs.
- *Blunting* of the *posterior costophrenic sulcus* seen on the upright lateral radiograph.
- Radiographs made with the patient in the lateral *decubitus* (side-lying) position are more sensitive because a *fluid–air level* becomes obvious over the lung field. As little as 50 mL of fluid can be detected in this projection.

The Lung Field Is Abnormally Black

Pneumothorax

Pneumothorax is air in the pleural cavity. It commonly occurs spontaneously (especially in tall, slim males), following a

penetrating chest wound, or following barotrauma (as can occur in scuba divers). It can also be associated with chronic lung pathologies or as a consequence of a medical procedure, such as the insertion of a central venous catheter or mechanical ventilation.

Pneumothoraces are divided into *tension* and *nontension* pneumathoraces. A tension pneumothorax is potentially fatal. Air accumulates in the pleural space with each inspiration but cannot escape, similar to a one-way valve. Positive pressure builds up, which produces a massive shift of the mediastinum *away* from the affected lung. The intrathoracic vessels become compressed and left-side cardiac venous return is obstructed. This emergency situation requires immediate relief of the pressure with insertion of a chest tube (Fig. 10-25). In contrast, a non–tension pneumothorax is a less severe pathology because there is no ongoing accumulation of air and thus no increasing pressure on the mediastinum (Fig. 10-26). It may require no treatment other than oxygen therapy and monitoring.

Most pneumothoraces are unilateral. Radiographic findings of pneumothorax may include the following:

- The lung field on the affected side will appear blacker due to absence of the lung vasculature.
- Within the blacker lung field, look for the *visceral pleural line,* or the lung edge, which normally is not visible.
- The *deep sulcus sign* present at the costophrenic angle (the angle is abnormally deep).
- A *mediastinal shift away* from the radiolucent lung field due to positive pressure in the affected hemithorax.

Chronic Obstructive Pulmonary Disease

Chronic obstructive pulmonary disease (COPD) is a diagnosis that includes a group of diseases with the common characteristic of airflow obstruction. *Emphysema* and *chronic*

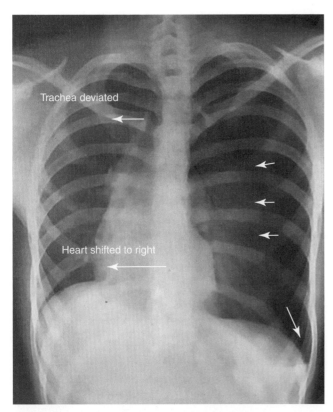

Figure 10-25 Tension pneumothorax in the left lung has pushed the heart, trachea, and entire mediastinum into the right hemithorax. Can you see the air-filled trachea displaced to the right? In the left hemithorax note that the edge of the left lung is marked by the short arrows. Air fills the widened pleural cavity between the arrows and the costal margin. The *deep sulcus sign* is indicated by the long arrow, which points to the characteristic deepened sulcus seen in pneumothorax. *(Image courtesy of http://www.xray2000.co.uk.)*

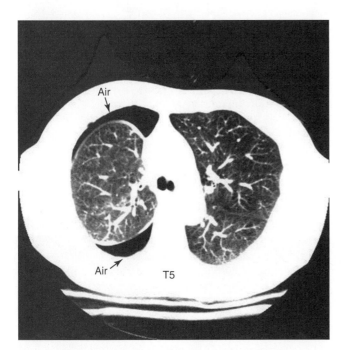

Figure 10-26 Axial CT at the level of the carina (see the right and left primary bronchus at midline). Air is evident in the pleural cavity anterior and posterior to the right lung.

bronchitis are the two most common types of COPD. Emphysema is the enlargement of the airspaces distal to the terminal bronchiole with destruction of the alveolar walls. This destruction reduces the surface area available for gas exchange with the bloodstream. Chronic bronchitis is inflammation of the airway walls with increased production of mucus. Inflammation leads to scarring and remodeling, which thickens the walls and results in narrowing of the vessels and restricted airflow. Patients often have both emphysema and chronic bronchitis, both of which are primarily caused by smoking.

Radiographically, the primary finding of COPD is hyperinflation of both lungs (Fig. 10-27). This hyperinflation results in the following:

- Increased radiolucency (blacker) of the lung fields
- Bullae (pockets of trapped air)
- Increased vertical height of the lungs
- Flattening or even scalloping of the diaphragm
- Narrowed mediastinum with a narrowed cardiac image
- Airspace below the heart
- Increased retrosternal airspace on the lateral radiograph

Advanced stages of COPD may result in *cor pulmonale* or pulmonary (right side) heart disease. The chest radiograph will show decreased vascular markings in the peripheral lung fields, and cardiomegaly due to right ventricular enlargement, right atrial dilatation, and a prominent pulmonary artery.

The Mediastinum Is Abnormally Wide

Aortic Dissection

Aortic dissection develops when a tear in the inner layer of the aorta permits a column of blood to separate (dissect) the inner and middle layers of the vessel. If the blood-filled channel ruptures through the outer aortic wall, aortic dissection is usually fatal. The most common site of aortic dissection is in the ascending aorta. Most dissections are preceded by *aortic aneurysm,* a weakness in the arterial wall that allows for abnormal dilation.

The predominant symptom is severe chest pain; this must be differentiated from a myocardial infarct. Treatment options include controlling the hypertension, interventional catheterization to place abdominal intraluminal stent grafts to prevent rupture, and open heart surgery to replace the dissected aorta with a synthetic graft.

Radiographic findings for aortic dissection may include (Fig. 10-28) the following:

- A *widened mediastinum*
- *Obliteration of the normal shape of the aortic arch*
- *Downward slant of the left mainstem bronchus* due to aortic compression
- *Tracheal deviation to the right* due to aortic compression

However, the chest radiograph may appear normal in some cases of aortic dissection and sensitivity is otherwise moderate, since many other conditions can widen the mediastinum. Diagnosis is confirmed with transesophageal echocardiography, CT angiography, or MR angiography, all which have high sensitivity and specificity (Fig. 10-29).

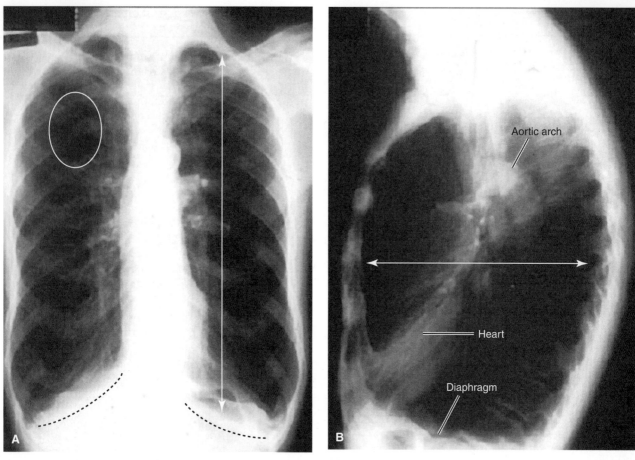

Figure 10-27 (A) PA radiograph of a patient with advanced COPD. Note the hyperinflation of the bilateral lungs fields (increased radiolucency), increased vertical dimension (arrow), scalloped diaphragms (dotted line), narrowed mediastinum, and diffuse bullae, with one most prominent in the right upper lobe. **(B)** Lateral radiograph shows the increased thoracic diameter known as "barrel chest" (arrow), hyperinflation, increased retrosternal air, and scalloped shape of the diaphragm.

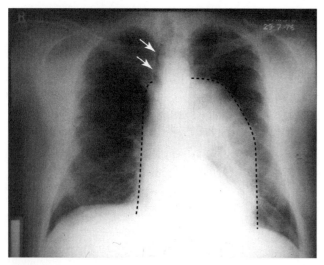

Figure 10-28 Aortic dissection. This 60-year-old man came to the emergency room with pain in the chest radiating to his back. Findings include a wide mediastinum due to a massive enlargement of the posterior portion of the arch and descending aorta (dotted). The enlargement extends from diaphragm to the hilum. The trachea is displaced (arrows). The lungs appear grossly normal with no visible pleural collection.

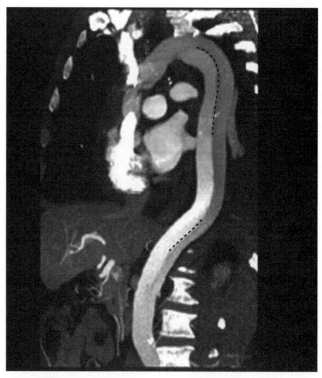

Figure 10-29 CT angiography, sagittal reconstruction of aortic dissection. Note the dual-chamber appearance of the aorta, extending from the aortic arch distal to the abdomen (dotted line).

Mediastinal Lymphadenopathy

Mediastinal lymphadenopathy is enlargement of the lymph nodes located within the mediastinum. Mediastinal nodes drain the thoracic viscera, including the lungs, heart, thymus, and thoracic esophagus. Mediastinal lymphadenopathy is usually a sign of serious underlying disease. Additionally, enlargement of the lymph nodes themselves may be life threatening, since they can cause obstruction of the airway or great vessels. There are many causes of mediastinal lymphadenopathy, including infections (tuberculosis is most common), malignancies (lymphoma, metastatic cancers), and sarcoidosis (common in young adults).

Chest radiographs and CT scanning have become the standard techniques for demonstration of intrathoracic lymphadenopathy (Figs. 10-30 and 10-31).

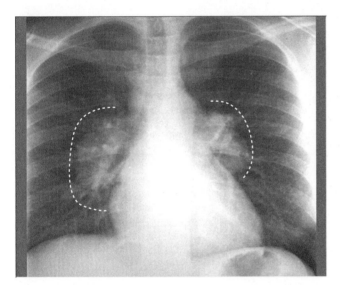

Figure 10-30 Mediastinal lymphadenopathy secondary to sarcoidosis, a granulomatous disorder of unknown cause affecting multiple organ systems and leading principally to bilateral hilar adenopathy and pulmonary infiltrates. The dotted lines surround the lobulated rounded masses characteristic of hilar lymph node enlargement.

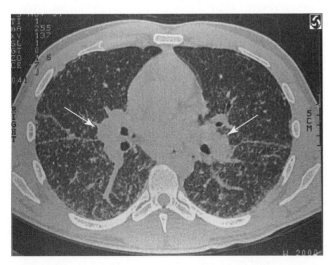

Figure 10-31 High-resolution computed tomography (HRCT) confirms miliary-like nodules in the bilateral hila and in a bronchovascular distribution. (*Miliary* means a pattern of widespread diffuse micronodules.) Arrows point to the lobulated rounded masses characteristic of hilar lymph node enlargement.

Radiographic findings of mediastinal lymphadenopathy depend upon which nodes are enlarged:

● Enlargement of the right upper paratracheal nodes causes uniform or lobular *widening of the right paratracheal stripe,* and an *increase in density of the superior vena cava* whose *border may become convex* to the lung.
● Enlargement of the aortopulmonary nodes may cause a *bulge in the angle between the aortic arch and the main pulmonary artery.*
● Enlargement of nodes below the carina will *increase the opacity of the subcarinal space* on the PA radiograph.
● Enlargement of the anterior mediastinal nodes will *increase the opacity of the retrosternal space* on the lateral view.
● Enlargement of hilar lymph nodes will cause *bilateral hilar enlargement* and a *rounded mass* in a portion of the hilum (this is in contrast to enlargement of hilar vessels which retain their branching pattern when enlarged).

The Heart Is Abnormally Shaped

Congestive Heart Failure

Congestive heart failure (CHF) occurs when the heart is unable to pump out adequate amounts of blood. CHF is a syndrome caused by diseases that weaken the heart muscle (e.g., coronary artery disease, myocardial infarct, and cardiomyopathy) or diseases that increase oxygen demand beyond the capability of the heart to deliver (e.g., hypertension, valve disease, thyroid disease, kidney disease, diabetes, or heart defects present at birth). In addition, heart failure can occur when several conditions are present at once.

Failure of the left side of the heart causes congestion of the pulmonary vasculature; fluid then backs up into the pulmonary veins and lungs, resulting in *pulmonary edema.* Fluid seeps out into the interstitium first, then eventually into the alveoli and pleural space. Failure of the right side of the heart leads to congestion of systemic capillaries and results in dependent peripheral *pitting edema and ascites* (fluid accumulation in the abdominal cavity), and *hepatomegaly* (enlargement of the liver).

Characteristics of CHF on the chest radiograph include the following (Fig. 10-32):

● *Cardiomegaly* (an enlarged heart)—based on the cardiothoracic ratio
● *Vascular redistribution* (blood vessels in the upper lobes become larger than those in the lower lobes)—an inverse of normal
● *Kerley B lines*-small horizontal white lines that extend to the pleura, caused by fluid accumulated in the interlobular septa as a result of pulmonary edema
● *Peribronchial cuffing*-bronchi seen head on are surrounded by fluid, a sign of pulmonary edema
● *Pleural effusion*
● *Bat-wing or butterfly pattern*-the replacement of lower lobe airspace in the lungs with fluid produces white lung fields, leaving the air-filled upper lobes dark; the bilateral dark areas are in the shape of wings on the PA radiograph

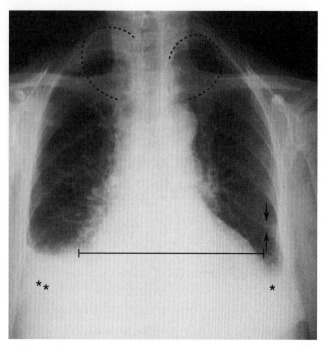

Figure 10-32 Congestive heart failure. Note the enlarged heart width (line) which exceeds the normal cardiothoracic ratio. A pleural effusion is seen filling the costophrenic recess on the right (two stars) and blunting the costophrenic angle on the left (one star). A bat-wing pattern is of airspace is seen in the upper lobes (dotted lines). The short horizontal white line extending to the pleura is a Kerley B line (arrows); it represents fluid in an interlobular septum.

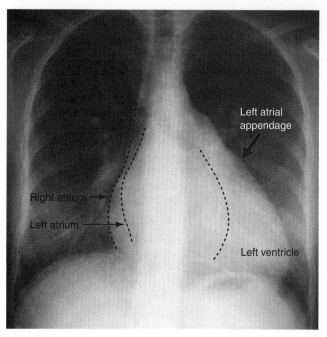

Figure 10-33 Mitral valve disease results in an enlargement of the left atrium, creating a double-line density on the right heart border (dotted lines) and a convexity on the left heart border at the atrial appendage (arrow). The left ventricle is also enlarged. *(Source of image: http://www.xray2000.co.uk.)*

Heart Valve Disease

Two types of problems can affect the heart valves. *Valve stenosis* is narrowing of the valve that results in resistance to blood flow, causing the heart to work harder. *Valve insufficiency,* also known as *valve incompetence,* means the valve does not close properly and blood leaks backward in the wrong direction. The heart has to work harder to pump the same blood out again. Possible causes of heart valve disease include congenital defects in the valve, rheumatic fever in childhood, cardiomyopathy (the thickened muscle obstructs blood flow), or age-related changes in the valves.

Symptoms of heart valve disease vary depending on which valve is affected and how severely. Symptoms can range from shortness of breath and fatigue to congestive heart failure as described above. People with heart valve disease are susceptible to *endocarditis,* an infection of the valve, and usually take prophylactic antibiotics prior to any surgeries.

Chest radiographs, echocardiograms, electrocardiograms, and CT angiograms are used to confirm the diagnosis of heart valve disease.

The radiographic findings of *mitral valve stenosis* may include the following (Fig. 10-33):

- A *straightening or bulging of the left heart border* at the atrial appendage, where it is normally concave
- A *double line density on the right heart border* representing the enlarged left atrium, which projects through the right atrium
- *Prominence of the upper lobe veins* due to increased pulmonary venous pressure

- *Kerley B lines,* small horizontal white lines that extend to the pleura, caused by fluid accumulated in the interlobular septa as a result of pulmonary edema

Advanced Imaging

Cardiac Ultrasound: Echocardiography

An echocardiogram is a noninvasive ultrasound test that has been a mainstay of cardiology since the 1960s. The value of this study is that it can provide specific information on abnormalities in the pattern of blood flow, cardiac output and ejection fractions, function of the valves, thickness and motion of the heart wall, the presence and severity of coronary artery disease, and the state of the pericardium. The different types of echocardiograms are the following:

- *Transthoracic echocardiography (TTE).* This is the standard method of performing an echocardiogram. The transducer is placed on the chest and images are taken through the chest wall.
- *Transesophageal echocardiography (TEE).* This is an alternate method of performing an echocardiogram. The transducer is passed into the patient's esophagus. Much clearer images are obtained as the ultrasound signal has only millimeters to travel without the interference of intervening bone and lung tissue. The disadvantage is the testing requires preliminary fasting and sedation (Fig. 10-34).
- *Stress echocardiography.* This study is performed before and after exercise on a treadmill or stationary bike. The patient is monitored by electrocardiography (ECG) during

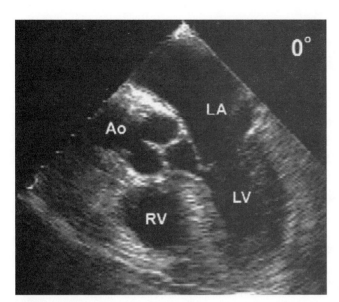

Figure 10-34 Transesophageal echocardiogram demonstrating the chambers of the heart. LA = left atrium, LV = left ventricle, RV = right ventricle, and Ao = aorta.

the test. The primary purpose is to compare blood flow to heart muscle at rest and again under stress to assess *ischemia* due to coronary artery disease. Stress may also be induced by intravenous administration of drugs that increase heart rate.

● *Doppler echocardiography.* This part of the echocardiogram study uses the Doppler principle to measure the velocity and direction of the blood flow within the heart.

These measurements allow assessment of valve function, abnormal communications between the left and right sides of the heart, any leaking of blood through the valves, and calculation of the cardiac output. Studies are viewed in color or black and white.

● *Three-dimensional (3D) echocardiography.* The emerging field of 3D echocardiography has now been shown to have several advantages over two-dimensional echocardiography, particularly for precise volume measurements, visualization of septal defects, and whole-valve evaluation. As application systems become easier to integrate into established hardware, 3D echocardiography and perhaps even virtual reality holographic images will become part of routine echocardiographic examinations (Fig. 10-35).

Nuclear Medicine

Ventilation/Perfusion Scan of the Lungs

The *ventilation/perfusion scan* is a pair of nuclear scan tests so named because it studies both airflow (ventilation) and blood flow (perfusion) in the lungs. The test is referred to as a *V/Q scan* for the initials V/Q, used in the mathematical equations that calculate airflow and blood flow respectively.

A V/Q scan is most often performed to detect a *pulmonary embolus* (blood clot in a pulmonary artery). It is also used to evaluate lung function in advanced pulmonary disease such as COPD and also as a tool for the quantification of lung performance before and after lung lobectomy surgery.

For the ventilation test, the patient inhales radioactive xenon gas. Multiple images of the chest are taken by a

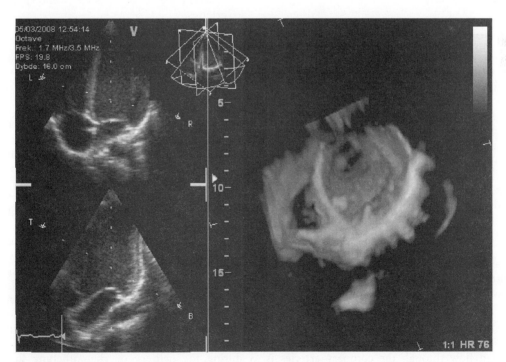

Figure 10-35 This is a still-capture of a GIF animation showing a moving echocardiogram; a 3D loop of a heart viewed from the apex, with the apical part of the ventricles removed and the mitral valve clearly visible. Because of missing data, the leaflets of the tricuspid and aortic valves are not clearly visible, but the openings are. To the left are two standard two-dimensional views taken from the 3D dataset. *(Image courtesy of http://www.wikipedia.org. It can be viewed at http://en.wikipedia.org/wiki/File:Apikal4D.gif.)*

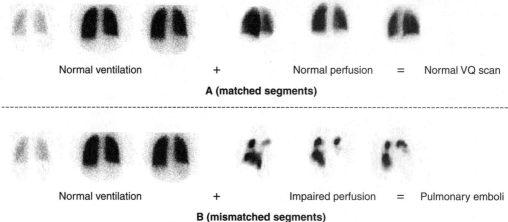

Normal ventilation　　　＋　　　Normal perfusion　　＝　　Normal VQ scan

A (matched segments)

Normal ventilation　　　＋　　　Impaired perfusion　　＝　　Pulmonary emboli

B (mismatched segments)

Figure 10-36 V/Q scans. **(A)** The lung scan is normal when both the ventilation and perfusion scans show "matching" amounts of radioactive tracer uptake in each lung segment. **(B)** A pulmonary emboli is probable when the ventilation scan tracer uptake does not "match" the perfusion scan uptake. Characteristic of pulmonary emboli are the multiple "defects" or reduced areas of tracer uptake on the perfusion scan.

gamma camera, which detects the segments of the lungs the gas has reached. For the perfusion test, technetium 99m, a radioisotope that attaches to red blood cells, is injected intravenously. The same images of the chest are again acquired by the gamma camera. The study is evaluated by comparing the two sets of chest images and matching lung segment to lung segment. A pulmonary embolus is diagnosed by observing a segment of lung that has *normal airflow,* but *decreased blood flow.* Criteria exists for how probable a pulmonary embolus is based on how many lung segment are "mismatched" between the ventilation and perfusion scans (Fig. 10-36).

Nuclear Perfusion Studies of the Heart

Nuclear perfusion studies use radioisotopes in conjunction with stress tests to detect the presence of coronary artery disease. These studies are commonly referred to as *nuclear stress tests* or *thallium or cardiolite stress tests.* (In contrast, a regular treadmill *stress test* uses *electrocardiography,* which translates the electrical activity of the heart into waveforms read on a monitor or paper strip.)

A radioisotope tracer (e.g., thallium, cardiolite) specific for the cells of the myocardium is injected intravenously. The patient's heart rate is increased either by treadmill exercise or induced by a pharmacological agent that increases the heart rate. The gamma camera scans the uptake of the tracer at rest, after exercise, and at rest again a few hours later. Complete studies evaluate all the walls of the heart from multiple axes and thus display dozens of images. Only a small sample is shown here (Fig. 10-37).

A comparison of the scans at both rest and exercise reveals any obstruction in the coronary arteries. Typically there are four possible results:

- *Normal perfusion during both exercise and rest* implies that the blood flow through the coronary arteries is unobstructed.
- *Normal perfusion at rest but decreased perfusion during exercise* implies that there is some degree of blockage in

one or more coronary arteries. This is called a *reversible defect.*

- *Decreased perfusion during both exercise and rest* implies a complete blockage of one or more coronary arteries, obstructing blood flow to that area of the heart at all times. This is a *nonreversible defect.* Even if blood flow were restored, that area of the heart muscle is permanently damaged from a prior myocardial infarct and cannot recover.
- A *combination of reversible and nonreversible defects* is common in patients with coronary artery disease, since different degrees of blockages will be present in different arteries.

Multigated Acquisition (MUGA) Scan

A *multigated acquisition (MUGA) scan* is a nuclear medicine test used to evaluate the function of the heart's ventricles. It is also known as *nuclear ventriculography.* The radioisotope technetium 99m is injected intravenously, and the gamma camera obtains a series of images of the heart (usually 16), from the *end-diastolic volume* (when the heart is completely filled) to the *end-systolic volume* (when the heart has ejected the blood). These multiply acquired pictures are put together into a movie of the heart beating.

These images are analyzed on a computer to calculate useful clinical parameters of heart function. This scan is the most accurate and reproducible way of measuring and monitoring the ejection fraction of the left ventricle, which is one of the most important metrics in assessing heart performance (Fig. 10-38). The advantage of MUGA is that it is more accurate than an echocardiogram while still being noninvasive.

A common clinical situation in which repeated MUGA scans are useful is in following a patient's cardiac function during the delivery of chemotherapy for cancer. Some chemotherapeutic agents can be toxic to the heart muscle. The MUGA scan can detect subtle, early changes in cardiac function that might be missed by other modalities.

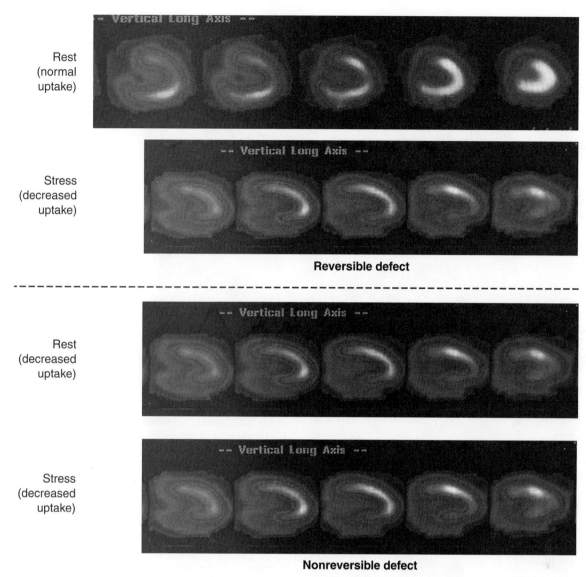

Figure 10-37 Nuclear perfusion study of the heart muscle. The amount of uptake of the radioisotope is compared at exercise stress and rest. The reversible defect shows normal perfusion at rest and decreased perfusion upon stress. The nonreversible defect shows decreased perfusion at both rest and stress.

Conventional Angiography

Angiography is a study of the blood vessels and can be performed in any organ system to assess blood flow, obstruction of blood flow usually caused by stenosis (abnormal narrowing), or aneurysms. There are several different techniques of angiography for assessing the cardiopulmonary system. The following are *conventional* angiographic procedures. An iodine-based contrast medium is delivered via a catheter inserted at the groin in the femoral vein and threaded up into the heart. The images are viewed via fluoroscopy:

- *Digital subtraction angiography*—a technique for viewing any following procedure. Images are produced by subtracting a "precontrast image" from images made after the contrast has been injected. Only the vessels are seen, not the surrounding anatomy.

- *Coronary angiography*—contrast is delivered into the left heart to evaluate the coronary arteries. This study is included under a group of *cardiac catheterization* procedures that include both diagnostic evaluation and interventional treatment (e.g., *balloon angioplasty, stent placement*) (Fig. 10-39).
- *Pulmonary angiography*—contrast is delivered through the right side of the heart and into the pulmonary artery to diagnose pulmonary embolism. *Aortic angiography* via left heart catheterization is used to assess aortic regurgitation, coarctation, patent ductus arteriosus, and dissection. These procedures have for the most part been replaced by CT angiography.
- *Ventriculography*—used to visualize ventricular wall motion and ventricular outflow and to calculate ejection fractions.

These conventional techniques are invasive and carry some risk. It is not unrealistic to surmise they will be

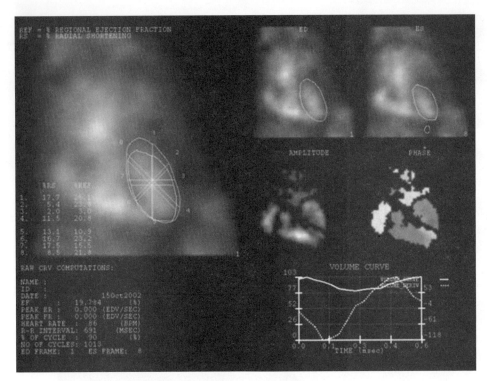

Figure 10-38 MUGA scan of the heart. At top right, end-diastolic volume (ED) shows the heart filled and end-systolic volume (ES) shows the heart after blood is ejected. At left is the comparison of the wall motion (arrow). At lower left, the ejection fraction is calculated at 19.7% (normal is greater than 50%, high risk is less than 35%). At lower right is a volume curve over time. A normal curve is shown in red. The patient's volumes are in white.

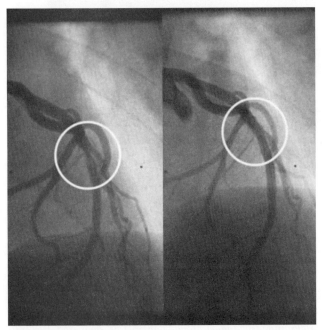

Figure 10-39 Coronary angiogram. A 38-year-old female was admitted with chest pain. An angiogram revealed double-vessel disease with 80% stenosis in the proximal left anterior descending, just beyond the origin of a large first diagonal artery (left). The lesion was dilated and a 3.0- by 11-mm stent was implanted with good angiographic results and no complications (right). *(Image courtesy of Greg Starke, MD.)*

guide transluminal interventions. As for pulmonary angiography, there is an evolving consensus that CT angiography is the primary imaging modality to diagnosis pulmonary emboli with higher sensitivity than V/Q scans and conventional angiography.

Computed Tomography Pulmonary Angiography

Computed tomography pulmonary angiography (CTPA) was introduced in the 1990s as an alternative to V/Q scanning. The contrast is injected through a peripheral vein, not through a catheter, as in conventional angiography.

In CTPA, the pulmonary vessels are filled with contrast and appear white. Any obstructions in the vessel (embolus or fat) appear darker (Fig. 10-40). Generally, the scan should be complete before the contrast reaches the left side of the heart and the aorta, which could result in artifacts. CTPA is possible only because of the high speed of modern scanners.

CTPA is typically only requested if pulmonary embolism is suspected clinically or based on the chest radiograph. After initial concern that CTPA would miss smaller emboli, a 2007 study comparing CTPA directly with V/Q scanning found that CTPA identified more emboli without decreasing the risk of long-term complications.

Magnetic Resonance Angiography

Magnetic resonance angiography (MRA) is a general term describing a diverse group of MRI pulse sequences used to generate a signal from flowing blood. (Remember, in conventional MRI, flowing blood has no signal and appears black.)

replaced someday by noninvasive CT and MR angiography. However, at present, coronary angiography remains the "gold standard" for depicting the anatomy and the severity of obstructive coronary artery disease. Moreover, it is needed to

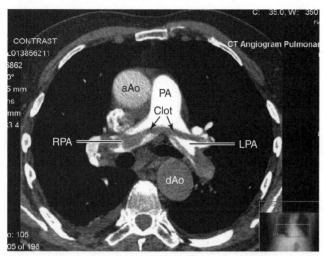

Figure 10-40 A CTPA, demonstrating a pulmonary embolus. This "saddle" embolus is named after the shape of the clot as it straddles the bifurcation of the pulmonary artery. The pulmonary arteries are filled with contrast and appear white. Any mass-filling defects, such as the clot here, appear gray. The anatomy is PA = pulmonary artery, aAo = ascending aorta, dAo = descending aorta, LPA = left pulmonary artery, RPA = right pulmonary artery. *(Source of image: http://www.en .wikipedia.org/wiki/CT_pulmonary_angiogram.)*

Clinically, MRA has been successful in studying the arteries of the cerebrovascular system as well as the aorta and its major branches, the renal arteries, and the lower extremities (Fig. 10-41). For the coronary arteries, however, MRA has been less successful than CT angiography or invasive catheter angiography.

However, MRA has important attributes that make it a promising technology in the assessment of the vascular system. Compared with CT angiography and conventional angiography, it is noninvasive, with no exposure to ionizing radiation or iodinated contrast. Compared to ultrasound, it is not operator-dependent. The current drawbacks of MRA are its comparatively high cost and somewhat limited spatial resolution; it is also generally less likely to be available in the emergency setting.

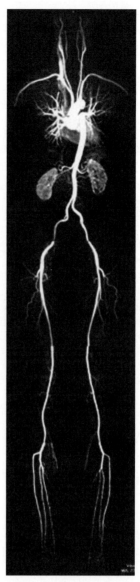

Figure 10-41 Normal whole-body MRA. After manual injection of intravenous contrast, the scan took 73 seconds to "run off" into the distal lower extremities. *(Image courtesy of Anil N. Shetty, Ph.D., Chief, MR Physics, William Beaumont Hospital, Royal Oak, MI.)*

Summary of Key Points

1. The chest radiograph is the first imaging study in cardiopulmonary assessment because it can help to (a) separate cardiac from pulmonary disease, (b) define many pathologies sufficiently to initiate treatment, or (c) narrow the differential diagnoses and direct the subsequent imaging investigation.

2. The routine radiographic examination of the chest includes two projections:
   ➤ Posteroanterior—demonstrates the lung fields, the mediastinum (trachea, heart, great vessels, esophagus), and bony thorax.

   ➤ Lateral—usually a left lateral, demonstrating the heart, left lung, retrosternal space, anterior and posterior mediastinum, and thoracic spine.

3. The *cardiothoracic ratio* is an estimate of heart size on the PA radiograph. In adults, the width of the heart should be less than half the width of the chest.

4. The *silhouette sign* helps to localize water-based lesions to a specific lobe of the lung. This sign refers to a *loss* of the normal heart or diaphragm border when a lesion is in a lobe adjacent to it.

5. The *air bronchogram sign* indicates that an airspace disease is present. The normally invisible terminal airway vessels become visible as they become outlined by abnormal fluid in the airspaces.

6. The diaphragm is normally at the 10th pair of posterior ribs. It may become abnormally elevated or flattened as a characteristic of specific pathologies. The right hemidiaphragm is higher because of the underlying liver; the left hemidiaphragm overlies the stomach and a gastric air bubble is usually present.

7. Pathology on radiograph can be divided into the following:
   ➤ *Lung fields abnormally white* (e.g., pneumonia, atelectasis, pleural effusion)
   ➤ *Lung fields abnormally black* (e.g., pneumothorax, COPD)
   ➤ *Mediastinum abnormally wide* (e.g., aortic dissection, lymphadenopathy)
   ➤ *Heart abnormally shaped* (e.g., CHF, mitral valve stenosis)

8. *Echocardiography* is an ultrasound study of the heart valuable for assessing blood flow, cardiac output, ejection fraction, valve function, heart wall motion, and the pericardium.

9. *Ventilation/perfusion (V/Q) scans* are nuclear medicine studies that use radioisotopes to evaluate the flow of air and blood to all segments of the lungs. A "mismatch" between the ventilation of air and the perfusion of blood in a lung segment usually indicates a pulmonary emboli.

10. *Nuclear perfusion studies* of the heart use a radioisotope to define the perfusion of blood in the myocardium at rest and under stress. This detects the presence and severity of coronary artery disease.

11. A *multigated acquisition (MUGA) scan* uses radioisotopes to evaluate the function of the heart ventricles. The result can be displayed as a movie of the beating heart and give accurate measurements of ejection fractions to monitor subtle changes in cardiac function.

12. *Angiography* is a study of blood flow in blood vessels. *Coronary angiography* is achieved via *cardiac catheterization. Computed tomography pulmonary angiography (CTPA)* is achieved via peripheral intravenous injection and is currently the study of choice to diagnose pulmonary emboli. *Magnetic resonance angiography (MRA)* is a noninvasive method and can be used to evaluate the vascular system in whole-body scans.

CASE STUDY

Pneumonia

History

The patient is a 47-year-old male with history of asthma. He experienced 5 days of dyspnea (shortness of breath) and fever. After seeing his physician, he was diagnosed with pneumonia and placed on an antibiotic. However, the following day, the patient experienced severe dyspnea and went to the emergency room. Upon initial examination, adventitious (abnormal) breath sounds were heard over both lower lobes and oxygen saturation was 84%. Blood tests revealed elevated *BUN (blood urea nitrogen)*, indicating renal impairment, and a normal *D-dimer* test, ruling out the likelihood of a deep venous thrombosis or pulmonary embolism. Patient underwent several imaging studies and was admitted to the intensive care unit.

Imaging Findings

A chest radiograph and a ventilation/perfusion (V/Q) scan were ordered. The V/Q scan was utilized to rule out pulmonary embolism and confirm ventilatory changes. The V/Q scan revealed reduced ventilation and perfusion of blood to the right and left lower lobes and the lingula on the left (Fig. 10-42). Radiographs revealed considerable consolidation of the right and left lower lobes and lingula (inferomedial portion of the left upper lobe bordering on the heart) (Fig. 10-43). A diagnosis of pneumonia was made, followed by the administration of intravenous (IV) antibiotics, nebulizer bronchodilators, and supplemental oxygen (3 L O$_2$/min). Oxygen saturation improved to 90% with this treatment.

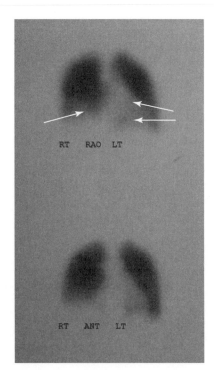

Figure 10-42 Two images from a V/Q scan demonstrating reduced ventilation and perfusion to both lower lobes and the lingula (arrows).

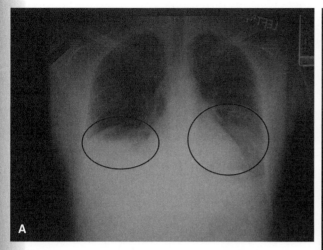

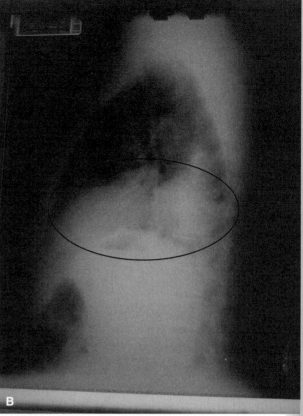

Figure 10-43 (A) AP and **(B)** lateral chest radiographs showing areas of consolidation in both lower lobes (circled).

Physical Examination and Treatment

On the second day in the hospital, the patient was seen by a physical therapist for chest physical therapy and mobilization. The patient's chief complaints were dyspnea, pain with breathing, and poor endurance.

Auscultation of the lungs revealed adventitious breath sounds over the bilateral lower lobes. Oxygen saturation was 88% on 3 L O_2/min via nasal cannula as monitored via a portable pulse oximeter device. Sitting resting heart rate was 108 beats per minute, blood pressure of 132/84 mm Hg, and respiratory rate 24 breaths per minute. Airway clearance techniques were performed over both lower lobes and the lingula. Approximately 10 mL of a mucopurulent exudate was collected and oxygen saturation became 92% on 3 L O_2/min, with reduction in adventitious sounds over all affected lobes. Upon standing, patient's heart rate went to 114 beats per minute, blood pressure to 136/80 mm Hg, respiratory rate to 28 breaths per minute; oxygen saturation remained at 92% without any symptoms of light-headedness. Patient was encouraged to ambulate 30 feet with contact guard, whereupon heart rate went to 134 beats per minute, blood pressure to 138/80 mm Hg, and respiratory rate to 32 breaths per minute; oxygen saturation dropped to at 86% with increasing symptoms of dyspnea and a productive cough. Patient's oxygen was increased to 4 L O_2/min and oxygen saturation returned to 92%, whereupon oxygen delivery was reduced back to 3 L O_2/min. Patient was shown how to use incentive spirometer and encouraged to spend as much time sitting and moving as possible.

Outcome

The next day, the patient's symptoms were significantly reduced and patient ambulated in the hallway 100 feet independently without desaturation of oxygen (which remained at 95%). Patient was encouraged to continue to increase his independent activity level while in the hospital and was subsequently discharged from physical therapy. Patient was discharged from the hospital 5 days after being admitted. Follow-up radiographs a week later revealed significant clearing of the consolidation (Fig. 10-44).

Discussion

Physical therapy examination corroborated medical findings. Airway clearance techniques helped to clear a significant amount of exudate, which improved oxygen saturation. Activity in this patient revealed increasing dyspnea and desaturation of oxygen in even mild exertion, which accompanies this extensive of a pneumonia. Early mobilization of patients with community-acquired pneumonia has been shown to be beneficial and cost-effective in reducing overall length of hospital stay without increasing the threat of adverse outcomes.

From Mundy LM, Leet, TL, Darst, K, et al: Early mobilization of patients hospitalized with community-acquired pneumonia. Chest 124(3):883, 2003.

continued

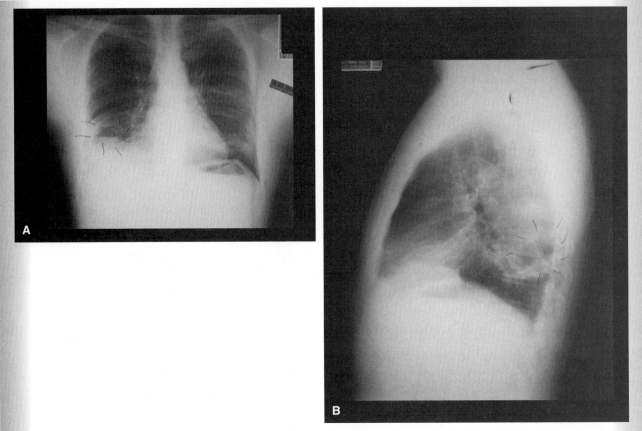

Figure 10-44 (A) AP and **(B)** lateral chest radiographs 2 weeks after treatment for pneumonia. The consolidation has mostly cleared. The radiologist has marked some remnant areas of concern to observe in follow-up radiographs.

References

1. Weber, EC, Vilensky JA, and Carmichael, SW: Netter's Concise Radiologic Anatomy. WB Saunders, Philadelphia, 2008.
2. Corne, E: Chest X-Ray Made Easy, ed. 2. Churchill Livingstone, New York, 2002.
3. Bontrager, KL: Textbook of Radiographic Positioning and Related Anatomy, ed. 6. Mosby, St. Louis, MO, 2005.
4. Frank, E, Smith, B, and Long, B: Merrill's Atlas of Radiographic Positions and Radiologic Procedures, ed. 11. Elsevier Health Sciences, Philadelphia, 2007.
5. Squires, LF, and Novelline, RA: Fundamentals of Radiology, ed. 4. Harvard University Press, Cambridge, MA, 1988.
6. Kelley, LL, and Peterson, CM: Sectional Anatomy for Imaging Professional, ed. 2. Mosby, St. Louis, MO, 2007.
7. Lazo, DL: Fundamentals of Sectional Anatomy: An Imaging Approach. Thomson Delmar Learning, Clifton Park, NY, 2005.
8. Erkonen, W, and Smith, W: Radiology 101: The Basics and Fundamentals of Imaging, ed. 2. Lippincott Williams & Wilkins, Philadelphia, 2004.
9. Daffner, RH: Clinical Radiology: The Essentials, ed. 3. Lippincott Williams & Wilkins, Baltimore, 2007.
10. Bax, J: Cardiovascular Imaging: A Handbook for Clinical Practice. Blackwell, Oxford, UK, 2005.
11. Ouellette, H, and Tetreault, P: Clinical Radiology Made Ridiculously Simple. MedMaster, Miami, 2003.
12. American College of Radiology (ACR): Practice Guideline for the Performance of Pediatric and Adult Chest Radiography. Revised 2006. Available at http://www.acr.org/SecondaryMainMenuCategories/quality_safety/guidelines/dx/Chest/chest_radiography.aspx.
13. ACR: Practice Guideline for the Performance of Pediatric and Adult Thoracic Computed Tomography (CT) Available at http://www.acr.org/SecondaryMainMenuCategories/quality_safety/guidelines/dx/Chest/ct_thoracic.aspx.
14. ACR: Practice Guideline for the Performance of Computed Tomography (CT) for the Detection of Pulmonary Embolism in Adults. Revised 2006. Available at http://www.acr.org/SecondaryMainMenuCategories/quality_safety/guidelines/dx/Chest/ct_pulmonary.aspx.
15. ACR: Practice Guideline for the Performance of High-Resolution Computed Tomography (HRCT) of the Lungs in Adults. Revised 2006. Available at http://www.acr.org/SecondaryMainMenuCategories/quality_safety/guidelines/dx/Chest/hrct_lungs.aspx.
16. ACR: Practice Guideline for the Performance of Pediatric and Adult Body Magnetic Resonance Angiography (MRA). Revised 2006. Available at http://www.acr.org/SecondaryMainMenuCategories/quality_safety/guidelines/dx/cardio/body_mra.aspx.
17. ACR: Practice Guideline for the Performance of Pediatric and Adult Cerebrovascular Magnetic Resonance Angiography (MRA). Revised 2006. Available at http://www.acr.org/SecondaryMainMenuCategories/quality_safety/guidelines/dx/cardio/cerebrovascular_mra.aspx.
18. ACR: Practice Guideline for the Performance and Interpretation of CT Angiography (CTA). Revised 2006. Available at http://www.acr.org/SecondaryMainMenuCategories/quality_safety/guidelines/dx/cardio/ct_angiography.aspx.
19. ACR: Practice Guideline for the Performance and Interpretation of Cardiac Magnetic Resonance Imaging (MRI) Revised 2006. Available at http://www.acr.org/SecondaryMainMenuCategories/quality_safety/guidelines/dx/cardio/mri_cardiac.aspx.
20. ACR: Practice Guideline for the Performance and Interpretation of Cardiac Computed Tomography (CT). Revised 2006. Available at http://www.acr.org/SecondaryMainMenuCategories/quality_safety/guidelines/dx/cardio/ct_cardiac.aspx.
21. ACR: Appropriateness Criteria for Acute Chest Pain Low Probability of Coronary Artery disease. Revised 2008. Available at http://www.acr.org/SecondaryMainMenuCategories/quality_safety/app_criteria/pdf/ExpertPanelonCardiovascularImaging/AcuteChestPainNoECGorEnzymeEvidenceofMyocardialIschemiaInfarctionDoc1.aspx.
22. ACR: Appropriateness Criteria for Acute Chest Pain Suspected Aortic Dissection. Revised 2008. Available at http://www.acr.org/SecondaryMainMenuCategories/quality_safety/app_criteria/pdf/ExpertPanelonCardiovascularImaging/AcuteChestPainSuspectedAorticDissectionDoc2.aspx.
23. ACR: Appropriateness Criteria for Acute Chest Pain Suspected Pulmonary Emboli. Revised 2008. Available at http://www.acr.org/SecondaryMainMenuCategories/quality_safety/app_criteria/pdf/ExpertPanelonCardiovascularImaging/AcuteChestPainSuspectedPulmonaryEmbolismUpdateinProgressDoc4.aspx.
24. ACR: Appropriateness Criteria for Chronic Chest Pain High Probability of Coronary Artery Disease. Revised 2006. Available at http://www. acr.org/SecondaryMainMenuCategories/quality_safety/app_criteria/pdf/ExpertPanelonCardiovascularImaging/ChronicChestPainNoEvidenceofMyocardialIschemiaInfarctionUpdateinProgressDoc7.aspx.
25. ACR: Appropriateness Criteria for Chronic Chest Pain Low to Intermediate Probability of Coronary Artery Disease. Revised 2008. Available at http://www.acr.org/SecondaryMainMenuCategories/quality_safety/app_criteria/pdf/ExpertPanelonCardiovascularImaging/ChronicChestPainSuspectedCardiacOriginUpdateinProgressDoc8.aspx.
26. ACR: Appropriateness Criteria for Congestive Heart Failure. Revised 2006. Available at http://www.acr.org/SecondaryMainMenuCategories/quality_safety/app_criteria/pdf/ExpertPanelonCardiovascularImaging/CongestiveHeartFailureDoc10.aspx.
27. ACR: Appropriateness Criteria for SOB Suspect Cardiac Origins. Revised 2006. Available at http://www.acr.org/SecondaryMainMenuCategories/quality_safety/app_criteria/pdf/ExpertPanelonCardiovascularImaging/ShortnessofBreathSuspectedCardiacOriginDoc15.aspx.
28. ACR: Appropriateness Criteria for Suspected Bacterial Endocarditis. Revised 2006. Available at http://www.acr.org/SecondaryMainMenuCategories/quality_safety/app_criteria/pdf/ExpertPanelonCardiovascularImaging/SuspectedBacterialEndocarditisDoc17.aspx.
29. ACR: Appropriateness Criteria for Suspected Congenital Heart Disease in Adults. Revised 2007. Available at http://www.acr.org/SecondaryMainMenuCategories/quality_safety/app_criteria/pdf/ExpertPanelonCardiovascularImaging/SuspectedCongenitalHeartDiseaseintheAdultUpdateinProgressDoc18.aspx.
30. ACR: Appropriateness Criteria for Suspected Lower Extremity Deep Vein Thrombosis. Revised 2005. Available at http://www.acr.org/SecondaryMainMenuCategories/quality_safety/app_criteria/pdf/Vascular/SuspectedLowerExtremityDeepVeinThrombosisDoc19.aspx.
31. ACR: Appropriateness Criteria for Acute Respiratory illness. Revised 2008. Available at http://www.acr.org/SecondaryMainMenuCategories/quality_safety/app_criteria/pdf/ExpertPanelonThoracicImaging/AcuteRespiratoryIllnessDoc1.aspx.
32. ACR: Appropriateness Criteria for Routine Chest Radiograph. Revised 2006. Available at http://www.acr.org/SecondaryMainMenuCategories/quality_safety/app_criteria/pdf/ExpertPanelonThoracicImaging/RoutineChestRadiographDoc7.aspx.
33. ACR: Appropriateness Criteria for Dyspnea. Revised 2006. Available at http://www.acr.org/SecondaryMainMenuCategories/quality_safety/app_criteria/pdf/ExpertPanelonThoracicImaging/DyspneaDoc3.aspx.
34. ACR: Appropriateness Criteria for Hemoptysis. Revised 2006. Available at http://www.acr.org/SecondaryMainMenuCategories/quality_safety/app_criteria/pdf/ExpertPanelonThoracicImaging/HemoptysisDoc4.aspx.
35. ACR: Appropriateness Criteia for Pulmonary Metastases. Revised 2006. Available at http://www.acr.org/SecondaryMainMenuCategories/quality_safety/app_criteria/pdf/ExpertPanelonThoracicImaging/ScreeningforPulmonaryMetastasesDoc9.

SELF-TEST

Image A

1. What projection is this?

2. What medical devices are seen?

3. What can you say about the cardiothoracic ratio?

4. What word describes the size of this heart?

5. A costophrenic angle cannot be seen on the left. What is the probable reason?

6. What is a likely diagnosis?

Image B

7. What projection is this?

8. What can you say about the cardiothoracic ratio?

9. How would you describe the width of the mediastinum?

10. How would you describe the look of the lung fields?

11. What can you say about the position and contours of the diaphragm?

12. What can you say about the heart and its position relative to the diaphragm?

13. What is a likely diagnosis?

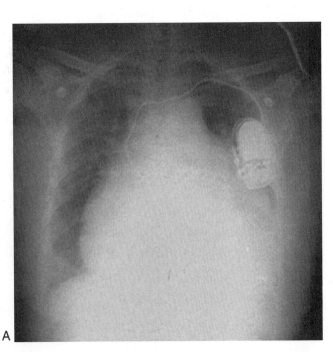

A

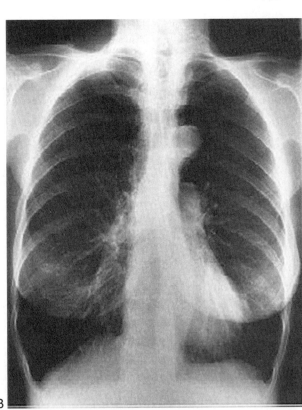

B

Chapter 11

RADIOLOGIC EVALUATION OF THE LUMBOSACRAL SPINE AND SACROILIAC JOINTS

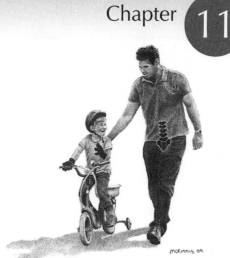

mcKinnis 09

The lumbar spine, lumbosacral articulation, and sacroiliac joints are prone to numerous dysfunctions related to mechanical stresses and degenerative changes. Additionally, this region is vulnerable to acute trauma from falls or heavy lifting and chronic strain from repetitive movements, ligamentous laxity, and poor posture. Those with resultant low back and buttock pain syndromes are among the most frequently treated patients seen in the clinic. It is essential that the clinical evaluation include knowledge of the underlying degenerative changes in the spine as revealed on radiographs. The degree of degeneration will affect the ability of the spine to withstand trauma, assume postural changes, and make functional gains in mobility and movement patterns.

Review of Anatomy

Osseous Anatomy[1–9]

Lumbar Spine

The five lowest vertebrae of the spinal column make up the lumbar spine (Fig. 11-1). The fifth lumbar vertebra is joined to the sacrum via the articulation of the inferior articular processes of L5 to the superior articular processes of the sacrum and, additionally, the L5–S1 intervertebral disk. These articulations define the lumbosacral junction (Fig. 11-2). The transformation of the lumbar lordosis to the convexity of the sacrum at this junction defines the lumbosacral angle. The caudal end of the sacrum articulates with the coccyx.

Lumbar vertebrae are characterized by large *bodies* that increase in size from the first to the fifth lumbar vertebra (Fig. 11-3). Short *pedicles* project posteriorly from the body and give rise to paired *superior and inferior articular processes*. Short, broad *laminae* unite in midline to form large, blunt, horizontally inclined *spinous processes. Transverse processes* are slender in the lumbar spine. *Spinal nerves* exit the *intervertebral foramen* bounded by coadjacent pedicles. *Zygapophyseal joints* (more commonly known as *facet joints*) articulate in a more nearly sagittally oriented plane than those of the thoracic spine with the exception of the inferior articular facets of L5. The lumbosacral facet joints lie in a more frontal plane of orientation. The intervertebral disks of the lower two lumbar segments and especially the lumbosacral junction

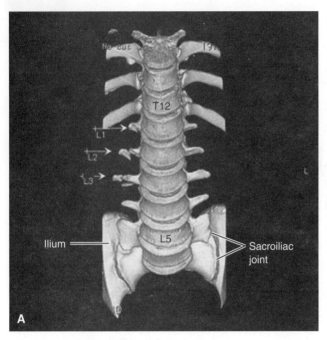
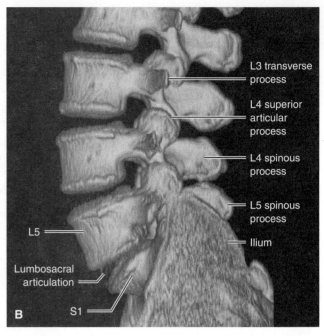

Figure 11-1 A three-dimensional (3D) reformatted CT scan of the lumbar spine and sacrum. **(A)** is an anterior coronal view The spine is normal with the exception of fractures at the tips of the right side transverse processes of L1, L2, and L3. These injuries were sustained by a professional football player during a regular season game as he jumped to catch the ball and was struck in the low back while tackled. An advantage of 3D CT imaging is the ability to visualize difficult-to-see structures that may not lie in cardinal planes. *(Image courtesy of Tom Hunkele, MPT, ATC.)* **(B)** is a sagittal view, showing normal anatomy of the lower lumbar vertebrae and lumbosacral articulation.

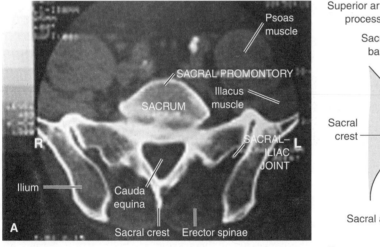
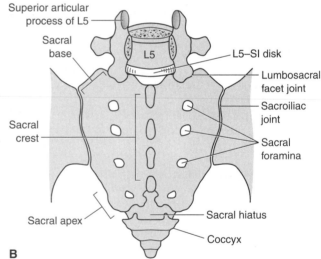

Figure 11-2 (A) Axial CT image of the sacrum and sacroiliac joints. **(B)** Posterior view of the lumbosacral articulation, sacrum, coccyx, and sacroiliac articulations. The L5 laminae and spinous process are cut away to show the L5 vertebral body and L5–S1 disk.

possess greater anterior than posterior height and exhibit a wedge-like shape.

Sacrum

The sacrum represents the fusion of five sacral bodies into a single bone. The superior end of the sacrum is its base and the inferior end is its apex. The large masses of bone lateral to the first sacral body segment are the alae, or wings, of the sacrum. The anterior surface of the sacrum is concave, smooth, and marked by four pairs of anterior sacral foramina. The rough, irregular, convex posterior surface is marked by a midline

sacral crest, representing the fused spinous processes; four pairs of posterior sacral foramina, corresponding with the anterior pairs; and large auricular surfaces that articulate with surfaces on the ilium, forming the sacroiliac joints. The failure of the fifth sacral laminae to unite leads to the development of the sacral hiatus (see Fig. 11-2), which is sometimes used as a portal for injection into the epidural space.

Sacroiliac Joint

The sacroiliac joints are formed primarily by the upper three sacral vertebrae. The articular surfaces are irregularly shaped

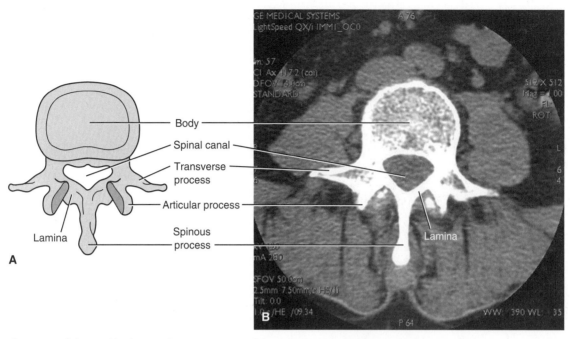

Figure 11-3 **(A)** Typical lumbar vertebra, superior view. **(B)** Axial CT image of lumbar vertebra.

but fit snugly into corresponding irregularities on the ilia; this contributes to the inherent stability of the joint. The joint itself lies in an oblique orientation to the frontal plane, with variations in angulation and shape.

Coccyx

The coccyx represents the fusion of three to five segments of bone into a single bone. The superior end of the coccyx is its base, and the inferior end is the apex. The coccyx articulates to the sacrum in such a way that it lies continuous with the dominant curve of the sacrum, and its tip points anteriorly toward the symphysis pubis.

Ligamentous Anatomy

Lumbar Spine

The vertebral column ligaments (Figs. 11-4 and 11-5), which arise in the upper cervical region and extend downward, reach their termination at the sacrum. The anterior longitudinal ligament extends from the atlas to the sacrum and increases in width as it descends, providing a strong anterior support in the lumbar spine. The posterior longitudinal ligament extends from the axis to the sacrum and decreases in width as it descends, providing less certain posterior support for the lumbar intervertebral disks. The remaining posterior ligaments—including the ligamenta flava and supraspinous, interspinous, intertransverse, and articular facet capsules—function similarly in the lumbar spine as in the cervical and thoracic regions, providing restraints to excessive flexion and rotation.

Lumbosacral Spine

The iliolumbar ligament (Fig. 11-6) extends from the transverse processes of the fifth lumbar vertebra to the posterior

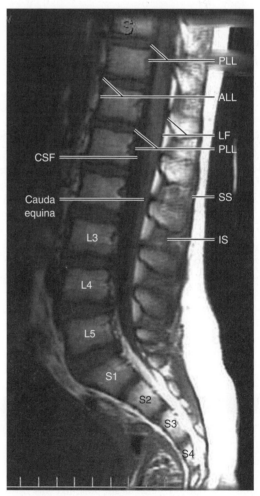

Figure 11-4 Lumbosacral spine, sagittal T1-weighted MR image identifying the anterior longitudinal ligament (ALL), posterior longitudinal ligament (PLL), ligamentum flavum (LF), supraspinous ligament (SS), and interspinous ligament (SS). CSF is cerebrospinal fluid.

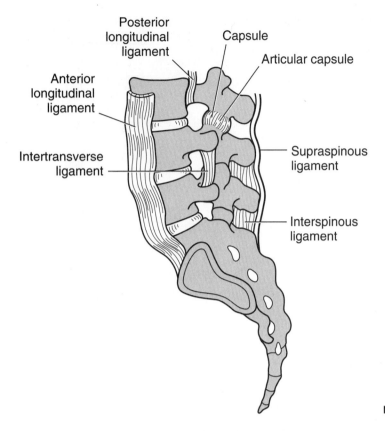

Figure 11-5 Ligaments of the lumbar spine.

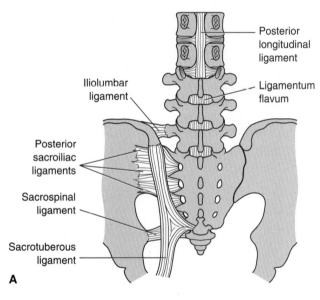

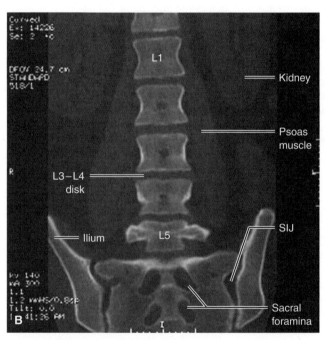

Figure 11-6 **(A)** Lumbosacral ligaments. The first and second lumbar vertebrae are cut away through the pedicles in order to view the posterior longitudinal ligament. **(B)** Coronal CT image of the lumbosacral spine.

iliac crests, providing a major restraint against excessive shear between L5 and the sacrum. The lumbosacral joint receives additional ligamentous support, like any other vertebral segment, from the anterior longitudinal ligament and the posterior ligaments, as described earlier.

Sacroiliac Joint

The primary ligamentous stabilizer of the sacroiliac joint is the interosseous ligament, extending between the sacrum and each ilium. Posterior support is provided by the posterior sacroiliac ligaments and anterior support by the anterior sacroiliac ligaments. Additional extrinsic support is provided by the sacrospinal ligament, extending from the ischial spine to the lower side of the sacrum and coccyx, and the sacrotuberous ligament, extending from the ischial tuberosity to the back of the sacrum and the posterosuperior iliac spine.

Joint Mobility

Lumbar Spinal Segments

The lumbar facet joints L1–L4 are vertically oriented in a sagittal plane. This orientation facilitates flexion and extension and somewhat limits rotation and lateral flexion. The mechanics of the lumbosacral joint, L5–S1, are unique. The change of facet orientation into a more frontal plane, the degree of inclination of the lumbosacral angle, and the articulation of the sacroiliac joints all directly affect the amount of mobility and the resistance to shear forces at this segment. The anteriorly directed shear forces that are imposed by normal upright posture have been estimated to be at least half of the total body weight. This tremendous amount of joint stress predisposes this segment to degenerative conditions and complications when fractured.

Sacroiliac Joint

The type and amount of movement at the sacroiliac joints is controversial; values differ according to various researchers. Despite the differing theories on where the axes of joint motion are located, it is generally accepted that (1) movement at the sacroiliac joints occurs in response to movement at adjacent bones or body segments and that (2) the cartilaginous, irregularly shaped articular surfaces permit adaptive deformation to a variety of imposed stresses. Thus, movement at the sacroiliac joint occurs not in isolation but in combination with and as a result of extrinsic movement. Trunk flexion, for example, incurs a reversal of lumbar lordosis, pelvic rotation about the hip joints, flaring of the posterior ilia, and a counternutation of the sacrum. These smoothly coordinated joint movements, acting in concert and including sacroiliac motion, are referred to in a functional sense as the lumbopelvic rhythm.

The sacroiliac joint is in part a synovial joint that undergoes marked changes in adulthood. Fibrous and bony ankylosis uniting the joint surfaces are normal aging changes that begin in late middle age. Women and men differ in the amount of mobility that remains preserved in this joint, and numerous factors influence this difference, including the lumbosacral articulation, configuration of the pelvic bones, and ligamentous laxity promoted by pregnancy and childbirth.

Growth and Development

Ossification of the Lumbar Vertebrae

Ossification of the lumbar vertebrae begins in the sixth week of fetal life. At birth, the bodies of the vertebrae are ossified and at least three ossification centers are present at each vertebral level to continue development of the body and posterior structures (Fig. 11-7). Fusion of the neural arches to the spinous processes occurs by age 2 or 3, and these posterior elements fuse to the vertebral body from ages 3 to 6. At puberty, secondary centers of ossification appear at the vertebral endplates and the spinous, transverse, and articular processes. These structures complete ossification by age 25.

Radiographic Appearance of the Neonatal Spine

At birth the shape of the thoracic and lumbar bodies is rounded. Radiographically the superior and inferior aspects of the vertebral bodies show dense calcification, appearing as clearly defined white margins with relatively darker, more radiolucent bodies. Occasionally the opposite will be seen, and the centrum of the bodies will appear densely calcified, causing a "bone within bone" radiographic image. The middle anterior aspects of the vertebral bodies will also show indentations, which are grooves for vertebral veins. Single or double grooves may also be seen on the posterior aspects of the vertebral bodies, and these may persist into adulthood.

Ossification of the Sacrum

The sacrum of the newborn is not fused; the individual sacral bodies, separated by intervertebral disk spaces, are evident on the lateral radiograph. Ossification centers are present for each sacral vertebral body, neural arch, and transverse process. The transverse (costal) processes fuse to the neural arches by age 5. The arches fuse to the body 2 or 3 years later. The arches unite posteriorly between ages 7 and 10. The secondary centers of ossification that join the wings of the sacrum on either side do not appear until 15 to 18 years of age; they fuse in the early twenties. Before their appearance, the sacroiliac joints look wider than one would expect. This appearance is normal.

The dorsal convexity of the sacrum is a primary spinal curvature that is present in utero and at birth (see Fig. 7-13). The secondary spinal curve of *lumbar lordosis* begins development with the onset of active prone extension, standing, and ambulatory skills. The development of the lumbar lordosis over the base of the sacrum also develops the lumbosacral angle. The inclination of this angle affects the amount of shear force the lumbosacral joint sustains during erect postures.

Ossification of the Coccyx

At birth the coccyx usually exhibits ossification of the first segment, and the remaining cartilaginous segments ossify from the top down, at varying points in time between birth and puberty. The segments generally fuse from the bottom up, and this time frame is highly variable. These variations make the interpretation of coccygeal abnormalities difficult. The coccyx is more freely movable in girls and women and is less likely to be fused to the sacrum. The first segment often fails to fuse to the second segment.

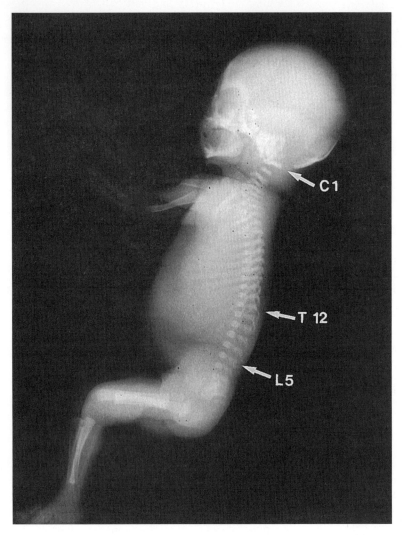

Figure 11-7 Normal radiographic appearance of a healthy 6-month-old infant. On this lateral view, the oval-shaped vertebral bodies and the individual sacral bodies are demonstrated.

Routine Radiologic Evaluation[10–19]

Practice Guidelines for Lumbar Spine Radiography in Children and Adults

The American College of Radiology (ACR), the principal professional organization of radiologists in the United States, defines the following practice guidelines as an educational tool to help practitioners provide appropriate radiological care for their patients.

Goals

The goal of radiographic examination of the lumbar spine is to identify or exclude anatomic abnormalities or disease processes.

Indications

The indications for radiologic examination include but are not limited to pain radiating into the legs; evaluation of scoliosis and kyphosis; osteoporosis and compression fractures; in children, hip pain, limping, or refusal to bear weight; trauma involving the spine; limitation in motion; planned or prior surgery; evaluation of primary and secondary malignancies; arthritis; suspected congenital anomalies and syndromes associated with spinal abnormality; evaluation of spinal abnormality seen on other imaging studies; follow-up of known abnormality; and suspected spinal instability.

Recommended Projections

The routine radiologic examination includes anteroposterior and lateral views. Additional views may be needed in some clinical circumstances and include right and left oblique views and a coned lateral view of the lumbosacral articulation, L5–S1.

Basic Projections and Radiologic Observations

The routine evaluation of the lumbar spine is similar to that of the cervical spine in that right and left oblique views are usually obtained. However, whereas the oblique views of the cervical spine visualize the *intervertebral foramina*, oblique views in the lumbar spine visualize the *facet joints*. Refer to Table 1-6 for a summary of radiographic views visualizing intervertebral foramina versus those of the facet joints in the various spinal regions.

Radiographic evaluation of the sacroiliac joint is separate from that of the lumbar spine. The orientation of the joint planes necessitates a separate examination, consisting of an anteroposterior (AP) axial view and right and left oblique views. Both sacroiliac joints are viewed simultaneously on the axial AP projection and each joint is viewed individually on the oblique projections.

The sacrum is visualized on a basic lumbar spine series but can also be radiographed as a separate examination if it is the area of interest. Specific radiographic evaluation of the sacrum includes an AP and a lateral view, extending from L5 to the coccyx. Similarly, if the coccyx is the area of interest, a basic radiographic evaluation includes an angled AP, to avoid superimposition of the symphysis pubis, and a lateral view, demonstrating the normal anterior curvature of the coccyx.

The usual examination procedure is to image the lumbosacral region with the patient in recumbent positions. Some clinical entities are better served by radiographic examination in erect, weight-bearing positions. To obtain the positioning desired, "non–weight-bearing" or "weight-bearing" must be specified in the radiologic requisition. Radiographs made in weight-bearing positions will be labeled as such. If no labels exist, it can be assumed that the radiographs were made without weight-bearing.

(Continued on page 310)

Routine Radiologic Evaluation of the Lumbar Spine

Anteroposterior

This view demonstrates the lumbar vertebral bodies, pedicles, spinous and transverse processes, and intervertebral disk spaces. A variation in the scope of the AP view depends on the size of the image receptor used. If a smaller image receptor is used, the five lumbar vertebrae are primarily visualized (lumbar spine view). If a larger image receptor is used, the five lumbar vertebrae, sacrum, and possibly coccyx are visible (lumbosacral view).

Radiologic Observations

The important observations are:

1. The patient may be positioned supine with the knees *straight*, preserving a lumbar lordosis, or with the knees *flexed*, eliminating the lordosis. The different positions produce slightly different images. In the former, the joint spaces undergo some distortion owing to the lordosis. In the latter, the joint spaces are in neutral. The choice between positions depends on a facility's or radiologist's preference.
2. The alignment of the vertebral bodies forms a vertical column with well-preserved intervertebral joint spaces.
3. The pedicles are oval densities on either side of teardrop–shaped spinous processes. The pedicles are spaced equidistantly from midline spinous processes. Interpedicular distance (*a* in Fig. 11-8) is normally 25 mm in L1–L3 and 30 mm in L4–L5. Misalignment in the relationship of these structures may indicate a fracture–dislocation. Remember that the distance between a pair of pedicles represents the transverse diameter of the spinal canal. A decrease in this space may compromise the spinal cord.
4. Intervals between consecutive spinous processes (*b* in Fig. 11-8) are relatively equal in the upper lumbar segments. An increased interval at one level may indicate a torn posterior ligament complex. The lower lumbar segments may exhibit decreased intervals as a result of positioning. If the patient's knees are flexed, the lordosis is flattened, so the interspinous intervals appear equal in the lower lumbar segments. If the patient's legs are straight, the lumbar lordosis is present, so the interspinous intervals appear decreased secondary to distortion.

Basic Projections

- **AP**
- Lateral
- Right and left obliques
- Lateral L5–S1

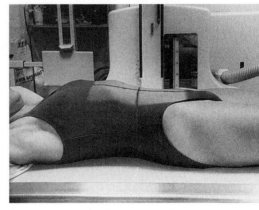

Setting up the Radiograph

Figure 11-9 Patient position for AP projection of the lumbar spine.

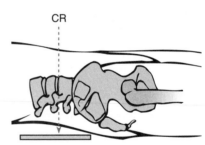

Figure 11-10 The central ray is perpendicular to the image receptor and passes through L3–L4.

5. The spinous processes are normally in the midline, at equal distances from the vertebral borders (*c* in Fig. 11-8).
6. The articular processes cast a butterfly-shaped shadow over the vertebral body (*d* in Fig. 11-8). Although the facet joints themselves are not visible, the alignment of the articular processes is. Misalignment is an indication of fracture–dislocation.
7. The upper margins of the proximal sacral foramina are identified as paired sharp arcuate lines in the paramedian area of the sacrum. Interruption of the smooth contour of these images could represent fracture. Absence of these images could indicate bone destruction.
8. The sacroiliac joints lie in an oblique plane, so this AP view does not reveal the true joint space. However, some general limited information on joint margin appearance and joint space thickness can be compared bilaterally.
9. The shadow of the psoas muscle can be visualized extending from the transverse processes and anterolateral vertebral bodies diagonally.

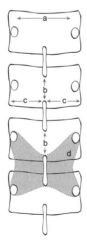

Figure 11-8 Radiographic spatial relationships on the AP view of the lumbar spine.

What Can You See?

Look at the radiograph (Fig. 11-11) and try to identify the radiographic anatomy. Trace the outlines of structures using a marker and transparency sheet. Compare results with the book tracing (Fig. 11-12). Can you identify the following:

- Lumbar vertebral bodies
- Spinous processes
- Pedicles
- Transverse processes
- Superior and inferior articular processes
- Sacrum
- Psoas shadow

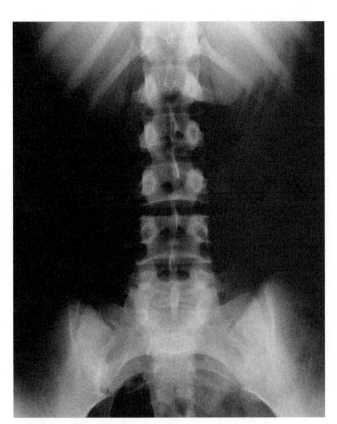

Figure 11-11 Anteroposterior radiograph of the lumbar spine.

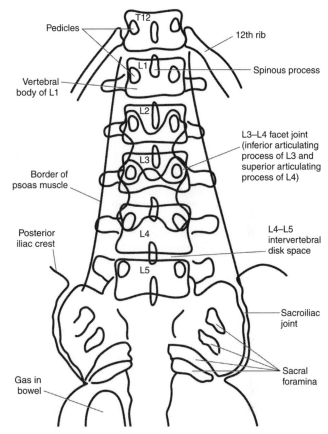

Figure 11-12 Tracing of AP radiograph of the lumbar spine.

Routine Radiologic Evaluation of the Lumbar Spine

Lateral

This view demonstrates the lumbar vertebral bodies, intervertebral disk spaces, pedicles, spinous processes, intervertebral foramina, and lumbosacral articulation.

Radiologic Observations

The important observations on the lateral view are:

1. As observed in the cervical and thoracic spines, normal alignment of the vertebrae is verified by identifying three roughly parallel lines (Fig. 11-13A):

   - *Line 1:* The anterior vertebral body line, representing the connected anterior borders of the vertebral bodies, forms a continuous lordotic curve.
   - *Line 2:* The posterior vertebral body line, representing the connected posterior borders of the vertebral bodies, forms a continuous curve parallel to line 1.
   - *Line 3:* The spinolaminar line, representing the junctions of the laminae at the spinous processes, forms a continuous curve parallel to lines 1 and 2.

   The spatial relationship of these three lines will remain constant during any amount of lumbar flexion or extension. Disruptions in these parallel lines may indicate fracture, dislocation, or spondylolisthesis. Remember that the spinal canal lies between lines 2 and 3; compromise of this space seriously threatens the integrity of the neurovascular structures.

2. The vertebral bodies are box-like, with distinct, smoothly curved osseous margins. Note any osteophyte formation at the joint margins, indicating degenerative changes.

3. The intervertebral disk space height is largest in the lumbar spine because of the thickness of the lumbar disks. Note the normal wedge shape of the disk spaces in the lowest lumbar segments and especially in L5–S1.

4. The pedicles are superimposed as a pair at each level.

5. A gravity line can be drawn through the center of the body of L3 and extended inferiorly, as shown in Figure 10-13B. Normally the vertical line will pass through the anterior third of the sacrum. If the line falls more

Basic Projections

- AP
- **Lateral**
- Right and left obliques
- Lateral L5–S1

Setting up the Radiograph

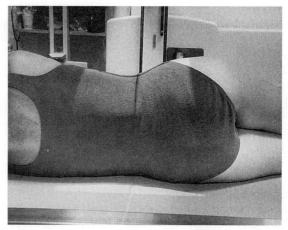

Figure 11-14 Patient position for lateral projection of the lumbar spine.

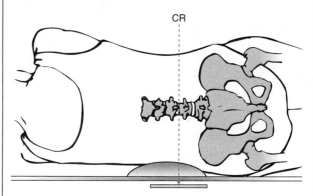

Figure 11-15 The central ray is perpendicular to the image receptor and passes through L3–L4.

than 1 to 2 cm anterior to the sacrum, this observation suggests anterior weight-bearing, with increased shear stress on the lower lumbar disks and facet joints. The value of this observation is more meaningful in erect, standing films; the side-lying position has the potential to alter the lordosis.

6. The intervertebral foramina image as radiolucent ovals. The foramina of L1–L2 through L4–L5 are best seen. The foramina of L5–S1 are less easily visualized because of the transitional anatomy at this level. Additionally, the L5–S1 foramina are typically smaller than those at the other lumbar levels; this feature is important to recognize in order to prevent or avoid a misleading interpretation of foraminal stenosis.

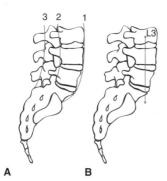

Figure 11-13 (A) Normal vertebral alignment is evidenced by the spatial relationships of three lines. **(B)** A gravity line extends from the body of L3 inferiorly and normally intersects the anterior third of the sacral base.

What Can You See?

Look at the radiograph (Fig. 11-16) and try to identify the radiographic anatomy. Trace the outlines of structures using a marker and transparency sheet. Compare results with the book tracing (Fig. 11-17). Can you identify the following:

- Three lines that reference vertebral alignment
- Vertebral bodies

- Intervertebral foramina
- Pedicles, laminae, and spinous processes

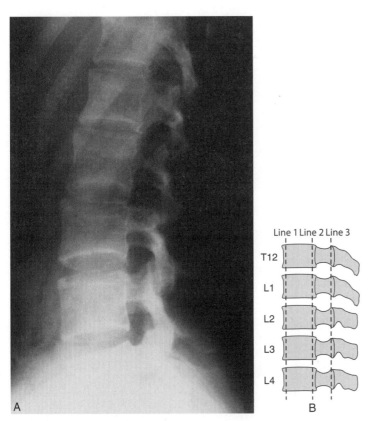

Figure 11-16 (A) Lateral radiograph of the lumbar spine. **(B)** Three parallel curves showing spinal alignment in thoracolumbar region.

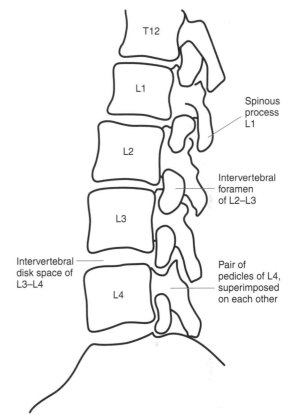

Figure 11-17 Tracing of lateral radiograph of the lumbar spine.

Routine Radiologic Evaluation of the Lumbar Spine

Right and Left Posterior Oblique

These views demonstrate the facet joints, the superior and inferior articular processes, the pars interarticularis (the small expanse of bone located between the superior and inferior articular facets), and the pedicles. Both right and left oblique projections are included in a lumbar spine study. The right posterior oblique (RPO) demonstrates right-side structures, and the left posterior oblique (LPO) demonstrates left-side structures. The posterior oblique views image the "downside" facet joints, closest to the image receptor. Alternatively, the anterior oblique positions may be used. Anterior obliques image the "upside" facet joints, farther from the image receptor. The results of the images are similar and cannot be readily distinguished on the radiograph. The radiograph is marked "right" or "left" in reference to what *structures* are being demonstrated.

Radiologic Observations

1. The articulation of two adjacent vertebrae produces a radiographic pattern that looks somewhat like a Scottie dog. The significance of clearly realizing this image is that the viewer is assured that the articulating processes and facet joints, as well as the pars interarticularis, are well demonstrated.

2. The configuration of the "Scottie dog" body parts represents these anatomic landmarks (Fig. 11-18): nose = transverse process; eye = pedicle; ear = superior articular process; neck = pars interarticularis; foreleg = inferior articular process; body = lamina and spinous process; tail = superior articular process of opposite side; hind leg = inferior articular process of opposite side.[17]

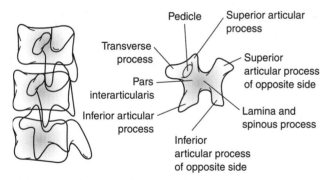

Figure 11-18 The image of a "Scottie dog" as seen on an oblique radiograph of the lumbar spine.

Basic Projections

- AP
- Lateral
- **Right and left obliques**
- Lateral L5–S1

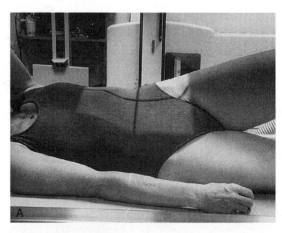

Setting up the Radiograph

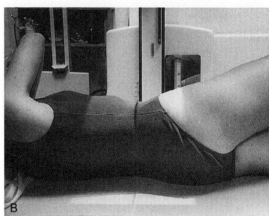

Figure 11-19 Patient position for **(A)** RPO and **(B)** LPO projection of the lumbar spine.

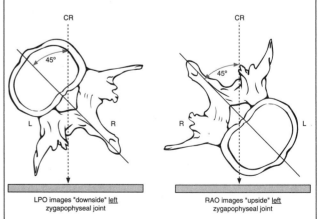

LPO images "downside" <u>left</u> zygapophyseal joint

RAO images "upside" <u>left</u> zygapophyseal joint

Figure 11-20 Examination of the facet joints may be obtained by using either anterior obliques (LAO and RAO) or posterior obliques (LPO and RPO).

What Can You See?

Look at the radiographs (Fig. 11-21) and try to identify the radiographic anatomy. Trace the outlines of structures using a marker and transparency sheet. Compare results with the book tracings (Fig. 11-22). Can you identify the following:

- Image of the "Scottie dog" at one level
- Pedicles
- Superior and inferior processes
- Facet joints

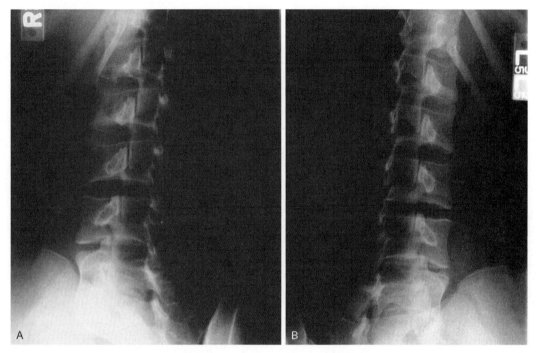

Figure 11-21 Radiographs of **(A)** right posterior oblique projection of lumbar spine, **(B)** left posterior oblique projection of lumbar spine.

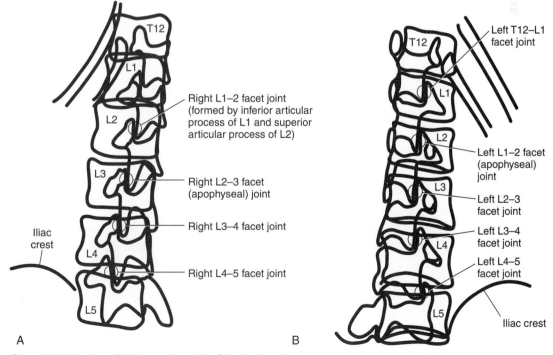

Figure 11-22 Tracings of oblique radiographs of the lumbar spine.

Routine Radiologic Evaluation of the Lumbar Spine

Lateral L5–S1

This view is a closeup, or *coned,* view of the lumbosacral junction. The term *coned* refers to the cone-shaped aperture that limits the x-ray field. The radiographic exposure is adjusted to visualize L5–S1 optimally through the superimposed density of the ilia.

Radiologic Observations

The important observations are:

1. The three parallel lines of vertebral body alignment, as described for the lateral lumbar spine view, continue to hold true in this spot film of the lumbosacral junction. Extensions of the lines now include the sacral body:

   - The anterior vertebral body line, extending from L4 to the anterior body of the sacrum, is normally smooth and continuous, including the area of transition at the lumbosacral junction. Step-offs in this line may be an indication of fracture, subluxation, dislocation, or retro- or anterolisthesis.
   - The posterior vertebral body line, extending from L4 to the posterior body of the sacrum, is likewise evaluated for abnormal step-offs.
   - The spinolaminar line, extending from L4 to the crest of the sacrum, is likewise evaluated for step-offs.

2. The L4–L5 and L5–S1 intervertebral disk spaces are observed for well-preserved potential spaces. Narrowing of the joint spaces, sclerotic joint margins, osteophyte formation, or lucency indicating a vacuum phenomenon are all indicators of degenerative disks.

3. Different methods exist to define the characteristics of the lumbosacral angle. Two of these are shown in Figure 11-23:

   (a) *Barge's angle:* On a weight-bearing lateral view, a line is drawn along the sacral base. A second line is drawn

Basic Projections

- AP
- Lateral
- Right and left obliques
- **Lateral L5–S1**

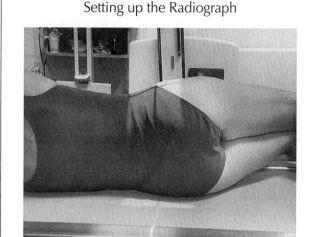

Figure 11-24 Patient position for a lateral L5–S1 spot film projection.

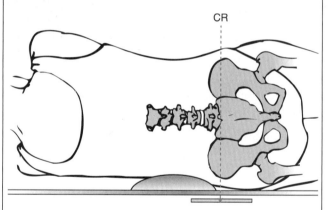

Figure 11-25 The central ray is perpendicular to the image receptor, passing through L5–S1.

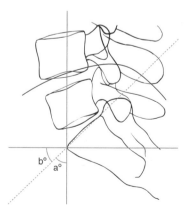

Figure 11-23 Barge's angle *(a)* and Ferguson's angle *(b)* quantify characteristics of the lumbosacral angle.

parallel to the vertical edge of the image. The inferior angle of intersection averages 53 degrees, with a standard deviation of 4 degrees.

   (b) *Ferguson's angle:* On a weight-bearing lateral view, a line is drawn along the sacral base. A second line is drawn horizontal to the edge of the image. The inferior intersecting angle averages 41 degrees, with a standard deviation of 2 degrees.

Smaller Barge's angles and larger Ferguson's angles are associated with increased compressive forces at the facet joints or transverse shearing forces at the disk. Larger Barge's angles and smaller Ferguson's angles are associated with increased axial loading of the disk and facet joints.

What Can You See?

Look at the radiograph (Fig. 11-26) and try to identify the radiographic anatomy. Trace the outlines of structures using a marker and transparency sheet. Compare results with the book tracing (Fig. 11-27). Can you identify the following:

- Lumbar vertebral bodies
- Pedicles, laminae, and spinous processes
- Intervertebral disks at L4–L5 and L5–S1
- Sacrum

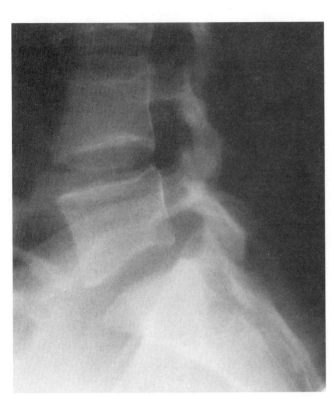

Figure 11-26 Coned lateral radiograph of L5–S1.

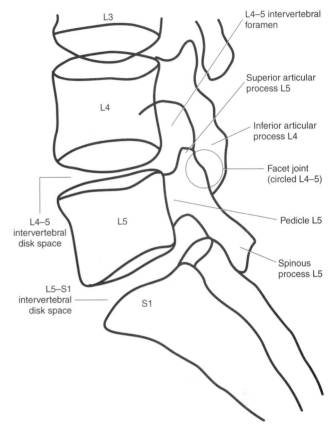

Figure 11-27 Tracing of lateral radiograph of L5–S1.

Routine Radiologic Evaluation of the Sacroiliac Joint

AP Axial

This view demonstrates the bilateral sacroiliac joints (SIJ). It is projected anteroposteriorly and angled in an inferior-to-superior direction, so that the greatest surface area of the joints is exposed. Because of the irregular topography and multiple planes of the joint surfaces, the entire SIJ cannot be visualized on a single view.

Radiologic Observations

The important observations (Fig. 11-28) are:

1. The articular surfaces are superimposed on each other, so each sacroiliac joint images as two radiolucent joint lines.
2. The articular surfaces are evaluated for smooth osseous margins.
3. The bilateral sacroiliac joints are evaluated for symmetry.
4. The L5–S1 articulation also lies in the plane of the central ray and can be evaluated on this view.
5. The coccyx may be visible.

Basic Projections

- AP axial
- **Right and left obliques**

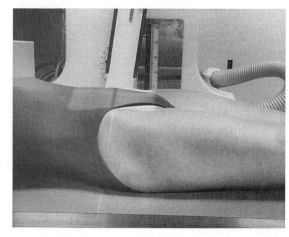

Setting up the Radiograph

Figure 11-29 Patient position for an AP axial projection of the bilateral sacroiliac joints.

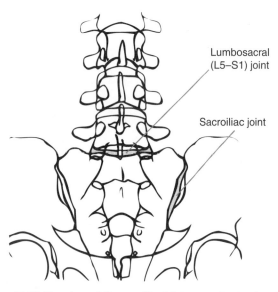

Figure 11-28 The plane of the sacroiliac joints approximates the plane of the lumbosacral joint in an AP axial view.

Lumbosacral (L5–S1) joint

Sacroiliac joint

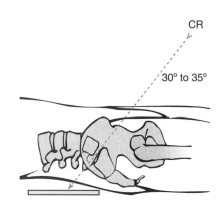

CR

30° to 35°

Figure 11-30 The central ray is angled 30 to 35 degrees, passing through the plane of the lumbosacral and sacroiliac joint articulations.

What Can You See?

Look at the radiograph (Fig. 11-31) and try to identify the radiographic anatomy. Trace the outlines of structures using a marker and transparency sheet. Compare results with the book tracing (Fig. 11-32). Can you identify the following:

● Body of L5
● Body of the sacrum, including the sacral spinous tubercles and foramina
● Sacroiliac joints
● Coccyx

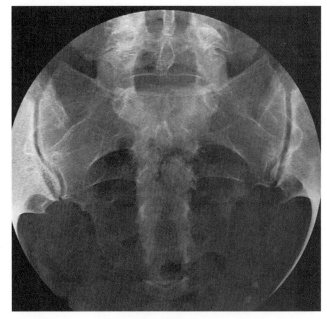

Figure 11-31 AP axial radiograph of the sacroiliac joints.

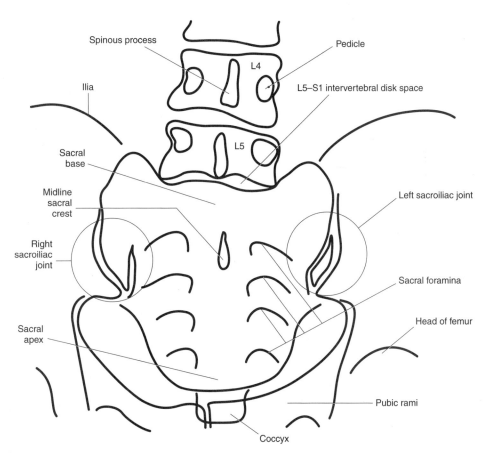

Figure 11-32 Tracing of AP axial radiograph of the sacroiliac joints.

Routine Radiologic Evaluation of the Sacroiliac Joint

Right and Left Obliques

Each oblique demonstrates an individual sacroiliac joint. These views are projected anteroposteriorly, with the pelvis rotated 30 degrees to prevent superimposition of the ilia over the sacroiliac joint. Both right and left posterior obliques are done for comparison purposes. (Anterior obliques are alternative positions.)

Radiologic Observations

The important observations are:

1. The obliquity of the projection permits visualization of the margins of the joint space along its entirety (Fig. 11-33).
2. The joint spaces are evaluated for preserved joint space.
3. The joint spaces are evaluated for degenerative changes, normally evident beginning in late middle age. Degenerative changes prominent in men include fibrosis and bony ankylosis across the joint space.

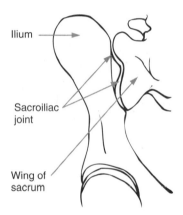

Figure 11-33 The obliquity of the projection permits visualization of the margins of the SIJ.

Basic Projections

- AP axial
- **Right and left obliques**

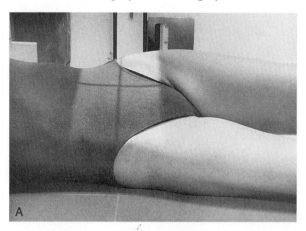

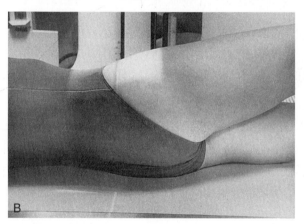

Figure 11-34 Patient position for **(A)** RPO projection of the right SIJ and **(B)** LPO projection of the left SIJ.

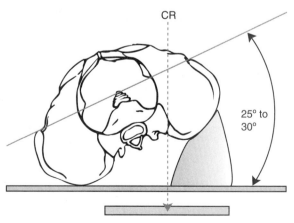

Figure 11-35 The patient is rotated 25 to 30 degrees so that the central ray passes through the SIJ and strikes the image receptor perpendicularly.

What Can You See?

Look at the radiographs (Figs. 11-36) and try to identify the radiographic anatomy. Trace the outlines of structures using a marker and transparency sheet. Compare results with the book tracings (Figs. 11-37). Can you identify on each oblique view the following:

- Ilium
- Wing of the sacrum
- Sacroiliac joint

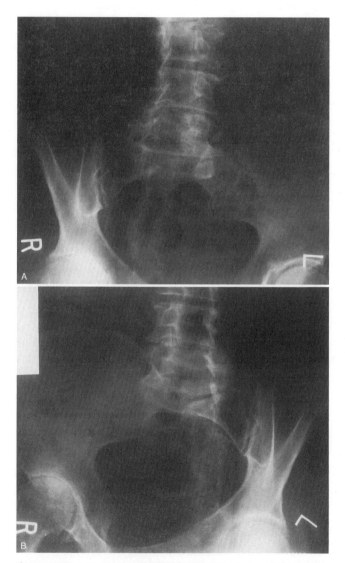

Figure 11-36 Radiographs of **(A)** oblique view of the right sacroiliac joint; **(B)** oblique view of the left sacroiliac joint.

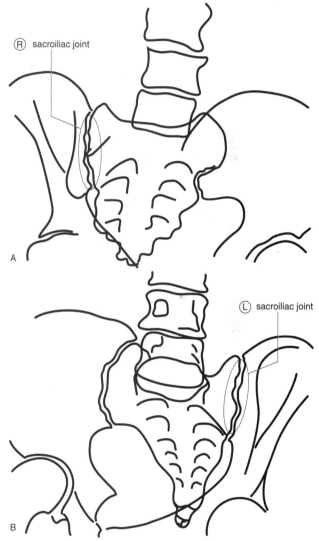

Figure 11-37 Tracings of radiographs of an oblique view of the **(A)** right sacroiliac joint and **(B)** left sacroiliac joint.

Trauma at the Lumbar Spine[18,20–42]

Diagnostic Imaging for Trauma of the Lumbar Spine

Computed tomography (CT) is now the imaging procedure of choice for evaluating trauma patients. The literature discusses the value of assessing the spine for fractures by using reformatted images from the thorax–abdomen–pelvis (TAP) body scan. The literature has not addressed the value of reformatted images compared with axial images for detecting thoracolumbar fractures, although there is agreement that reformatted images should be performed, since this involves no additional cost or radiation exposure and may improve characterization of alignment. Radiographs (AP and lateral) may still be obtained to help localize injuries. Magnetic resonance imaging (MRI) is not indicated if the CT exam is normal because isolated ligamentous injuries are rare in the lumbar spine. If there is neural compromise, MRI is indicated to evaluate cord edema, cord contusion, epidural hematoma, ligamentous disruption, or nerve root involvement.

Fractures of the Lumbar Spine

Fractures and fracture–dislocation injuries in the lumbar spine share similar mechanisms of injury and similar radiographic appearances as the corresponding injuries in the lower thoracic spine. The thoracolumbar junction, T11–L2, is the predominant site of vertebral fractures because these vertebrae are the transitional region between the relatively fixed thoracic spine and the mobile lumbar spine and forces are often dissipated here. Figure 11-38 exemplifies this—the patient lands on his feet from a great height, fractures his hindfoot, and the force continues up the kinetic chain and dissipates as a fracture in the thoracolumbar vertebrae.

Refer to Chapter 9 for details on vertebral compression fractures and to Table 9-2 for the common thoracolumbar vertebral injury patterns.

Spondylolysis

Spondylolysis is a defect at the pars interarticularis (Figs. 11-39 and 11-40). The defect may be congenital (rare), traumatic, or, as is most common, due to a stress fracture caused by chronic strain. L4–L5 and L5–S1 are most often affected. Spondylolysis may occur bilaterally or unilaterally.

Mechanism of Injury

Traumatic or stress fractures of the pars interarticularis are highly associated with repetitive mechanical loading of the back, especially in trunk extension. Work that involves heavy, high lifting or overhead lifting is such an example. In athletics, three types of sports are associated with spondylolysis: weight-loading sports such as weight lifting; repetitive trunk rotation sports such as tennis, baseball, or golf; and sports that involve hyperextension of the back, such as seen in diving, gymnastics, swimming, football (especially for linemen), and volleyball. There is also evidence that individuals with more *frontally* oriented facet joints (as opposed to the usual sagittal orientation) or those with facet joint plane assymmetries (*facet tropism*) are at greater risk for developing spondylolysis.

Clinical Presentation

The patient typically presents with nonradiating, unilateral low back pain. Pain is exacerbated with loading at the site, as would occur with trunk extension and rotation, or with upright single-leg standing.

Radiologic Findings

The oblique view visualizes the pars interarticularis without superimposition. The classic radiologic finding is a radiolucent line across the pars (Fig. 11-41), referred to as a "collar on the Scottie dog." Radiographs may be negative, however, if the stress fracture site has not separated.

Advanced Imaging

The optimal advanced imaging modality to diagnose spondylolysis is controversial. Bone scans are sensitive but cannot offer detailed anatomy information. Axial CT scans have high sensitivity and anatomic detail, but the level must be known first, and getting images of the pars is technically challenging. Reformatted multiplanar CT images and three-dimensional reconstructions have increased the reliability and value of CT. MRI can detect early lesions by identifying edema, but the spectrum of findings has not yet been fully validated. Single photon emission computed tomography (SPECT) demonstrates excellent accuracy in defining spondylolysis but is expensive and not readily available in all areas.

Theoretically, a combination of conventional radiographs and bone scans can determine whether a fracture is new or old. Acute fractures would have both a positive radiograph and a positive bone scan, indicating active healing with a good prognosis for bony union. The combination of a positive radiograph and a negative bone scan indicates the absence of healing activity, as seen in an old fracture united with fibrous union.

Treatment

Healing of a spondylolysis requires several weeks to several months. Activities that load the spine must be curtailed until the patient is pain free, and then gradually resumed over a length of time. For most patients this takes 3 to 6 months.

Rehabilitation is important to correct poor posture, teach appropriate body mechanics for daily activities, strengthen and stretch imbalanced or weak musculature, and provide appropriate bracing if needed. Bracing is controversial but can be useful to teach reduction of excessive lordotic posture or protect the correct posture when activities that may aggravate the condition are being performed.

Complications

Nonunion is a common complication. The long-term prognosis is good even with continuation of sporting activities.

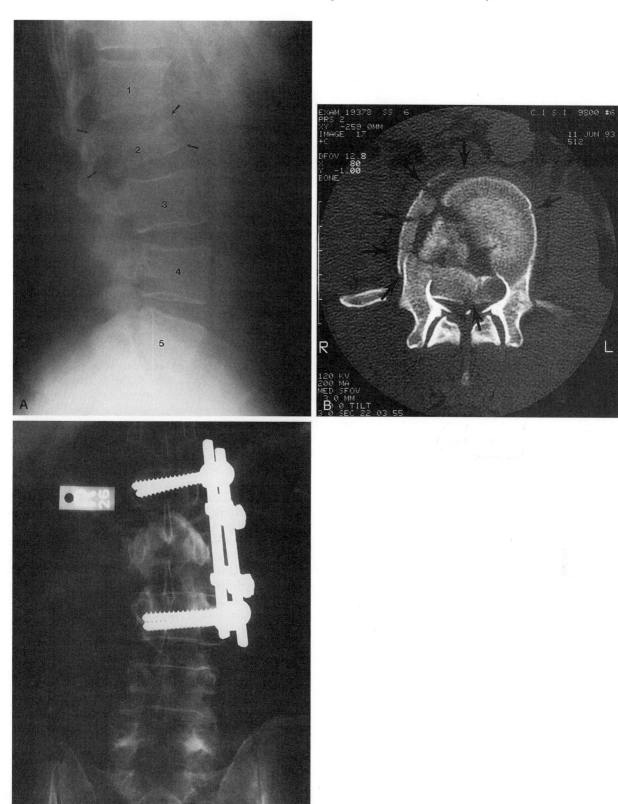

Figure 11-38 Burst fracture of L2. This 46-year-old man fractured his second lumbar vertebra when he fell 20 feet out of a tree as he was hanging Christmas lights (see Figs. 9-39 and 14-50 for additional rib and hindfoot fractures sustained from this fall). **(A)** Lateral plain film shows the compression deformity of the second lumbar vertebra (arrows). **(B)** Axial CT image of L2 demonstrates a comminuted burst fracture of the body (arrows indicate multiple fracture sites). **(C)** Anteroposterior plain film made postoperatively demonstrates internal fixation.

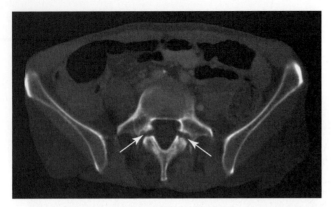

Figure 11-39 Bilateral spondylolysis of L5. This axial CT image demonstrates the defects of the pars interarticularis in both the right and left sides, interrupting what is normally a complete ring between the anterior and posterior elements of the vertebra. *(Image courtesy of Laughlin Dawes, MD.)*

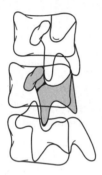

Figure 11-40 The radiologic sign of spondylolysis is an image of a "collar on the Scottie dog" as seen on the oblique view. The "collar" is the radiolucent cleft that results from separation of bone at the fracture site.

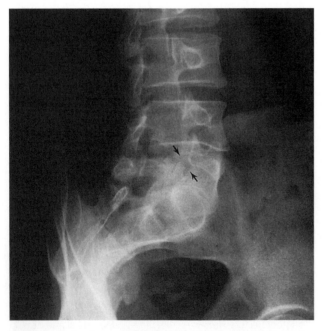

Figure 11-41 Lumbar spondylolysis. This oblique view of the lumbar spine demonstrates spondylolysis, a defect in the pars interarticularis. The arrows bracket the extent of the defect. The radiolucent line image caused by the defect has been referred to as "a collar on the Scottie dog." No associated spondylolisthesis is apparent on this view.

Spondylolisthesis is a consequence of nonunion of spondylolysis. Bilateral spondylolysis is more commonly associated with spondylolisthesis, but a unilateral spondylolysis can also cause the vertebrae to slip forward asymmetrically. In that case the spinous process will rotate to the side of the slip. The rotation of the spinous process can be palpated or be demonstrated on the AP view of the lumbar spine.

Spondylolisthesis

Spondylolisthesis is the forward displacement of one vertebra upon the stationary vertebra beneath it. The term is derived from the Greek *spondylo* (vertebra) and *listhesis* (slide on an incline). Although spondylolisthesis is synonymous with *forward displacement*, an alternative term for that is *anterolisthesis*. Additionally, the term *retrolisthesis* defines the posterior displacement of a vertebra.

Incidence

Approximately 5% to 10% of people have a spondylolisthesis. Children and adolescents are typically affected by spondylolisthesis; it is more apparent in those involved in athletic activities. The increased athletic activities in adolescence or physical labor in adulthood are often the instigating factors that cause low back pain. The lower lumbar levels, L4–L5 and L5–S1, are most often involved.

Etiology

Spondylolisthesis can be a consequence of spondylolysis (Fig. 11-42). However, spondylolisthesis is not only associated with defects of the pars interarticularis. Spondylolisthesis can also result from congenital or developmental aberrations, pathological processes, or degenerative changes.

Congenital or developmental aberrations include elongation of the pedicles and a defective, dissolved, or stretched pars interarticularis. These conditions may favor the development of multiple fatigue or stress fractures of the pars interarticularis.

Degenerative spondylolisthesis is due to degenerative changes in the intervertebral disk and facet joints. Loss of optimal articulation results from decreased disk height and laxity of joint ligaments and joint capsules. Not associated with fractures or osseous defects of any kind, degenerative spondylolisthesis is sometimes referred to as *pseudospondylolisthesis* (Fig. 11-43).

Clinical Presentation

The patient complains of pain after athletic activities or physical labor. Lumbar flexion, which reduces the displacement, usually reduces or abates the pain.

Palpation of the spinous processes can reveal either a rotation or a deep depression. Rotation of the spinous process is correlated with an asymmetrical slip as would result from a unilateral spondylolysis. A palpable depression over the spinous process, or step-off, in palpation is the classic clinical sign of spondylolisthesis. This *spinous process sign* is correlated with radiologic findings to determine the type of spondylolisthesis present.

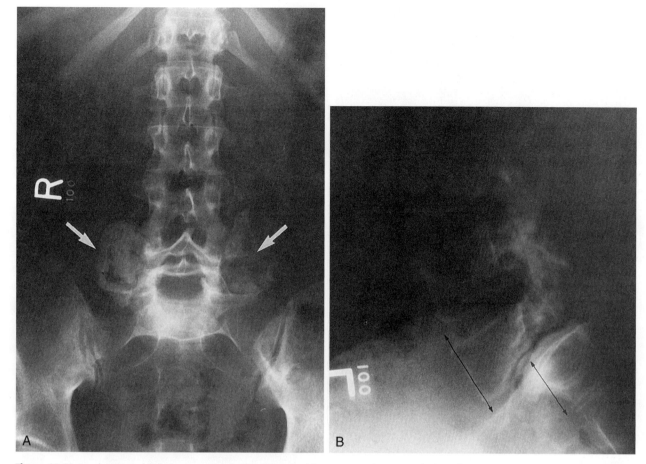

Figure 11-42 Lumbar spondylolisthesis, grade 3. This 32-year-old woman underwent a fusion of L4 to L5 in order to correct a severe anterolisthesis. The procedure failed over time. **(A)** Bone grafts are noted on the anteroposterior film (white arrows). **(B)** Lateral spot film of the lumbosacral junction shows a grade 3 spondylolisthesis of L5–S1 (line arrows).

Radiologic Findings

Spinous Process Sign

The radiologic presentation of the spinous process sign distinguishes between degenerative spondylolisthesis and fracture spondylolisthesis (Fig. 11-44).

In degenerative spondylolisthesis, the entire vertebra slips forward as a unit. The step-off of the spinous process is *below the level of the slip*. For example, if L4 slips forward as a unit, the spinous process slips forward with it; thus the step-off is at L4–L5.

In fracture spondylolisthesis, bilateral spondylolysis results in the forward slip of the vertebral body, pedicles, and superior articular processes while the inferior articular processes, laminae, and spinal process remain in normal position. The step-off is *above the level of the slip*. For example, if L4 is fractured, the vertebral body slips forward while the spinous process remains in normal position; thus the step-off is at L3–L4.

Grading Spondylolisthesis

Spondylolisthesis is evaluated on the lateral view. The amount of forward slippage is graded in quarters, in reference to the extent the vertebral body surpasses the normal anterior vertebral body line (Fig. 11-45):

- Grade 1: 25% of the involved vertebral body overhangs the subjacent vertebra.
- Grade 2: 50%
- Grade 3: 75%
- Grade 4: 100%
- Grade 5 (spondyloptosis): The vertebral body has completely fallen off.

In degenerative spondylolisthesis, the amount of displacement may not be obvious on routine films.

Stress radiographs may reveal the actual stability or instability of the involved segment. Stress radiographs in the lumbar spine are similar to those made in the cervical spine. Lateral flexion and extension radiographs are taken at the end ranges of each of these movements to stress the supporting ligaments and evaluate their ability to check excessive joint motion.

Treatment

Conservative measures include physical therapy and restriction of activites that load the spine in extension. Stretching

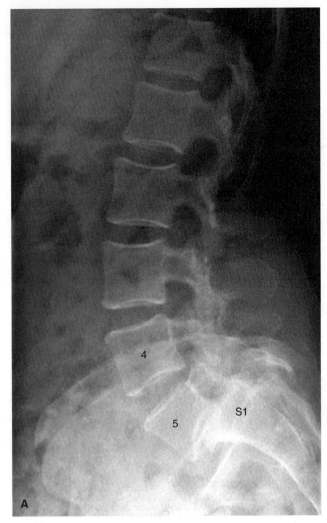

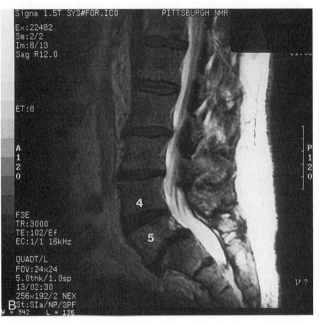

Figure 11-43 Degenerative spondylolisthesis of L5 on S1, grade 2, in a 60-year-old man. **(A)** Lateral plain film of the lumbosacral junction. **(B)** Sagittal T1-weighted MRI of the lumbosacral spine. In contrast to the lateral radiograph made with the patient standing, there is minimal compromise of the spinal canal. Advanced imaging is made with the patient *non–weight-bearing*. So remember that a functional problem, made worse with the patient upright, may not be fully appreciated with advanced imaging.

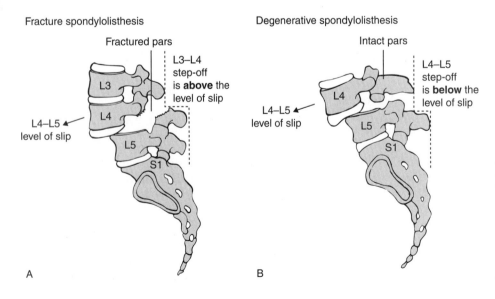

Figure 11-44 (A) Fracture spondylolisthesis can be differentiated from **(B)** degenerative spondylolisthesis by the "spinous process sign." In (A), the forward slippage of the anterior portion of the vertebra creates a palpable step-off of the spinous processes at the interspace *above* the level of the slip. In (B), the intact vertebra slips forward as a unit, creating a step-off at the interspace *below* the level of the slip. (*Adapted from Greenspan,*[17] *pp. 10–42.*)

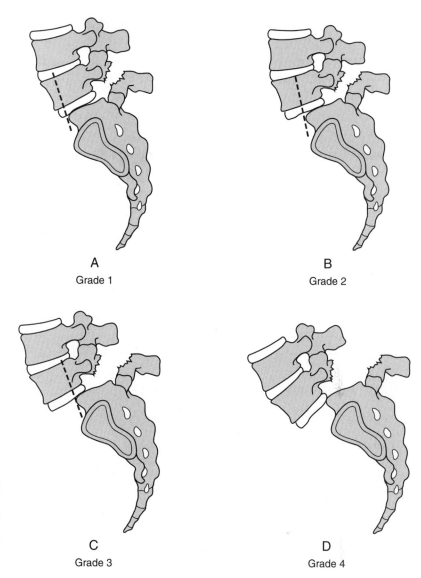

A
Grade 1

B
Grade 2

C
Grade 3

D
Grade 4

Figure 11-45 Grades of spondylolisthesis, based on the amount of vertebral body surpassing the normal anterior vertebral border line. **(A)** In grade 1, 25% of the vertebral body has subluxed forward; **(B)** grade 2, 50%; **(C)** grade 3, 75%; **(D)** grade 4, 100% of the vertebral body has surpassed the normal anterior vertebral body line. *(Adapted from Greenspan,*[17] *pp. 10–45.)*

the lumbar joints into flexion can be a self-reduction maneuver and give considerable pain relief. Analgesics and bracing that reduces loads to the lumbar spine can be helpful during acute phases.

Surgical fusion with instrumentation such as screws or cages is indicated in cases of neurological compromise or persistent pain that does not respond to conservative measures.

Degenerative Conditions at the Lumbar Spine[18,43–66]

Degenerative conditions in the lumbar spine have similar radiographic characteristics as those same conditions seen in the cervical spine. Degenerative joint disease (DJD), degenerative disk disease (DDD), spondylosis deformans, and diffuse idiopathic skeletal hyperostosis (DISH) present the same radiologic findings in the lumbar spine as discussed earlier in Chapter 7 for the cervical spine. Table 11-1 presents an overview of the radiologic characteristics of these degenerative conditions.

Some characteristics of degeneration are more often associated with the lumbar spine region than with other regions of the spine. *Spinal stenosis* and *intervertebral disk herniations* are degenerative pathological conditions typically associated with the lumbar spine.

Clinical Considerations of the Degenerative Spine

Degenerative processes are slow to form, and the body generally has time to adapt. Eventually, however, the body may reach limits in its ability to adapt. The spine may become symptomatic to even minor trauma. The normal, nondegenerative spine has a margin of safety in its elastic capsules, resilient and flexible ligaments, hydrated and cushioning disks and cartilage, and wide-open foramina. The degenerative spine, in contrast, has lost its margin of safety and, in trauma, suffers greater dysfunction and requires longer time to heal. A review of the acute patient's radiographs, with special observation of the underlying chronic degenerative changes, is important in

TABLE 11-1 ● *Degenerative Conditions at the Spine: Characteristics and Radiologic Findings*

	Characteristics	Radiologic Findings
Degenerative Disk Disease (DDD)	• Dehydration of the disk • Nuclear herniation • Annular protrusion • Fibrous replacement of annulus • Intravertebral herniation of nuclear material • Accumulation of nitrogen gas in fissures of disk	• Decreased disk space height • Osteophytes at vertebral endplates • Schmorl's nodes • Vacuum phenomenon
Degenerative Joint Disease (DJD)	• Affects zygapophyseal (facet) joints • Articular cartilage thinning • Subchondral bone sclerosis • Eburnation • Osteophytosis	• Decreased zygapophyseal joint space • Sclerosis • Osteophytosis at joint margins
Spondylosis	• Formation of osteophytes at the vertebral endplates in response to degenerative disk disease	• Osteophytes visible as radiodense irregularities at vertebral joint margins
Spondylosis Deformans	• Anterior or anterolateral disk herniation resulting in anterior or anterolateral vertebral endplate osteophytosis	• Claw-like spurs cupping toward intervertebral disk—present at more than one level, but distinguish from DISH
Diffuse Idiopathic Skeletal Hyperostosis (DISH)	• Rheumatological abnormality characterized by proliferation of bone at osseous sites of ligamentous and tendinous attachments, notably at the anterior longitudinal ligament of the spine	• Flowing ossification of at least four contiguous vertebrae • Preservation of disk height and absence of DDD findings • Absence of sacroiliitis or zygapophyseal joint DJD

appreciating the patient's pain pattern and assists in developing a comprehensive treatment plan.

Degenerative changes cannot be reversed. However, the surrounding environment of the joints can be optimized to modify pain and preserve functional range of motion. Rehabilitation can include (1) segmental mobilization techniques to restore joint mobility, (2) therapeutic exercise to balance muscle strength and flexibility to promote optimal posture, (3) patient education to teach occupational and leisure activity accommodations that decrease stressful postures or maladaptive behaviors, and (4) therapeutic modalities to provide pain relief.

Lumbar Stenosis

Spinal stenosis is defined as a narrowing or constriction of the spinal canal secondary to adjacent soft tissue or bony enlargement (Fig. 11-46). The essential structures in the spinal canal that can be compromised by spinal stenosis are the spinal cord, the thecal sac enclosing the cerebrospinal fluid, and the dural membranes that enclose the thecal sac.

Classification

Spinal stenosis is classified either by etiology or by the anatomic region involved. Etiologically, spinal stenosis is divided into congenital and acquired types (Table 11-2). Anatomically, spinal stenosis is divided into the following three regions:

1. Stenosis of the central spinal canal
2. Stenosis of the intervertebral foramen
3. Stenosis of the subarticular or lateral recesses (distance between the thecal sac and intervertebral foramen)

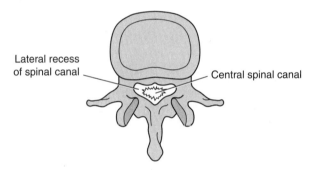

Figure 11-46 (A) Spinal stenosis is a constriction of the spinal canal. The location of lumbar stenosis is divided into three anatomic locations: (1) stenosis of the central spinal canal, (2) stenosis of the intervertebral foramina, and (3) stenosis of the lateral recesses.

More than one region may be involved at the same segment. The combination of intervertebral foramen and lateral recess stenosis is sometimes referred to as *peripheral stenosis*. All three regions in combination act to constrict the spinal canal concentrically.

Incidence

Valid data on incidence and prevalence are difficult to obtain because of the lack of specific diagnostic criteria for spinal stenosis. Additionally, most patients with mild spinal stenosis are asymptomatic; the absolute frequency can only be estimated. Some studies report CT and MRI evidence of spinal stenosis in up to one-fourth of the asymptomatic population under age 40. Other studies suggest that most patients older than age 60 manifest some degree of spinal stenosis.

In general, symptomatic spinal stenosis seems to affect more men than women, appearing at first in the 40- to 50-year-old age range and increasing with age. Spinal stenosis

TABLE 11-2 ● *Conditions Associated With Spinal Stenosis*

Congenital
- Achondroplasia (dwarfism)
- Morquio's syndrome (mucopolysaccharidosis)
- Down's syndrome
- Idiopathic stenosis (developmentally narrow canal dimension)

Acquired
- Prior surgery: laminectomy, fusion, chemonucleolysis
- Spondylolisthesis: spondylolitic or degenerative
- Infection: diskitis, vertebral osteomyelitis
- Tumor: metatstatic disease
- Spinal deformity secondary to trauma
- Bulging of annulus
- Herniation of intervertebral disk posterolaterally
- Posterior longitudinal ligament thickening
- Posterior longitudinal ligament ossification
- Hypertrophy of zygapophyseal joints
- DJD of zygapophyseal joints
- Hypertrophy of ligamentum flavum
- Epidural fat deposition
- Spondylosis of vertebral joint margins
- Uncovertebral joint hypertrophy (cervical spine)
- Metabolic/endocrine disorders: Paget's disease, acromegaly, calcium pyrophosphate dihydrate deposition disease (CPPD), which thickens spinal ligaments

associated with degenerative spondylolisthesis, however, is more common in women. Overall, spinal stenosis is most common in the cervical and lumbar spinal regions. Central canal narrowing is most prevalent at L4.

Etiology

Acquired spinal stenosis is often a complication or advanced stage of degenerative processes at the intervertebral segment. Numerous structures altered by degenerative changes may contribute to the constriction: osteophytes at joint margins, bony hypertrophy of the pedicles, laminae, and zygapophyseal joints, intervertebral disk bulging, or displacement of the entire vertebra itself in the case of degenerative spondylolisthesis or thickening of the ligamenta flava.

The severity of these degenerative processes, the possible combinations of degenerative processes, and how much constriction is symptomatic is highly variable among individuals.

Normally, the anteroposterior diameter of the spinal canal in normal adult men is as follows:

- Cervical spine C3–C5: 17 to 18 mm
- Cervical spine C5–C7: 12 to 14 mm
- Thoracic spine: 12 to 14 mm
- Lumbar spine: 15 to 27 mm

Cervical spine stenosis is associated with anteroposterior diameters of less than 10 mm. Thoracic spine stenosis is associated with anteroposterior diameters less than 10 to 13 mm. Lumbar spine stenosis is associated with anteroposterior diameters less than 10 to 12 mm.

Clinical Presentation

Severe cases of spinal stenosis can result in significant disability. In the cervical spine, the most serious complication of spinal stenosis is central cord syndrome. This incomplete cord lesion is associated with hyperextension injuries and results in a proportionately greater loss of motor function to the upper extremeties than the lower extremities, with variable sensory sparing. Cervical spine stenosis is also associated with long tract and radicular signs, headaches, pain, and radiating electric-like shock sensations elicited with cervical spine flexion. Concurrent cervical and lumbar spinal stenosis can present with gait disturbance, myelopathy, and radiculopathy, resembling multiple sclerosis, amyotrophic lateral sclerosis, or other motor neuron diseases.

In the lumbar spine, the most serious complication of spinal stenosis is the cauda equina syndrome. This cord lesion presents as loss of rectal tone, urinary retention, saddle anesthesia, and loss of bulbocavernosus reflex with sacral sparing. These conditions are surgical emergencies requiring decompression to prevent permanent loss of function.

Mild and moderate cases of spinal stenosis present with varying degrees of vascular and neurogenic compression symptoms. Lumbar spine stenosis presents with diffuse unilateral or bilateral low back and/or lower extremity pain, numbness, and weakness. Symptoms are often aggravated with standing and walking and relieved with sitting. Lumbar extension, in general, will narrow the canals and exacerbate the symptoms, while lumbar flexion opens the available space and provides some relief. Patients often report that they can shop for long periods of time without pain if they can lean their forearms on a shopping cart. This posture of trunk, hip, and knee flexion is known as the *simian stance*.

Neurogenic claudication is congestion of the blood vessels at a stenotic level. This congestion inhibits nerve conduction and results in poorly defined leg pain, numbness, and weakness. Neurogenic claudication is differentiated from vascular claudication by the aggravating factors. Neurogenic claudication is exacerbated by standing and spinal extension. Vascular claudication is exacerbated by exercise and is improved with standing.

Disk herniation can also be differentiated clinically by aggravating factors. Pain from disk herniation is aggravated by sitting, flexion, lifting, and Valsalva maneuvers and is often relieved with walking. Pain from spinal stenosis is not affected by any of those maneuvers and is aggravated with walking.

Radiologic Findings

Radiographically, stenosis is suggested by the location of severe degenerative changes at a spinal segment. However, because of gender, race, and age differences, radiographic measures of the spinal canal or intervertebral foramen lack specificity.

Conventional radiographs are significant for the exclusion or assessment of conditions often associated with spinal stenosis (see Table 11-2).

Advanced Imaging

CT scans are widely used for the evaluation of spinal stenosis, providing both axial and three-dimensional information regarding encroachment of the spinal canal (Fig. 11-47). Myelography will show the amount of actual constriction of the thecal sac (Fig. 11-48). MRI is valuable in the assessment of the thecal sac and contents. SPECT is valuable for discriminating stenosis from medical disease, infections, and tumors.

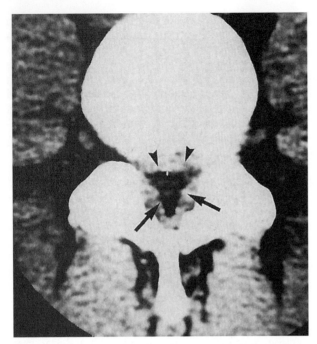

Figure 11-47 Transverse axial CT image of stenosis. The thickened ligamentum flavum (arrows) narrows the spinal canal significantly. There is also a posterior disk bulge (arrowheads). The dorsal sac is compromised by *stenosis* from both of these abnormalities. *(From Yochum and Rowe,[18] p. 308, with permission.)*

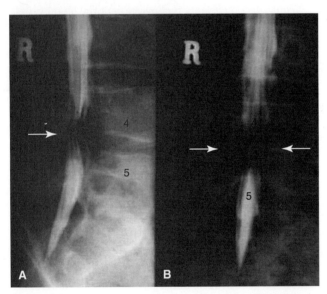

Figure 11-48 Lumbar spine myelogram, (A) lateral and (B) AP views. An almost complete constriction of the opacified thecal sac is noted at the L4–L5 stenotic interspace (arrows). *(Image courtesy of Nick Oldnal, http://www.xray2000.uk.co.l.)*

Treatment

Mild and moderate spinal stenosis is managed with analgesic medications, nonsteroidal anti-inflammatory drugs (NSAIDs), epidural steroid injections, and physical therapy for strengthening and flexibility exercises.

Surgical options for the treatment of severe spinal stenosis widen the spinal canal by removing, trimming, or realigning offending structures. Procedures include decompressive laminectomy, foraminectomy, facetectomy, diskectomy, and microendoscopic laminectomy; fusion is sometimes required to stabilize the segment. The quest for an artificial intervertebral disk replacement, as a motion-preserving answer to fusion techniques, began in the 1950s. Clinical application began in the 1980s in Europe. In the United States, a lumbar artifical disk was approved for use on one segment, either L4–L5 or L5–S1, in 2004. This technology, although in its infancy, represents a move toward more physiologically correct stabilization techniques in the field of spinal surgery. A benefit of preserving motion in any joint is the minimization of degenerative changes in adjacent joints (Fig. 11-49).

Intervertebral Disk Herniations

Intervertebral disk herniation is defined as an extension of the nucleus pulposus through the annulus fibrosis and beyond adjacent vertebral margins.

Incidence

Intervertebral disk herniations are among the most frequent pathologies affecting the diskovertebral junction. Intervertebral disk herniation is most common in the 25- to 45-year-old age group. Men are more frequently affected than women. There is a predominance of occurrence in individuals who smoke, are obese, or are exposed to vehicular vibration. Many risk factors have been suggested, but it is difficult to discriminate between factors that are causative and factors that exacerbate symptoms from an existing herniation.

Intervertebral disk herniations are most common at the lumbar spine. Ninety percent occur at L4–L5. A small percentage occurs at L3–L4; rarely are the L1 or L2 levels involved. Thoracic spine intervertebral disk herniations are rare; when they do occur, they are likely to be posterocentral and result in myelopathy rather than radiculopathy. Cervical spine intervertebral disk herniations occur with a 90% frequency at the C5–C6 level and result in radiculopathy. Myelopathy develops more often in the cervical spine than in the lumbar spine.

Etiology

Injury to the intervertebral disk may result from degenerative changes in the vertebral joints that impose excessive axial, shear, or rotational forces on the disk. These forces contribute to the degeneration of the annulus fibrosus. Injury to the intervertebral disk may also be due to acute trauma, such as a vertebral compression fracture or endplate fracture.

Injury to the annulus fibrosus is manifested by tears or fissures within its structure. These disruptions provide a pathway for herniation of the nucleus pulposus. Studies suggest the nucleus must also be injured for herniation to occur. In a healthy disk, natural properties of cohesiveness appear to contain the nucleus, in spite of experimentally created annular fissures.

Herniations of nuclear material through the confines of the annulus fibrosus may occur *anteriorly, intravertebrally,* or *intraspinally* (Fig. 11-50):

- *Anterior disk herniations may* be due to acute compression injuries or to a weakness in the attachment of the annulus to the vertebral rim via Sharpey's fibers. Protrusion of the

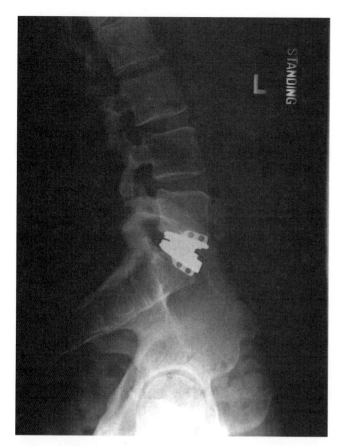

Figure 11-49 Artificial intervertebral disk replacement at L5–S1. This radiograph was made with the patient standing. An appreciation of the inherent mobility of the device is seen in the segmental extension of L5–S1. *(Image courtesy of Greg Hughes.)*

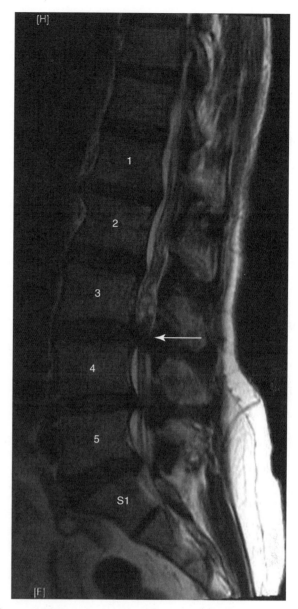

Figure 11-51 Posterior intravertebral disk herniations. This midline sagittal T2-weighted MRI shows a bunched and wavy cauda equina above the large L3–L4 posterior disk herniation (arrow) and a straight cauda equina below it. There are also mild posterior disk herniations at L1–L2, L2–L3, L4–L5, and L5–S1. There is loss of disk high signal consistent with disk dessication due to the herniation of nuclear material. *(Image courtesy of Laughlin Dawes, MD.)*

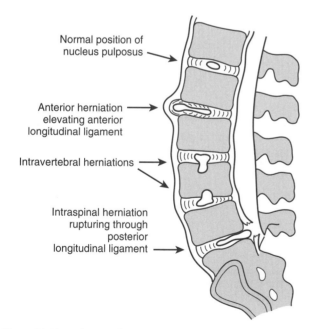

Normal position of nucleus pulposus

Anterior herniation elevating anterior longitudinal ligament

Intravertebral herniations

Intraspinal herniation rupturing through posterior longitudinal ligament

Figure 11-50 Various configurations of intervertebral disk herniations.

nucleus may elevate the anterior longitudinal ligament and lead to osteophyte formation at the anterior and lateral vertebral joint margins (Fig. 11-51). This condition is known as *spondylosis deformans*.

- *Intravertebral disk herniations* may be due to acute trauma or, more commonly, due to a weakening of the vertebral endplate, as in osteoporosis or Scheuermann's disease. Protrusion of nuclear material into the vertebral body may lead to the formation of small osseous cavities known as Schmorl's nodes. Protrusion of nuclear material at the anterior edge of the vertebral body that causes a triangular fragment of bone to be separated from the body is called a *limbus vertebra*.

- *Intraspinal disk herniations* are posterior or posterolateral protrusions of nuclear material that have the potential to compromise the spinal canal and neural elements, presenting significant symptomology often requiring therapeutic or medical intervention. Intraspinal herniations may result from acute trauma, such as falls or heavy lifting, or from pre-existing degenerative conditions that weaken the elasticity and resiliency of the annulus and the posterior ligaments, rendering the disk unable to withstand normal stresses. The physical characteristics of an intraspinal herniation are variable, as is the degree of symptoms that may appear.

Clinical Presentation

Anterior and intravertebral disk herniations, by themselves and excluding associated trauma, are usually devoid of clinical symptomatology.

Intraspinal disk herniations cause low back pain and referred or radicular pain. Symptoms are typically exacerbated with active flexion, prolonged sitting, and Valsalva maneuvers. Nerve root pressure can result in loss of muscle strength, decreased muscle stretch reflexes (deep tendon reflexes), and paresthesias. In rare cases, cauda equina syndrome can develop and is a surgical emergency.

Terminology

Terminology to describe the various degrees of disk herniations has not been standardized within the literature. Some more commonly used descriptions are the following (Fig. 11-52):

- *Posterior prolapse:* The nucleus pulposus is displaced posteriorly within the confines of the annulus fibrosus, causing a distortion of the posterior boundaries of the annular ring. The annulus may or may not protrude into the spinal canal.
- *Contained disk herniation:* Radial tears extend to the posterolateral corner of the annulus; a portion of the nucleus displaces to the extent of the tear, but it remains contained under the posterior longitudinal ligament.
- *Uncontained or extruded disk herniation:* Pressure of the herniation forces the nucleus through the annulus and causes the posterior longitudinal ligament to protrude into the spinal canal.
- *Sequestered disk:* A portion of the nucleus has separated and migrated into the spinal canal.

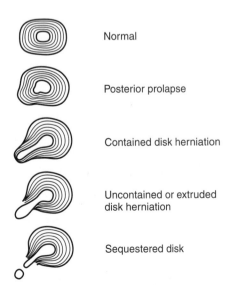

Normal

Posterior prolapse

Contained disk herniation

Uncontained or extruded disk herniation

Sequestered disk

Figure 11-52 Schematic to define various degrees of posterior disk herniations as viewed in cross section.

Radiologic Findings

No Imaging Can Be Prudent

In general, it is widely accepted that imaging studies to investigate a suspected disk herniation are unnecessary in the first 4 to 6 weeks following the onset of symptoms. Central to this philosophy is the fact that 20% to 35% of *asymptomatic* individuals have disk herniations, as determined by MRI, CT, and myelography.[26] Many patients with diskogenic pain patterns improve significantly with conservative treatment in 4 to 6 weeks. Imaging in the early stages of an acute episode may reveal pre-existing abnormalities that are not related to the current acute episode. This information may confuse the situation, present a dire picture for the patient, eliminate chances for conservative management, and instigate premature or unnecessary surgical consultation.

Imaging Is Prudent When . . .

Imaging studies are indicated when conservative treatment fails and other treatment options need to be explored. Exceptions to this practice are those patients who exhibit signs of impending cauda equina syndrome; immediate imaging is necessary in such cases.

Conventional radiographic evaluation for disk herniation is of little value and will read normal except for pre-existing degenerative changes such as joint space alterations, spondylosis, osteophytosis, vacuum sign, or Schmorl's nodes (Fig. 11-53).

Advanced Imaging

Advanced imaging techniques—including myelography, CT myelography, diskography, CT, and MRI—are used alone or as complementary investigative studies to diagnose and determine a treatment plan.

Myelography was the original study of choice to define disk pathology. See Figure 1-30 for a myelogram study of a posterior disk herniation in the lumbar spine. Myelography is now considered inferior to both MRI and CT. However, CT myelography can provide anatomic detail that surpasses both MRI and CT. CT myelography is most often used to diagnose disk pathology in the cervical and thoracic regions.

MRI is excellent in providing information on the morphological changes in the disk as well as physiological and chemical changes within the disk. See Figure 7-47 for an MRI study of a disk herniation in the cervical spine.

Discography images the morphology of the disk via the injection of radiopaque dye into the nucleus. The dye disperses through the nucleus and any fissures present in the annulus. The value of discography is that it is also a provocation test that can help determine whether the patient's pain is due to disk pathology. The dye causes distention of the annulus; if the patient's pain is reproduced, the disk can be considered the source.

Treatment

In general, intervertebral disk herniations have a good prognosis with conservative management. The natural healing processes of the disk include cicatrization (healing by scar formation) and retraction. It is also theorized that the epidural blood supply facilitates phagocytosis of the

Figure 11-53 Degenerative disk disease of the lumbar spine in a 66-year-old woman. **(A)** Lateral film demonstrates decreased disk space height at all lumbar segments and lower thoracic segments. Spondylosis deformans (osteophyte formation in response to degenerative disk disease) is evident at all vertebral margins, both anteriorly and posteriorly (see all arrows). The L4–L5 disk space is greatly diminished, and a radiolucency is seen paralleling the endplate. This is known as the *vacuum sign* and is thought to represent a collection of nitrogen gas from adjacent extracellular fluid that has seeped into the discal fissures. In movements of the spine that produce a decrease of pressure in the disk, such as extension, nitrogen is released from the adjacent extracellular fluid and, because of the pressure gradient, accumulates in the fissures of the disk. This collection of gas can be made to disappear with spinal flexion and reappear with extension. Studies have shown this vacuum sign to be a common sign of disk aging and degeneration, with an incidence of 2% to 3% in the general population. The large arrow indicates the vacuum sign. **(B)** An AP view of the spine demonstrates marginal spurs, a scoliosis, and, again, the vacuum sign in the L4–L5 interspace.

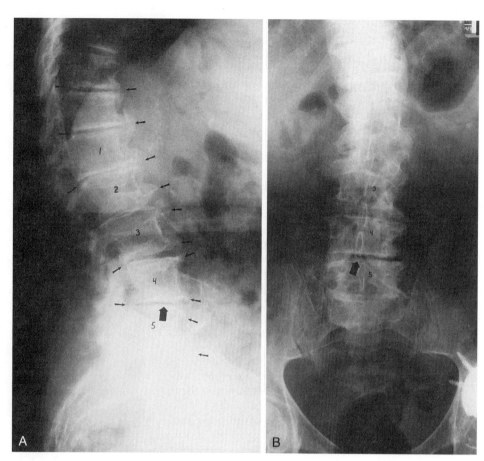

herniated material. Conservative measures include physical therapy, analgesics, short-term bedrest, and restricted activities. Only a small percentage of patients require surgery. Surgery is most successful on patients who have exhausted all other options.

Sacroiliac Joint Pathology[18,67–72]

The sacroiliac joints cannot accurately be assessed on conventional radiographs until after the changes of normal growth and development have completed the ossification of the sacrum, between ages 15 and 18. Until then the sacroiliac joints appear wider than would normally be expected. This developmental process must be taken into account in viewing radiographs of adolescents and young adults.

Ligamentous Injury

The characteristics of motion at the sacroiliac joints remain controversial, so it follows that the characteristics of injury patterns sustained by the joints are also controversial.

Subluxation hypotheses and various types of strain and sprain attributed to the sacroiliac joints are debated for their role in low back pain syndromes as well as coccygeal dysfunction. The extreme stability of the joints afforded by the topographical anatomy discourages hypermobility theories, while the fact that the joints are synovial and innervated strongly supports joint susceptibility to painful ligamentous

strain, inflammation, hypo- or hypermobility, and degenerative changes.

Conventional radiographic examination of the sacroiliac joints cannot evaluate sacroiliac joint stability or instabilities. However, the presence of acute inflammation or degenerative changes that may accompany sacroiliac joint dysfunction are evident on radiographs. These conditions are discussed next.

Degenerative Joint Disease

Degenerative joint disease (DJD) at the sacroiliac joint manifests the same radiographic hallmarks as seen in any synovial joint: decreased joint space, subchondral sclerosis, and osteophyte formation at joint margins. In advanced cases, the joint space may not be well visualized because osteophytes bridge the joint space.

Radiographically, only the lower halves of the joint space image represent the synovial portion of the joints. The upper portions of the joints are syndesmotic. Thus, evaluation of DJD is confined to the lower half of the radiographic joint space.

Sacroiliitis

Sacroiliitis is inflammation of the synovial portions of the sacroiliac joints. It may involve one or both joints. Etiology may comprise inflammatory disorders, arthritides of rheumatoid type, infections, or early degenerative processes.

Radiographically, the lower half of the joint space will appear wide, secondary to progressive inflammatory erosions. In later subacute stages the joint spaces will be narrowed and exhibit other changes typical of degenerative joint disease (Fig. 11-54).

Ankylosing Spondylitis

Ankylosing spondylitis is a chronic, progressive inflammatory arthritis characterized by joint sclerosis and ligamentous ossification. The disease usually manifests first in stiffness of the sacroiliac joints and later extends to the lumbar and thoracic spines. Numerous extra-articular features—including pulmonary fibrosis and cardiac insufficiencies—may complicate the disease. Men are affected seven times more often than women, with onset predominantly in the 20s. Early diagnosis is confirmed by laboratory studies.

Radiographic evidence of the disease often appears first in abnormal narrowing of the upper half of the sacroiliac joints. Fusion of the joint spaces eventually occurs (Fig. 11-55). Squaring-off of the anterior borders of the vertebral bodies is another early radiographic indicator of the disease. In later stages, syndesmophytes form, bridging the vertebral bodies. Additionally, facet joints and intervertebral joints fuse, and the entire spine then exhibits the hallmark radiographic image of the disease known as the "bamboo spine."

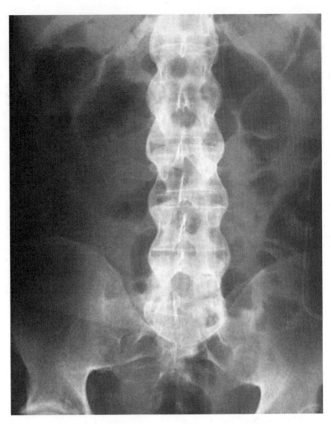

Figure 11-55 Late-stage ankylosing spondylitis with characteristic "bamboo spine," a result of progressive fusion of the facet and intervertebral joint spaces as well as syndesmophytes bridging the vertebral bodies. Note the location of the sacroiliac joints are barely discernible due to bony fusion across the joint spaces. (*Image courtesy of John Hunter, MD.*)

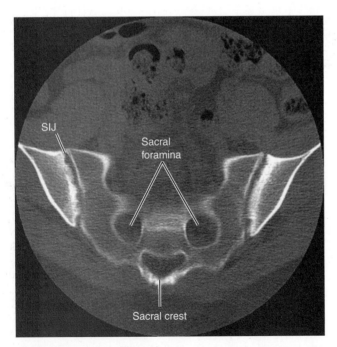

Figure 11-54 Degenerative joint disease of the sacroiliac joints. This axial CT slice across the upper sacrum demonstrates narrowing of both sacroiliac joint spaces with sclerosis of the subchondral bone, pronouced on the iliac side of the joints. Without any further information and based on this image alone, the possible differential diagnoses for this patient include psoriatic arthritis, Reiter's syndrome, infection, and ankylosing spondylitis.

Lumbosacral Anomalies[6,18,39,40]

Congenital or developmental anomalies frequently occur at the junctions of the spinal curvatures. The lumbosacral junction is often the site of vertebral anomalies.

Anomalies are generally related to a structure's (1) failure to develop, (2) arrested development, or (3) development of accessory bones. Spinal anomalies may occur in isolation or in combination with other spinal, visceral, or soft tissue malformations.

The descriptions of block vertebrae, butterfly vertebrae, hemivertebrae, and Schmorl's nodes, as presented in Chapter 9 in connection with thoracic spine anomalies, hold true for their appearance in the lumbar spine (Fig. 11-56). Refer to Table 9-3 for characteristics of these anomalies.

Common anomalies appearing with greatest frequency at the lumbosacral junction include *facet tropism, aberrant transitional vertebrae,* and *spina bifida.*

Facet Tropism

Facet *tropism* ("turning in") consists of asymmetry of the planes of the facet joint articulations at one spinal level. One of the facet joints at L5–S1, for example, may be oriented to a more nearly sagittal plane than the other (Fig. 11-57).

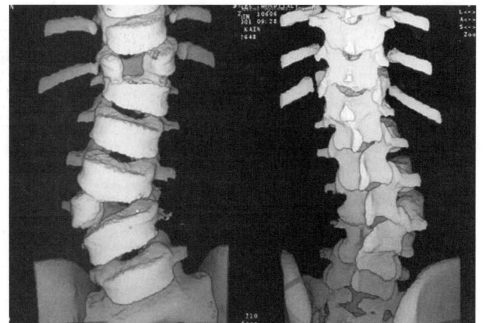

Figure 11-56 Hemivertebra seen on a 3D reformatted CT scan. Anterior coronal view is on the left and posterior coronal view is on the right. How many lumbar vertebrae are present, including the hemivertebra? Surgical removal of the hemivertebra will restore normal alignment to the spine and negate the scoliosis. *(From the Scoliosis Research Society, with permission.)*

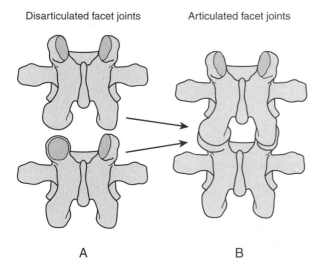

Disarticulated facet joints   Articulated facet joints

A   B

Figure 11-57 Facet tropism. The left facet joint is oriented in a frontal plane, while the right facet joint at the same level is oriented in a more nearly sagittal plane. (A) Disarticulated view of the vertebrae. (B) View of articulated vertebrae.

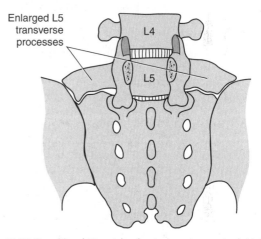

Enlarged L5 transverse processes

L4

L5

Figure 11-58 Transitional L5 vertebra (posterior cutaway view). Note the enlarged transverse processes forming articulations with the sacrum and iliac crests.

Clinical considerations focus on the altered joint biomechanics. Asymmetrical movements will occur at that segment, and adjacent segments will likely accommodate with excessive compensatory motion. Degenerative joint disease of the involved segment and the adjacent segments may be accelerated.

Radiographically, one facet joint space will appear normally radiolucent while the involved facet joint space appears absent because it is not in the normal plane of evaluation.

Aberrant Transitional Vertebrae

Aberrant transitional vertebrae are vertebrae that have adopted morphological characteristics of vertebrae from an adjacent spinal region. The cervicothoracic and thoracolumbar areas may exhibit aberrant transitional vertebrae, but the lumbosacral area is the most common region of occurrence.

In the lumbosacral region, aberrant transitional vertebrae have sometimes been described by terms such as "lumbarization of S1" or "sacralization of L5." Lumbarization of S1 means that S1 has lumbar-like features, and at first glance it may appear that six lumbar vertebrae are present on the AP radiograph. Sacralization of L5 means that L5 appears to be part of an elongated sacrum.

Most commonly seen is the adoption of sacral characteristics by the L5 vertebra (Figs. 11-58 and 11-59). The transverse processes of L5 expand in width and height, appearing more similar in size to parts of the sacral ala than to normal lumbar processes. These enlarged transverse processes may form accessory joints, either unilaterally or bilaterally, with the ilia. The body of L5 usually remains normal in size, although the L5–S1 intervertebral disk is generally vestigial.

Clinically, a lumbar aberrant transitional vertebra is thought to be insignificant, with no evidence of predisposition

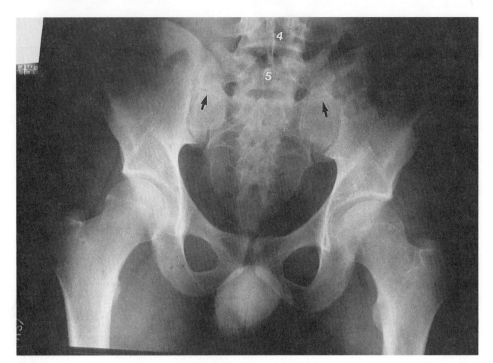

Figure 11-59 Sacralization of L5. Note the enlarged transverse processes of L5, expanded in width and height, appearing more in size like the sacral ala than like normal lumbar transverse processes. Additionally, the inferior aspects of the enlarged transverse processes of L5 appears to have formed articulations with the ala of the sacrum (arrows).

to low back pain or role in prolonging low back pain. It is reasonable to assume, however, that the decreased mobility caused by accessory articulations and the vestigial disk would cause the adjacent freely moving segments to compensate and predispose those segments to degenerative changes. Furthermore, if the accessory articulations at the transitional segment are unilateral, resultant altered biomechanics of both the transitional segment and adjacent segments may predispose the joints to accelerated degenerative changes.

Radiographically, the AP view will show the enlarged transverse processes, the presence of accessory articulations of the transverse processes to the ilia, and the narrowed disk space at L5–S1.

Spina Bifida[5,8,18,21,22]

Spina bifida is a failure of the posterior vertebral arches to fuse (Fig. 11-60). It is the most common congenital anomaly of the spine. Clinically, variations of this anomaly range from no clinical significance to associated paralysis.

Spina Bifida Occulta

Spina bifida occulta (*occulta* meaning "hidden") is the most benign manifestation and is often discovered on radiograph as a purely incidental finding (Fig. 11-61). Spina bifida occulta is the failure of the laminae to fuse at midline and form a spinous process. There is no associated neurological involvement and the architecture of the vertebra is not weakened. Although uninformed patients may be alarmed at this radiographic finding, it usually holds no clinical significance.

Radiographically, the AP view will show a radiolucent cleft between the laminae, with an absent or diminutive spinous process.

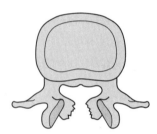

Figure 11-60 Spina bifida is a failure of the posterior vertebral arches to unite.

Spina Bifida Vera

Spina bifida vera (*vera* meaning "true") or spina bifida manifesta (*manifesta* meaning "known") is the more serious expression of this anomaly, in which the defect in posterior arch fusion is large enough to allow protrusion of the spinal cord and its coverings outside of the spinal canal. The sac that forms outside of the body is called a meningocele if it contains only cerebrospinal fluid, spinal cord coverings, and nerve roots and the spinal cord remains within the canal. The neurological deficits are variable in this case and may not be evident at birth but develop in later childhood. A meningomyelocele is a sac that contains the meningocele structures plus the spinal cord itself. Complications include serious neurological deficits, deformities, and hydrocephalus. The most devastating version of spinal cord herniation is the myelocele. In this case the herniation of the cord and related structures is completely outside and without protective covering of the dura or even skin. Infection often leads to infant death.

Radiographically, the AP view will show a wide interpedicular distance, representing the failure of arches to develop. On the lateral film a water-density mass may be evident posterior to the bony defect, representing the cerebrospinal fluid within the sac (Fig. 11-62).

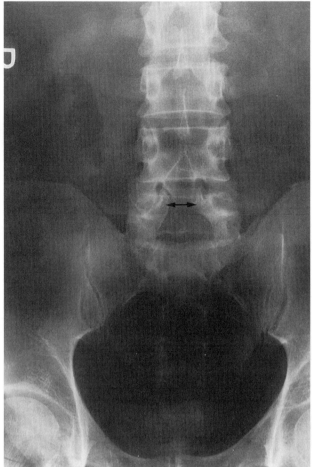

Figure 11-61 Spina bifida occulta. An incidental finding in a routine lumbar series in this 41-year-old man was a large radiolucent cleft at L5, representing a failure of the laminae to unite and form a spinous process. The lined arrow extends over the width of the cleft. No clinical symptoms were related to this finding.

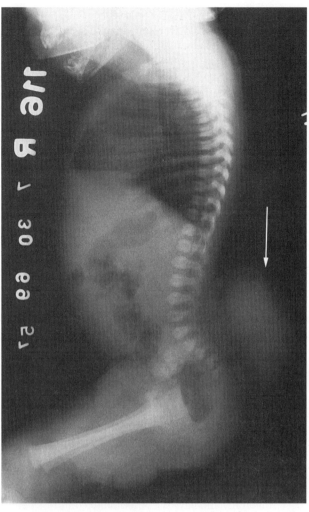

Figure 11-62 Myelomeningocele. A large lumbar myelomeningocele is demonstrated on this lateral view of a 2-day-old infant boy.

Summary of Key Points

Routine Radiologic Evaluation

1. The routine radiologic evaluation of the lumbar spine includes five projections:

   ➤ *Anteroposterior* demonstrates all five lumbar vertebral bodies.
   ➤ *Lateral* demonstrates alignment of the lumbar vertebrae and the intervertebral disk spaces.
   ➤ *Right and left obliques* demonstrate the facet joint articulations. The "Scottie dog" image is seen on this projection.
   ➤ *Lateral L5–S1 spot film* demonstrates, in greater close-up detail, the lumbosacral junction.

2. The routine radiologic evaluation of the sacroiliac joint includes three projections:

   ➤ *Anteroposterior axial projection* demonstrates both joints simultaneously.

   ➤ *Right and left oblique projections* demonstrate each sacroiliac joint individually through the oblique plane of the joint.

Trauma

3. Compression fractures of the vertebral bodies are common injuries at the thoracolumbar (T11–L2) region.

4. Spondylolysis is a defect at the pars interarticularis. The defect may be congenital, degenerative, traumatic, or a stress fracture due to chronic strain. It may occur unilaterally or bilaterally.

5. Spondylolysis is diagnosed on the oblique radiograph as a radiolucent streak across the pars interarticularis, often referred to as a "collar on the Scottie dog."

6. Spondylolisthesis may be a consequence of spondylolysis. Spondylolisthesis is the anterior displacement of one vertebra upon the stationary vertebra beneath it.

Degenerative Conditions

7. Spondylolisthesis may result from degenerative joint changes. In the absence of a fracture, this condition is called degenerative spondylolisthesis or pseudospondylolisthesis.

8. Fracture spondylolisthesis can be differentiated from degenerative spondylolisthesis by the spinous process sign, either clinically or on the lateral radiograph.

9. Spinal stenosis is a narrowing of the spinal canal caused by degenerative joint and disk changes. A spinal stenosis can be classified into three anatomic regions: (1) stenosis of the central canal, (2) stenosis of the intervertebral foramen, and (3) stenosis of the lateral or subarticular recesses. More than one region may be involved at the same intervertebral level.

10. Radiographically, stenosis is suggested by the location of the degenerative changes. Additional studies such as myelography, CT, and MRI can define the amount of encroachment and thecal sac constriction.

Intervertebral Disk Herniations

11. Intervertebral disk herniation is a protrusion of the nuclear disk material through the confines of the annulus fibrosus. Herniations may occur anteriorly, intravertebrally, or intraspinally.

12. Anterior disk herniations may elevate the anterior longitudinal ligament, instigating osteophyte formation at the anterior and lateral joint margins; this is known as spondylosis deformans. Intravertebral disk herniations may protrude through the vertebral endplates and form osseous cavities known as Schmorl's nodes. Intraspinal herniations generally protrude posterolaterally and have the potential to compress neural elements.

13. Conventional radiographs are of little value in the demonstration of intervertebral disk herniations, other than to identify pre-existing degenerative changes.

14. CT myelography is excellent for demonstrating anatomic detail. MRI is excellent for demonstrating the morphological and physiochemical changes in the annulus. Discography is a contrast media study of the disk that also serves as a provocation test to identify the disk as a source of the patient's pain.

Sacroiliac Joint Pathology

15. The sacroiliac joints cannot be accurately assessed on radiograph till the sacrum is fully ossified at ages 15 to 18. Until then, an abnormally wide joint space can be expected.

16. Radiography is helpful in the evaluation of sacroiliac joint pathologies such as degenerative joint disease and sacroiliitis. The radiographic assessment is directed to the lower halves of the joints, which are synovial articulations.

17. Ankylosing spondylitis is a progressive inflammatory arthritis characterized by joint sclerosis and ligamentous ossification. The disease usually manifests first in the sacroiliac joints and later ascends through the lumbar and thoracic spines. Early radiographic indicators include abnormal narrowing of the upper halves of the sacroiliac joints and squaring off of the anterior borders of the vertebral bodies. In later stages syndesmophytes form, bridging vertebral bodies and presenting the characteristic "bamboo spine" image on radiographs.

Lumbosacral Anomalies

18. Anomalies appear with some frequency at the lumbosacral spine and are often incidental findings, without significant clinical implications.

19. Aberrant transitional vertebrae are often named by the predominant characteristics. Sacralization of L5 is the most common anomaly at this region.

20. Other common anomalies include spina bifida occulta and facet tropism. Usually incidental findings, such anomalies can result in clinical pathology if asymmetrical articulations are present.

 Please refer to the text's enclosed CD-ROM for the American College of Radiology's current Musculoskeletal Appropriateness Criteria for the following topic: *Suspected Spine Trauma.*

CASE STUDIES

Case Study 1

Low Back Pain

The patient is a 47-year-old male accountant who enjoys playing racquetball and lifting weights. He was referred to physical therapy for conservative management of low back pain.

History

The patient reported that he has experienced episodes of low back pain intermittently since his mid-20s. Until now, the pain had always been isolated to the lumbar region and usually resolved on its own within a few days of onset. The current episode started at the end of a day in which he had worked at his desk longer than usual and then gone to the gym to lift weights. While dressing after his shower, he began to experience central low back pain and burning pain into his right buttock and posterior thigh. Concerned by the new symptoms, he saw his primary care physician 2 days later, who prescribed a nonsteroidal anti-inflammatory drug (NSAID) and asked the patient to return for a follow-up appointment in 2 weeks.

Initial Imaging

At the follow-up appointment the patient reported no change in his symptoms. The physician ordered conventional radiographs and magnetic resonance imaging (MRI) of the lumbar spine and also referred the patient to physical therapy.

Physical Therapy Examination

Patient Complaint

The patient's initial physical therapy appointment took place 3 weeks after onset of the current episode. The imaging results were not yet available.

The patient continued to complain of central low back, right buttock, and right posterior thigh pain. He was not experiencing any saddle paresthesias or bowel or bladder changes. His back pain worsened with prolonged sitting at his desk and in his car. He said that the pain in both the back and right lower extremity would improve when he stood up and walked around a little.

Physical Examination

The neurological screening examination revealed normal and symmetrical lower extremity muscle stretch reflexes, muscle strength, and sensation. Straight leg raise testing on the right reproduced the buttock and thigh pain at 50 degrees. The patient's posture was unremarkable other than a slightly decreased lumbar lordosis in standing.

Physical Therapy Intervention

The physical therapist designed a treatment plan based on a working hypothesis of diskogenic low back pain with referral into the buttock and posterior thigh. The therapist was confident that the patient's condition would improve, given that his symptoms responded to changes in position. The plan included joint mobilization, extension exercises and body mechanics training, including spinal stabilization activities and avoidance of flexion postures.

Imaging Results

The patient brought the imaging reports to his second physical therapy appointment. The conventional radiographs were unremarkable for any degenerative or pathological abnormalities. The MRI report noted, "moderate right posterolateral herniation of the L5–S1 intervertebral disk. There is evidence of L5–S1 degenerative disk changes. Moderate compression of the corresponding nerve root is noted" (Fig. 11-63).

Outcome

The patient's physician had already been in contact with the patient prior to his second appointment with the therapist. The physician recommended referral to a neurosurgeon to discuss possible surgical interventions. The therapist phoned the physician and persuaded him to allow the patient to continue with physical therapy for 3 weeks before seeing the neurosurgeon.

After 3 weeks, the patient's thigh and buttock pain had resolved and his central low back pain was reduced by 50%. He felt he was making good progress and was performing a modified resistive exercise program at the gym. The patient elected not to see a neurosurgeon.

Discussion

This case exemplifies a common situation that arises with patients who experience low back pain and seek medical intervention. These patients are often referred prematurely for a surgical consult based on the results of MRI findings *without an adequate trial of conservative management first*. Significant findings on MRI should not dominate patient management. Rather, integration of this

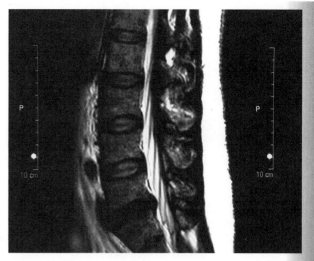

Figure 11-63 The report from this MR image noted "moderate right posterolateral herniation of the L5–S1 intervertebral disk," "evidence of L5–S1 degenerative disk changes," and "moderate compression of the corresponding nerve root."

information with the overall clinical presentation of signs, symptoms, and pain pattern should direct treatment.

In this patient's case, the MR image did help to confirm the therapist's suspicion of intervertebral disk pathology. However, the clinical picture did not completely fit with MRI findings of nerve root compression. The buttock and posterior thigh pain may be explained by compression or irritation of the S1 nerve root, but these symptoms were intermittent. The patient *did not* have other neurological signs or symptoms of S1 nerve root compression, such as numbness/tingling in the foot, muscle weakness, or diminished reflexes. Therefore referral to a neurosurgeon, whose primary task is to determine whether the patient is a surgical candidate, was premature and eventually not necessary in the patient's management.

The case is summarized in Figure 11-64.

CRITICAL THINKING POINTS

1. The prevalence of disk herniations determined by MRI, computed tomography (CT), and myelography in asymptomatic individuals is estimated to be between 20% and 35%.

2. In the absence of clinical signs of severe nerve root compression, imaging studies are not usually necessary in the acute phase of low back pain because the results will not likely alter the treatment plan or outcome.

3. Conservative management of low back pain should be given an adequate length of time (several weeks) prior to radiologic investigation or surgical consultation.

CASE STUDY 2

Spinal Stenosis

The patient is a 58-year-old man complaining of bilateral lower extremity pain with activity.

History

The patient's internal medicine physician referred him to physical therapy after ruling out vascular claudication via Doppler arterial flow studies.

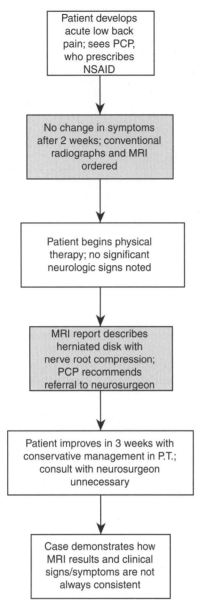

Figure 11-64 Pathway of case study events. Imaging is highlighted.

Physical Therapy Examination

Patient Complaint

The patient had been experiencing gradually increasing pain in both calves over the past month. He said that his pain increased some with standing and especially after walking for 5 minutes or more. He stated that sitting relieved his pain. As a result, he had not been as active as he used to be, forgoing his usual mile-long walks with his wife.

Physical Examination

Examination of the lower extremities was normal for strength, sensation, muscle stretch reflexes, and range of motion. His dorsalis pedis and posterior tibial pulses were strong. Lumbar active range of motion was within normal limits, with complaints of moderate low back pain with lumbar extension. Treadmill walking at a comfortable pace began to reproduce his lower extremity pain after 4 minutes.

Imaging

The therapist contacted the internal medicine physician to discuss the possibility of spinal stenosis as a source of the patient's lower extremity symptoms. The physician agreed to order a CT myelogram. The myelogram (Fig. 11-65) demonstrated significant blockage of the contrast material in the thecal sac at the L4–L5 level, confirming the suspicion of central spinal stenosis. The CT myelogram demonstrated narrowing of the spinal canal, particularly at L4–L5, due to a combination of degenerative factors, including intervertebral disk bulging at the L4–L5 level and a grade 1+ degenerative spondylolisthesis.

Intervention

The patient was managed conservatively in physical therapy. Treatment included joint mobilization above the level of the spondylolisthesis, stretching of the lumbar spine into flexion, strengthening of abdominal muscles, back stabilization exercises, postural retraining, and patient education.

Outcome

The patient showed some improvement over the next few months. He experienced a reduction in the intensity of lower extremity pain during ambulation and could walk for longer distances before onset of the symptoms. He continued to experience calf pain but was satisfied enough with his progress that he elected not to pursue surgical intervention.

Discussion

In some cases, the physical therapist may be more familiar with advanced imaging modalities for musculoskeletal problems than the referring physician is. In this case, the internal medicine physician ruled out peripheral vascular disease but did not follow up specifically on the possibility of spinal stenosis.

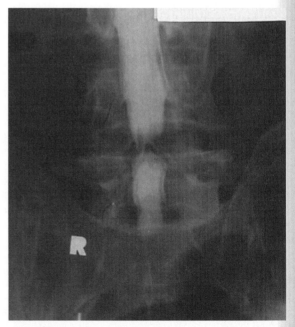

Figure 11-65 Myelogram showing evidence of constriction of the thecal sac at L4–L5.

The suggestion of a CT myelogram was appropriate based on the clinical presentation. The confirmation that this imaging provided permitted the therapist to (1) design an approriate treatment plan, (2) mobilize safely at a specific spinal level, and (3) provide definitive information to the patient. The patient was then able to understand his pain, restrict activities judiciously, and make the choice to live with it without fear of the unknown.

The case is summarized in Figure 11-65.

CRITICAL THINKING POINT

Not all primary care physicians are knowledgeable about orthopedic conditions. Radiologists are the best resource for the selection of imaging modalities. However, to make the appropriate selection, radiologists must first be provided with the full clinical picture. In daily clinical practice, this is not practical. The radiologist cannot be consulted on every patient the physician refers to imaging.

Physical therapists, as health-care professionals, should be knowledgeable about which imaging modalities are appropriate to confirm or rule out the common diagnoses they would see in their specific patient population. In this case, CT myelography was an appropriate suggestion for the therapist to make.

Case studies adapted by J. Bradley Barr, PT, DPT, OCS.

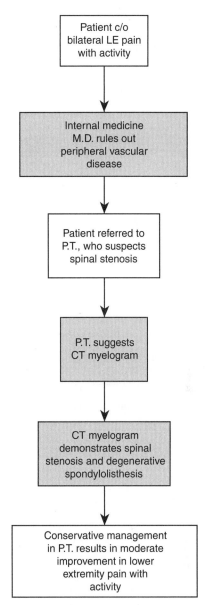

Figure 11-66 Pathway of case study events. Imaging is highlighted.

References

Anatomy

1. Netter, FH: Atlas of Human Anatomy, ed. 4. WB Saunders, Philadelphia, 2006.
2. Yochum, TR, and Rowe, LJ: Essentials of Skeletal Radiology, ed. 3. Williams & Wilkins, Baltimore, 2004.
3. Nordin, M, and Frankel, VH: Basic Biomechanics of the Musculoskeletal System, ed. 3. Lippincott Williams & Wilkins, Philadelphia, 2001.
4. Whiting, W, and Zernicke, R: Biomechanics of Musculoskeletal Injury, ed. 2. Human Kinetics, Champaign, IL, 2008.
5. Gehweiler, JA, et al: The Radiology of Vertebral Trauma. WB Saunders, Philadelphia, 1980.
6. Meschan, I: An Atlas of Normal Radiographic Anatomy. WB Saunders, Philadelphia, 1960.
7. Weber, EC, Vilensky, JA, and Carmichael, SW: Netter's Concise Radiologic Anatomy. WB Saunders, Philadelphia, 2008.
8. Magee, DJ: Orthopedic Physical Assessment, ed. 5. WB Saunders, Philadelphia, 2007.
9. Kapandji, IA: The Physiology of the Joints. Vol. 3, The Trunk and Vertebral Column. Churchill Livingstone, New York, 1974.

Routine Exam

10. American College of Radiology: Practice Guideline for the Performance of Spine Radiography in Children and Adults. 2007 (Res. 39). Accessed May 18, 2008 at http://www.acr.org.
11. Frank, E, Smith, B, and Long, B: Merrill's Atlas of Radiographic Positions and Radiologic Procedures, ed. 11. Elsevier Health Sciences, Philadelphia, 2007.
12. Bontrager, KL: Textbook of Radiographic Positioning and Related Anatomy, ed. 6. Mosby, St. Louis, MO, 2005.
13. Chew, FS: Skeletal Radiology: The Bare Bones, ed. 2. Williams & Wilkins, Baltimore, 1997.
14. Fischer, HW: Radiographic Anatomy: A Working Atlas. McGraw-Hill, New York, 1988.
15. Wicke, L: Atlas of Radiologic Anatomy, ed. 5. Lea & Febiger, Malvern, PA, 1994.
16. Weir, J, and Abrahams, P: An Atlas of Radiological Anatomy. Yearbook Medical, Chicago, 1978.
17. Squires, LF, and Novelline, RA: Fundamentals of Radiology, ed. 4. Harvard University Press, Cambridge, MA, 1988.
18. Greenspan, A: Orthopedic Radiology: A Practical Approach, ed. 4. Lippincott, Williams & Wilkins, Philadelphia, 2004.
19. Whitley, A: Clark's Positioning in Radiography, ed. 12. Hodder Arnold, 2005.

Trauma

20. Denis, F: The three-column spine and its significance in the classification of acute thoracolumbar spinal injuries. Spine 8:817, 1983.
21. American College of Radiology: Appropriateness Criteria: Clinical Condition: Suspected Spine Trauma. Available at http://www.acr.org/Secondary MainMenuCategories/quality_safety/app_criteria/pdf/ExpertPanelonMus culoskeletalImaging/SuspectedCervicalSpineTraumaDoc22.aspx.
22. El-Khoury, GY: New trends in imaging of thoraco-lumbar spine trauma. Virtual Hospital, University of Iowa, Iowa City, 2003. Accessed November 5, 2003 at http://www.vh.org/adult/provider/radiology/thoracolumbarspinetrauma/.
23. Kelley, LL, and Peterson, CM: Sectional Anatomy for Imaging Professional, ed. 2. Mosby, St. Louis, MO, 2007.
24. Lazo, DL: Fundamentals of Sectional Anatomy: An Imaging Approach. Thomson Delmar Learning, Clifton Park, NY, 2005.
25. Ip, D: Orthopedic Traumatology: A Resident's Guide. Springer, New York, 2006.
26. McConnell, J, Eyres, R, and Nightingale, J: Interpreting Trauma Radiographs. Blackwell, Oxford, UK, 2005.
27. Bernstein, MR, Mirvis, SE, and Shanmuganathan, K: Chance-type fractures of the thoracolumbar spine: Imaging analysis in 53 patients. Am J Roentgenol 187:859, 2006.
28. Levi, AD, et al: Neurologic deterioration secondary to unrecognized spinal instability following trauma—A multicenter study. Spine 31(4):451, 2006.
29. Sava, J, et al: Thoracolumbar fracture in blunt trauma: Is clinical exam enough for awake patients? J Trauma 61(1):168, 2006.
30. Dai, LY, et al: Thoracolumbar fractures in patients with multiple injuries: Diagnosis and treatment—A review of 147 cases. J Trauma 56(2):348, 2004.
31. Diaz, JJ, et al: Practice management guidelines for the screening of thoracolumbar spine fracture. J Trauma 63(3):709, 2007.

32. Berry, GE, et al: Are plain radiographs of the spine necessary during evaluation after blunt trauma? Accuracy of screening torso computed tomography in thoracic/lumbar spine fracture diagnosis. J Trauma 59(6):1410, 2005.
33. Berquist, TH: Imaging of Orthopedic Trauma, ed. 2. Raven Press, New York, 1989.
34. Bucholz, RW, Heckman, J, and Court-Brown, C (eds): Rockwood and Green's Fractures in Adults, ed. 6. Lippincott Williams & Wilkins, Philadelphia, 2005.
35. McCort, JJ, and Mindelzun, RE: Trauma Radiology. Churchill Livingstone, New York, 1990.
36. Drafke, MW, and Nakayama, H: Trauma and Mobile Radiography, ed. 2. FA Davis, Philadelphia, 2001.
37. Koval, KJ, and Zuckerman, JD: Handbook of Fractures, ed. 3. Lippincott Williams & Wilkins, Philadelphia, 2006.
38. Eiff, M, et al: Fracture Management for Primary Care. WB Saunders, Philadelphia, 2003.
39. Marsharawi, YM, et al: Lumbar facet orientation in spondylolysis: A skeletal study. Spine 32(6):E176, 2007.
40. Masci, L, et al: Use of one-legged hyperextension test and MRI in the diagnosis of active spondylolysis. Br J Sports Med 40(11):940, 2006.
41. Krupski, W and Majcher, P: Radiologic diagnostic of lumbar spondylolysis. Ortop Tramatol Rehabil 6(6):809, 2004.
42. Dunn, AJ, et al: Radiologic findings and healing patterns of incomplete stress fractures of the pars interarticularis. Skel Radiol 37(5):443, 2008.

Degenerative Conditions

43. Daffner, RH: Clinical Radiology: The Essentials, ed 3. Williams & Wilkins, Baltimore, 2007.
44. Marchiori, DM: Clinical Imaging with Skeletal, Chest, and Abdomen Pattern Differentials, ed. 2. Mosby, St. Louis, MO, 2004.
45. Herzog, RJ: The radiologic assessment for lumbar disc herniation. Spine 21(Suppl 24):19, 1996.
46. Jensen, M, et al: Magnetic resonance imaging of the lumbar spine in people without back pain. N Engl J Med 2(331):69, 1994.
47. van Rijn, J, et al: Observer variation in MRI evaluation of patients suspected of lumbar disk herniation. Am J Roentgenol 184:299, 2005.
48. Kalichman, L, and Hunter, DJ: Diagnosis and conservative management of degenerative lumbar spondylolisthesis. Eur Spine J 17(3):327, 2008.
49. Saal, JS: General principles of diagnostic testing as related to painful lumbar spine disorders: A critical apprisal of current diagnostic techniques. Spine 27(22):2538, 2002.
50. Rubinstein, SM, and van Tulder, M: A best-evidence review of diagnostic procedures for neck and low-back pain. Best Pract Res Clin Rheumatol 22(3):471, 2008.

Stenosis

51. Saint-Louis, LA: Lumbar spinal stenosis assessment with computed tomography, magnetic resonance imaging, and myelography. Clin Orthop Relat Res (384):122, 2001.
52. Zeifang, F, et al: Gait analysis does not correlate with clinical and MR imaging parameters in patients with symptomatic lumbar spinal stenosis. BMC Musculoskel Disord 9(1):89, 2008.
53. Sirvanci, M, et al: Degenerative lumbar spinal stenosis: Correlation with Oswestry Disability Index and MR imaging. Eur Spine J 17(5):679, 2008.
54. Willen, J, et al: Surgical results in hidden lumbar spinal stenosis detected by axial loaded computed tomography and magnetic resonance imaging: An outcome study. Spine 33(4):E109, 2008.
54. Geissner, MR, et al: Spinal canal size and clinical symptoms among persons diagnosed with lumbar spinal stenosis. Clin J Pain 23(9):780, 2007.

DDD

55. Modic, MT, and Ross, JS: Lumbar degenerative disk disease. Radiology 245(1):43, 2007.
56. O'Neill, C, et al: Accuracy of MRI for diagnosis of discogenic pain. Pain Physician 11(3):311, 2008.
57. Valat, JP: Evolution of the concepts about nonspecific low back pain. Rev Prat 58(3):261, 2008.
58. Bellaiche, L, and Petrover, D: Imaging in chronic low back pain: Which one and when? Rev Prat 58(3):273, 2008.
59. Auerbach, JD, et al: Streamlining the evaluation of low back pain in children. Clin Orthop Relat Res 466(8):1971, 2008.
60. Buttermann, GR: The effect of spinal steroid injections for degenerative disc disease. Spine 4(5):495, 2004.
61. Beattie, PF: Current understanding of lumbar intervertebral disc degeneration: A review with emphasis upon etiology, pathophysiology, and lumbar magnetic resonance imaging findings. J Orthop Sports Phys Ther 38(6):329, 2008.

Artificial Disks

62. Griffith, SL, et al: A multicenter retrospective study of the clinical results of the LINK SB Charite intervertebral prosthesis. The initial European experience. Spine 19(16):1842, 1994.

63. Thalgott, JS, et al: A new classification system for degenerative disc disease of the lumbar spine based on magnetic resonance imaging, provocative discography, plain radiographs, and anatomic considerations. Spine J 4(6 Suppl):167S, 2004.

64. Freeman, BJ, and Davenport, J: Total disc replacement in the lumbar spine: A systematic review of the literature. Eur Spine J 15(Suppl 3):S439, 2006.

65. David, T: Long-term results of one-level lumbar arthroplasty: Minimum 10 year follow-up of the CHARTE artificial disc in 106 patients. Spine 32(6):661, 2007.

66. Lehman, RA Jr, and Lenke, LG: Long-segment fusion of the thoracolumbar spine in conjunction with a motion-preserving artificial disc replacement: Case report and review of the literature. Spine 32(7):E240, 2007.

SIJ

67. Hancock, MJ, et al: Systematic review of tests to identify the disc, SIJ, or facet joint as the source of low back pain. Eur Spine J 16(10):1539, 2007.

68. Hansen, HC, et al: Sacroiliac joint intervention: A systematic review. Pain Physician 10(1):165, 2007.

69. Frey, ME, et al: Efficacy and safety of percutaneous sacroplasty for painful osteoporotic sacral insufficiency fractures: A prospective, multicenter trial. Spine 32(15):1635, 2007.

70. Braun, J: Ankylosing spondylitis. Lancet 369(9570):1379, 2007.

71. Zochling, J, et al: Magnetic resonance imaging in ankylosing spondylitis. Curr Opin Rheumatol 19(4):346, 2007.

72. Song, IH: Diagnosing early ankylosing spondylitis. Curr Rheumatol Rep 9(5): 367, 2007.

SELF-TEST

Radiograph A

1. Identify this *projection*.

2. Which intervertebral disk spaces are narrowed?

3. The three curving parallel lines that indicate *normal vertebral alignment* are disrupted. Identify which vertebra is not in normal alignment.

4. Describe the altered *position* of this vertebra.

5. What altered bony characteristics are present along the *anterior margins* of several vertebrae? What are some possible clinical or pathological significances of these alterations?

Radiograph B

6. Identify this *projection*.

7. Describe the *anomaly* present. What are some possible *clinical* or *pathological* significances of this anomaly?

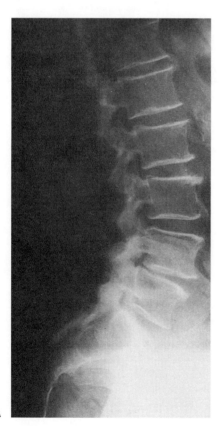

A

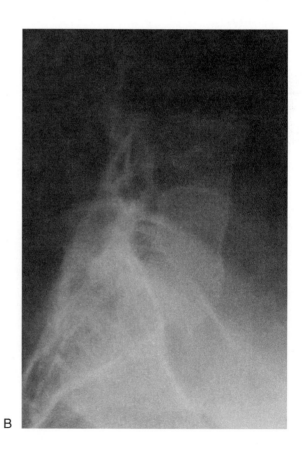

B

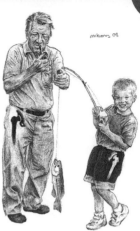

RADIOLOGIC EVALUATION OF THE PELVIS AND HIP

The *pelvis* is the keystone of the skeleton, a link between the weight forces from the trunk and upper body and the ground forces transmitted by the lower body. The structural strength of the pelvis is provided by its substantial osseous components and its relatively rigid ring-like architecture. Trauma to the pelvis requires great force, and fractures here are often associated with serious vascular and visceral complications.

The *femur* is the largest bone in the body. The proximal ends of the femurs articulate with the pelvic acetabula to form the *hip joints*. The hip joints have great structural and ligamentous stability yet permit a wide range of motion. The primary function of the hip joints is to transmit ground forces in the erect skeleton, allowing for maintenance of upright posture and ambulation. In radiology, the hip joints are most often evaluated to assess degenerative processes that manifest here as well as the fractures sustained here. Rehabilitation is important in the restoration of functional and ambulatory skills after the hip is compromised.

Review of Anatomy[1–6]

Osseous Anatomy

Pelvis

The pelvis consists of four bones: two coxal or innominate bones, the sacrum, and the coccyx. The ilium, ischium, and pubis make up each coxal bone. The fusion of these three components forms the cup-shaped acetabulum, which accepts the head of the femur to form the hip joint (Figs. 12-1 and 12-2).

Ilium

The superior portion of each coxal bone is the *ilium*. The flared, thin upper portion of the ilium is the *ala*, or wing. The upper margin of the ala is the *iliac crest*, extending from the *anterosuperior iliac spine (ASIS)* to the *posterosuperior iliac spine (PSIS)*. Less prominent landmarks include the *anteroinferior iliac spine (AIIS)*, inferior to the ASIS, and the

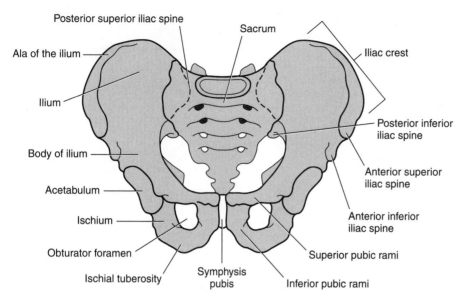

Figure 12-1 The bony pelvis.

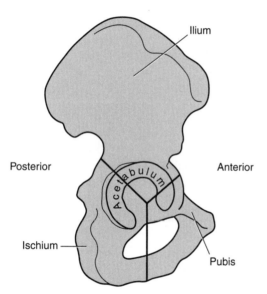

Figure 12-2 Each innominate bone is formed by the fusion of the ilium, ischium, and pubis bones. The cup-shaped acetabulum is formed at the junction of these three components.

posteroinferior iliac spine (PIIS), inferior to the PSIS. The inferior portion of the ilium is the *body*, which includes the upper two-fifths of the acetabulum.

Ischium

The *ischium* is the inferior and posterior portion of each coxal bone. The upper portion of the ischium is the *body*; it forms the posterior two-fifths of the acetabulum. The lower portion is the *ramus*, ending caudally at the *ischial tuberosity*.

Pubis

The *pubis* is the inferior and anterior portion of each coxal bone. The *body* of the pubis makes up the anteroinferior one-fifth of the acetabulum. The *superior rami* extend anteriorly and medially from each body to form the midline *symphysis pubis joint*. The inferior rami extend posteriorly and inferiorly from the symphysis pubis and join with the rami of the ischia.

Proximal Femur

The hip joint is the articulation between the acetabulum and the proximal femur. The proximal femur is composed of four parts: the head, neck, greater trochanter, and lesser trochanter (Figs. 12-3 and 12-4).

Femoral Head

The head is spherical in shape, covered with cartilage, and has a central depression or *fovea* for attachment of the *ligamentum teres (capitis femoris ligament)*. The head articulates with the acetabulum to form the *hip joint*.

Femoral Neck

The head joins the neck at the *subcapital sulcus*. The neck is pyramidal in shape and contains prominent pits for the entrance of blood vessels. The neck connects the head to the *shaft* of the femur. The angle formed at the junction of the neck to the shaft is the *angle of inclination* and measures in the range of 125 to 135 degrees in adults. The neck is also angled anteriorly on the shaft, approximately 15 degrees in adults. This is called *anteversion*.

Greater and Lesser Trochanters

The greater trochanter is a large quadrilateral projection marking the upper lateral end of the femoral shaft. The lesser trochanter is a smaller conical projection marking the junction of the inferior medial neck to the femoral shaft. The *intertrochanteric crest* joins the trochanters posteriorly. The *intertrochanteric line* on the anterior aspect of the femur represents the junction of the neck to the shaft and the site of attachment of the hip joint *capsule*.

Ligamentous Anatomy

Hip Joint

The hip joint is a synovial ball-and-socket joint. The spherical femoral head articulates with the acetabulum, which is deepened by a fibrocartilaginous labrum. The strong fibrous joint capsule extends from the bony rims and labrum of the acetabulum to the intertrochanteric line just superior to the intertrochanteric crest.

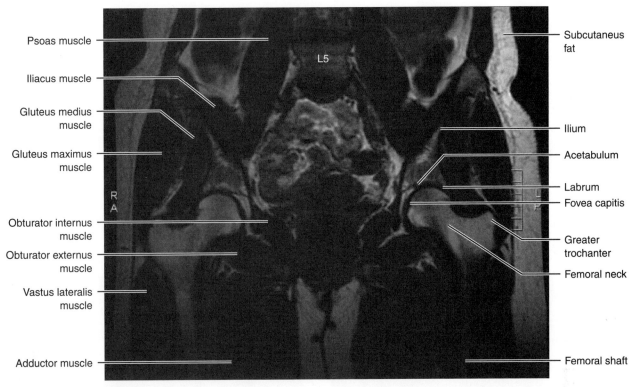

Figure 12-3 Coronal T1-weighted MRI of bilateral hips.

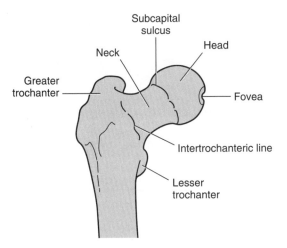

Figure 12-4 The proximal femur.

Three ligaments or thickenings of the joint capsule provide stability to the hip joint (Fig. 12-5).

1. The *iliofemoral ligament* lies anteriorly and extends from the AIIS to the intertrochanteric line. It is taut in full extension and promotes stabilization of the pelvis on the femur in erect posture.
2. The *pubofemoral ligament* lies medially and inferiorly and extends from the inferior acetabular rim to the inferior femoral neck. It helps to limit abduction and extension.
3. The *ischiofemoral ligament* forms the posterior margins of the capsule and extends from the ischial portion of the acetabulum to the superior femoral neck. Additionally, the *ligamentum teres* acts in providing

joint stabilization. Extending from the fovea on the femoral head to the acetabular notch, the ligamentum teres limits adduction.

Joint Mobility

Mobility at the pelvis occurs at the articulations of the sacroiliac joints and by associated deformation of the fibrocartilaginous *interpubic disk* at the symphysis pubis.

Mobility at the hip takes places in all three planes. In the sagittal plane approximately 0 to 140 degrees of flexion and 0 to 15 degrees of extension are possible. Abduction ranges from 0 to 30 degrees, and adduction ranges from 0 to 25 degrees. When the hip is flexed, 0 to 90 degrees of external rotation and 0 to 70 degrees of internal rotation are possible. Circumduction, or a combination of movement through the elemental planes, is also freely available at the hip joints. The articular surfaces glide upon each other as component movements during all of these motions.

Growth and Development

Pelvis

At birth, a large portion of the pelvis is ossified, but the upper ilium, majority of the acetabulum, lower end of the ischium, and medial end of the pubis are cartilaginous. The junction of the cartilaginous portions of the ilium, ischium, and pubis forms the triradiate cartilage, which makes up the acetabular fossa. By age 10, most of the cartilage has ossified in the coxal bones, although the triradiate

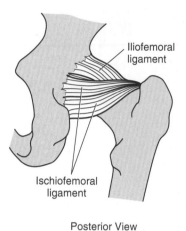

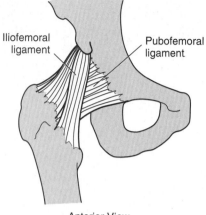

Posterior View   Anterior View

Figure 12-5 Ligament of the hip joint.

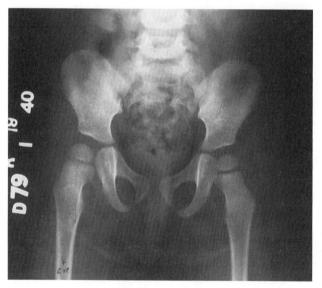

Figure 12-6 Normal radiographic appearance of the pelvis of a healthy 2-year-old girl. The majority of the pelvis is ossified, except the acetabulum which is primarily cartilaginous. Note the normal appearance of very wide sacroiliac joints and the unfused sacral bodies. At the femur, the epiphysis for the femoral head is well ossified; the epiphyses for the greater and lesser trochanters will not appear for several more years. Note also the large femoral neck to femoral shaft angle of almost 170 degrees. This angle will progressively decrease with growth and development of the femur to approximately 130 degrees.

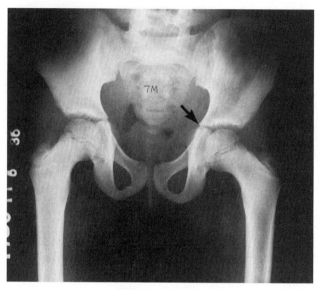

Figure 12-7 Normal radiographic appearance of the pelvis of a healthy 7-year-old boy. The innominate bones are ossified, with the exception of the triradiate cartilage (arrow) of the acetabular fossa. At the sacrum, the bodies, neural arches, and costal processes have fused over the previous 2 years and the sacrum now appears in its gross adult form. The sacroiliac joints remain wide in appearance. At the femurs, the epiphyses for the greater trochanters, which had appeared approximately 2 years earlier, are now well developed and ossified. The epiphyses for the lesser trochanters will appear in another 2 or 3 years. Note the decrease in the angles of inclination of the femoral necks to the femoral shafts compared to the radiograph at age 2.

cartilage remains (Figs. 12-6 and 12-7). Secondary centers of ossification appear at puberty. The triradiate cartilage fuses at about age 17, whereas the remaining coxal epiphyses may not fuse until the early 20s.

The shape of the pelvis is similar in boys and girls until puberty. At that time distinct differences begin, and development is modified according to sex (Fig. 12-8). The adult male pelvis is usually narrower and less flared, exhibiting an oval or heart-shaped pelvic inlet, and the angle of the public arch is less than 90 degrees. The adult female pelvis, adapted for childbirth, is usually broader, exhibits a round pelvic inlet, and the angle of the pubic arch is greater than 90 degrees.

Proximal Femur

The shaft of the femur is ossified at birth. Ossification extends to the neck soon after birth. The epiphysis for the head of the femur initiates ossification between 3 and 6 months of age. The epiphysis for the greater trochanter appears between 4 and 5 years of age and the epiphysis for the lesser trochanter between 9 and 11 years of age. All of these secondary ossification centers fuse in the late teens (Figs. 12-6 and 12-7).

The angles of inclination of the femoral neck to the shaft are quite large at birth and decrease with development. At birth the neck-to-shaft angle is approximately 175 degrees.

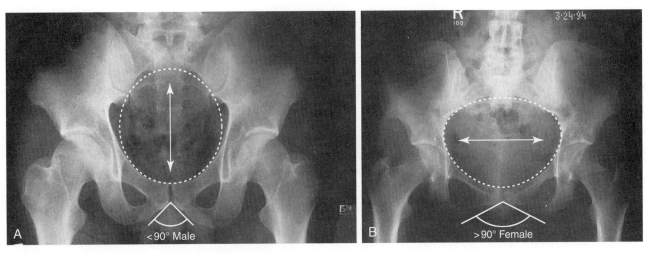

Figure 12-8 In general, the adult male pelvis **(A)** is narrower, with an oval-shaped inlet and angle of pubic arch less than 90 degrees; in contrast, **(B)** the adult female pelvis is broader, with a rounder inlet and greater angle of pubic arch.

Subsequent growth of the femur decreases the angle to approximately 125 degrees in the adult. Additionally, approximately 40 degrees of anteversion is present at birth, decreasing to approximately 15 degrees in adulthood. Consequently, the acetabulum adapts its obliquity to accommodate the growing femur, exhibiting a 10-degree difference in horizontal orientation from birth to maturity.

Routine Radiologic Evaluation[7–18]

Practice Guidelines for Extremity Radiography in Children and Adults

The American College of Radiology (ACR), the principal professional organization of radiologists in the United States, defines the following practice guidelines as an educational tool to assist practitioners in providing appropriate radiologic care for patients.

Goals

The goal of the hip radiographic examination is to identify or exclude anatomic abnormalities or disease processes.

Indications

The indications for radiologic examination include but are not limited to trauma; osseous changes secondary to metabolic disease, systemic disease, or nutritional deficiencies; neoplasms; infections; arthropathies; preoperative, postoperative, and follow-up studies; congenital syndromes and developmental disorders; vascular lesions; evaluation of soft tissue (e.g., suspected foreign body); pain; and correlation of abnormal skeletal findings on other imaging studies.

Recommended Projections

Anteroposterior (AP) and lateral projections are recommended for the hip. The osseous pelvis is evaluated with an AP projection.

Basic Projections and Radiologic Observations

Pelvis

The basic radiologic evaluation of the pelvis includes, by proximity, a basic evaluation of the bilateral hip joints. Thus, the AP radiograph of the pelvis provides an AP view of both hip joints. This is advantageous for bilateral comparison purposes of the hips or to scout for trauma and identify the need for a unilateral hip radiograph.

Hips

The AP radiograph of the pelvis is sometimes adequate for evaluation of the hips; at other times it is not. To obtain an AP pelvic radiograph, the central ray is centered at midline over the pelvis; this can result in subtle distortion of anatomy at the periphery of the radiograph as well as loss of detail. Therefore when the hip or proximal femur is the specific area of clinical interest, a unilateral hip radiograph is made with the central ray centered over the femoral neck.

The basic projections that evaluate the hip are the unilateral AP radiograph and the *lateral frog-leg radiograph*. These views provide greater radiographic detail of the proximal femur, acetabulum, and joint space.

The term *frog-leg* is a reference to the position the patient's leg is placed in to provide a lateral view of the proximal femur. The frog-leg position defines a supine patient with a flexed, externally rotated, and laterally abducted hip joint combined with knee flexion. The radiograph is taken from an AP direction, but the beam actually travels through the medial to lateral aspect of the proximal femur. Thus, a lateral view of the femur, rotated 90 degrees from its position in the AP radiograph, is obtained.

For patients who cannot rotate their leg to the frog-leg position, such as those who have sustained trauma to the hip and should not be moved unnecessarily, an *axiolateral inferosuperior projection* (also known as a *groin-lateral projection* or *cross-table lateral*) is substituted. This true lateral is also used for postsurgical evaluation. The involved leg is able to stay in a neutral position for this view.

Routine Radiologic Evaluation of the Pelvis

Anteroposterior

This view demonstrates the entire pelvis, the sacrum, the coccyx, the lumbosacral articulation, and both proximal femurs and hip joints.

Radiologic Observations

The important observations are:

1. The general architecture of the pelvic girdle should appear symmetrical on each side of midline (Fig. 12-9). If the patient is correctly positioned, without rotation, this symmetry is evidenced by equal size of the iliac alae (*a* in Fig. 12-9) and obturator foramina (*b* in Fig. 12-9). Asymmetry in these structures can indicate improper positioning of the patient or rotation of the innominates. Possibilities are:
   - A narrowed iliac ala combined with a wider obturator foramen on the ipsilateral side can indicate external rotation of the innominate bone.
   - A wider iliac ala combined with a narrower obturator foramen on the ipsilateral side can indicate internal rotation of the innominate bone.
2. The iliac alae normally become more radiolucent at their anterolateral borders because the bony mass is thinner there.
3. The interpubic cartilaginous disk of the symphysis pubis is represented by a radiolucent potential space.
4. The sacrum and coccyx are aligned with the symphysis pubis (*d* in Fig. 12-9).
5. The sacroiliac joints and their potential joint spaces are visible (see the discussion of the AP axial view of the sacroiliac joint in Chapter 11 for further details).
6. The hip joints are normally articulated in a ball-and-socket configuration.
7. The femoral necks are visible in their full extent, because they have been positioned in a plane parallel to the image receptor.
8. The femurs should exhibit symmetrical *angles of inclination* from the femoral neck to the femoral shaft. The normal range is 125 to 135 degrees. Angles less than this are varus deformities; angles greater than this are valgus deformities. Asymmetry may be a sign of femoral fracture.
9. The landmarks of the acetabulum and related structures are referenced by several radiographic lines (Fig. 12-10). Disruptions in these line images may indicate fracture or other abnormality.
   - The *acetabular roof* (*a* in Fig. 12-10) represents the superior cortical aspect of the acetabular cup, which corresponds to the major weight-bearing portion of the acetabulum.
   - The *anterior acetabular rim* (*b* in Fig. 12-10) represents the anterior margins of the acetabular cup.
   - The *posterior acetabular rim* (*c* in Fig. 12-10) represents the posterior cortical rim of the acetabular cup.

Basic Projection

- AP

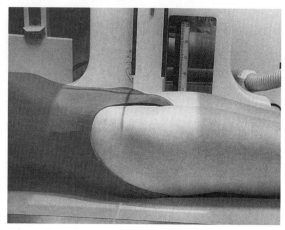

Figure 12-11 Patient position for AP pelvis radiograph.

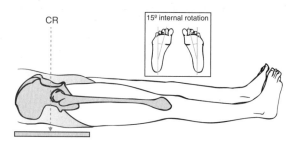

Figure 12-12 The central ray is perpendicular to the image receptor, and is directed midway between the levels of the ASIS and the symphysis pubis. The lower extremities are internally rotated 15 to 20 degrees to place the femoral neck plane parallel to the image receptor.

- The *iliopubic* (or *iliopectineal* or *arcuate*) line (*d* in Fig. 12-10) is a line from the sciatic notch to the pubic tubercle. It represents the limit of the anterior column of the acetabulum.
- The *ilioischial line* (*e* in Fig. 12-10) is a line from the iliac notch to the inner surface of the ischium, representing the posteromedial margin of the quadrilateral surface of the iliac bone, and the limit of the posterior acetabular column. Normally this line is tangential to or intersects the radiographic teardrop.
- The *radiographic teardrop* (*f* in Fig. 12-10) is an image seen on the medial aspect of the acetabulum, formed by the cortical surfaces of the pubic bone and ischium, representing the anteroinferior aspect of the acetabulum.

What Can You See?

Look at the radiograph (Fig. 12-13) and try to identify the radiographic anatomy. Trace the outlines of structures using a marker and transparency sheet. Compare results with the book tracing (Fig. 12-14). Can you identify the following:

- Two coxal bones
- L5 vertebra, sacrum, and coccyx
- Proximal femurs
- Acetabulum
- Acetabular roof, anterior and posterior rims
- Iliopubic, ilioischial, and teardrop lines

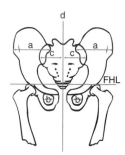

Figure 12-9 Radiographic spatial relationships of pelvic alignment.

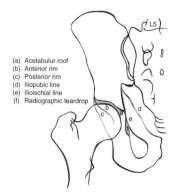

(a) Acetabular roof
(b) Anterior rim
(c) Posterior rim
(d) Iliopubic line
(e) Ilioischial line
(f) Radiographic teardrop

Figure 12-10 Radiographic landmarks that designate intact borders of the acetabulum.

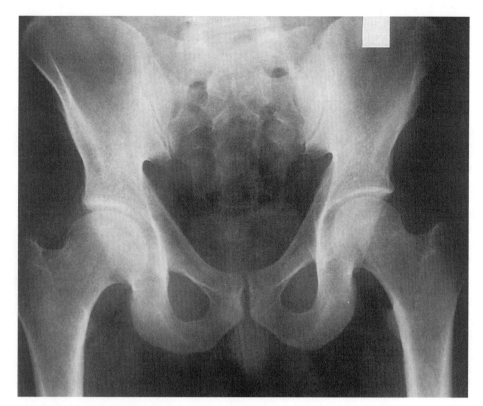

Figure 12-13 Anteroposterior radiograph of the pelvis.

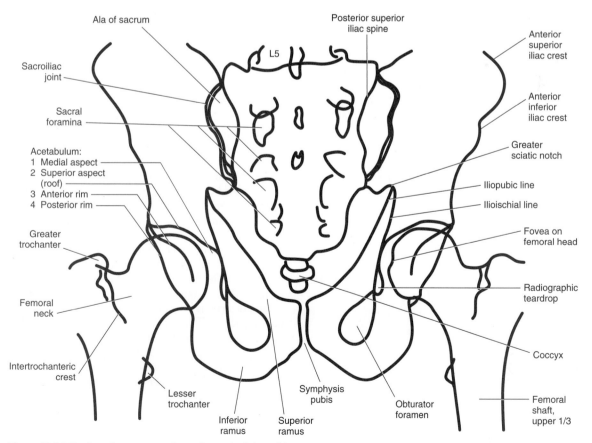

Figure 12-14 Tracing of anteroposterior radiograph of the pelvis.

Routine Radiologic Evaluation of the Hip and Proximal Femur

Anteroposterior

This view demonstrates the acetabulum, femoral head, neck, and proximal third of the shaft, the greater trochanter, and the angle of inclination of the femoral neck to the shaft.

Radiologic Observations

The important observations are:

1. The patient is positioned supine with the legs straight and the involved lower extremity internally rotated 15 to 20 degrees. This amount of rotation compensates for the normal anteversion of the femoral neck and allows the neck to be visualized parallel to the image receptor. In correct positioning the lesser trochanter is obscured, or only its tip is showing.
2. Correct position of the femoral head in the acetabulum as well as correct alignment of the femoral head to the femoral shaft can be assessed by identifying these line images and spatial relationships (Fig. 12-15):

   - *Shenton's hip line* (*a* in Fig. 12-15): It should be possible to draw a smooth curve along the medial and superior surface of the obturator foramen to the medial aspect of the femoral neck.
   - The *iliofemoral line* (*b* in Fig. 12-15): It should be possible to draw a smooth curve along the outer surface of the ilium that extends inferiorly along the femoral neck.
   - *Femoral neck angle* (*c* in Fig. 12-15): This angle is formed by the intersection of a line drawn through the center of the femoral shaft and a line drawn through the center of the femoral neck. Normally this angle averages 130 degrees. Angles less than this are termed *coxa vara;* angles greater than this are termed *coxa valga.*

   Disruptions in these lines are associated with hip dislocation, femoral neck fracture, and slipped femoral capital epiphysis. Disruptions in the femoral neck angle may be a clue to femoral neck fracture; in this case, the terms *varus deformity* and *valgus deformity* refer to the angle of displacement.

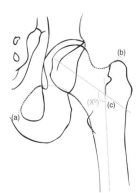

Figure 12-15 Radiographic spatial relationships of normal position of the proximal femur.

Basic Projections

- **AP**
- Lateral frog-leg

Setting up the Radiograph

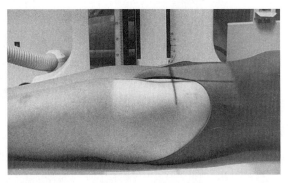

Figure 12-16 Patient position for an anteroposterior radiograph of the left hip.

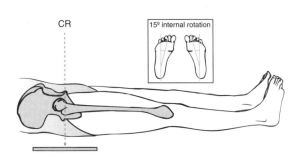

Figure 12-17 The central ray is perpendicular to the image receptor and passes through the femoral neck.

---

3. The hip joint radiographic joint space should be well preserved. Narrowing of the space is associated with degeneration of the articular cartilage. Widening of the joint space is associated with joint effusion.
4. The osseous margins of the femoral head and acetabular cup should be smooth and clearly defined. Sclerotic subchondral areas, narrowed joint space, and osteophytes at the joint margins are associated with degenerative joint disease.
5. The ball-and-socket configuration of the hip joint should be obvious. Destruction of normal joint congruity may be caused by various pathologies including avascular necrosis, rheumatoid arthritis, degenerative joint disease, and destructive tumors.
6. The increased density of the cortex of the femoral shaft is normally quite pronounced. Thinning or evaporation of this radiodense image indicates that an abnormal metabolic process is in effect, such as osteoporosis.
7. Trabecular markings of the head and neck normally appear clear and sharp. A washed-out or demineralized appearance may indicate that an abnormal metabolic process is present.

What Can You See?

Look at the radiograph (Fig. 12-18) and try to identify the radiographic anatomy. Trace the outlines of structures using a marker and transparency sheet. Compare results with the book tracing (Fig. 12-19). Can you identify the following:

- Acetabulum (roof, anterior, and posterior rims)
- Proximal femur (head, neck, and shaft)

- Greater and lesser trochanter and intertrochanteric crest
- Increased cortical densities of the femoral shaft

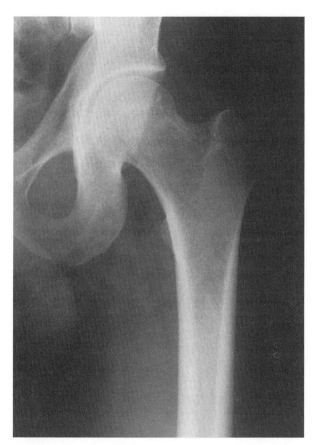

Figure 12-18 Anteroposterior radiograph of the left hip.

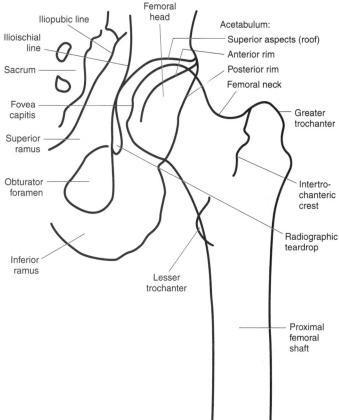

Figure 12-19 Tracing of anteroposterior radiograph of the hip.

Routine Radiologic Evaluation of the Hip and Proximal Femur

Lateral Frog-Leg

This view demonstrates the femoral head, neck, and proximal third of the femoral shaft and the greater and lesser trochanters from the *medial* aspect.

Radiologic Observations

The important observations are:

1. The hip of the supine patient has been positioned in flexion, external rotation, and lateral abduction. This rotates the femur 90 degrees from the AP hip projection.
2. For patients who cannot rotate a leg to this position, an *axiolateral inferosuperior projection* (also known as a *groin-lateral projection* or *cross-table lateral*) is substituted (Fig. 12-20).
3. The femur is now viewed from a medial-to-lateral aspect. The lesser trochanter is now anterior, and the greater trochanter is now posterior. The greater trochanter is thus superimposed behind the neck, and the lesser trochanter is superimposed in front of the neck and extends slightly below the medial border of the femur.
4. The expanse of the femoral head is well exposed.
5. The radiographic image of the acetabulum is unchanged from the AP view.
6. The angle of inclination of the femoral neck to the shaft is not visible, and the angle of anteversion is distorted; therefore, neither is evaluated on this view.

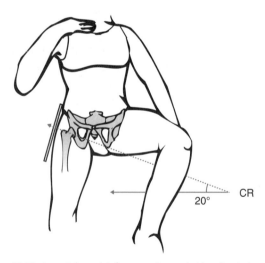

Figure 12-20 An axiolateral inferosuperior projection (groin-lateral) is made by flexing the uninvolved extremity up out of the way and directing the central ray through the femoral neck at an inferosuperior angle.

Basic Projections

- AP
- **Lateral frog-leg**

Setting up the Radiograph

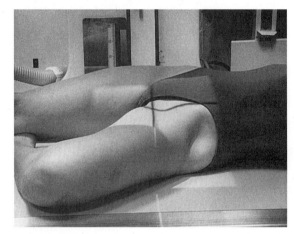

Figure 12-21 Patient position for lateral frog-leg radiograph.

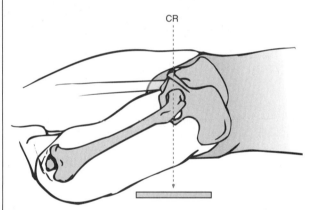

Figure 12-22 The central ray passes in a mediolateral direction through the femoral neck, striking the image receptor perpendicularly.

What Can You See?

Look at the radiograph (Fig. 12-23) and try to identify the radiographic anatomy. Trace the outlines of structures using a marker and transparency sheet. Compare results with the book tracing (Fig. 12-24). Can you identify the following:

- Acetabulum
- Proximal femur (head, neck, and shaft)
- Greater trochanter, superimposed behind the femoral neck
- Lesser trochanter as it projects beyond the lower margin of the femur

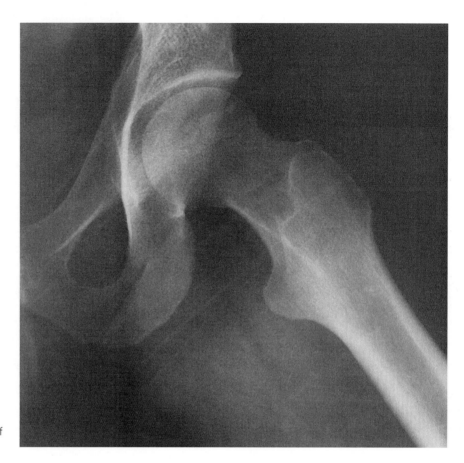

Figure 12-23 Lateral frog-leg radiograph of the left hip.

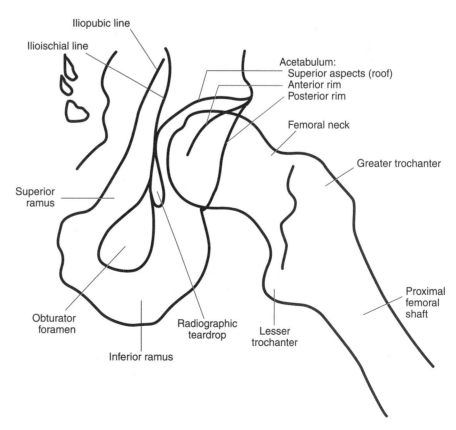

Figure 12-24 Tracing of lateral frog-leg radiograph of the hip.

Trauma at the Pelvis and Hip[10,19–36]

Diagnostic Imaging for Trauma of the Pelvis and Hip

Trauma to the pelvis and hip can be divided into *low-energy injuries,* such as avulsions or individual bone fractures, and *high-energy injuries,* which disrupt the pelvic ring.

Low-Energy Injuries

In low-energy injuries, the AP pelvic radiograph is obtained first to assess for location of injuries. If further investigation is needed to define the extent of an injury more clearly, various special projections can be performed to demonstrate specific anatomy. Most common are oblique views of the pelvis, commonly known as Judet views (Fig. 12-25). These anterior or posterior oblique views are used to demonstrate the columns of the acetabulum free of superimposition. Additionally, conventional tomography or computed tomography (CT) is useful in diagnosing fracture characteristics in areas of complex topography.

Other optional projections to assess the pelvis are variations on the AP view. Angling the central ray 40 degrees caudad results in an *AP axial pelvic inlet view,* which demonstrates the pelvic inlet in its entirety. Angling the central ray approximately 30 degrees cephalad results in the *AP axial pelvic outlet view,* which demonstrates the superior and inferior pubic rami and the ischium well.

At the hip, the AP and axiolateral (groin-lateral, cross-table lateral) views define the characteristics of most fractures of the proximal femur.

High-Energy Injuries

In high-energy injuries a more extensive trauma survey is necessary. This is because the magnitude of force sufficient to disrupt the pelvic ring usually causes multiple associated injuries. Fractures of the pelvis are often accompanied by life-threatening visceral injuries involving major blood vessels, nerves, and the bladder and urinary tract. Modern trauma centers use high-speed CT scanners to obtain a *thorax-abdomen-pelvis (TAP)* series, which can quickly assess injuries of the trauma patient in one examination.

Fractures of the Pelvis

Mechanism of Injury

The majority of pelvic fractures are a result of motor vehicle accidents. The remainder is caused by falls or pedestrian or motorcycle accidents.

Classifications

Various classifications of pelvic fractures exist, based on configuration, force mechanisms, or inherent stability. The broadest categorization identifies *stable* versus *unstable* fractures. Determination of the stability of the pelvic ring is the significant factor in the orthopedic treatment, prognosis, and rehabilitation of the patient. The pelvic ring is defined as the continuous osseous cage formed by the paired coxal bones and the sacrum, including the relatively rigid articulations at the sacroiliac joints and the symphysis pubis.

Stable Fractures

Stable pelvic fractures do not disrupt any of the joint articulations (Fig. 12-26). Stable fractures include the following:

1. Avulsion fractures of the ASIS, AIIS, or ischial tuberosity, commonly seen in athletes owing to forceful or repetitive muscle contraction of the sartorius, rectus femoris, or hamstring attachments, respectively
2. Iliac wing fractures
3. Sacral fractures
4. Ischiopubic ramus fractures

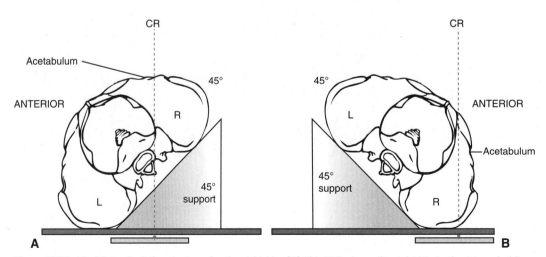

Figure 12-25 *AP oblique (Judet) projections for the right hip.* **(A)** This LPO places the right hip in the *internal oblique* position and demonstrates the iliopubic column and posterior rim of the right acetabulum. **(B)** This RPO places the right hip in the *external oblique* position and demonstrates the ilioischial column and the anterior rim of the acetabulum.

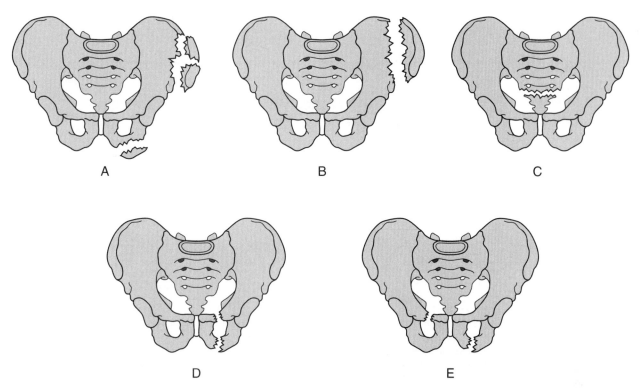

A   B   C

D   E

Figure 12-26 Examples of *stable* pelvic fractures include **(A)** avulsions of the ASIS, AIIS, or ischial tuberosity; **(B)** iliac wing fractures; **(C)** sacral fractures; and **(D)** ipsilateral and **(E)** contralateral pubic rami fractures.

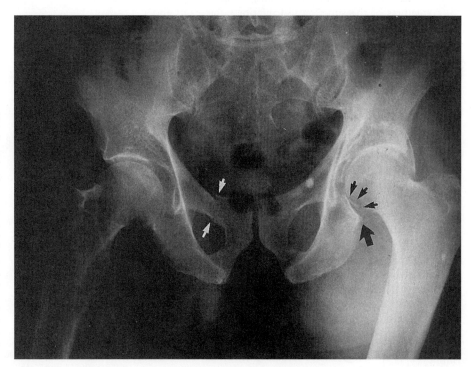

Figure 12-27 Stable pelvic fractures. This 55-year-old woman was injured in a motor vehicle accident. She sustained a complete transverse fracture of the right superior pubic ramus (white arrows), and on the left side an impaction fracture of the femoral head (small black arrows) and a fracture of the inferior acetabular rim (large black arrow). Note the great amount of swelling at the left hip and upper thigh evidenced by the increased radiodensity of the soft tissues. These types of fractures at the hip are commonly referred to as "dashboard fractures" because a common mechanism of injury is when the knee strikes the dashboard in a collision resulting in forces transmitted up the femur and into the acetabulum. An incidental and common finding on radiographs of the pelvis is the pebble-like radiodensity located over the left superior rami. This could represent a calcified kidney stone, gall stone, or valve in a vein.

The last three types of fractures are usually the result of lateral compression forces or vertical shear forces and falls. Ischiopubic ramus fractures are quite common and constitute almost half of all pelvic fractures (Fig. 12-27).

Unstable Fractures

Unstable fractures result from disruption at two or more sites on the pelvic ring and are frequently associated with internal hemorrhage. Unstable fractures include the following (Fig. 12-28):

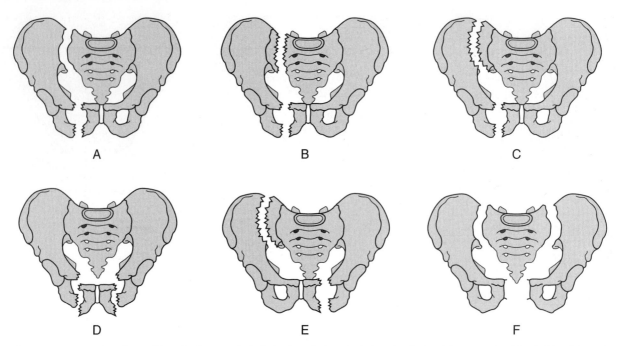

Figure 12-28 Examples of *unstable* pelvic fractures include (A, B, and C) vertical shear (Malgaigne) fractures, involving ischiopubic rami and disruption of an ipsilateral sacroiliac joint, be it **(A)** through the joint itself, **(B)** through a fracture of the sacral wing, or **(C)** a fracture on the iliac bone; **(D)** straddle fractures, involving all four ischiopubic rami; **(E)** bucket handle fractures, involving both ischiopubic rami on one side and the contralateral sacroiliac joint; and **(F)** dislocations involving one or both sacroiliac joints and the symphysis pubis.

1. *Vertical shear* or *Malgaigne* fractures, involving unilateral fractures of the superior and inferior pubic rami and disruption of the ipsilateral sacroiliac joint (the damage at the sacroiliac joint may be through the joint itself or via fracture of the nearby sacral wing or iliac bone)
2. *Straddle fractures,* involving all four ischiopubic rami
3. *Bucket handle fractures,* involving an ischial ramus, the ipsilateral pubic ramus, and the contralateral sacroiliac joint (Fig. 12-29)

The mechanism of these fractures is often vertical shear, sometimes combined with AP or lateral compression forces (Fig. 12-30).

Dislocations

Dislocations are also considered unstable injuries. Dislocations at the pelvis may occur unilaterally, involving one sacroiliac joint and the symphysis pubis, or bilaterally, involving both sacroiliac joints and the symphysis pubis. The bilateral pelvic dislocation is commonly referred to as a *sprung pelvis.* The precipitating force is usually an AP compression that in effect springs open the pelvis as in opening a book.

Dislocation of the symphysis pubis, also referred to as a *diastasis* or separation, can occur in isolation, as seen in cases of acute trauma, or related to pregnancy or delivery (Fig. 12-31).

Radiologic Evaluation

Most fractures of the pelvis are demonstrated on the AP pelvis radiograph. Optional views used to demonstrate anatomy further without superimposition include the pelvic oblique views and the AP axial inlet view and the AP axial outlet view. CT is useful to identify location of fragments, assess joint spaces, and evaluate comminuted fractures.

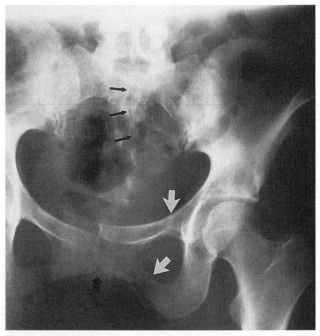

Figure 12-29 Unstable pelvic fractures. This 30-year-old woman was injured in a motor vehicle accident. She sustained a vertical fracture through the body of the sacrum (three black arrows), a left-side transverse superior pubic ramus fracture with superior displacement, a left-side comminuted inferior pubic ramus fracture (white arrows), and a diastasis of the symphysis pubis (large black arrow). These injuries constitute an unstable pelvic fracture pattern because more than two sites of the pelvic ring are disrupted.

Complications

The mortality rate from pelvic fractures is substantial, ranging from 5% to 15%. Acute hemorrhage and visceral damage present life-threatening complications.

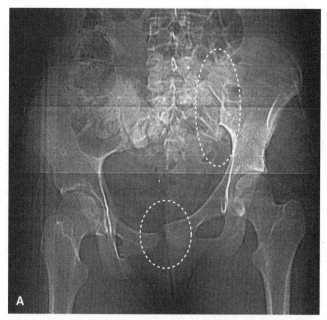

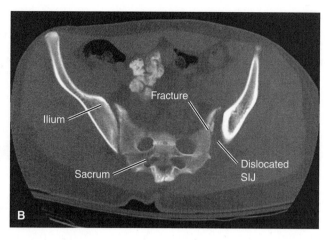

Figure 12-30 Vertical shear fracture–dislocation of the pelvis. **(A)** This *scout film* is produced by the CT scanner to identify location of the scan slices to follow. The elevation of the hemipelvis is a classic appearance of a dislocated sacroiliac joint with pubic symphysis disruption. Note the right side pubic rami fractures. **(B)** Axial CT scan showing the dislocated sacroiliac joint space evidenced by the wide joint space and asymmetrical ilium due to its elevated position. *(Image courtesy of John C. Hunter, MD, University of California, Davis School of Medicine.)*

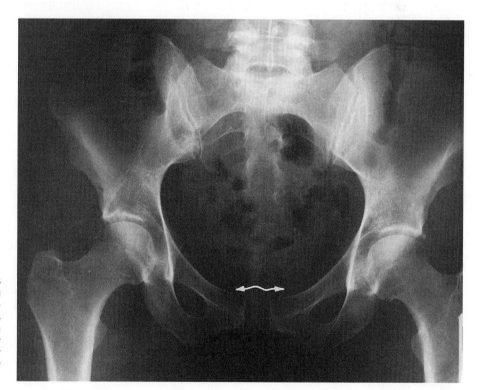

Figure 12-31 Diastasis of the symphysis pubis in a 35-year-old woman following childbirth. The susceptibility of the ligamentous structures of the symphysis pubis to the increase in ligament-relaxing estrogen hormones during pregnancy and during labor may have been a factor in this condition. The wavy white arrow marks the separation of the joint.

Other complications associated with pelvic fractures include infection, thromboembolism, malunion, and posttraumatic arthritis.

Treatment

Stable Fractures

Stable fractures are treated with a brief period of bed rest, analgesics, and range-of-motion exercises as tolerated. Rehabilitation focuses on progressive mobility and ambulation with adaptive devices to limit weight bearing on the affected side. Avulsion-type fractures in the young athlete require crutch-assisted ambulation and rehabilitation to regain full strength and range of motion. Return to full function may require 6 to 12 weeks. Excessive callus formation at the site of avulsion may result in prolonged symptoms.

Unstable Fractures

Unstable fractures of the pelvic ring are treated with internal fixation, external fixation, skeletal traction, or combinations of these. Internal fixation devices include compression screws and plates. A common external fixator is a rectangular frame design mounted on two to three 5-mm pins spaced 1 cm apart along the anterior iliac crest. The external frame is used for 8 to 12 weeks, and the patient is ambulatory, based on radiographic evidence of stability and healing.

Rehabilitation focuses on restoration of ambulation in the healing phase and return to full strength and function after bony union is complete.

Dislocations

Dislocations of the sacroiliac joints are surgically stabilized with posterior cancellous screws or anterior sacroiliac plate fixation. Diastasis of the pubic symphysis is surgically stabilized with plate fixation.

Fractures of the Acetabulum

Fractures of the acetabulum are sometimes difficult to evaluate on the routine AP views because of superimposition of the femoral head and the configuration of the acetabular cup itself. For this reason, anterior and posterior oblique or Judet projections are obtained to complete the trauma evaluation. Conventional tomography or CT may supplement the conventional radiographs, as in evaluation of the pelvis. Note, however, that the first indication of fracture on the AP pelvic projection may be a disruption in one or more of the six radiographic line images normally visible on that view (see Fig. 12-10).

Mechanism of Injury

Acetabular fracture results from impaction of the femoral head into the acetabular cup. The configuration of the fracture depends on the position of the hip at the time of impaction. If the hip is in neutral position, an impaction through the greater trochanter will result in a transverse fracture of the acetabulum. If the hip is flexed, an impaction through the femur will result in a posterior fracture of the acetabulum.

Classification

Classification of acetabular fractures is related to anatomic position. The pelvis is divided into anterior and posterior columns (Fig. 12-32). The anterior column is composed of the iliopubic area; the posterior column is composed of the ilioischial area. These divisions meet at the midline of the acetabulum. Fractures occurring at the acetabulum are thus defined as the following:

1. Anterior-column fractures
2. Posterior-column fractures
3. Transverse fractures, involving both columns
4. Complex fractures, involving a T-shaped configuration

The terms *anterior-* or *posterior-lip* fractures refer to fractures at the acetabular rims without extension into the pubic or ischial bones. Posterior-lip fractures and posterior-column fractures are the most common acetabular fractures and are frequently associated with femoral head impaction or femoral head posterior dislocation (Fig. 12-33). These fractures are often referred to as "dashboard" fractures because they result from the knee striking the dashboard in a motor vehicle accident (see also Fig. 12-27).

Radiologic Evaluation

The landmark lines that designate the intact borders of the acetabulum are well demonstrated on the AP pelvic radiograph. Also, the oblique pelvic views can be used to demonstrate the anterior or posterior columns of the acetabulum without superimposition. CT scans are valuable for identifying the fracture configuration (Fig. 12-34).

Complications

Complications include infection, nerve injury (sciatic, femoral, or superior gluteal nerves), heterotopic ossification, avascular necrosis, malunion, and posttraumatic arthritis.

Treatment

Nondisplaced acetabular fractures with good congruity of the hip joint are often treated with skeletal traction and close monitoring to ensure that the fracture site does not subsequently displace.

Displaced and unstable acetabular fractures can be difficult for the surgeon to treat; these fractures are often comminuted and are intra-articular, requiring near-perfect reduction for good functional outcome. Surgical decision making and applied techniques are complex.

Rehabilitation focuses on maintaining range of motion and progressive ambulation with protected weight-bearing.

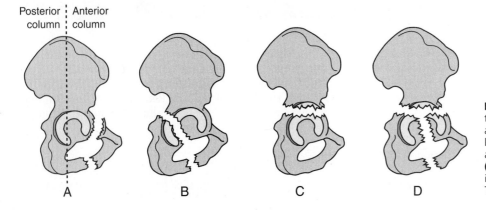

Posterior column : Anterior column

A   B   C   D

Figure 12-32 The innominate bone and the acetabulum are divided into *anterior* and *posterior columns* to reference the location of trauma. Classification of acetabular fractures: **(A)** anterior column, **(B)** posterior column, **(C)** transverse, involving both columns, **(D)** complex or T-shaped, involving both columns.

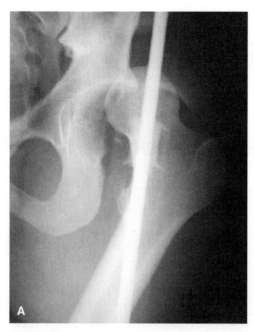
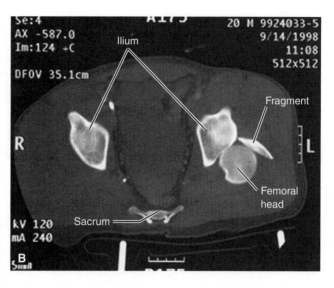

Figure 12-33 Femoral head posterior dislocation with posterior wall acetabular fracture. **(A)** AP radiograph of the dislocated left hip. The metal bar is first-aid splint device. **(B)** Axial CT scan shows the femoral head posterior to the ilium, with an adjacent large fracture fragment from the acetabulum that has moved superiorly with the femoral head. *(Image courtesy of John C. Hunter, MD, University of California, Davis School of Medicine.)*

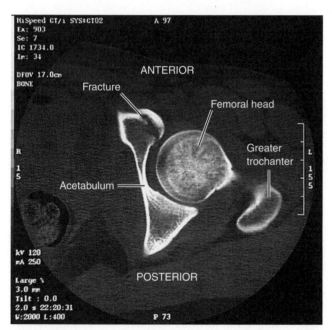

Figure 12-34 Axial CT scan of the left hip reveals an anterior column fracture of the acetabulum. Note on this slice the greater trochanter seems separate from the proximal femur; this appears so because the slice is just above the level of the femoral neck. On the next few slices the femoral neck would be visible.

Fractures of the Proximal Femur

Incidence and Mechanism of Injury

More than 300,000 hip fractures occur in the United States annually. The average age of occurrence is 77 years for women, 72 years for men. The majority of these patients are female and have mild to severe osteoporosis. Falls are the most frequent cause of fracture, although the bone may fracture first, precipitating the fall.

Proximal femur fractures due to trauma are uncommon in children and young adults because of the inherent strength of this bone. Great force is required to fracture the proximal femur in these age groups, and motor vehicle accidents are the usual precipitating mechanism.

Stress fractures in the proximal femur may be seen in young adults; these are usually associated with cyclical loading stresses as seen in distance runners, military recruits, and ballet dancers (Fig. 12-35).

Radiologic Evaluation

The radiographic evaluation of proximal femur fractures is usually complete on the AP and lateral views (either a mediolateral frog-leg view or the axiolateral groin–lateral view).

CT, magnetic resonance imaging (MRI), or radionuclide bone scans may supplement the radiographs. These modalities are especially valuable in the detection of subtle or impacted fractures or in confirming the presence of a fracture when conventional radiographs are negative but the index of suspicion is high. MRI is currently the choice of study for diagnosing stress fractures.

Classification

Proximal femur fractures are commonly referred to as "hip" fractures. Although the term is not exactly incorrect, it is too general to be useful for clinical management decisions. Proximal femur fractures can be broadly divided into intracapsular and extracapsular fractures (Fig. 12-36). The distinction in these two groups is not only in anatomic location but also in potential for vascular disruption and healing complications. These two groups of fractures have very different surgical treatment choices and prognoses.

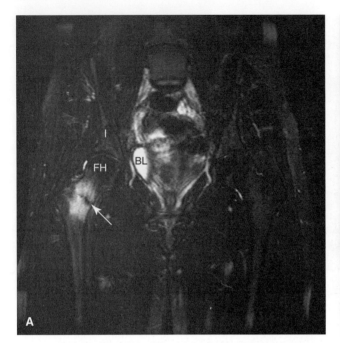
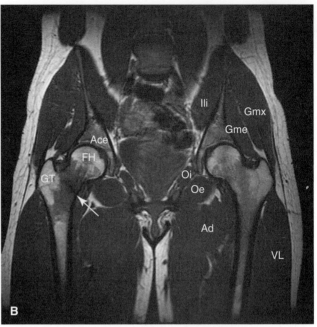

Figure 12-35 Stress fracture of the femoral neck in a 20-year-old female runner seen on two sequences. **(A)** Coronal T2-weighted MRI of the hip demonstrates a linear band of low signal (arrow) with adjacent area of high signal . Stress fractures are readily seen on T2 sequences, as the low signal fracture line will be surrounded by the bright high signal of adjacent bone edema. Fluid is bright on T2, so the urine in the bladder *(Bl)* is also high signal. **(B)** Coronal T1-weighted MRI also demonstrates the fracture line as low signal and the surrounding edema as an intermediate signal. Other structures are FH, femoral head; GT, greater trochanter; Ace, acetabulum; Oi, obturator internus; OE, obturator externus; Ad, adductor; VL, vastus lateralis; Gmx, gluteus maximus; Gme, gluteus medius.

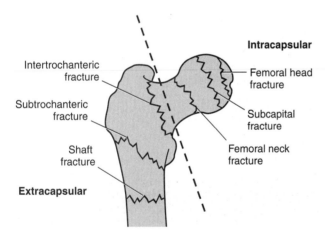

Figure 12-36 Fractures of the proximal femur are broadly divided into *intracapsular* and *extracapsular* sites. Intracapsular fractures are especially vulnerable to posttraumatic vascular complications because of the injury potential of blood vessels in close proximity.

Intracapsular Fractures

Intracapsular fractures of the proximal femur are located within the hip joint capsule. These include the *femoral head, subcapital,* and *femoral neck* regions. The femoral neck can also be subdivided into *transcervical* and *basicervical* regions.

Complications Intracapsular fractures are fraught with complications because of the frequently associated tearing of the *circumflex femoral arteries.* These vessels form a ring at the base of the neck, and ascending branches supply the femoral neck and head. Only a minor blood supply is

available through the foveal artery in the ligamentum teres at the femoral head. The primary blood supply to the neck and head is dependent on the integrity of these vessels. The proximity of the vascular configuration is readily susceptible to injury when this region is fractured. Posttraumatic complications include avascular necrosis, delayed union, and nonunion (Fig. 12-37).

Treatment Surgical treatment varies depending on the amount of displacement, stability of the fracture site, and additional factors including age, health, and prior functional status of the patient.

Impacted, nondisplaced fractures have up to a 20% probability of subsequently displacing. These fractures are often fixated with three cancellous screws. Displaced fractures in young adults are also usually treated with multiple screw fixation.

Femoral neck fractures in elderly patients are usually treated with some type of prosthetic replacement, either bipolar or unipolar hemiarthroplasty, or total hip arthroplasty. The advantages of prosthetic replacement over internal fixation for this age group include quicker full weight-bearing ambulation and elimination of the risks of nonunion, avascular necrosis, failure of fixation, and subsequent need for a second surgery.

Rehabilitation involves progressive ambulation skills and restoration of range of motion and strength.

Extracapsular Fractures

Extracapsular fractures of the proximal femur occur below the distal attachment of the joint capsule at the trochanteric region.

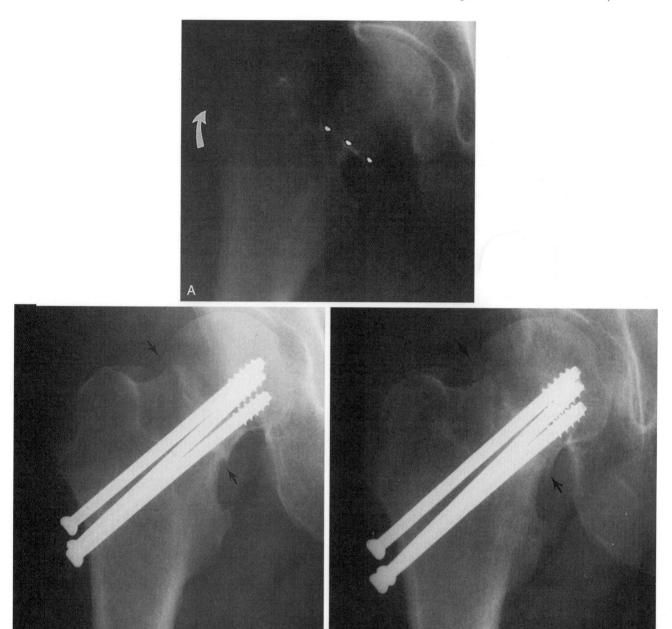

Figure 12-37 Femoral neck fracture. This 52-year-old man injured his hip in a fall off a truck bed as he was unloading furniture. **(A)** Anteroposterior view of the right hip shows a complete fracture of the femoral neck with superior displacement. The open arrows mark the borders of the femoral neck just proximal to the fracture site. **(B)** Restoration of alignment and good compression is obtained via fixation with three compression screws. The arrows mark the extent of the fracture line. **(C)** Follow-up films 9 weeks later show no evidence of healing. The fracture line remains radiolucent and no new bone growth is noted. The delayed union of this fracture is most likely caused by the damage sustained by the major blood vessels in this region. All intracapsular fractures are susceptible to complications in healing because of the frequently associated tearing of the circumflex femoral arteries. It can be assumed that the major displacement of the fracture fragments at the time of injury contributed to the severity of the damage to the vessels.

Extracapsular fractures are divided into two subgroups: *intertrochanteric* and *subtrochanteric* fractures. Intertrochanteric fractures are located in the region between the greater and lesser trochanters, often extending diagonally from one to the other (Fig. 12-38). Intertrochanteric fractures account for 50% of all fractures of the proximal femur. Subtrochanteric fractures occur below the intertrochanteric line, at the level of the lesser trochanter or immediately distal to it.

Complications In contrast to intracapsular fractures, this region's blood supply is not precarious or prone to injury. The trochanteric region is supplied by branches from the circumflex artery and also from nearby muscle attachments. Posttraumatic complications such as avascular necrosis or nonunion are rare.

Complications associated with intertrochanteric fractures are related to fixation failure leading to a varus deformity.

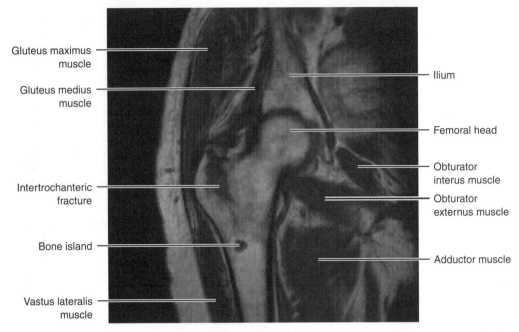

Figure 12-38 Intertrochanteric hip fracture as seen on a coronal T1-weighted MRI of the hip.

Treatment options are acceptance of the deformity (in patients who are marginal ambulators or poor surgical risks) or revision with prosthetic replacement.

Treatment Surgical internal fixation includes angled plate and sliding hip screw combinations or intermedullary rods. Rehabilitation involves protected weight-bearing ambulation in the early healing phases, followed by progressive restoration of strength, range of motion, and functional skills.

Hip Dislocation

Hip dislocations are due to high-energy trauma such as motor vehicle accidents or falls from heights. The hip can dislocate anteriorly, posteriorly, or centrally through the acetabulum. About 90% of hip dislocations occur posteriorly and are associated with concomitant fractures. Fractures of the acetabulum, femoral head, and patella are most often involved.

Radiologic Evaluation

On the AP pelvic radiograph, the heads of the femurs should normally be equal in size. In posterior hip dislocations the affected femoral head appears smaller. In anterior dislocations the affected femoral head appears larger because it is further from the image receptor and undergoes magnification.

Oblique views may be obtained to ascertain the presence of osteochondral fragments and assess the integrity of the acetabulum.

CT scans are usually obtained after closed reduction to assess the femoral head and congruency of joint surfaces, to screen for the possibility of intra-articular fragments, and to rule out associated fractures of the femoral head and acetabulum (see Fig. 12-33).

Complications

The prognosis for a good functional outcome after hip dislocation is best in those patients who do not have associated fractures at the hip. Posttraumatic arthritis is the most frequent long-term complication of hip dislocation, resulting in a painful and degenerative joint. Incidence is significantly higher with associated acetabular or femoral head fractures.

Avascular necrosis is a complication that may result from (1) the acute injury, (2) the prolonged period of time the hip remained dislocated prior to reduction, or (3) repeated attempts at reduction. It may become clinically apparent up to 5 years after the original injury.

Sciatic nerve injury complicates 10 to 20% of posterior hip dislocations. Injury to the femoral nerve and artery is associated with anterior dislocations.

Heterotopic ossification occurs in 2% of patients; incidence rises with surgery.

Thromboembolism risk necessitates prophylactic treatment.

Treatment

Closed reduction via longitudinal traction is achieved under general anesthesia or intravenous sedation. Open reduction is necessary when closed reduction fails or when fracture of the acetabulum or femur requires fragment excision or internal fixation. Rehabilitation involves protected weight-bearing and progressive ambulation, range of motion, and strengthening.

Pathological Conditions at the Hip[10,19–21,37–60]

Degenerative Joint Disease of the Hip

Degenerative joint disease (DJD), also referred to as *osteoarthritis*, is the most common disease affecting the hip joints.

Etiology

The etiology of DJD at the hip may be primary, developing without a clear precursor, or secondary, directly related to some predisposing trauma or pathological condition. Secondary, osteoarthritis in the hip may be due to a variety of preexisting conditions such as fracture, Paget's disease, epiphyseal disorders, congenital dislocation, avascular necrosis, or other inflammatory arthritides.

Clinical Presentation

Progressive pain and loss of joint motion are the clinical features of DJD. Ambulation becomes impaired from loss of joint congruity as well as from the increased pain upon weight-bearing.

Radiologic Findings

The radiographic hallmarks of DJD at the hip joint include (Fig. 12-39):

- Joint space narrowing
- Sclerotic subchondral bone
- Osteophyte formation at the joint margins

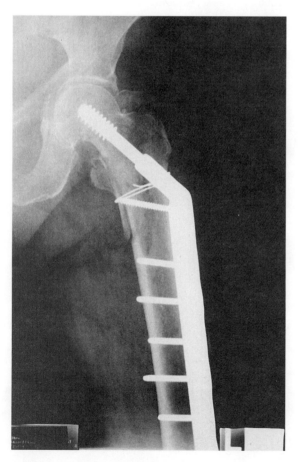

Figure 12-39 Intertrochanteric fracture of the hip. This postoperative film demonstrates fracture fixation via a side plate and screw combination device. The fracture line is evident, extending diagonally through the intertrochanteric region to the proximal femoral shaft. Some comminution is evident, and a large fragment on the medial shaft is noted. The imposed added densities of swelling in the soft tissues are seen.

- Cyst or pseudocyst formation
- Migration of the femoral head

The first three findings are common in the degenerative changes of any joint. The last two findings are more characteristic of the hip joint.

Cysts are the result of degeneration of the articular cartilage. Loss of the buffering effect afforded by the articular cartilage results in microfractures in the subchondral bone. These fractures permit intrusion of joint synovial fluid into periarticular bone. As a result, cysts are formed, which show up radiographically as distinctive subarticular radiolucent lesions. In the acetabulum these cysts are called *Egger's cysts* (see Fig. 2-42).

Another feature of DJD in the hip joint is the migration of the femoral head. Destruction of the articular cartilage alters normal joint congruity between the femoral head and the acetabulum. The most common pattern of altered surface relationship is for the femoral head to migrate to or articulate in a superomedial position relative to its normal position.

As in other joints affected by DJD, the severity of degenerative changes evident on radiograph does not always correlate with the severity of the clinical symptoms. Pain, stiffness, and loss of function may be of a greater degree than radiographic evidence would seem to justify, and conversely, symptoms may be moderate in the presence of severe radiographic changes.

Treatment

Conservative treatment of hip joint DJD is designed with the goals of decreasing pain, restoring flexibility and strength, and preserving functional activities and ambulation with assistive devices as needed to unload the joint from full weight-bearing stresses.

Surgical treatment is necessary in severe cases of DJD and may include wedge osteotomy to alter joint biomechanics and promote weight bearing on an uninvolved surface of the femoral head; femoral head and neck resection; *hemiarthroplasty* to replace a degenerative femoral head; or *total hip arthroplasty* to replace the degenerative femoral head and degenerative acetabulum. *Hip resurfacing* is a more recent modification of joint replacement, offered to younger patients with good bone density (Figs. 12-40, 12-41, and 12-42).

Functional Leg Length

Rehabilitation after surgical treatment focuses on a restoration of functional range of motion and functional strength and should also include equalization of functional leg length. Some surgical procedures may temporarily lengthen the lower extremity when the musculature is tightened to obtain joint stability; this effect is usually temporary, and the leg will "shorten" over a period of months. Some surgical procedures do result, in some patients, in a shorter lower extremity.

Radiographic evaluation is the only method to obtain *true leg length* measurements. However, in postsurgical rehabilitation, obtaining the multiple radiographs needed to assess true leg length measurements is *not* important. Knowing true leg length is not necessary to treat the functional leg length difference, which is not a fixed measurement.

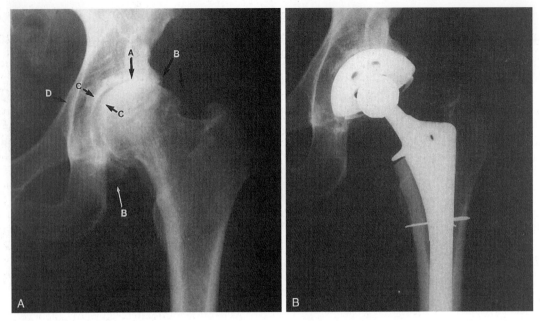

Figure 12-40 Total hip replacement. **(A)** The preoperative film of this severely degenerative hip joint of a 44-year-old man demonstrates the classic signs of degenerative joint disease: *A,* Narrowed joint space with superior migration of the femoral head; *B,* osteophyte formation at the joint margins of both the acetabulum and the femoral head; *C,* sclerosis of subchondral bone on both sides of the joint surface; *D,* acetabular protrusion, a bony outpouching of the acetabular cup in response to the progressive superior and medial migration of the femoral head. **(B)** Postoperative film shows a total hip arthroplasty. Both the acetabular and the femoral portions of the joint have been resected and replaced with prosthetic components.

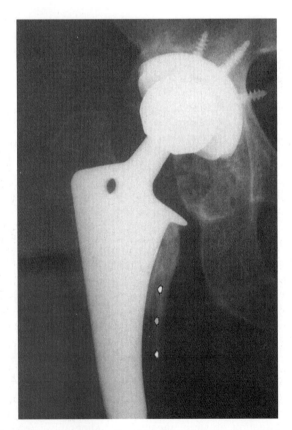

Figure 12-41 Loosening of a total hip prosthesis. The radiolucent streak paralleling the medial aspect of the stem of the femoral component (open arrows) represents space within the shaft of the femur caused by unwanted movement of the femoral prosthesis.

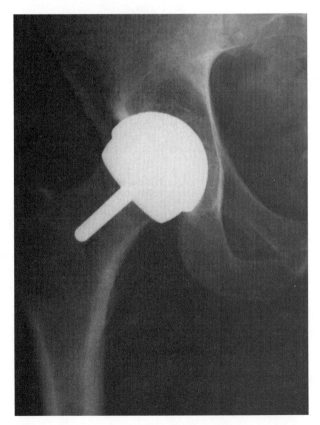

Figure 12-42 Hip resurfacing. This alternative to conventional total hip arthroplasty is usually performed on younger patients with good bone density. A metal coating is cemented over the femoral head, and a metal liner is impacted into the acetabulum. This liner has a coating to promote ingrowth of bone to further stabilize it. Long-term risks include femoral neck fracture and metal-on-metal wear debris.

Functional leg length takes into account not only the length of the bones but multiple other factors, both static and dynamic, that can affect the level of the iliac crests when the patient is *standing*. Factors that affect functional leg length can include the following:

- Pelvic obliquity
- Lumbosacral scoliosis
- Hip flexion contractures
- Hip adductor contractures
- Knee flexion contractures
- Knee varus or valgus deformities
- Asymmetrical foot pronation
- DJD at the ankles
- DJD of the knees
- DJD of the contralateral hip joint
- Degenerative processes at the lumbar spine
- Joint arthroplasty of either knee or of the contralateral hip

Some of these factors are related to degenerative processes; others may be related to compensatory maneuvers that have occurred in the body over a period of years to adapt to the progressively degenerative hip joint or other degenerative joints. Unconscious adaptations in the kinetic chain of the body occur to position the *face forward and eyes level to the horizon*. Surgically reconstructing the hip joint will abruptly alter these relationships inherent in the kinetic chain of the body.

The physical or occupational therapist must assess functional leg length, in standing, throughout the course of rehabilitation and make necessary adjustments with heel or shoe lifts to obtain a level pelvis. The expense of a permanent shoe lift should be delayed until the positive changes of rehabilitation (reduced contractures, strengthened muscles) are sufficient and further change is unlikely. Temporary lifts inside the shoe, or unmatched shoes, can suffice for the interim.

A level pelvis will not only enhance normal gait, balance, and strength potential but will help align the spine so that the eyes are level to the horizon, negating the need for compensatory (and possibly painful) measures elsewhere in the lower extremity joints or spine.

Rheumatoid Arthritis of the Hip

Rheumatoid arthritis is a progressive, systemic, autoimmune inflammatory disease primarily affecting synovial joints. Incidence is three times greater in women, and onset is most common in young adulthood.

Clinical Presentation

The clinical features of rheumatoid arthritis are morning joint stiffness, bilateral and symmetrical swelling of the joints, pain and functional disability, rheumatoid nodules, positive rheumatoid factor test, and radiographic changes consistent with rheumatoid arthritis.

Radiologic Findings

Rheumatoid arthritis at the hip is characterized by:

- Osteoporosis of periarticular areas, becoming more generalized with advancement of the disease
- Symmetrical and concentric joint space narrowing

- Articular erosions, located either centrally or peripherally in the joint
- Synovial cysts located within nearby bone
- Periarticular swelling and joint effusions
- Axial migration of the femoral head
- Acetabular protrusion

In the hip joint, osteoporosis is often first seen at the femoral head. Concentric joint space narrowing will promote an axial migration of the femoral head into the acetabulum, sometimes causing *acetabular protrusion,* an expansion of the acetabulum into the pelvis (Fig. 12-43). Articular erosions become evident when the joint surfaces lose their optimal congruity. The spherical shape of the femoral head becomes distorted, and the acetabulum loses its cuplike appearance. Synovial cysts may be located in proximity to the joint, at the acetabulum or femoral head. Joint effusions may be difficult to identify on plain radiographs and are best demonstrated on MRI.

A distinct difference between DJD and rheumatoid arthritis is that rheumatoid arthritis has minimal or absent reparative processes. Thus, radiographic features such as sclerotic subchondral bone and osteophyte formation, hallmarks of DJD, are not features of rheumatoid arthritis. The radiograph may show characteristics of both processes, however, because both processes may occur at a joint as separate entities. Remissions and exacerbations are typical in rheumatoid arthritis. Destructive changes from a prior exacerbation can cause mechanical stresses that predispose the joint to secondary degenerative processes while the joint is in remission from the rheumatoid arthritis.

Treatment

Conservative treatment addresses both pain and disability. Pharmacological treatments include nonsteroidal antiinflammatory drugs as well as more aggressive corticosteroids, gold salts, and immunosuppressive drugs. Rehabilitation focuses on pain relief modalites, splinting, adaptive functional and ambulatory devices, and exercise to promote strength and range of motion and minimize deformity.

Surgical treatment in advanced cases is total hip joint arthroplasty. Rehabilitation after joint arthroplasty is the same as described for joint arthroplasty due to DJD. Restoration of functional range of motion and strength and equalization of functional leg length are critical for pain-free mobility.

Avascular Necrosis of the Proximal Femur

Avascular necrosis (AVN) of the proximal femur is a complicated disease process initiated by an interruption of blood supply to the femoral head, causing bone tissue death. AVN can have different presentations. If an infarction affects a local segment of bone, it is called *osteochondritis dissecans.* This is most often seen in weight-bearing bones. An infarction that affects an entire epiphysis in a growing child is called *epiphyseal ischemic necrosis.* The proximal femur is the most common location for this occurrence.

Etiology

The etiology of femoral head avascular necrosis is diverse. Although avascular necrosis can develop idiopathically, most

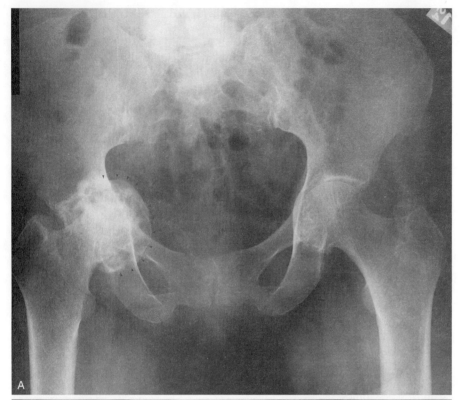

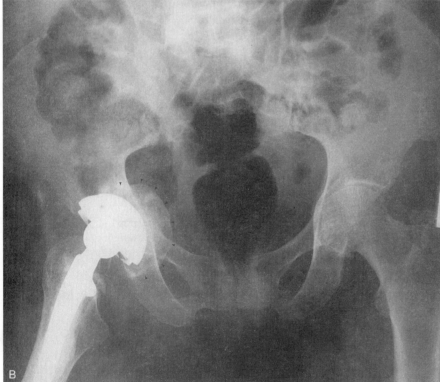

Figure 12-43 Acetabular protrusion. **(A)** The hip joints of this 79-year-old woman with rheumatoid arthritis also show characteristics of osteoarthritis; both processes may occur at a joint as separate entities. Additionally, destructive changes from a prior rheumatoid exacerbation can cause mechanical stresses that predispose the joint to secondary osteoarthritic processes while the joint is in remission from the rheumatoid arthritis. The striking feature of this film, however, is the large acetabular protrusion of the right hip joint (outlined with small black triangles). This bony pouching of the acetabulum into the pelvis is a result of concentric joint space narrowing and axial migration of the femoral head through osteoporotic periarticular bone. **(B)** After total hip arthroplasty, the deformity of acetabular protrusion is still evident.

conditions that disrupt the blood supply to a segment of bone can be divided into three categories:

- Conditions that result in external blood vessel compression or disruption near or within the bone, such as *trauma, infection,* or *steroid administration* (Fig. 12-44).

- Conditions that result in blood vessel occlusion because of thickening of the vessel wall, such as *radiation therapy, systemic lupus erythematosus,* or *giant cell arteritis.*
- Conditions that result in blood vessel blockage from a thomboembolic process, such as *alcoholism, diabetes,* or *sickle cell disease.*

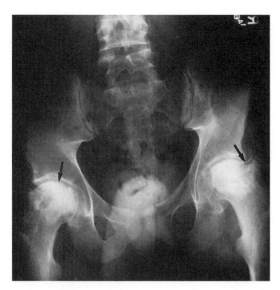

Figure 12-44 AVN of bilateral femoral heads with crescent sign. This 38-year-old man had been on steroid therapy for the management of chronic obstructive lung disease for several years prior to the development of AVN bilaterally in the femoral heads. This radiograph shows the late stages of AVN with advanced deformities. Note the loss of the ball-and-socket configuration of the hips secondary to progressive collapse of the bone. The left hip shows greater deformity than the right. The arrows point to the crescent sign, a radiolucent line paralleling the articular surface, which represents collapse of necrotic subchondral bone.

Posttraumatically, avascular necrosis is commonly associated with femoral neck fractures (Fig. 12-45). The greater the severity and displacement of the fracture, the greater the chance of avascular necrosis developing. Other direct traumas to the joint, such as contusions or dislocations, are less frequently associated with avascular necrosis but have the potential to develop avascular necrosis if the blood vessels become torn or sustain prolonged compression in the injury.

Epiphyseal ischemic necrosis at the femoral head can appear unilaterally or bilaterally. This expression of AVN is known as *Legg-Calvé-Perthes* disease. This disease is seen predominantly in young boys, the average age being about 6 years (Fig. 12-46). The literature either refers to this condition as an idiopathic avascular necrosis or associates it with subtle trauma, synovitis, infection, or metabolic bone disease.

Clinical Presentation

The earliest clinical signs of AVN at the femoral head are related to the synovitis or inflammatory response of the joint. Nonspecific dull pain in the joint, thigh, or leg is often reported. Adults eventually exhibit limited joint motion and a progressive painful limp. Children often exhibit a painless, slowly evolving limp. If the epiphyses are affected bilaterally, a waddling-type gait may be seen.

Radiologic Findings

Radiographic evaluation in the initial stages of AVN may appear normal for several weeks. One of the first radiographic signs, appearing as early as 4 weeks postinjury, is a radiolucent crescent image, representing the collapse of the necrotic subchondral bone of the femoral head (see Fig. 12-44). This crescent sign appears parallel to the superior rim of the femoral head, subjacent to the articular surface.

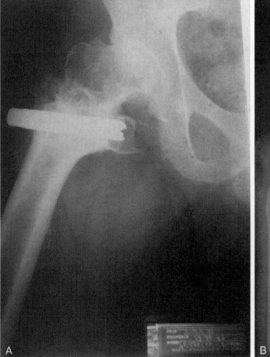
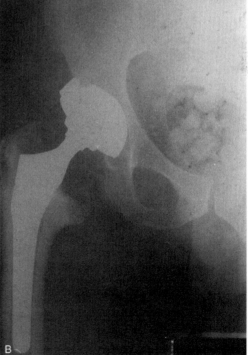

Figure 12-45 Advanced AVN of the femoral head, resected. **(A)** This 72-year-old man underwent a hip pinning several years earlier to fixate a femoral neck fracture. Healing was complicated by vascular interruption. The femoral head became necrotic and, over the years, progressively collapsed until the hip joint was no longer functional and ambulation was severely impaired. **(B)** The femoral head was resected and a total hip arthroplasty performed. The postoperative film shows the femoral component articulated in the acetabular cup. *(From Richardson and Iglarsh,[15] pp. 653 and 673, with permission.)*

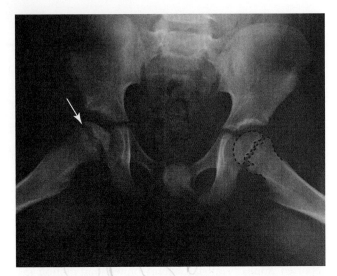

Figure 12-46 Legg–Calvé–Perthes disease. Necrosis of the secondary epiphysis of the femoral head developed idiopathically in this 7-year-old boy. Note the flattening and irregularity of the right side femoral head (arrows). The left femoral head and growth plate has been outlined to show a normal configuration.

Sclerosis and cyst formation at the femoral head are other characteristic signs of the initial necrotic processes and healing attempts taking place. These radiographic signs can be distinguished from the similar characteristic signs of osteoarthritis by the normal preservation of the radiographic joint space, which is not involved in the necrotic process.

In advanced stages of AVN, the femoral head will collapse, or appear flattened, because of structural weakness and impaired ability to withstand weight-bearing forces. The entire femoral head and neck will become more radiodense because of new bone attempting to heal the microfractures of the trabeculae and because of calcification of necrotic marrow. Eventually the progressive collapse of the femoral head will alter joint surface congruity and involve the acetabulum. At this advanced stage the joint space will be markedly compromised.

Radiologists identify the stages of progression of the disease by the presence of the foregoing signs. Table 12-1 provides a summary of the radiologic staging of avascular necrosis of the femoral head.

Advanced Imaging

Radionuclide bone scans identify increased uptake at the site of the lesion soon after injury. Currently, however, MRI is considered the most appropriate study for early sensitivity and specificity in diagnosing AVN (Fig. 12-47).

Treatment

Successful healing with conservative treatment is common in younger patients. Generally, the prognosis is better in younger patients because they possess a healthier, more adaptable blood supply. Revascularization of the femoral head is often achieved with conservative treatment, which may include prolonged avoidance of weight-bearing, traction, bracing, casting, and exercise.

The prognosis in adults is more variable and may or may not require surgical intervention. The course and prognosis

TABLE 12-1 ● Radiologic Staging of Avascular Necrosis of the Femoral Head	
Stage	**Criteria**
0	Normal x-ray film, normal bone scan, and MRI
I	Normal x-ray film, abnormal bone scan, or MRI A. Mild (under 15%) B. Moderate (15%–30%) C. Severe (over 30%)
II	Sclerosis and/or cyst formation in femoral head A. Mild (under 15%) B. Moderate (15%–30%) C. Severe (over 30%)
III	Subchrondral collapse (crescent sign) without flattening A. Mild (under 15%) B. Moderate (15%–30%) C. Severe (over 30%)
IV	Flattening of head *without* joint narrowing or acetabular involvement A. Mild (under 15% of surface *and* under 2 mm depression) B. Moderate (15%–30% of surface *or* 2–4 mm depression) C. Severe (over 30% of surface *or* over 4 mm depression)
V	Flattening of head *with* joint narrowing and/or acetabular involvement A. Mild B. Moderate (determined as above plus estimate of acetabular involvement) C. Severe
VI	Advanced degenerative changes

From Steinberg, ME (ed.): The Hip and Its Disorders. WB Saunders, Philadelphia, 1991, p. 634.

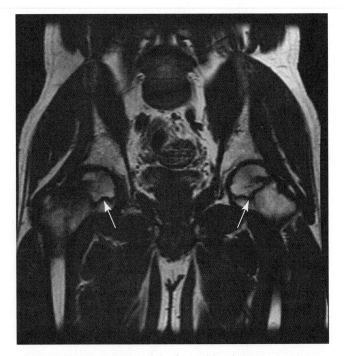

Figure 12-47 Bilateral AVN of the femoral heads in a young woman who has been on long-term corticosteroid therapy for systemic lupus erythematosus (SLE). Coronal T1-weighted MRI of the hips shows serpiginous (wavy) lines of low signal intensity bilaterally with intermediate signal at the right femoral neck and shaft representing edema.

of this AVN at the femoral head is highly variable. The events from initial avascularity through revascularization, reossification, and remodeling may take several years, if not arrested at any stage. Surgical intervention is often necessary in older patients and may include drilling into the femoral head to hasten revascularization; grafting healthy bone into the drill holes to assist the repair process; varus derotation osteotomy to provide a viable weight-bearing surface on the femoral head; or, as a last resort, osteotomy and replacement arthroplasty.

Slipped Femoral Capital Epiphysis

Slipped femoral capital epiphysis (SFCE) is a posteromedioinferior displacement of the proximal femoral epiphysis that occurs during childhood or adolescence. This condition is the most common disorder of the hip in adolescence.

Etiology

A weakening of the epiphyseal plate at the junction of the femoral neck and head allows the head to displace. The etiology of this weakness is unknown but is theorized to be related to an imbalance between growth hormone and the sex hormones, which weaken all epiphyseal plates. The extreme shear and weight-bearing forces inherent to the functioning of the hip joint render the epiphysis vulnerable to displacement.

Other etiologies have been implicated, including trauma, obesity, vertical orientation of the epiphyseal plate, retroversion of the proximal femur, renal osteodystrophy, and physical activity.

Clinical Presentation

Clinical symptoms include vague patterns of pain in the hip or knee area, limited hip range of motion, antalgic gait, and limb length shortening. The onset is insidious and often coincides with growth spurts at puberty. The disorder appears twice as often in boys; obesity and delayed maturation are common characteristics in affected individuals of either sex.

Radiologic Findings

Radiographic abnormalities will coincide with the amount of slippage present. Radiographic signs on the AP projection include a blurring and widening of the physis and a decreased height of the epiphysis relative to the contralateral hip. The lateral frog-leg projection best demonstrates the amount of epiphyseal displacement (Fig. 12-48).

Treatment

Conservative treatment is not generally successful, and surgical fixation is usually necessary to prevent further slippage and stabilize the physis. In situ pinning is the most common treatment.

Developmental Dysplasia of the Hip

Developmental dysplasia of the hip (DDH) is a malformation of the hip joint found at birth or in young children beginning to walk. This condition is also referred to as *developmental*

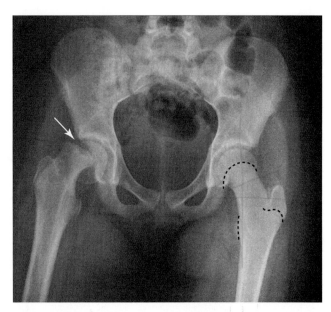

Figure 12-48 Slipped femoral capital epiphysis. This lateral frog-leg view of the right hip of a 13-year-old girl demonstrates the posterior, medial, and inferior displacement of the epiphysis of the femoral head that is characteristic for this condition. The weakness of the epiphyseal plate that permits this displacement is theorized to be related to an imbalance between growth hormone and sex hormones.

dislocation of the hip (still *DDH*). The older terminology for this condition was *congenital hip dysplasia* or *congenital hip dislocation*. The change in terminology reflects a shift in the literature toward developmental, rather than congenital, etiologies.

Etiology

Proposed theories for etiology include genetic, hormonal, or mechanical (related to the fetus position in utero) causes. DDH usually affects the left hip, is more predominant in girls, and has a familial tendency. Risk factors include firstborn children and children born in a breech position.

Clinical Presentation

The presentation of the disorder is variable. The difference between dysplasia and dislocation is the amount of the malformation of the joint.

DDH may be evident upon newborn physical examination via Ortolani's or Barlowe's orthopedic maneuvers or by the physical characteristics of uneven thigh skin folds, uneven leg lengths, and less mobility at the hip on the affected side. DDH may also be subtle and not clinically evident until later. Well-baby checkups routinely reassess the hip joints because of this possibility. Some mild cases of dysplasia may not even become apparent until adulthood.

Radiologic Findings

The head of the femur is not ossified in the infant, and the ossification center for the femoral head epiphysis does not appear until 3 to 6 months of age. Therefore the radiographic evaluation of this disorder is not assessed by

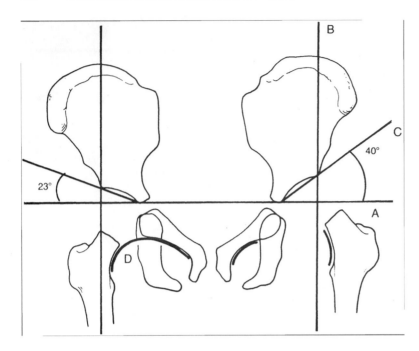

Figure 12-49 Radiological measurements in assessment of developmental dysplasia of the hip. A horizontal line **(A)** is drawn through the junctions of the iliac, ischial, and pubic bones at the center of the acetabulum (Hilgenreiner's line). A perpendicular line **(B)** is drawn through the outer border of the acetabulum (Perkins's line). The secondary ossification center of the femoral head (or, in its absence, the medial metaphyseal beak of the proximal femur) should lie within the inner lower quadrant formed by the intersection of these lines. The acetabular index, a measure of acetabular depth, can be estimated by inscribing a line **(C)** joining the inner and outer edges of the acetabulum. The angle formed by this line and line A is normally less than 30 degrees, as on the left. Increased angles, as on the right, indicate acetabular hypoplasia. Shenton's line **(D)** is inscribed along the inferior border of the femoral neck and inferior border of the superior pubic ramus. It is ordinarily smooth and unbroken. Proximal displacement of the femoral head in congenital hip dislocation results in interruption of line D.

direct visualization but by evaluating a series of drawn lines and intersecting angles relating the ossified portions of the pelvis to the ossified femoral shaft. From these measurements the depth of the acetabulum and the orientation of the cartilaginous femoral head are determined (Fig. 12-49).

MRI or ultrasound is very valuable in the assessment of DDH in the infant; the deformity of the acetabulum and femoral head can be well visualized prior to ossification.

Treatment

Early diagnosis and treatment is necessary in infancy, prior to ambulation, to promote normal joint development and prevent the debilitating consequences of later disabling deformity (Figs. 12-50 and 12-51).

Treatment in the newborn consists of a soft positioning harness to maintain reduction of the joint and allow normal articulation to develop. Beyond 6 months of age, treatment options include closed reduction under anesthesia, application of a hip spica body cast to maintain the reduction and allow the ligaments to shorten adaptively and stabilize the joint, or surgical intervention, including acetabular or intertrochanteric osteotomy, inverted labrum removal, or adductor tenotomy, also followed by cast application (Fig. 12-52).

Rehabilitation needs are extensive and include strengthening, stretching, positioning, and functional skill development.

Femoroacetabular Impingement With Labral Pathology

Femoroacetabular impingement describes a mechanical pathology that results from abutment of the femoral head with the acetabulum. The fibrocartilaginous labrum,

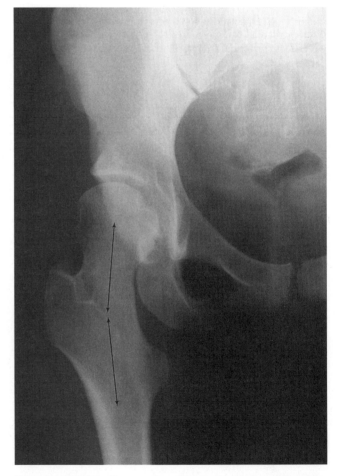

Figure 12-50 DDH with coxa valga. Abnormalities in the configuration of the acetabulum in the proximal femur are seen in this 20-year-old woman. Note the abnormally wide angle of inclination of the femoral neck to the femoral shaft (line arrows measuring 170 degrees), described as *coxa valga*.

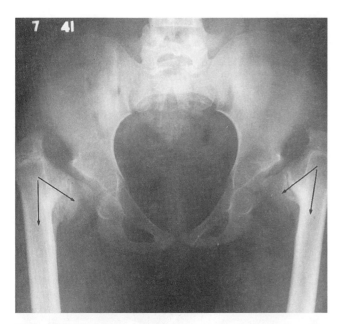

Figure 12-51 DDH with coxa vara. Abnormalities in the configuration of the acetabulum and proximal femur are present bilaterally in this teenager. The extremely small angles of inclination (line arrows measuring 50 degrees) of the femoral heads to the femoral shafts are described as *coxa vara* deformities.

attached to the acetabular rim, provides some structural resistance to movement of the femoral head within the acetabulum; as such, it is vulnerable to injury when normal joint arthrokinematics are compromised.

Etiology

Femoroacetabular impingement is associated with any predisposing factors that alter normal osseous anatomy at the hip. Factors include prior slipped femoral capital epiphysis, avascular necrosis, altered femoral head to neck junction configuration, acetabular retroversion, or developmental hip dysplasias. The abnormal hip anatomy will lead to painful symptoms when the patient performs activities that require repetitive extreme ranges of motion, or even when the patient performs normal ranges of motion over time.

Two types of impingement have been described: *cam* and *pincer*. Cam impingement occurs when the femoral head–neck junction is offset and the femoral head cannot fully clear the acetabular rim. Pincer impingement is due to "overcoverage" of the femoral head by the acetabulum, due to conditions such as a deep socket (coxa profunda), acetabular protrusion, and acetabular retroversion. Many patients have a combination of both types of impingement.

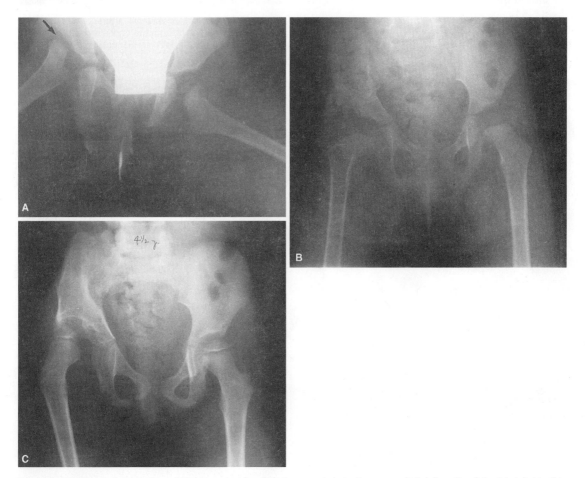

Figure 12-52 Surgical correction of DDH in a toddler. **(A)** Arrow points to the congenital deformity of the hip joint in this 16-month-old boy. For comparison, note the configuration of the normal left hip joint. This film was made preoperatively. **(B)** This follow-up film was made at 22 months of age. The child had undergone a posterior iliac osteotomy to create an acetabular fossa. Note the delay in the ossification of the femoral capital epiphysis on the right. **(C)** Follow-up film made when the child was 4½ years of age shows relatively satisfactory results. The proximal femur is adequately articulated in the surgically sculpted acetabulum, and the hip is functional for all ambulatory activities.

Clinical Presentation

Patients often present with snapping, clicking, limited hip range of motion, hip flexion contractures, and, most indicting, painful provocation tests. Anterior impingement is reproduced when the hip is passively moved to end range flexion, adduction, and internal rotation. Posterior impingement is reproduced with hip extension and external rotation. True hip locking is highly associated with labral tears.

Radiologic Findings

Pelvic and hip radiographs are assessed for alteration in proximal femur anatomy including head-to-neck angle, neck-to-shaft angle, and acetabular configuration. Characteristic findings for impingement include an osseous bump on the head-to-neck junction of the femur. This abnormal anatomic shape of the femoral head is coined the "pistol grip" deformity and associated with cam-type impingement, because the offset femoral head will not clear the acetabular rim adequately. The "figure eight" or "crossover" sign of the acetabulum represents an anterior rim that covers over too much of the femoral head, leading to pincer-type impingement. This sign is seen when the anterior and posterior acetabular rims do not meet superiorly as they should but instead cross over each other more distally (Fig. 12-53).

MR arthrography is the diagnostic modality of choice for visualizing labral tears (Fig. 12-54).

Treatment

The surgical goal is to restore normal head-to-neck junction offset and clearance of the femoral head within the acetabulum. This is achieved with bony resection at the

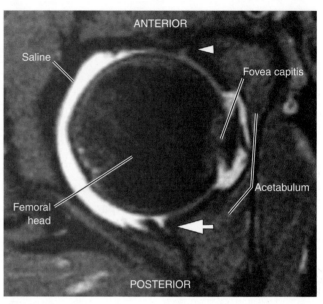

Figure 12-54 Labral tears. Axial MR arthrogram of the hip shows a posterior labral detachment from the underlying acetabular rim (arrow), as well as a blunting of the normally triangular anterior labrum (arrowhead).

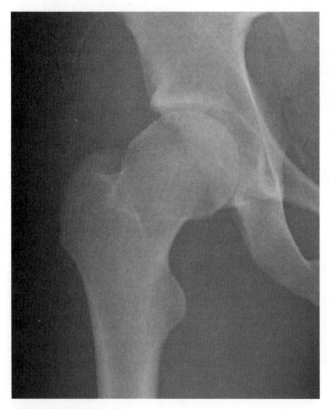

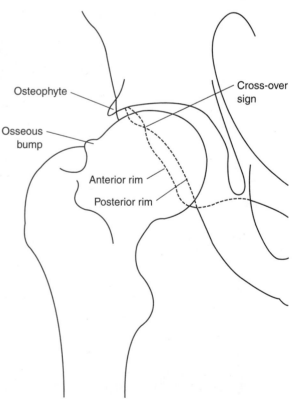

Figure 12-53 Radiographic signs of femoroacetabular impingement. The osseous bump on the subcapital area of the femoral head results in a convex shaped area instead of a normal concave shaped femoral head-to-neck junction. This is known as a "pistol grip" deformity and is associated with cam type impingement of the femoral head into the acetabulum. The "crossover" or "figure eight" sign refers to retroversion of the acetabulum. Normally the anterior and posterior rims of the acetabulum meet superiorly. In this case the anterior rim is lateral to the posterior rim and the lines of the rims are seen to cross more distally. This suggests an "overcoverage" of the femoral head by the acetabulum and is cause for anterior impingement.

head-to-neck junction and/or rim resection, resuturing healthy labral tissue back to the rim as possible. These surgeries are usually performed arthroscopically.

Interestingly, recent evidence supports a hypothesis that so-called primary osteoarthritis of the hip is actually secondary to femoroacetabular impingement rather than excessive contact stress. The implication is that surgical attempts to restore normal anatomy to avoid femoroacetabular impingement may be performed early, before major cartilage damage requires total hip arthroplasty.

Summary of Key Points

Routine Radiologic Evaluation

1. The routine radiographic evaluation of the *pelvis* is one projection: The *anteroposterior,* which demonstrates the entire pelvis, sacrum, coccyx, and lumbosacral articulation as well as both hip joints. Six lines reference the normal position of the acetabulum: the radiographic teardrop, the iliopubic line, the ilioischial line, the anterior acetabular rim, the posterior acetabular rim, and the acetabular roof. Disruptions in these line images may indicate fracture, dislocation, or pathology.

2. The routine radiographic evaluation of the unilateral hip includes two projections:
   ➤ *AP:* The normal ball-and-socket configuration of the hip joints is seen. Destruction of normal joint congruity may be caused by various pathologies including avascular necrosis, rheumatoid arthritis, degenerative joint disease, and destructive tumors.
   ➤ *Lateral frog-leg:* This view demonstrates the proximal femur from a mediolateral aspect so that the lesser trochanter is seen in profile. Correct position of the femoral head in the acetabulum is assessed by identifying the iliofemoral line, Shenton's hip line, and femoral neck angle.

Trauma Radiography

3. In low-energy injuries, the *AP pelvic* view is obtained to locate injuries. Additional views used to demonstrate specific anatomy are the following:
   ➤ *Oblique or Judet views of the pelvis:* These views demonstrate the columns of the acetabulum free of superimposition.
   ➤ *AP axial pelvic inlet view:* This view demonstrates the pelvic inlet.
   ➤ *AP axial pelvic outlet view:* This view demonstrates the superior and inferior pubic rami and ischia.
   ➤ *Axiolateral (groin-lateral) view of the proximal femur:* This view demonstrates most fractures of the proximal femur.
   ➤ *Computed or conventional tomography:* These are useful in diagnosing fracture characteristics in areas of complex topography.

4. In high-energy injuries, a *trauma survey* is necessary because the magnitude of force sufficient to disrupt the pelvic ring usually causes multiple associated injuries. The standard trauma survey includes AP views of the chest, abdomen, and pelvis and a lateral view of the cervical spine. Where available, high speed CT can evaluate all these areas at once on a *thorax-abdomen-pelvis (TAP)* series.

Fractures

5. *Fractures of the pelvis* are broadly classified as stable fractures or unstable fractures, in which two or more articulation sites on the pelvic ring are disrupted.

6. Stable *ischiopubic ramus fractures* comprise half of all pelvic fractures.

7. *Acetabular fractures* are most common at the posterior column or posterior rim of the cup and are frequently associated with femoral head impaction or posterior dislocation.

8. *Proximal femoral fractures* are classified as *intracapsular fractures,* often complicated by vascular disruption potentially progressing to avascular necrosis, and *extracapsular fractures,* in which vascular complication is rare.

Pathological Conditions at the Hip

9. *Degenerative joint disease (DJD)* at the hip joints is diagnosed on radiographs by (1) joint space narrowing, (2) sclerotic subchondral bone, and (3) osteophyte formation at joint margins, (4) radiolucent cysts known as Egger's cysts, and (5) superior migration of the femoral head secondary to articular cartilage loss and altered joint surface relationships. Note that the amount of radiographic evidence of degenerative joint disease may not always correlate with the severity of clinical symptoms.

10. Rehabilitation after joint arthoplasty restores range of motion, strength, and *functional leg length.* Functional leg length is the result of many static and dynamic factors affecting the overall kinetic chain of the body in standing.

11. *Rheumatoid arthritis* at the hip joints is evidenced radiographically by the bilateral presence of (1) demineralization of the femoral head, (2) concentric joint space narrowing, (3) axial migration of the femoral head into the acetabulum, sometimes causing acetabular protrusion, and (4) articular erosion loss of the ball-and-socket joint configuration. Reparative processes signified by subchondral sclerosis and osteophyte formation (hallmarks of DJD) are minimal or absent.

12. *Avascular necrosis (AVN)* of the proximal femur is the result of interrupted circulation to the femoral head. It is associated posttraumatically with intracapsular hip fractures but can also be seen idiopathically in both children and adults. Earliest detection is by radionuclide bone scans or MRI. Radiographic diagnosis is not conclusive until several weeks into the disease process.

13. *Slipped femoral capital epiphysis (SFCE)* is the most common disorder of the hip in adolescence, appearing twice as frequently in boys. Weakening of the epiphyseal plate at the junction of the femoral head and neck allows the femoral head to displace posteriorly, medially, and

interiorly. The frog-leg projection best demonstrates the amount of displacement.

14. *Developmental dysplasia of the hip (DDH)* is a malformation of the hip found at birth or young childhood. Radiographic evaluation measures lines and intersecting angles relative to the ossified portions of the pelvis and femoral shaft. MRI or ultrasound studies can provide direct visualization of the hip.

15. *Femoroacetabular impingement* describes a mechanical pathology that results from abutment of the femoral head with the acetabulum. Standard radiographs can show anatomic abnormalites of the proximal femur or acetabulum that contribute to maladaptive joint arthrokinematics. MR arthrography is most appropriate for diagnosing associated labral pathology.

 Please refer to the text's enclosed CD-ROM for the American College of Radiology's current Musculoskeletal Appropriateness Criteria for the following topics: *Avascular Necrosis of the Hip, Chronic Hip Pain, Imaging after Total Hip Arthroplasty.*

CASE STUDIES

CASE STUDY 1

Heterotopic Ossification After Femoral Fracture

The patient is a 30-year-old man participating in rehabilitation in physical therapy following open reduction and internal fixation of a midshaft fracture of the femur.

History of Trauma

The patient was a restrained passenger in a car struck from the side by a truck that ran a red light. Having an obvious open fracture to the femur, along with abrasions, he was immediately transferred by ambulance to the nearest hospital's emergency department.

Initial Imaging

Conventional radiographs ordered in the emergency department revealed a comminuted, displaced, and overriding midshaft femur fracture.

Intervention

The patient's fracture was reduced in the operating room the same day. The femur was stabilized with an intramedullary rod through the femoral shaft.

Physical Therapy Management

The patient began rehabilitation in physical therapy as an inpatient, and continued as an outpatient after hospital discharge. At 4 weeks postsurgery, the patient had progressed to partial weight-bearing ambulation with crutches. However, he continued to complain of severe pain at the fracture site, which was exacerbated with knee motion. Palpation of the soft tissues over the fracture site demonstrated increased warmth and swelling. Progress in knee flexion had halted at 70 degrees with a hard end feel. The therapist phoned the orthopedic surgeon and voiced concerns regarding these factors; the possibility of heterotopic ossification (HO) was discussed.

Additional Imaging

The patient was reevaluated by the orthopedic surgeon, and radiographs were ordered (Fig. 12-55). A diagnosis of heterotopic ossification surrounding the healing fracture site was confirmed.

Discussion

The physical therapist recognized that the patient's progress in rehabilitation was being limited by an unknown factor. The clinical signs of limited range of motion, localized warmth and swelling at the fracture site, and acute pain not commensurate with this subacute stage of healing could represent many abnormal conditions, including infection and thrombophlebitis. However, the probability of heterotopic ossification was greater, given the provocation of pain when the knee was flexed (stretching the involved soft tissues at the site of ossification). Additionally, key risk factors of heterotopic ossification were present: history of trauma, an open fracture with internal fixation, and the time frame (the time since surgery coincided with the time it normally takes for a mass to develop).

The physical therapist acted correctly in contacting the physician as soon as it became apparent that the course of rehabilitation

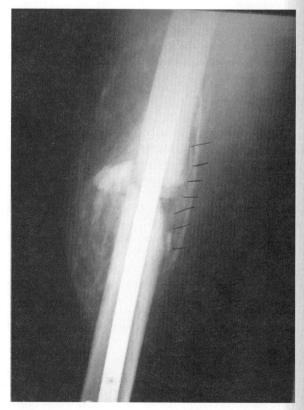

Figure 12-55 AP radiograph of the femur showing heterotropic bone formation at the fracture site 4 weeks after open reduction and internal fixation with an intermedullary rod.

was adversely affected and that imaging or laboratory studies were necessary to evaluate the new situation.

The case is summarized in Figure 12-56.

CRITICAL THINKING POINTS

Manifestation of heterotopic ossification is divided into three categories:

1. *Myositis ossificans progressiva* is a rare metabolic bone disease characterized by progressive metamorphosis of skeletal muscle to bone.

2. *Myositis ossificans circumscripta* is a localized soft tissue ossification after neurological injury or burns.

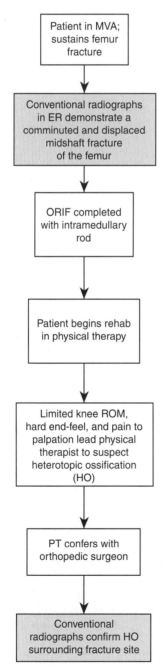

Figure 12-56 Pathway of case study events. Imaging is highlighted.

3. *Traumatic myositis ossificans* occurs from direct injury to muscle. This is the specific term for the type of heterotopic ossification seen in this case.

The reported incidence of traumatic myositis ossificans varies, but it is not uncommon. The incidence is highest in patients who undergo open reduction and internal fixation of a fracture. For instance, over half of patients with hip fracture develop myositis ossificans. The incidence increases to over 80% of patients if open reduction and internal fixation are performed.

Of all patients who develop heterotopic ossification, 10% to 20% will have significant functional deficits. The role of physical therapy is controversial. Some authors suggest that passive stretching causes microtrauma and predisposes the development of HO, whereas others stress the importance of stretching to retard fibrous ankylosis. Most of the literature supports the use of active and gentle passive range of motion exercises to maintain available joint range of motion and avoid progressive contracture.

Conventional radiographs are able to show evidence of heterotopic ossification 3 to 5 weeks postinjury. Bone scans detect early increases in vascularity and are a reliable indicator in making the earliest diagnosis.

CASE STUDY 2
Bone Infarct at the Proximal Femur

The patient is a 57-year-old man being treated by a physical therapist for management of low back, right buttock, and right posterior thigh pain.

History of Trauma

Prior to one of his physical therapy appointments, the patient's wife called to report that her husband had slipped and fallen on a wet floor while stepping out of the shower. She said he fell on his right hip and was experiencing increased thigh pain. The therapist requested that she bring him in to his appointment if he was able to walk.

Physical Therapy Reexamination

Patient Complaint

The patient reported an increase in the pain affecting his low back and the usual distribution of his thigh pain. He also noted new pain located at the greater trochanter, which he struck when he fell. He denied any other new symptoms.

Physical Examination

The patient was able to walk into physical therapy without assistance but with a slightly antalgic gait pattern, which had not been present previously. His lumbar active range of motion was limited slightly more than at prior appointments. All other testing with the physical examination was similar to previous exam findings with a few exceptions. The patient complained of hip pain at the end range of hip flexion, abduction, and combined flexion/adduction. He was very tender to palpation over the greater trochanter.

Additional Imaging

The physical therapist called the referring physician to report his findings. They agreed that the new clinical signs warranted radiographic examination. Conventional radiographs (Fig. 12-57) of the hip showed no evidence of fracture or other acute injury, but the radiologist's report noted a "lytic and sclerotic lesion in the subtrochanteric portion of the proximal right femur." The radiologist recommended magnetic resonance imaging (MRI) to determine the exact nature of the lesion.

The MRI was completed (Fig. 12-58), and the radiologist concluded that the lesion was a "remote bone infarction of the proximal right femur of doubtful clinical significance."

Outcome

The physical therapist and referring physician agreed that the bone infarction was probably not related to the patient's low back or posterior thigh symptoms, nor was it related to his new hip pain from the fall. The patient continued with treatment in physical therapy. His greater trochanter pain resolved in approximately 1 week, and his previous low back and posterior thigh symptoms improved gradually over the next 3 weeks.

Discussion

The physical therapist played an important role in this case by communicating quickly with the physician to obtain conventional radiographs for the patient after his fall. Serious acute injury was ruled out by the studies, but the unexpected finding in the proximal femur raised new concerns. The patient and his family feared the worst. Being familiar with radiography, the therapist was able to explain better the language in the radiologist's report to the family, helping to calm their fears until the MRI could be completed. Once the MRI report was available, the therapist again helped to educate the patient and his family about the report's meaning and redirected the patient's focus back to the management of his low back pain.

The case is summarized in Figure 12-59.

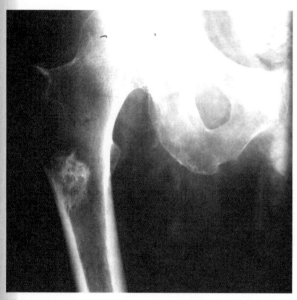

Figure 12-57 AP radiograph of the right femur. A lytic and sclerotic lesion is present at the subtrochanteric region.

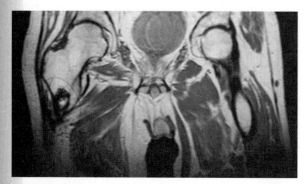

Figure 12-58 MR image demonstrating a remote bone infarct in the right proximal femur.

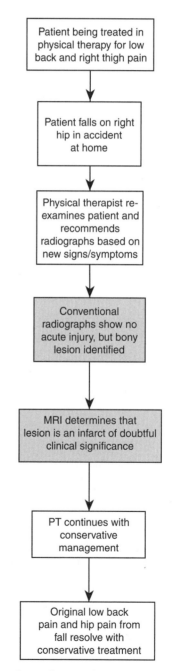

Figure 12-59 Pathway of case study events. Imaging is highlighted.

CRITICAL THINKING POINTS

This case illustrates a few important points:

1. A good working relationship between a physical therapist and referring physicians can expedite the diagnostic process when imaging is necessary to rule out significant injury after a new incident.

2. Incidental findings on diagnostic imaging, such as the bone infarct in this case, are not uncommon and must be considered as part of the entire clinical picture.

3. Incidental findings are not always easily identifiable as *incidental*. The professional collaboration between the three professionals enabled the incidental finding to be quickly and accurately devalued in this case.

4. Knowledge about diagnostic imaging helped the physical therapist to provide patient education to alleviate fear of the unknown.

Case studies adapted by J. Bradley Barr, PT, DPT, OCS.

References

1. Netter, FH: Atlas of Human Anatomy, ed. 4. Saunders, Philadelphia, 2006.
2. Nordin, M, and Frankel, VH: Basic Biomechanics of the Musculoskeletal System, ed. 3. Lippincott Williams & Wilkins, Philadelphia, 2001.
3. Whiting, W, and Zernicke, R: Biomechanics of Musculoskeletal Injury, ed. 2. Human Kinetics, Champaign, IL, 2008.
4. Norkin, CC, and Levangie, PK: Joint Structure and Function, A Comprehensive Analysis, ed. 2. FA Davis, Philadelphia, 1992.
5. Meschan, I: An Atlas of Radiographic Anatomy. WB Saunders, Philadelphia, 1960.
6. Weber, EC, Vilensky, JA, and Carmichael, SW: Netter's Concise Radiologic Anatomy. WB Saunders, Philadelphia, 2008.
7. American College of Radiology (ACR): Practice Guideline for the Performance and Interpretation of Magnetic Resonance Imaging (MRI) of the Hip and Pelvis for Musculoskeletal Disorders. 2006. Accessed July 22, 2008 at http://www.acr.org.
8. ACR: Practice Guideline for the Performance of Radiography of the Extremities. 2006. Accessed July 22, 2008 at http://www.acr.org.
9. Weissman, B, and Sledge, C: Orthopedic Radiology. WB Saunders, Philadelphia, 1986.
10. Greenspan, A: Orthopedic Radiology: A Practical Approach, ed. 4. Lippincott Williams & Wilkins, Philadelphia, 2004.
11. Bontrager, KL: Textbook of Radiographic Positioning and Related Anatomy, ed. 6. Mosby, St. Louis, MO, 2005.
12. Fischer, HW: Radiographic Anatomy: A Working Atlas. McGraw-Hill, New York, 1988.
13. Wicke, L: Atlas of Radiographic Anatomy, ed. 5. Lea & Febiger, Malvern, PA, 1994.
14. Frank, E, Smith, B, and Long, B: Merrill's Atlas of Radiographic Positions and Radiologic Procedures, ed. 11. Elsevier Health Sciences, Philadelphia, 2007.
15. Squires, LF, and Novelline, RA: Fundamentals of Radiology, ed. 4. Harvard University Press, Cambridge, MA, 1988.
16. Chew, FS: Skeletal Radiology: The Bare Bones, ed. 2. Williams & Wilkins, Philadelphia, 1997.
17. Weir, J, and Abrahams, P: An Atlas of Radiological Anatomy. Yearbook Medical, Chicago, 1978.
18. Krell, L (ed): Clark's Positioning in Radiology, Vol. 1, ed. 10. Yearbook Medical, Chicago, 1989.
19. ACR: Appropriateness Criteria for Chronic Hip Pain. 2003. Accessed July 22, 2008 at http://www.acr.org.
20. ACR: Appropriateness Criteria for Avascular Necrosis of the Hip. 2003. Accessed July 22, 2008 at http://www.acr.org.
21. ACR: Appropriateness Criteria for Imaging After Total Hip Arthroplasty. 2003. Accessed July 22, 2008 at http://www.acr.org.
22. Rockwood, CA, and Green, DP (eds): Fractures in Adults, ed. 5. Lippincott Williams & Wilkins, Philadelphia, 2002.
23. Beaty, J, and Kasar, J (eds): Rockwood and Wilkins' Fractures in Children, ed. 6. Lippincott Williams & Wilkins, Philadelphia, 2005.
24. Koval, KJ, and Zuckerman, JD: Handbook of Fractures, ed. 2. Lippincott Williams & Wilkins, Philadelphia, 2002.
25. Eiff, M, et al: Fracture Management for Primary Care. WB Saunders, Philadelphia, 2003.
26. Marchiori, DM: Clinical Imaging with Skeletal, Chest, and Abdomen Pattern Differentials. Mosby, St. Louis, MO, 1999.
27. Richardson, JK, and Iglarsh, ZA: Clinical Orthopedic Physical Therapy. WB Saunders, Philadelphia, 1994.
28. Yochum, TR, and Rowe, LJ: Essentials of Skeletal Radiology, ed. 3. Williams & Wilkins, Baltimore, 2004.
29. Kelley, LL, and Peterson, CM: Sectional Anatomy for Imaging Professional, ed. 2. Mosby, St. Louis, MO, 2007.
30. Lazo, DL: Fundamentals of Sectional Anatomy: An Imaging Approach. Thomson Delmar Learning, Clifton Park, NY, 2007.
31. IP, D: Orthopedic Traumatology: A Resident's Guide. Springer, New York, 2006.
32. McConnell, J, Eyres, R, and Nightingale, J: Interpreting Trauma Radiographs. Blackwell, Oxford, UK, 2005.
33. Berquist, TH: Imaging of Orthopedic Trauma, ed. 2. Raven Press, New York, 1989.
34. Bucholz, RW, Heckman, J, and Court-Brown, C (eds.): Rockwood and Green's Fractures in Adults, ed. 6. Lippincott Williams & Wilkins, Philadelphia, 2005.
35. McCort, JJ, and Mindelzun, RE: Trauma Radiology. Churchill Livingstone, New York, 1990.
36. Drafke, MW, and Nakayama, H: Trauma and Mobile Radiography, ed. 2. FA Davis, Philadelphia, 2001.
37. Smyth, JB: Complications of hip replacement: A long page. The Physiotherapy Site, Exeter, UK, 2003. Accessed October 4, 2004 at http://www.thephysiotherapysite.co.uk/hip/thr_complications.html.
38. Beaty, J (ed.): Rockwood and Wilkins' Fractures in Children, ed. 5. Lippincott Williams & Wilkins, Philadelphia, 1999.
39. Hofmann, AA, et al: Minimizing leg length inequality in total hip arthroplasty: Use of preoperative templating and intraoperative x-ray. Am J Orthop 37(1):18, 2008.
40. Sathappan, SS, et al: Effect of anesthesia type on limb length discrepancy after total hip arthroplasty. J Arthrop 23(2):203, 2008.
41. Lakshmanan, P, et al: Achieving the required medial offset and limb length in total hip arthroplasty. Acta Orthop Belg 74(1):49, 2008.
42. Zheng, Z, et al: Prevention and treatment of leg length discrepancy after total hip arthroplasty. Zhongguo Xiu Fu Chong Jian Wai Ke Za Zhi. 22(6):662, 2008.
43. D'Amico, M, et al: Balance lower limb loads and 3D spine modifications after total hip replacement: Effects of leg length discrepancy correction. Stud Health Technol Inform 123:409, 2006.
44. Rubash, HE, and Parvataneni, HK: The pants too short, the leg too long: Leg length inequality after THA. Orthopedics 30(9):764, 2007.
45. Murphy, SB, and Ecker, TM: Evaluation of a new leg length measurement algorithm in hip arthroplasty. Clin Orthop Relat Res 463:85, 2007.
46. Kim, RH, et al: Metal-on-metal total hip arthroplasty. J Arthrop 2008 (Epub ahead of print.). Accessed August 1, 2008 at http://www.ncbi.nlm.gov/pubmed.
47. Amstutz, HC, and Le Duff, ML: Eleven years experience with metal-on-metal hybrid hip resurfacing: A review of 1000 conserve plus. J Arthrop 23(6 Suppl 1):36, 2008. Accessed August 1, 2008 at http://www.ncbi.nlm.gov/pubmed.
48. Gomez, PF, and Morcuende, MD: Early attempts at hip arthroplasty, 1700s to 1950s. Iowa Orthop J 25:25, 2005.
49. Iagnocco, A, et al: Ultrasound imaging for the rheumatologist. Ultrasonography of the hip. Clin Exp Rheumatol 24(3):229, 2006.
50. Loder, RT, et al: Slipped femoral capital epiphysis. Instr Course Lect 57:473, 2008.
51. Richolt, FA, et al: Quantitative evaluation of angular measurements on plain radiographs in patients with slipped femoral capital epyphysis: A 3-dimensional analysis of computed tomography-based computer models of 46 femora. J Pediatr Orthop 28(3):291, 2008.
52. Tins, B, Cassar-Pullicino, V, and McCall, I: The role of pre-treatment MRI in established cases of slipped femoral capital epiphysis. Eur J Radiol 70(3):570, 2009.
53. Norton, K: Developmental dyplasia of the hip. Accessed July 22, 2008 at http://www.emedicine.com.
54. Grissom, L, et al: Imaging in the surgical management of developmental dislocation of the hip. Clin Orthop Relat Res 466(4):791, 2008.
55. Gunay, C, Atalar, H, Doqruel, H, et al: Correlation of femoral head coverage and Graf alpha angle in infants being screened for developmental dysplasia of the hip. Int Orthop 33(3): 761, 2009.
56. Stein-Zamir, C, et al: Developmental dysplasia of the hip: Risk markers, clinical screening and outcome. Pediatr Int 50(3):341, 2008.
57. Richards, PJ, Pattison, JM, Belcher, J, et al: A new tilt on pelvic radiographs: A pilot study. Skel Radiol 38(2):113, 2009.
58. Taunton, M: Femoroacetabular impingement. Orthopaedia 2007. Accessed August 1, 2008 at http://www.orthopaedia.com. Accessed August 1, 2008.
59. Ganz, R, et al: The etiology of osteoarthritis of the hip: An integrated mechanical concept. Clin Orthop Relat Res 466(2):264, 2008.
60. Larson, CM, et al: A review of hip arthroscopy and its role in the management of adult pain. Iowa Orthop J 25:172, 2005.

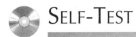

SELF-TEST

Radiograph A

1. Identify this *projection*.

2. Based on the bony configuration of the pelvis and the pelvic inlet, would you guess this patient is *male* or *female*?

Radiograph B

3. What is the most striking feature of the *bilateral hip joint spaces*?

4. Describe the *position* of the *femoral heads* in relation to the *acetabulum*.

5. What is the *term* used to describe the altered configuration of the *acetabulum*?

6. Does a *degenerative process* or an *inflammatory process* appear to be responsible for the changes visible at the hip joints?

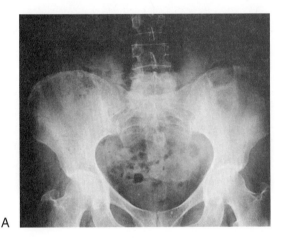

A

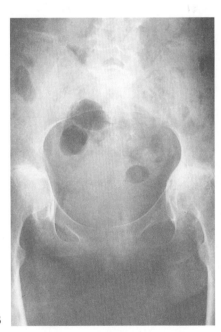

B

Chapter 13

RADIOLOGIC EVALUATION OF THE KNEE

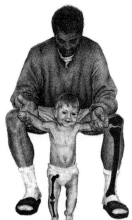

CHAPTER OUTLINE

The knee has been subjected to more clinical investigation and scientific research than any other joint in the body.[1] A reason for this may be the enormous number of patients with knee disorders—over 1.3 million annual visits to emergency departments in the United States are made because of knee trauma.[2]

The complex arthrokinematics of the knee allows for great stability combined with great mobility. This mechanical compromise enables the knee to withstand tremendous weight-bearing and load transmission forces while promoting ambulatory freedom. The knee's unique anatomy, combined with its exposed location between the two longest bones of the body, does, however, predispose it to various injuries, trauma, and other pathologies.

The knee is well demonstrated on the routine radiologic evaluation. Most fractures as well as nontraumatic disorders are adequately defined via conventional radiographs. Internal derangement of the joint and other soft tissue pathology is usually demonstrated best with magnetic resonance imaging (MRI).

Review of Anatomy[3–10]

Osseous Anatomy

The knee joint, or *femorotibial joint,* is formed by the articulation of the distal end of the femur to the proximal end of the tibia. Adaptive congruency of the articular surfaces is made possible by the interposed *menisci.* Associated with the knee joint are the *patellofemoral joint,* an articulation between the anterior aspect of the femur and the patella, and the *tibiofibular joint,* an articulation between the lateral aspect of the tibia and the fibular head (Figs. 13-1 and 13-2).

Distal Femur

The distal femur exhibits medial and lateral condyles, which are separated anteriorly by the patellar surface, also known as the trochlear groove or intercondylar sulcus.

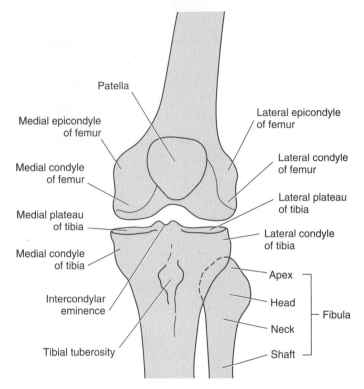

Figure 13-1 Knee, anterior aspect.

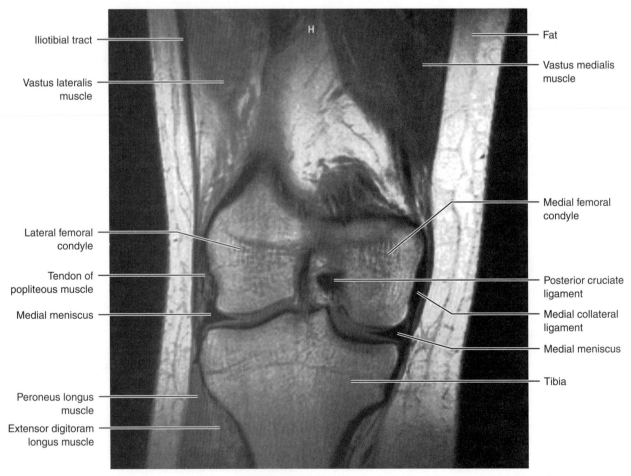

Figure 13-2 Coronal, T1-weighted MRI of the knee. *(Image courtesy of http://www.medcyclopaedia.com by GE Healthcare.)*

Posteriorly, the femoral condyles are divided by the deep intercondylar fossa. Medial and lateral epicondyles are prominences, proximal to the condyles, serving as sites of muscle attachment.

Patella

The patella is a large sesamoid bone embedded in the quadriceps tendon. Its smooth articular surface has multiple facets for efficient load-distribution mechanisms during its tracking actions on the trochlear groove. The outer anterior surface is convex and roughened. The broad superior surface is the base, and the pointed inferior surface is the apex of the patella.

Proximal Tibia

The proximal tibia exhibits medial and lateral condyles, which superiorly form the flared articular surface, the tibial plateau. Located between the condyles on the tibial plateau is the intercondylar eminence or tibial spine, composed of two small pointed prominences, the intercondylar tubercles. The lateral condyle has a facet on its posteroinferior surface for articulation with the head of the fibula. At the midline of the anterior proximal tibia, just distal to the condyles, is the tibial tuberosity, a prominence serving as the distal attachment of the patellar ligament. Beginning distally from this point is the anterior crest of the tibia. This sharp ridge represents the anterior surface of the tibial shaft and extends to the medial malleolus.

Fibula

The fibula is the non–weight-bearing bone of the lower extremity. The proximal end of the fibula is the head, which articulates with the tibia. The superior tip of the head is the apex or styloid process. The tapered region inferior to the head is the fibular neck. The long slender shaft of the fibula ends distally as the lateral malleolus at the ankle.

Ligamentous Anatomy

There are four major stabilizing ligaments of the knee joint (Fig. 13-3): the *medial collateral*, the *lateral collateral*, the *anterior cruciate*, and the *posterior cruciate*. Other various minor ligaments and the muscular complexes provide additional stability.

The *medial collateral ligament*, also known as the *tibial collateral ligament*, arises from the medial epicondyle of the femur and extends to the medial condyle and medial surface of the tibia. Fibers of the medial collateral ligament blend with the joint capsule and medial meniscus. The medial collateral ligament is the prime stabilizer against valgus stresses in either flexion or extension.

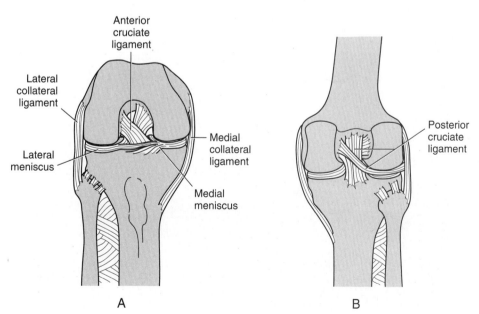

Figure 13-3 Major ligaments of the knee joint: **(A)** anterior view; **(B)** posterior view.

The *lateral collateral ligament,* also known as the *fibular collateral ligament,* arises from the lateral epicondyle of the femur and extends to the fibular head. The lateral collateral ligament is extra-articular in that it does not blend with the joint capsule or lateral meniscus. The lateral collateral ligament plays a role in defending the knee against varus stresses.

The *anterior cruciate ligament (ACL)* arises from the nonarticular area of the tibial plateau just anterior to the intercondylar eminence and extends to the posterior medial aspect of the lateral femoral condyle. The anterior cruciate lies entirely within the joint capsule but is extrasynovial. This ligament functions as the primary restraint against anterior tibial displacement.

The *posterior cruciate ligament (PCL)* is also extrasynovial but contained within the joint capsule. It arises from behind the intercondylar eminence and extends to the lateral aspect of the medial femoral condyle. The posterior cruciate is the primary stabilizer against posterior tibial displacement.

The *patellar ligament,* also referred to as the *patellar tendon,* extends from the apex of the patella to the tibial tuberosity (Fig. 13-4). The patellar ligament can be considered a continuation of the common tendon of the quadriceps muscle group.

Joint Mobility

The knee functions as a specialized hinge joint, permitting a wide range of flexion and extension movement in the sagittal plane. Accessory rotation mobility is present in the transverse plane.

Femorotibial Osteokinematics

Normal values for active motion range from 0 degrees of extension, or 10 degrees of hyperextension, to 145 degrees of flexion. Tibial rotation is possible to 45 degrees both medially and laterally when the knee is positioned in flexion. Abduction and adduction in the frontal plane are similarly affected by the amount of joint flexion, reaching a maximum of a few degrees each when the knee is flexed in the range of 0 to 30 degrees.

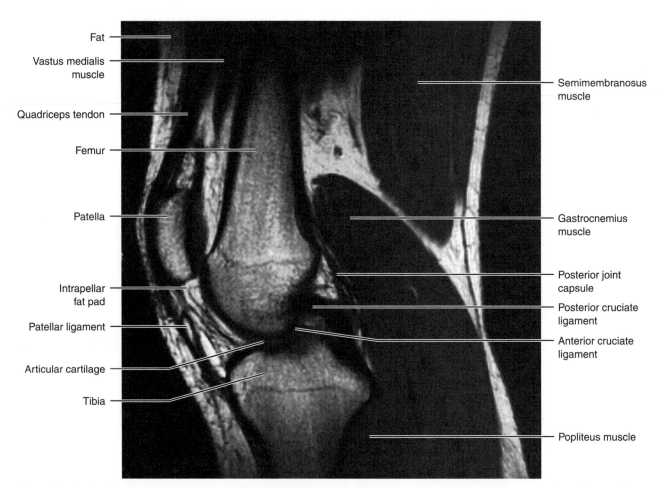

Figure 13-4 Sagittal T1-weighted MRI of the knee. The patella is embedded within the quadriceps tendon. The distal extension of the quadriceps tendon is the *patellar ligament. (Image courtesy of http://www.medcyclopaedia.com by GE Healthcare.)*

Femorotibial Arthrokinematics

The tibiofemoral joint arthrokinematics follow the orthopedic rules for convex–concave surfaces. That is, the motions of knee extension and flexion occur via a combined movement of rolling and gliding of the femoral convex surfaces relative to the tibial concave surfaces. The specific actions of the articular surfaces depend on whether the joint is functioning in a closed- or open-chain kinetic state and whether flexion or extension is occurring.

Patellofemoral Joint Biomechanics

The patellofemoral joint functions as a saddle type of joint. The primary motion is a gliding or tracking action along the trochlear groove. In knee extension the patella is positioned at the superior end of the trochlear groove, and during flexion the patella will track or glide caudally in the trochlear groove. The patella glides distally a distance of approximately 7 cm from full knee extension to flexion. Both medial and lateral patellar facets contact the femur at extension and through 90 degrees of flexion. Beyond 90 degrees the patella rotates, or tilts, and remains in contact with only the medial femoral condyle. At full knee flexion, the patella sits deep in the trochlear groove.

The Q Angle

The patellofemoral joint mechanics are mediated directly or indirectly by the pull of the quadriceps muscle on the patella. Proximally, the angulation of the hip joint, or distally, the mechanics of the foot, may alter the angle of pull of the quadriceps on the patella, known as the *Q angle* (Fig. 13-5). The Q angle is determined by the intersection of the line of pull of the quadriceps with the line connecting the center of the patella to the center of the tibial tuberosity. The normal Q angle is approximately 10 degrees, and values greater than this may indicate a predisposition to inadequate patellar tracking and resultant instability. The patella itself serves to lengthen the lever force arm of the quadriceps and allows for a wider distribution of femoral compressive forces. Maladaptive mechanics at the patellofemoral joint can lead to painful conditions and functional disability of the knee joint.

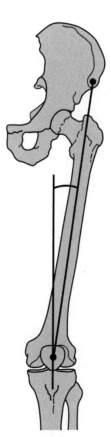

Figure 13-5 The direction of pull of the quadriceps on the patella is described in terms of the *Q angle,* the angle formed by the intersection of a line drawn from the center of the patella to the tibial tuberosity and a line drawn from the center of the patella to the anterosuperior iliac spine.

Tibiofibular Joint Biomechanics

The proximal tibiofibular joint is a gliding type of synovial joint. Limited movement is available between the lateral tibial condyle and the head of the fibula. Note that the distal tibiofibular joint is not synovial but a syndesmotic joint, which is only slightly movable.

Growth and Development

At birth, the secondary epiphyseal centers for the distal femur and the proximal tibia are present and can be identified as ossified structures on radiograph (Fig. 13-6). The secondary epiphyseal center for the head of the fibula does not appear until approximately 3 years of age. The patella is not visible on radiographs until it begins ossification at approximately 4 years of age. The physis of each long bone continues to grow progressively, and the epiphyseal plates finally fuse postpuberty at approximately 16 to 18 years of age (Fig. 13-7). Women generally show earlier skeletal maturity than men.

Routine Radiologic Evaluation[11–21]

Practice Guidelines for Knee Radiography in Children and Adults[11]

The American College of Radiology (ACR), the principal professional organization of radiologists in the United States, defines the following practice guidelines as an educational tool to help practitioners provide appropriate radiologic care for their patients.

Goals

The goal of the knee radiographic examination is to identify or exclude anatomic abnormalities or disease processes.

Indications

The indications for radiologic examination include but are not limited to trauma (including suspected physical abuse); osseous changes secondary to metabolic disease, systemic disease, or nutritional deficiencies; neoplasms; infections; non-neoplastic bone pathology; arthropathies; preoperative, postoperative, and follow-up studies; congenital syndromes and developmental disorders; vascular lesions; evaluation of soft tissue (such as a suspected foreign body); pain; correlation of abnormal skeletal findings on other imaging studies.

Basic Projections and Radiologic Observations[11–21]

The minimum recommended projections are an *anteroposterior (AP)* and *lateral* projection of the knee and patella, and a *tangential view* of the patella. A common additional view to most routine examinations is the *posterioanterior axial view of the intercondylar fossa*.

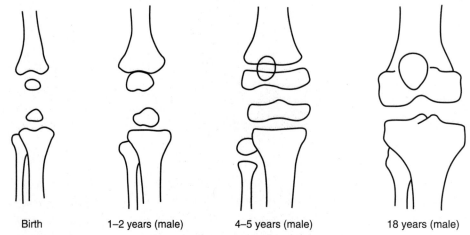

Birth   1–2 years (male)   4–5 years (male)   18 years (male)

Figure 13-6 Radiographic tracings of ossification of the knee at varying ages from birth through 18 years. *(Adapted from Meschan,[5] p. 218.)*

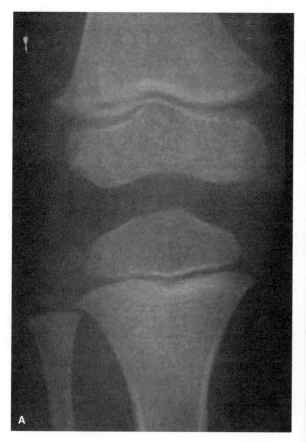

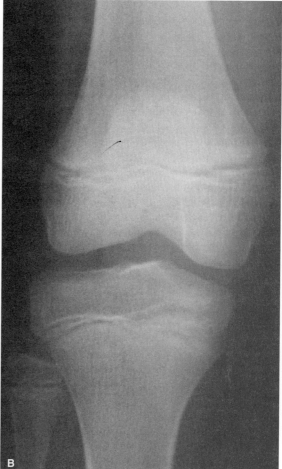

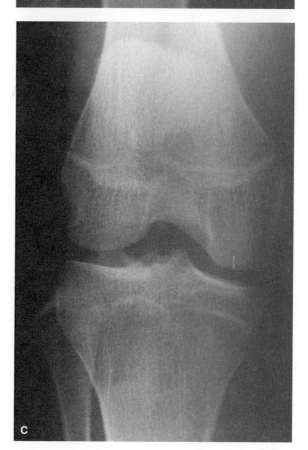

Figure 13-7 Normal growth and development. **(A)** At 3 years of age, the secondary epiphyses of the distal femur and proximal tibia are present, while the head of the fibula is barely visible as a pebble size ossification. **(B)** At 9 years of age, the secondary epiphyses have reached their normal adult shape. The growth plates are "open," as evidenced by radiolucent lines. **(C)** At age 16, the epiphyseal plates have completely fused, but the growth lines are still evident, especially across the proximal tibia.

Routine Radiologic Evaluation of the Knee

Anteroposterior

This view demonstrates the distal femur, proximal tibia, the femorotibial articulation, and head of the fibula.

Radiologic Observations

The important observations are:

1. The patella is superimposed over the distal femur. The inferior pole (apex) of the patella normally lies at the level of the joint line (*a* in Fig. 13-8) but does not cross it.
2. The femorotibial radiographic joint space is normally well defined in both the medial and lateral compartments. In a normal knee, these interspaces are of equal height (*b* in Fig. 13-8).
3. The articular surface of the tibial plateau is seen end-on, with only minimal surface area visualized.
4. The medial half of the fibular head is superimposed behind the tibia.
5. The long axes of the femur and tibia normally are in alignment (*c* in Fig. 13-8).
6. Normal radiographic contrast between the bones and soft tissues should be evident. Trabecular markings and cortical margins should appear distinct.

Basic Projections

- **AP**
- Lateral
- Posterioanterior (PA) axial "tunnel" view of the intercondylar fossa
- Tangential view of the patellofemoral joint

Setting up the Radiograph

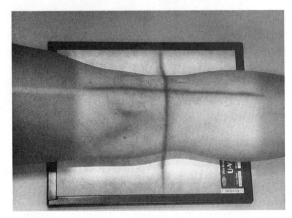

Figure 13-9 Patient position for AP radiograph of the knee.

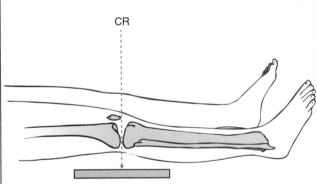

Figure 13-10 The central ray is directed inferior to the distal pole of the patella, passing through the femorotibial joint space.

What Can You See?

Look at the radiograph (Fig. 13-11) and try to identify the radiographic anatomy. Trace the outlines of structures using a marker and transparency sheet. Compare results with the book tracing (Fig. 13-12). Compare to the three-dimensional (3D) computed tomography (CT) image of the knee (Fig. 13-13). Can you identify the following:

- Distal femur (identify medial and lateral condyles)
- Proximal tibia (identify the medial and lateral condyles and intercondylar eminence)
- Femorotibial joint space (compare the height of the medial and lateral compartments)
- Patella
- Proximal fibula (identify head, neck, and shaft)

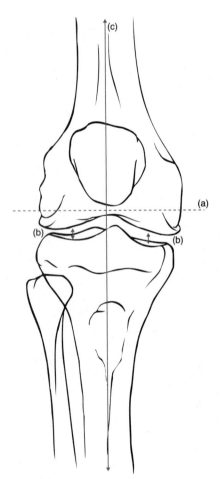

Figure 13-8 Radiographic spatial relationships in the normal knee: (*a*) the inferior pole of the patella does not cross the joint space, (*b*) the medial and lateral joint spaces are of equal height, and (*c*) the long axes of the femur and tibia are in alignment.

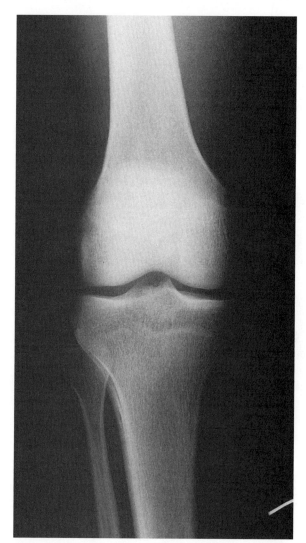

Figure 13-11 Anteroposterior radiograph of the right knee.

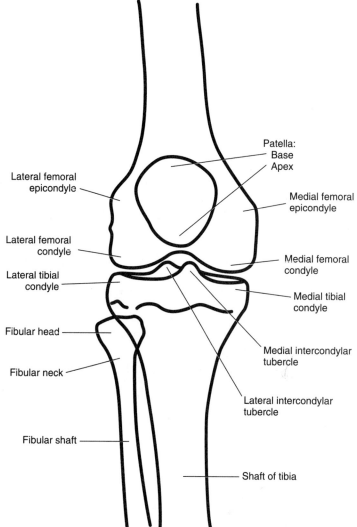

Figure 13-12 Tracing of radiograph of AP view of the right knee.

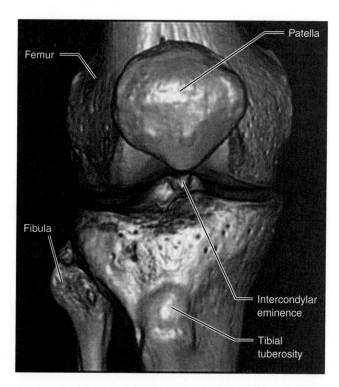

Figure 13-13 Three-dimensional CT image of the knee. *(Image courtesy of http://www.medcyclopaedia.com by GE Healthcare.)*

Routine Radiologic Evaluation of the Knee

Lateral

This view demonstrates the patellofemoral joint in profile, the suprapatellar bursa, the quadriceps tendon, and the patellar tendon. The patient is normally in a lateral recumbent position, lying on the side that is being examined.

Radiologic Observations

The important observations are:

1. The knee is flexed approximately 20 degrees for a standard lateral.
2. The x-ray beam is directed through the knee in a medial-to-lateral direction; thus a portion of the fibular head is superimposed behind the tibia.
3. In true lateral positioning, the femoral condyles will appear almost entirely superimposed over one another. However, magnification of the medial condyle will cause its line image to appear slightly inferior to the lateral condyle.
4. The tibial medial and lateral condyles are also superimposed on one another. The intercondylar eminence projects above the tibial plateau and is partly superimposed by the femoral condyles.
5. The relationship of the patella to the femur is examined. Abnormally superior positioning of the patella is termed *patella alta*. Abnormally inferior positioning of the patella is termed *patella baja*.
6. The relationship of the length of the patella (measure from its base to its apex, *a* in Fig. 13-14) to the length of the patellar ligament (measured from its attachment at the patellar apex to the tibial tuberosity, *b* in Fig. 13-14) is examined. These distances are normally approximately equal, and normal variance does not exceed 20%. More than 20% variation indicates an abnormal patellar position.

Basic Projections

- AP
- **Lateral**
- PA axial "tunnel" view of the intercondylar fossa
- Tangential view of the patellofemoral joint

Setting up the Radiograph

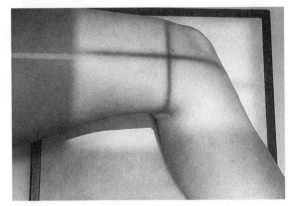

Figure 13-15 Patient postion for lateral radiograph of the knee.

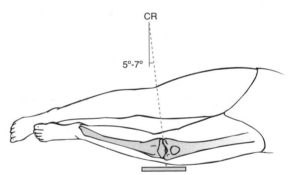

Figure 13-16 The central ray is directed to the knee joint and angled 5 to 7 degrees cephalad. This slight angulation will prevent the joint space from being obscured by the magnified image of the medial femoral condyle.

7. Normal radiographic contrast between the bones and soft tissues should be evident. The cortical margins of the long bones and the patella should be distinct.
8. The suprapatellar bursa normally images as a thin, radiolucent strip just posterior to the quadriceps tendon. The bursa becomes distended with joint effusion and images as an oval-shaped density in the presence of joint injury.
9. A fabella, a small sesamoid bone located in the posterior joint capsule at the insertion of the lateral head of the gastrocnemius muscle, is noted in up to 18% of the population. When present, it will be seen as a small, oval-shaped density in the posterior soft tissues. Abnormal conditions, such as joint effusion or arthritis, may displace the fabella.

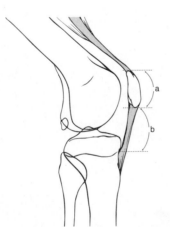

Figure 13-14 Radiographic spatial relationship of patellar position. Normally the length of the patella (*a*) equals the length of the patellar ligament (*b*) within a 20% variance.

What Can You See?

Look at the radiograph (Fig. 13-16) and try to identify the radiographic anatomy. Trace the outlines of structures using a marker and transparency sheet. Compare results with the book tracing (Fig. 13-17). Compare the ossoeous anatomy on the radiograph with the T1-weighted MRI (Fig. 13-19). Can you identify the following:

- Distal femur (identify the medial and lateral condyles)
- Proximal tibia (identify the tibial tuberosity, articular surface, and intercondylar eminence)
- Proximal fibula (identify head, neck, and shaft)
- Patella (measure and compare the length of the patella to the length of the patellar ligament)

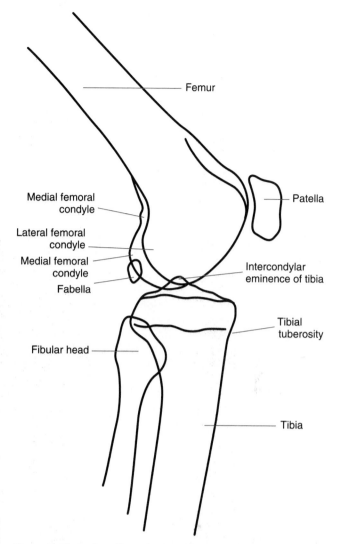

Figure 13-18 Tracing of lateral radiograph of the knee.

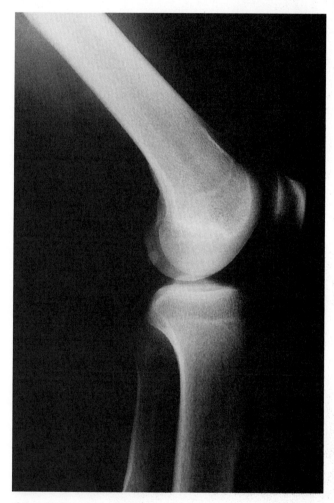

Figure 13-17 Lateral radiograph of the knee.

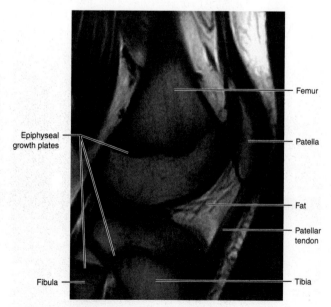

Figure 13-19 Sagittal T1-weighted MRI of the knee.

Routine Radiologic Evaluation of the Knee

Posteroanterior Axial "Tunnel" View of the Intercondylar Fossa

This view demonstrates the intercondylar fossa, the posterior aspects of the femoral and tibial condyles, the intercondylar eminence of the tibia, and the tibial plateaus. In the routine examination, this view is usually included to detect loose bodies in the joint, assess possible osteochondral defects, and observe any narrowing of the femorotibial joint space.

Radiologic Observations

The important observations are:

1. The patient is prone and the knee is flexed approximately 40 degrees in this projection. The x-ray beam enters from a posterior to anterior direction.
2. The normal appearance of the intercondylar fossa is similar to that of a railroad tunnel entrance (Fig. 13-20), hence the nickname "tunnel view" for this projection. Osteochondral defects or erosions secondary to blood in the joint may cause the fossa to assume a squared-off shape, instead of an inverted U.
3. The patella is superimposed behind the distal femur.
4. The intercondylar fossa should appear open and its surface well visualized.
5. The tibial articular surface should be partially visible. Both tibial spines of the intercondylar eminence should be visible.
6. The fibular head is partially superimposed over the proximal tibia.

Basic Projections

- AP
- Lateral
- **PA axial "tunnel" view of the intercondylar fossa**
- Tangential view of the patellofemoral joint

Setting up the Radiograph

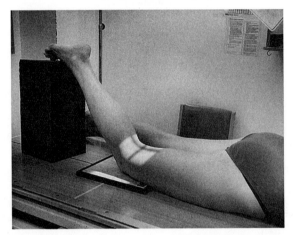

Figure 13-21 Patient position for axial view of the intercondylar fossa of the knee.

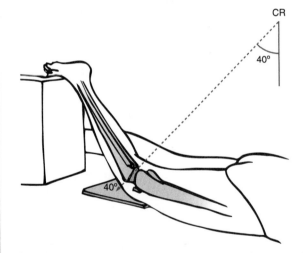

Figure 13-22 The central ray is angled caudad 40 degrees and directed posterioanteriorly through the joint.

What Can You See?

Look at the radiograph (Fig. 13-23) and try to identify the radiographic anatomy. Trace the outlines of structures using a marker and transparency sheet. Compare results with the book tracing (Fig. 13-24). Can you identify the following:

- Distal femur (identify the medial and lateral condyles and the intercondylar fossa)
- Proximal tibia (identify the medial and lateral condyles and the intercondylar eminence)
- Fibula
- Patella superimposed behind the femur

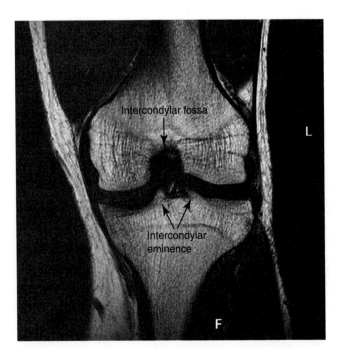

Figure 13-20 Coronal T1-weighted MRI of the tunnel-like intercondylar fossa.

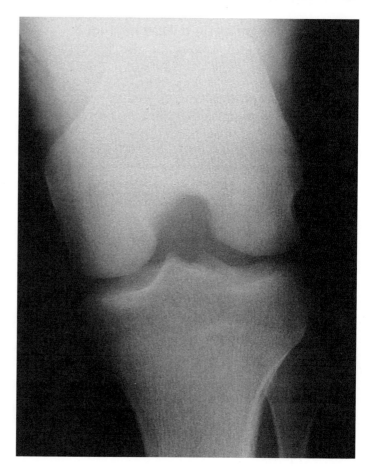

Figure 13-23 PAr axial radiograph of the intercondylar fossa of the right knee.

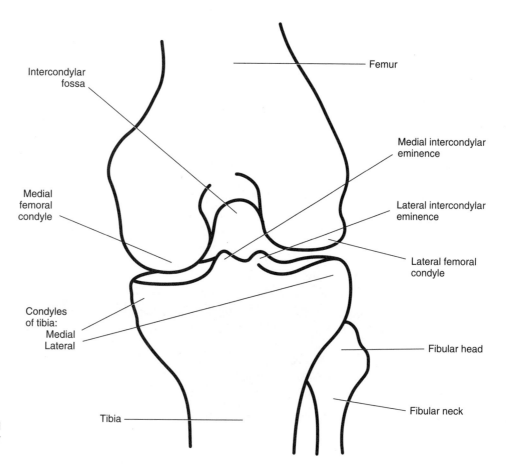

Figure 13-24 Tracing of PA axial radiograph of the intercondylar fossa of the knee.

Routine Radiologic Evaluation of the Knee

Tangential View of the Patellofemoral Joint

This view demonstrates an axial view of the patellofemoral joint space and the articular surfaces of the patella and the femur.

Radiologic Observations

The important observations are:

1. The patient is positioned supine and the knee is flexed 45 degrees. The x-ray beam enters parallel to the patellofemoral joint space or *tangentially* across the joint surface. The beam may enter in a superoinferior direction (the *Merchant view*) or, as demonstrated here, an inferosuperior direction.
2. The articular surface of the patella should be smooth and distinct. Two superimposed borders may be imaged because of the irregular topography of the articular surface.
3. On this view the medial and lateral facets of the patella are visible. The medial facet normally is larger than the lateral and may show a more steeply sloped contour.
4. The intercondylar sulcus is identified as the groove between the distal femoral condyles.
5. This view can be used to detect subtle subluxations of the patella. Alan C. Merchant described two measurements that can be used to determine normal positioning of the patella[13]:

   - *The sulcus angle (a* in Fig. 13-23) is the angle between lines drawn from the highest points of the femoral condyles to the deepest point of the trochlear groove. This angle has a normal value of 138 degrees plus or minus 6 degrees. Shallow sulcus angles (those with greater measurements) may be related to recurrent patellar dislocations.
   - *The congruence angle* helps to define the position of the patella within the intercondylar sulcus. First, a reference line is drawn bisecting the sulcus angle. A second line is drawn from the apex of the sulcus angle to the most posterior or lowest point on the patellar articular ridge. If the second line is *medial* to the reference line, the resultant congruence angle formed (*b* in Fig. 13-23) is assigned a *negative* value. If the second line is *lateral* to the reference line, the resultant congruence angle is assigned a *positive* value. Merchant's study found an average congruence angle of −6 degrees in normal subjects.[13] A congruence angle of +16 degrees or more was associated with lateral patellar subluxation or other patellofemoral disorders.

In evaluating the patellofemoral relationship, remember that this projection can provide information only specific to the position of knee flexion. A series of axial CT or MRI slices can provide more information on the entire patellofemoral joint surface congruity (Fig. 13-25). Any image, however, is static, and cannot provide information on the dynamic forces that govern patellar tracking. This information requires hands-on evaluation.

Basic Projections

- AP
- Lateral
- PA axial "tunnel" view of the intercondylar fossa
- **Tangential view of the patellofemoral joint**

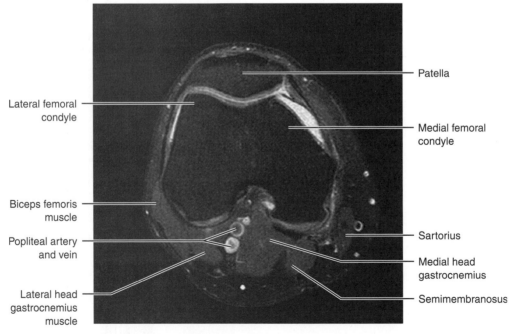

Figure 13-25 Axial T2-weighted MRI of the patellofemoral joint. Viewing all axial slices along the patellar articular surface will give valuable information on joint congruity.

Setting up the Radiograph

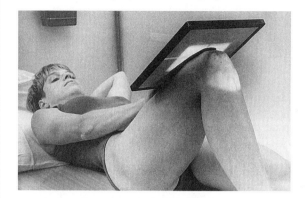

Figure 13-26 Patient position for tangential ("sunrise") radiograph of the patellofemoral joint.

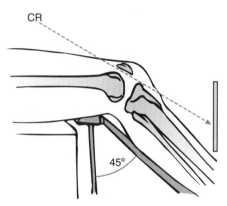

Figure 13-27 The central ray is directed through the patellofemoral joint space, parallel to the joint surfaces.

- Patella (identify the medial and lateral surfaces)
- Femoral condyles (identify the medial and lateral surfaces)
- Measurement of the sulcus angle
- Measurement of the congruence angle

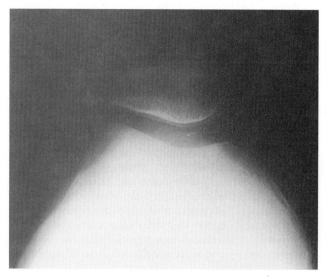

Figure 13-28 Tangential radiograph of the patellofemoral joint.

What Can You See?

Look at the radiograph (Fig. 13-28) and try to identify the radiographic anatomy. Trace the outlines of structures using a marker and transparency sheet. Compare results with the book tracing (Fig. 13-29). Can you identify the following:

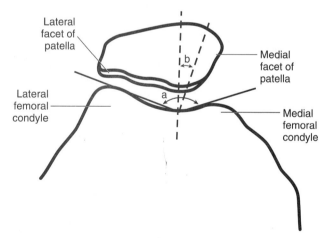

Figure 13-29 Tracing of tangential view of the patellofemoral joint.

Additional Views Related to the Knee

Oblique Views of the Knee

Oblique views of the knee are included in some facilities' routine series of the knee. For the internal oblique, the entire leg is internally rotated 45 degrees and the central ray is directed at the midjoint. This demonstrates the lateral femoral condyle without superimposition and more of the fibular head is visible. For the external oblique view, the entire leg is rotated 45 degrees externally, and the medial femoral condyle is viewed without superimposition (Fig. 13-30).

Trauma at the Knee[22-50]

In the course of the 1.3 annual emergency department visits for knee trauma mentioned in the introduction, over a million knee radiographs will be made. This makes radiographs of the knee the most comon radiographs performed for trauma—yet the knee radiograph has the lowest yield for diagnosisng clinically significant fractures. Only about 5% of those million patients will have a fracture. The rest will have soft tissue injuries that will not be diagnosed by radiographs. So why are unnecesssary radiographs routinely performed despite clear supporting data? Reasons cited include fear of lawsuits, failure to obtain an adequate history, lack of practitioner confidence in the clinical exam, and expectations on the part of patients.

Diagnostic Imaging for Trauma of the Knee

Researchers have been working to design protocols to reduce the number of radiographs used in the evaluation of extremity injuries. The *clinical decision rules* created in Ottawa and Pittsburgh are the best known guidelines for the appropriate use of radiographs in acute knee injuries. These similar guides have an excellent sensitivity for identifying fracture by applying simple predictive parameters. Radiographs *should* be ordered after trauma if there is any of the following present: joint effusion after a direct blow or fall, inability to walk without limping, palpable tenderness over the patealla

or fibular head, or inability to flex the knee to 90 degrees. Radiographs *should not* be ordered if a patient had a twisting injury but is able to walk and no effusion is present.

With guidelines correctly applied, conventional radiographs are adequate for identification and treatment of most of the fractures that do occur at the knee. Once the fracture has been identified, there are times that further imaging is required. *Computed tomography (CT)* can define the degree of fragmentation or depression of the articular surface, to assist preoperative planning.

In the case of suspected fracture but normal radiographs, *magnetic resonance imaging (MRI)* or *triple-phase bone scans* can identify occult or subtle fractures, or stress fractures. Both of these modalities are highly sensitive to fracture, but only MRI is specific to the anatomic location.

It is prudent to remember that fractures *known to be missed* are fractures of the patella, tibial plateau, tibial spine, and fibular head.

Of all the soft tissue injuries suffered at the knee, a twisting mechanism is the cause of three-fourths of them. MRI is essential in the evaluation of injuries to the menisci, the cruciate ligaments, the collateral ligaments, and the articular cartilage. Clinical decision rules for the evaluation of soft tissue injuries are not yet published.

Angiography or *magnetic resonance angiography (MRA)* is indicated in severe fractures or dislocation at the knee, because there is a high association of vascular disruption.

Fractures

Fractures of the Distal Femur

Mechanism

Fractures of the distal femur occur when great force is applied, as in motor vehicle accidents or falls from great heights. Low-level forces or minor falls can cause fracture if the bone is weakened by pre-existing osteoporosis or other pathology.

Classifications

Many classifications exist for the purpose of assisting in surgical decisions and tracking treatment outcome. A basic

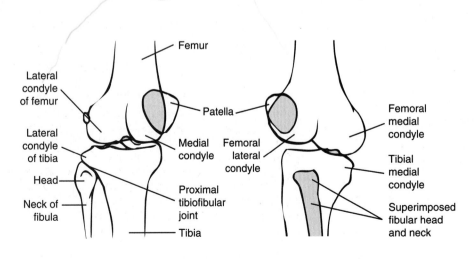

A. Internal oblique view of the knee   B. External oblique view of the knee

Figure 13-30 (A) Internal oblique view of the knee. **(B)** External oblique view of the knee.

classification of distal femur fractures is organized by location as supracondylar, intercondylar, or condylar fractures (Fig. 13-31).

Supracondylar fractures are fractures occurring at a site superior to the femoral condyles. Fracture patterns associated with supracondylar fractures are comminution, impaction, or linear, with or without displacement (Fig. 13-32).

Intercondylar fractures are located in the region between the medial and lateral femoral condyles. The fracture pattern appearing in this instance is commonly referred to as a "Y" fracture because the condyles are split apart from each other and from the shaft.

Condylar fractures are usually linear and involve only one femoral condyle.

Radiologic Evaluation

The radiographic assessment of distal femur fractures is usually complete on the routine AP and lateral projections of the knee. CT may assist in evaluating the depth and extent of the fracture lines.

Treatment

The objective of treatment in femoral fractures is not perfect anatomic reduction of the fracture site but restoration of the knee axis to a normal relationship with the hip and ankle.

Nonoperative treatment of distal femoral fractures may involve continuous skeletal traction via pinning through the tibial shaft, followed by casting at 3 to 6 weeks after injury. Good or excellent results are reported in over 80% of patients treated with nonoperative methods.

Open reduction with internal fixation is usually necessary with fractures that are open, associated with neurovascular damage, have displaced intra-articular fragments, pathological fractures, or the patient has marked obesity or ipsilateral leg fractures.

Rehabilitation begins early to maintain joint range of motion. Ambulation with partial weight bearing is progressed as radiographic evidence demonstrates healing. Patients are generally ambulating well with a device 4 weeks after injury and can expect return to normal activity within 3 to 4 months.

Complications

Complications include malunion, which may result in a rotated or shortened limb; joint and soft tissue adhesions; and posttraumatic degenerative joint disease.

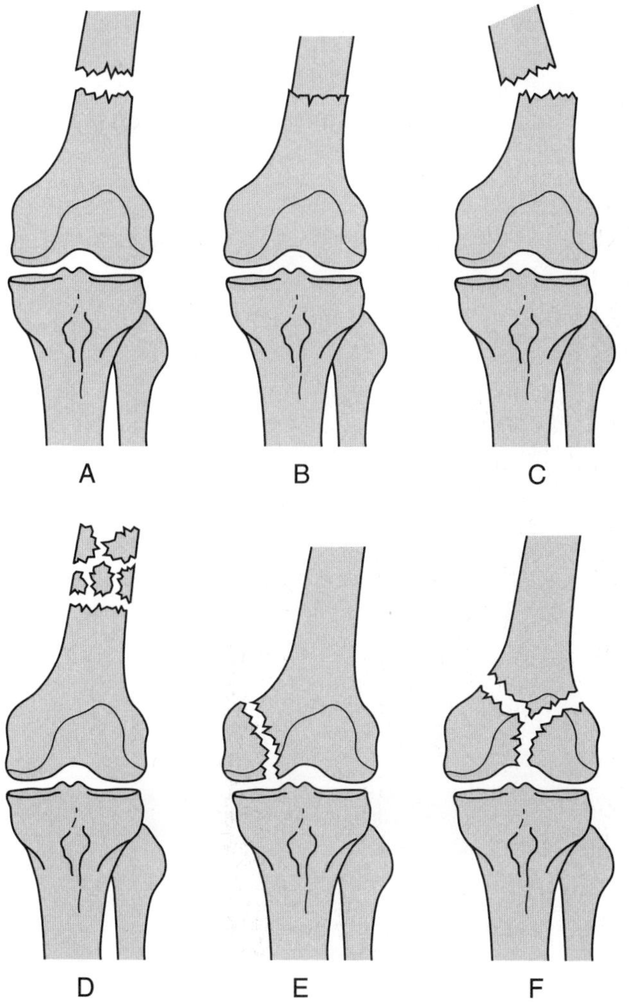

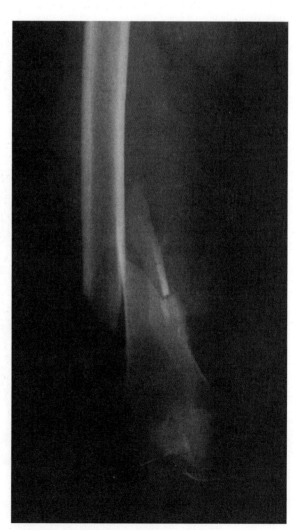

Figure 13-32 Supracondylar fracture of the distal femur. This 83-year-old woman was injured in a motor vehicle accident. The fracture is severely comminuted. The major fracture line extends obliquely through the lower third of the femoral shaft.

Figure 13-31 Fractures of the distal femur can be classified as supracondylar **(A)** nondisplaced, **(B)** impacted, **(C)** displaced, **(D)** comminuted, **(E)** condylar, or **(F)** intercondylar.

Fractures of the Proximal Tibia

Mechanism

Fractures of the proximal tibia in adults occur most frequently at the medial and lateral tibial plateaus, when varus or valgus forces combined with axial compression cause the hard femoral condyle to impact and depress the softer tibial plateau. A common mechanism of injury is a car–pedestrian accident in which the car's bumper strikes the pedestrian's knee (Fig. 13-33). Elderly patients with osteoporosis are more likely to sustain a tibial plateau fracture than a soft tissue injury after a twisting injury to the knee.

Proximal tibial fractures in children occur in entirely different patterns because of the uniqueness of growing bone. Areas predisposed to fracture are the epiphyseal growth plate and the metaphyseal region, which is composed of extensively remodeled new endosteal trabecular bone and more fenestrated laminar cortical bone, both of which predispose to compression injury (Fig. 13-34).

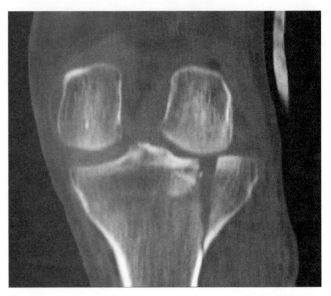

Figure 13-33 Coronal CT of the knee showing a vertical split fracture of the lateral tibial plateau. The fibula is not seen because this slice is anterior to it.

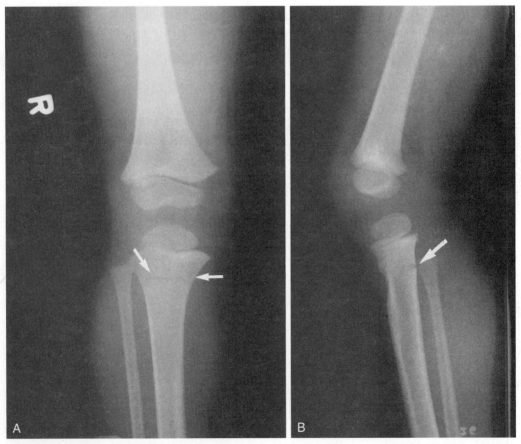

Figure 13-34 Proximal tibial fracture. In children, the areas of the proximal tibia most vulnerable to fracture are the epiphyseal growth plate and the metaphyseal region, which is composed of newly remodeled bone susceptible to compression injury. This 3½-year-old boy fell off a jungle gym and sustained a transverse, greenstick-type fracture through the metaphysis of the proximal tibia. **(A)** The AP view of the knee demonstrates the transverse linear fracture site (arrows). **(B)** The lateral view of the knee localizes the fracture site to the posterior margin of the proximal metaphysis. The fracture line breaks through the posterior cortex but does not extend to the anterior cortex (arrow). Although this fracture appears simple, any fracture in this region in growing bone can develop undesirable sequelae, namely angulation and deformity secondary to overgrowth at the healed fracture site. (It is interesting to note the absence of the image of the patella, which does not begin ossification until 4 years of age.)

Classification

The Hohl classification system of tibial plateau fractures identifies six common fracture patterns and their predisposing force mechanisms (Fig. 13-35):

- *Type I:* A nondisplaced vertical split fracture of the lateral tibial plateau caused by a pure valgus force
- *Type II:* A local depression of the lateral tibial plateau caused by a combination of axial and valgus forces
- *Type III:* A displaced vertical split fracture with depression at the lateral plateau caused by a combination of valgus and axial forces, often associated with proximal fibula fracture
- *Type IV:* A displaced depressed fracture of the medial plateau caused by varus and axial forces
- *Type V:* A vertical split fracture of the anterior or posterior aspect of the tibial plateau caused by axial forces
- *Type VI:* Displaced, comminuted fractures of both condyles caused by axial forces, often associated with proximal fibular fractures

Radiologic Evaluation

AP, lateral, and both oblique radiographs of the knee are usually obtained. The expanse of the tibial plateau necessitates the imaging of various depths, possible on reconstructed CT, to determine accurately the extent of the fracture line or the amount of depression present across the plateaus.

A *lipohemarthrosis* is commonly seen with tibial plateau fracture. Fat and blood escapes from the marrow space

through the fracture and mixes with synovial fluid in the joint. As fat is less dense than blood, it floats on the blood. This *parfait sign* can be seen on radiographs as well as CT and MRI. It is also known as the *FBI sign* (fat-blood interface) (Fig. 13-36).

Treatment

Treatment of tibial plateau fractures depends on the amount of tibial depression, comminution, and joint instability. Joint instability can happen when the varus or valgus forces acting on the knee rupture the collateral ligament contralateral to the fracture site. Also, significant depression of one plateau will also cause joint instability due to loss of the buttressing effect of the tibial plateau to the femoral condyle. This instability may occur despite intact ligaments.

Nonoperative treatment is indicated for minimally displaced fractures and, especially, in elderly patients with osteoporosis. The patient is non–weight-bearing for 4 to 6 weeks, then partially weight-bearing until solid bony union is radiographically evident, as should occur in another 4 to 6 weeks.

Operative treatment is indicated in patients with significant articular surface depression or displacement, open fractures, or ruptured ligaments. Internal fixation utilizes plates or screws and can involve elevating and internally fixating the depressed plateau and filling the underlying defect with bone grafts.

Complications

Possible complications include peroneal nerve injury; popliteal artery injury; avascular necrosis of small articular fragments, which may result in loose bodies in the joint; joint and soft tissue adhesions due to prolonged immobilization; and posttraumatic degenerative joint disease.

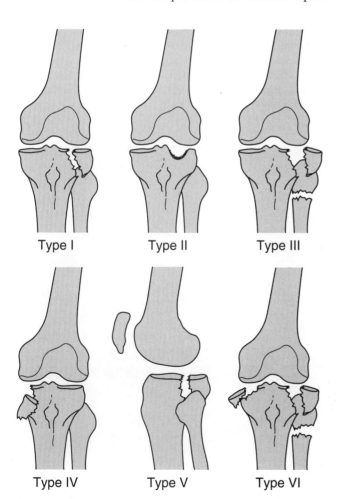

Figure 13-35 The Hohl classification of tibial plateau fractures.

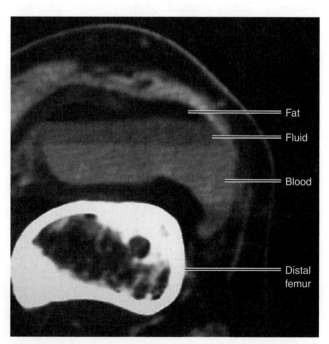

Figure 13-36 Axial CT image at the level of the suprapatellar pouch demonstrating a lipohemarthrosis. This *parfait sign* is caused by the layering of the fat and blood that has mixed with the joint fluid. The fat and blood has escaped from the marrow space through an articular fracture. Since fat is less dense than blood, it floats on the blood. This diagnostic sign of fracture can be seen on radiographs as well as CT and MRI. It is also known as the *FBI sign* (fat-blood interface).

Fractures of the Patella

Mechanism of Injury

The patella is vulnerable to two types of injury. Falls or dashboard impactions fracture the patella as it is compressed against the femur. Avulsion fractures occur when the patella is pulled apart by forceful contraction of the quadriceps coupled with passive resistance of the patellar ligament. This is seen in the attempt of a person to keep from falling after tripping.

Classification

Patellar fractures are described by the direction of the fracture line and whether the fracture is displaced or not. The most frequently seen fracture pattern is a transverse linear fracture line through the midregion of the bone (Fig. 13-37).

Radiologic Evaluation

Radiographic assessment of patellar fractures is generally complete on routine tangential, lateral, and oblique views.

Treatment

Nonoperative treatment is indicated in nondisplaced or minimally displaced fractures. Immobilization in a long leg cast for 4 to 6 weeks with full weight-bearing, crutch-assisted ambulation is typical and is often followed with a hinged knee brace for protected progressive return of knee motion.

Operative treatment is indicated for significant fragment displacement, articular incongruity, or open fractures. Multiple methods of fixation exist, including tension banding with wires or cancellous screws (Fig. 13-38). Range-of-motion exercises are initiated a fews days after surgery, and ambulation is progressive to partial and then full weight bearing by 6 weeks.

Partial patellectomy is indicated in some comminuted fractures to restore articular congruity. Severe comminution, with little hope of restoring a functional articular

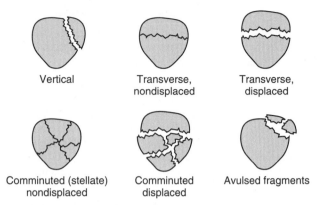

Vertical

Transverse, nondisplaced

Transverse, displaced

Comminuted (stellate) nondisplaced

Comminuted displaced

Avulsed fragments

Figure 13-37 Examples of patellar fractures.

surface, requires excision of the fracture fragments and reconstruction of the quadriceps expansion.

Complications

If the patella is present, complications include posttraumatic degenerative joint disease of the patellofemoral joint. If the patella has been excised, the patient may experience significant functional impairment. The loss of the patella as a pulley to increase the angle of pull of the quadriceps results in a chronic loss of knee extension strength.

Patellofemoral Subluxations

Acute traumatic dislocations of the patellofemoral joint are rare (Fig. 13-39). The usual mechanism is a direct blow to a flexed knee, as in a motor vehicle accident, or a powerful quadriceps contraction superimposed on a rotary or valgus force at the knee, as when a runner is cutting to the direction opposite his or her planted foot.

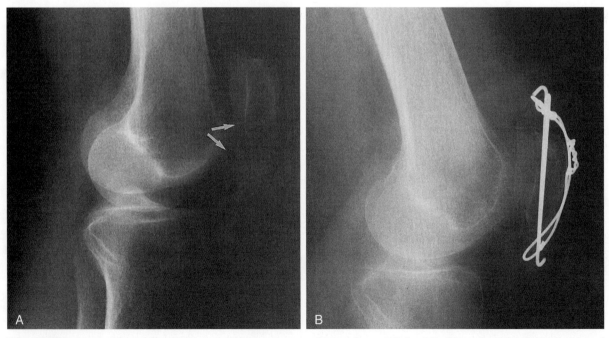

Figure 13-38 Fracture of the patella. This very active 68-year-old woman fractured her patella in a fall off her roller skates. **(A)** Lateral view of the knee demonstrates a transverse linear fracture line through the distal third of the patella. The white arrows indicate the wide displacement of the fracture fragments. **(B)** Follow-up films demonstrate pin-and-wire fixation devices and successful healing of the fracture site.

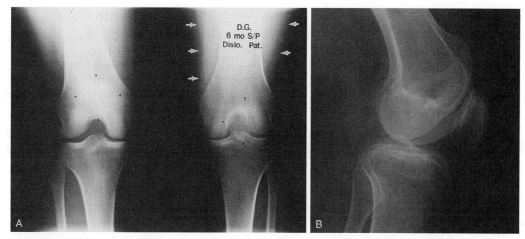

Figure 13-39 Dislocation of the patella. **(A)** This 16-year-old girl had dislocated her patella in a skateboarding accident. Follow-up films made 6 months after injury show patella baja, an abnormally inferior position of the patella, secondary to extensor mechanism insufficiency. The black triangles denote the abnormal position of the patella on the patient's left and the normal position of the patella on the patient's right. The white arrows indicate the diminished soft tissue shadow representing a decrease in the bulk of the quadriceps muscle group. Compare with the uninvolved right thigh shadow for normal soft tissue image. In addition to muscle atrophy, note the disuse atrophy of bone by comparing the increased radiolucency of the proximal tibia and distal femur on the involved extremity with that of the uninvolved extremity. This demineralization of bone is directly related to the prolonged disuse of the extremity. **(B)** Lateral view of the left knee demonstrates the abnormal inferior position of the patella.

Chronic subluxations of the patella are much more common than true dislocations. Extensive literature exists devoted to patellar tracking dysfunctions, extensor mechanism deficiencies, and pathognomonic biomechanical factors present at the patellofemoral joint or acting on the joint, all of which can contribute to the predisposition for the initial subluxation or dislocation and the susceptibility for recurrent subluxation or dislocation.

Radiologic Evaluation

Although the diagnosis of a chronically subluxing patellofemoral joint is clinically evident by history or physical examination, radiographs are necessary to determine whether osteochondral fragments or fractures are present, assist in the diagnosis of subtle subluxations, and provide information regarding the joint articular surfaces and joint congruity at different points in the range of motion.

The recommended projections for evaluating subluxation are not standard and vary among authors. Multiple tangential and lateral views made at varying degrees of flexion are suggested, as are weight-bearing AP and oblique views. Axial MRI and CT can provide information on joint congruity with the knee in extension (Fig. 13-40). A limitation of any imaging study is that the images are static while the disorder is dynamic; that is, the patella subluxes only during movement, when biomechanical forces are acting on it. Thus, in the clinical management of this condition, a correlation of imaging information and clinical examination best serves to aid clinical decision making.

Treatment

Conservative treatment focuses on minimizing the abnormal pathognomonic biomechanics that predispose the patellofemoral joint to subluxation. Strengthening and

stretching exercises, orthotics, patellar taping, and muscle reeducation are part of rehabilitation.

Surgical release of the lateral patellar retinaculum may be indicated for correction of patellar malalignment. Distal repositioning of the patellar tendon insertion is indicated for the correction of extensor mechanism malalignment or to reduce an excessive patellar Q angle.

Injury to the Articular Cartilage

Three separate traumatic conditions afflict the articular cartilage at the knee: *osteochondral fracture, osteochondritis dissecans,* and *spontaneous osteonecrosis.* These conditions have similar radiologic appearances; therefore the terms are often used interchangeably—incorrectly. However, these are separate conditions with distinct etiologies and treatments.

Osteochondral Fracture

Osteochondral fractures are commonly seen in young athletes. The femoral condyles, tibial plateaus, or patella may sustain an osteochondral fracture. The lateral femoral condyle is often involved, and may be related to a transient patellar dislocation. The severity of the injury may range from only a minor indentation of the articular cartilage to a portion of the articular cartilage becoming detached, often taking with it a piece of subchondral bone.

Mechanism

It is most often sports-related injuries involving combinations of shear, rotation, and impaction forces at the knee that damage the articular cartilage (then simply *chondral fracture*) or the articular cartilage and underlying subchondral bone (*osteochondral fracture*).

Radiologic Evaluation

A partially attached fragment is referred to as an *osteocartilaginous flap,* and a segment that is completely detached and floating freely about the joint is an *osteochondral fragment* (Fig. 13-41). A chondral fracture, involving only the cartilage, would not be seen on radiograph and would be demonstrated by MRI.

Treatment

Treatment depends on the stability of the fracture. If the fracture fragment is well attached to bone, immobilization and several weeks of non–weight-bearing may be adequate. Detached fragments and loose bodies may be removed arthroscopically. Large dime-sized fragments may be treated with arthroscopic drilling underneath the fragment to cause bleeding and stimulate new growth. Bioabsorbable pin fixation of fragments has shown good results. Transplants of non–weight-bearing articular cartilage to the defect are also possible.

Osteochondritis Dissecans (OCD)

This condition is seen in older children, teenagers, and young adults, particularly those active in sports. Dull pain and chronic joint effusions are exacerbated with weight-bearing activity. OCD has come to be considered a chronic form of osteochondral fracture. The non–weight-bearing medial femoral condyle is involved 85% of the time.

Mechanism

As in the case of osteochondral fracture, shearing and rotational forces act to detach a fragment of articular cartilage and subchondral bone.

Radiologic Evaluation

In the early stages of osteochondritis dissecans, radiographs will show no abnormalities. In the later stages, a radiolucent line is present separating the detached fragment from the femoral condyle. Loose bodies in the knee joint are a common finding.

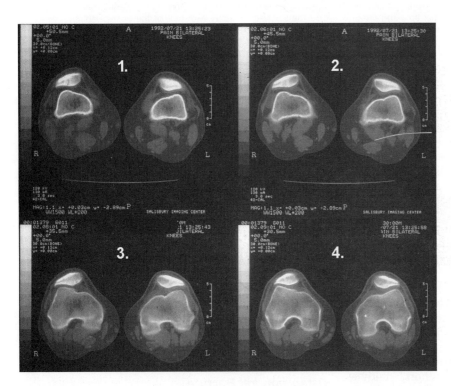

Figure 13-40 CT images showing poor congruency of the patellofemoral joint. Each image shows both knees; the right knee is to your left. These axial slices through the patella and trochlear sulcus of the femur, numbered 1 to 4, are made at 5-mm intervals from the superior aspect of the patella to its more inferior aspect. Note that the patellae articulate only with the lateral aspect of the trochlear sulcae and are tilted laterally (externally rotated). *(Image courtesy of Cliff Spohr, MD.)*

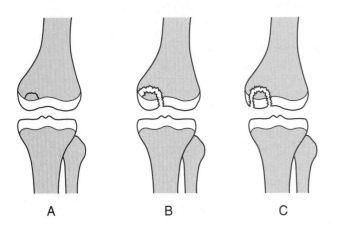

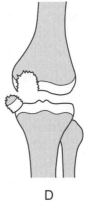

Figure 13-41 Examples of chondral fractures: **(A)** osteochondral body with intact articular cartilage; **(B)** osteocartilaginous flap; **(C)** detached osteochondral fragment; **(D)** detached osteochondral fragment in joint. Avascular necrosis of any of these lesions is termed *osteochondritis dissecans.*

MRI, in T1 or T2 sequences, will demonstrate the lesion early as an intermediate signal with a low signal line separating the lesion from surrounding healthy bone (Fig. 13-42A,B).

Treatment

Conservative treatment in young patients with nondisplaced fragments includes limitation of activity with the use of crutches and restricted range of motion for a trial of 3 to 6 months. If symptoms persist or failure to unite is observed, surgical treatment is recommended.

Many surgical options exist. Arthroscopy drilling of the defect may be performed, in the hope that revascularization will occur. Pinning or screw fixation may be performed to stabilize the fragment. Excision of the fragment and removal of loose bodies may be necessary. Osteochondral autograft or allograft transplantation (OATS) involves harvesting from other areas of the knee to reconstruct a weight-bearing surface. Autologous chondrocyte implantation (ACI) requires harvesting of a small amount of cartilage cells for cloning, and subsequent reimplantation. Bone grafting of the OCD crater is often necessary prior to implantation.

Spontaneous Osteonecrosis

This disorder affects older adults and has a predilection for the *weight-bearing* area of the medial femoral condyle.

Mechanism

Spontaneous osteonecrosis presents in older adults, usually female, as an acute pain without a history of trauma. Etiology is not clear but has been associated with steroids, administered either parenterally or by intra-articular injection. It is also associated with preexisting meniscal tears that may cause a concentrated area of stress between the femoral condyle and meniscal fragment. There is also suggestion that this disorder is actually a chronic stress fracture of the subchondral bone.

Radiologic Evaluation

Bone scans are most sensitive to the initial stages of this disorder. The first indication on routine radiographs will be a flattening of the affected femoral condyle. Some 1 to 3 months after the onset of pain, a radiolucent lesion is visible surrounded by a sclerotic marginal line representing attempts at repair. MRI will demonstrate the lesion as an intermediate signal with a low-signal line separating the lesion from surrounding healthy bone.

Treatment

Controversy exists regarding the best treatment of spontaneous osteonecrosis. The condition can be self-limiting with conservative care, respond to arthroscopic debridement and drilling for revascularization, or require a unicompartmental arthroplasty.

Meniscal Tears

Clinical Presentation

Meniscal tears are common sports-related injuries. Isolated tears present with intermittent clicking and eventually chronic blocking or locking of knee joint motion, accompanied by episodes of effusion and pain.

Mechanism of Injury

Meniscal tears occur during shear, rotary, and compression forces that abnormally stress the fibrocartilaginous tissues.

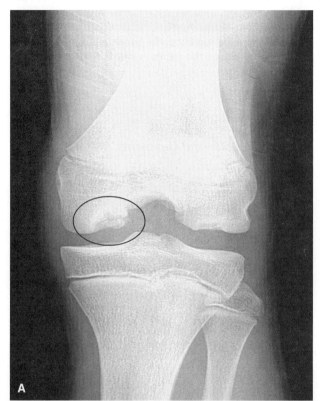

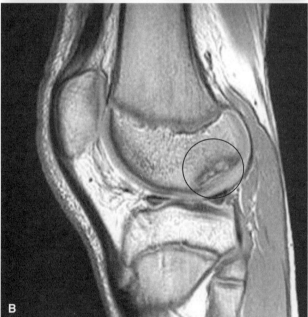

Figure 13-42 (A) Osteochondral defect on the medial aspect of the lateral femoral condyle (circled) in a 15-year-old soccer player. **(B)** Sagittal T1-weighted MR image demonstrating the defect within an intact articular cartilage. A 1-year rest from the aggravating activity of running was all that was required to allow this defect to resolve spontaneously without surgical intervention. *(Image courtesy of Travis Tasker.)*

The medial meniscus is more frequently injured than the lateral meniscus because of its greater peripheral attachment and decreased mobility, impairing its ability to withstand imposed forces.

The lateral meniscus is more prone to injury, however, if a developmental abnormality often referred to as a *discoid meniscus* is present. A discoid lateral meniscus is an enlarged, thickened meniscus, theorized to be caused by repetitive movements. An abnormally wide lateral radiographic joint space is evident on the AP knee projection if this condition exists.

Radiologic Evaluation

MRI is the standard modality for evaluating the menisci. The spectrum of injury characteristics is presented in Figure 13-43. On MRI, the menisci are seen as low signal intensity structures (dark) with a higher signal intensity (bright) tear that extends to the surface. A globular or linear focal increased signal intensity *within* the substance of the meniscus, that *does not* extend to the surface, is not a tear. These findings are thought to represent degeneration in the substance of the meniscus.

The most common meniscal tears are vertically oriented through the tissue; a longitudinal extension of a vertical tear is called a *bucket handle tear* (Fig. 13-44). Degenerative tears in the older age groups are usually horizontally oriented.

Treatment

Treatment involves surgical intervention, because the torn fragment will disrupt normal knee functioning. Total meniscectomies are uncommon unless the entire meniscus is involved. Partial meniscectomies excise the torn portion of the meniscus and preserve as much of the meniscus as possible. Surgical repair of tears is possible in peripherally located tears where good vascularity is present.

Rehabilitation generally involves an early phase of protected joint motion, isometric exercise, and partial weight bearing; an intermediate phase of progressive isotonic and isokinetic exercise and progressive ambulation; and a return to function phase involving full restoration of normal range of motion and plyometrics to prepare for joint-loading situations. Generally, the patient returns to full function in 4 to 5 months.

Injury to the Ligaments

Tears of the Collateral Ligaments

Clinical Presentation

The patient presents after an acute episode with pain, joint effusion, and instability upon physical examination via ligamentous stress testing.

Mechanism of Injury

The lateral collateral is injured from a varus force. The medial collateral ligament is typically injured as a result of a valgus force. The medial ligament is the more commonly injured collateral and is often associated with tears of the joint capsule and medial meniscus, to which it is firmly attached. Severe injuries will damage the anterior cruciate

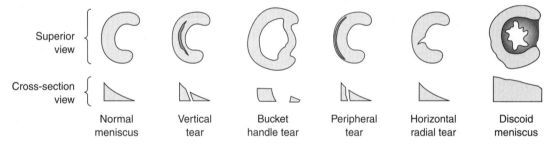

Figure 13-43 Examples of meniscal tears.

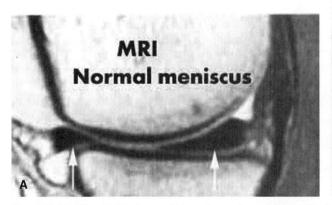

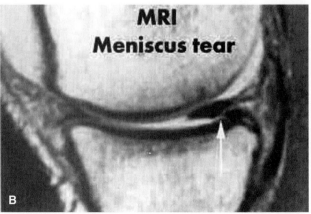

Figure 13-44 **(A)** Axial CT of normal triangular meniscus. **(B)** Axial CT of meiniscal tear. Note the high-intensity signal of the tear, which extends into the inferior surface of the meniscus (arrow).

ligament as well, and this combination of injuries is referred to as *O'Donoghue's terrible (or unhappy) triad* (Fig. 13-45).

Radiologic Evaluation

Radiographic assessment via stress films can demonstrate instability by application of a valgus force at the knee while an AP projection is made. Excessive widening of the medial joint space is consistent with a diagnosis of medial collateral ligament tear. Additionally, arthrography will demonstrate a leak of contrast material at the tear site, acutely; when the capsule seals the contrast will not leak even though the ligament remains disrupted. Chronic tears may heal and eventually ossify, and then the characteristic *Pellegrini-Stieda* lesion will be evident on the AP radiograph, diagnostic of the old injury.

MRI is the study of choice with T2-weighted sequences the most revealing (Fig. 13-46). Discontinuity of the low-signal-intensity ligament is best demonstrated on the coronal image.

Treatment

Treatment in the case of isolated collateral ligament tears may be conservative with controlled-motion bracing and extensive rehabilitation through progressive phases as noted previously for meniscus tears. Surgical repair is often required in more involved injuries, followed by extensive rehabilitation.

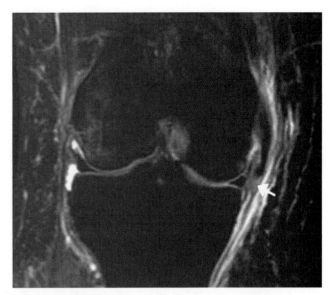

Figure 13-46 Coronal T2-weighted MRI showing complete rupture of the medial collateral ligament as an abrupt discontinuity of the low signal (dark) ligament (arrow).

Tears of the Cruciate Ligaments

Sports-related anterior cruciate ligament injuries occur at a rate of about 200,000 per year in the United States. Women are affected up to eight times more often than men participating in the same sports; factors implicated in this disparity include hormones, anatomic differences, and more upright posture during athletic activity. True incidence of the less common posterior cruciate ligament injury is not known.

Mechanism of Injury

Mechanisms of injury to the posterior cruciate ligament involve external forces that strike the anterior aspect of the knee, as in dashboard injuries (Fig. 13-47). Mechanisms of injury to the anterior cruciate ligament involve noncontact forces that place great valgus and rotary stresses on the knee, as when an athlete suddenly decelerates, turns, and hears the classic "pop" of a rupture (Fig. 13-48).

Knee dislocation, a rare occurrence caused by high-energy trauma, ruptures at least three of the four major ligamentous structures of the knee. Knee dislocations rupture the cruciates and cause, at varying degrees, injury to the collaterals, capsule, and menisci (Fig. 13-49).

Radiologic Evaluation

Radiographs are required to evaluate possible associated avulsion fractures at the site of cruciate ligament attachments. Sagittal MR images are best to demonstrate the cruciates. An indirect sign of anterior cruciate tear on MRI is known as "kissing contusions" or the *lateral femoral notch sign*, which represents the bone contusion that occurs as the anterior cruciate is torn (see Fig. 5-13 for an image of a bone bruise). This impaction of the lateral femoral condyle on the posterior tibial plateau occurs during the flexion–rotation–valgus mechanism of the injury. As the tibia displaces anteriorly, it hits the lateral femoral condyle, indenting in it. This contusion produces a bone marrow edema, which is seen as an area of high signal intensity.

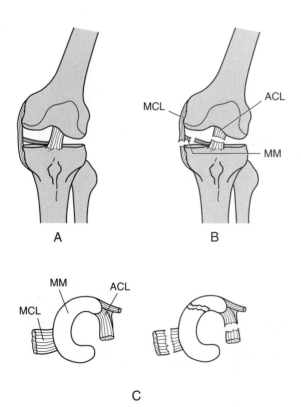

Figure 13-45 The "terrible triad," a combination of injuries to the medial meniscus (MM), medial collateral ligament (MCL), and anterior cruciate ligament (ACL), viewed from two different perspectives. **(A)** Intact ligaments stretched by valgus force. **(B)** Rupture of MCL, ACL, and MM. **(C)** Superior views: left, normal relationship of MCL, ACL, and MM; right, rupture of MCL, ACL, and MM.

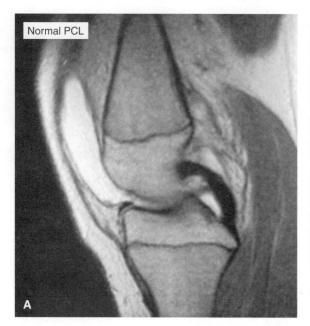

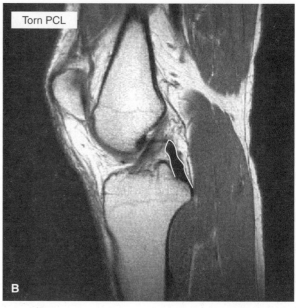

Figure 13-47 (A) Sagittal MRI demonstrating a normal posterior cruciate ligament seen as a low-signal continuous cord-like structure. **(B)** Sagittal MRI demonstrating a rupture of the posterior cruciate ligament seen as a interuption in the cord-like structure (outlined).

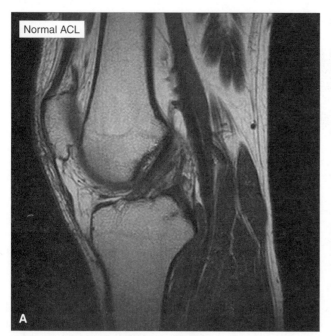

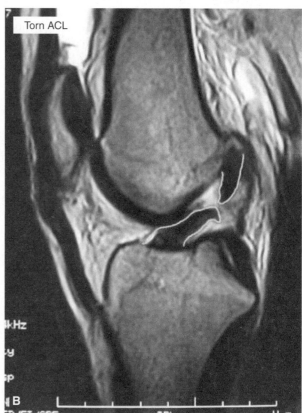

Figure 13-48 (A) Sagittal MRI demonstrating a normal anterior cruciate ligament extending from the anterior tibial plateau to the posterior femoral condyle. **(B)** Sagittal MRI demonstrating a complete midsubstance tear of the anterior cruciate ligament (outlined).

Treatment

Treatment depends on the amount of joint instability, the associated structural damage, and the patient's desired activity level.

Conservative treatment includes controlled-motion bracing and extensive strengthening rehabilitation. Surgical intervention may include direct, primary repairs to the injured tissues or reconstructive procedures using tendon grafts, followed by extensive rehabilitation in progressive phases. The patient usually returns to full normal activity within 4 to 6 months.

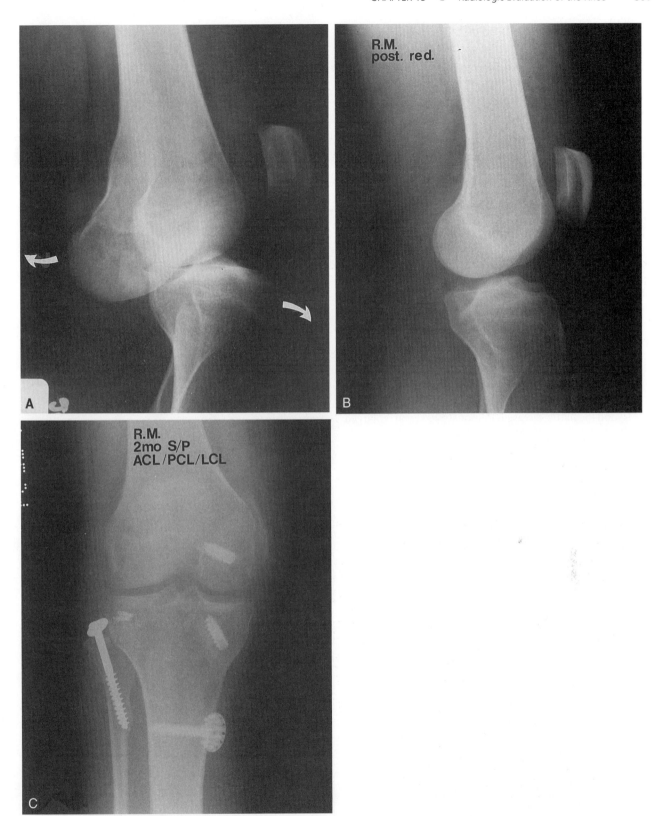

Figure 13-49 Anterior dislocation of the knee with rupture of ligaments. This 22-year-old man was injured when he was thrown from a horse he was trying to saddle-break and the horse fell on him. **(A)** Lateral view of the knee shows the anterior displacement of the tibia in relation to the distal femur. **(B)** Lateral film made after reduction demonstrates normal articulating relationships and absence of any fractures. Note the great amount of capsular effusion and soft tissue swelling. **(C)** Although the patient did not sustain any fractures, he did rupture several ligaments. This AP film demonstrates the hardware used to surgically fixate and reconstruct the attachments of the anterior cruciate ligament, posterior cruciate ligament, and lateral collateral ligament. This patient was fortunate in that he escaped neurovascular injury during the initial accident. About half of all knee dislocations involve some degree of damage to the popliteal artery or peroneal nerve.

Trauma at the Patellar Ligament

Two similar conditions related to repetitive trauma occur at the ends of the patellar ligament (Fig. 13-50). Both disorders present clinically with soft tissue swelling, pain, and localized tenderness. Adolescents, predominantly boys, are most frequently affected.

Sinding–Larsen–Johansson disease refers to the disorder at the proximal patellar attachment, and *Osgood–Schlatter* disease refers to the disorder at the distal patellar attachment.

Mechanism of Injury

These disorders are mechanical in etiology, possibly initiated by trauma such as a fall, and as such are not true disease processes. The repetitive irritation from tension forces generated by quadriceps activity postinjury is theorized to be a factor in the development of these *traction apophysitis* conditions. Chronic irritation from activities such as jumping and running on hard surfaces exacerbates these conditions.

Radiologic Evaluation

Sinding–Larsen–Johansson disease is demonstrated by fragmentation of the inferior pole of the patella (Fig. 13-51). Calcification and ossification often appear in the patellar ligament when the condition has become chronic.

Osgood–Schlatter disease is demonstrated by an enlarged and deformed tibial tubercle (Fig. 13-52).

The lateral radiograph usually establishes the diagnosis as bone fragmentation; ossification within the tendon is obvious at either location.

Treatment

Treatment consists of limited activity, modalities to control inflammation and pain, and protective padding to prevent further impact to the knee. Surgical excision of large calcified areas may be necessary.

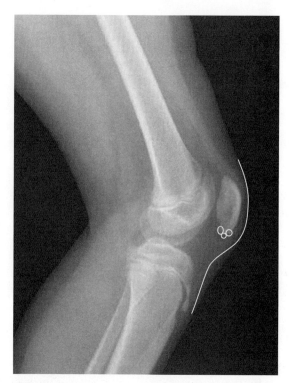

Figure 13-51 Sinding–Larsen–Johansson disease. On this lateral view of the knee, ossification and fragmentation within the patellar ligament is apparent just distal to the patella (circled calcifications). Note the corresponding bulge evident in front of the patellar ligament.

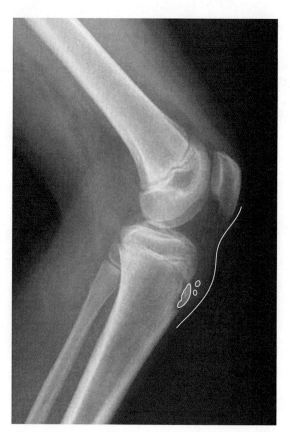

Figure 13-52 Osgood–Schlatter disease. This lateral radiograph of the knee demonstrates ossification and fragmentation with the patellar ligament at its attachment to the tibial tubercle (circled). Note the corresponding anterior bulge evident in front of the tibial tubercle.

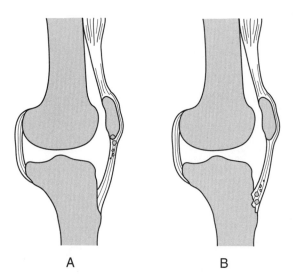

Figure 13-50 Representation of traction apophysitis with fragmentation in the patellar ligament **(A)** at the inferior patellar pole, known as *Sinding–Larsen–Johansson* disease, and **(B)** at the tibial tuberosity, known as *Osgood–Schlatter* disease.

Degenerative Joint Disease[2,7,8,18,19,20,30,32,51–53]

Degenerative joint disease (DJD), or osteoarthritis, of the knees is present radiographically to some degree in the majority of people over age 55. Repetitive mechanical and compressive stresses from occupational, recreational, athletic, and normal activities of daily living over many decades typically result in degenerative changes in the joints. Also, secondary degenerative changes are long-term sequelae of previous fracture, meniscal, or ligamentous injury.

Radiologic Evaluation

The characteristic radiographic signs of DJD at the knee may include the following:

1. Decreased radiographic joint space
2. Sclerosis of subchondral bone
3. Osteophyte formation at joint margins
4. Subchondral cyst formation
5. Varus or valgus joint deformity

The routine radiographic examination sufficiently demonstrates these changes (Fig. 13-53). Recurrent joint effusions are

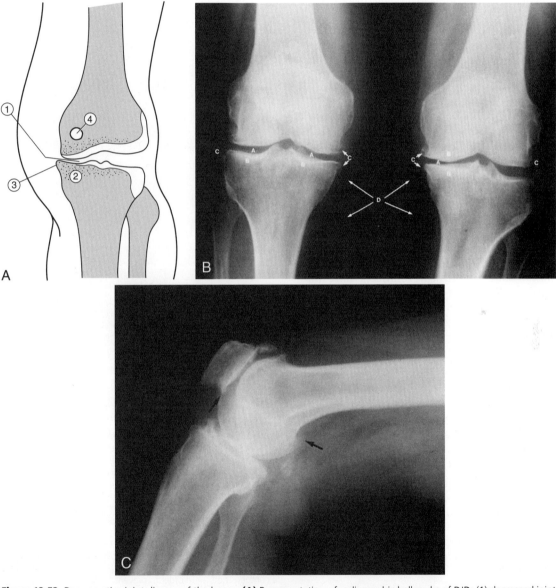

Figure 13-53 Degenerative joint disease of the knees. **(A)** Representation of radiographic hallmarks of DJD: (1) decreased joint space, (2) sclerotic subchondral bone, (3) osteophyte formation at joint margins, and (4) subchondral cyst formation. **(B)** AP weight-bearing view of bilateral knees in an elderly man demonstrates the characteristic hallmarks of advanced DJD: (a) narrowed joint spaces (note the extreme narrowing of the medial compartment of patient's left knee); (b) sclerosis of subchondral bone; (c) osteophyte formation at joint margins; (d) joint deformity secondary to loss of articular cartilage thickness and altered joint congruity. Note the soft tissue outline of both extremities, which shows a medial bulging at the joint line combined with a bowleg or varus deformity secondary to the medial angulation and slight rotation of the tibia. This deformity is more pronounced on the patient's left lower extremity. **(C)** On this lateral view of the knee, note DJD of the patellofemoral joint and femorotibial joint with flattening of the patellar articular surface and marked spur formation at the patella margins and the margins of the femoral condyles (arrows). The irregularly shaped density in the soft tissue of the popliteal fossa is the fabella. The large soft tissue mass hanging down from the popliteal space is the Baker's cyst.

a characteristic of exacerbations of both noninflammatory and inflammatory arthritides. A consequence of this is the formation of a popliteal cyst, known as a Baker's cyst, which is evident on the lateral radiograph.

Location of DJD

The location of DJD at the knee is described in terms of the knee's anatomic compartments. The medial compartment of the knee is the articulation between the medial femoral and tibial condyles. The lateral compartment of the knee is the articulation between the lateral femoral and tibial condyles. The patellofemoral articulation is also referred to as a compartment and is susceptible to degenerative changes as well.

Advanced DJD of the lateral or medial compartment alters the congruity of the articular surfaces and may cause a valgus- or varus-type deformity, respectively, visible both on films and clinically (Fig. 13-54).

Treatment

Nonsurgical treament of DJD includes rehabilitation for strengthening, restoration of functional leg length, ambulatory devices, bracing, and pain management via nonsteroidal anti-inflammatory drugs or intra-articular steroid injections.

Degenerative changes that cause significant debility may require surgical intervention. *Total joint arthroplasty (or total knee replacement)* is a surgical procedure that replaces the articular surfaces of the femur, tibia, and patella (Fig. 13-55). *Unicompartmental knee replacement* resurfaces only the affected compartment (Fig. 13-56A,B). Complications of either procedure include bone fracture, instability, infection, and loosening of the prosthesis.

Goals of rehabilitation after joint replacement are to restore functional strength, functional joint range of motion, and functional leg length. (See Chapter 12 for a discussion on functional leg length.)

Knee Anomalies[13,18,19,32]

Anomalies can generally be grouped into categories related to a structure's failure to develop, arrested development, or the development of accessory bones. At the knee an additional grouping is needed, regarding the deformity that may be present within the bone itself, as in the example of congenital limb bowing. Common examples of knee and lower extremity congenital deformities are *genu valgum*, *genu varum*, and *genu recurvatum*.

Genu Valgum

Genu valgum is the angular deformity of the lower extremities commonly referred to as "knock-knees." The distal ends of the tibia are spaced widely apart when the knees are approximated (Fig. 13-57A,B).

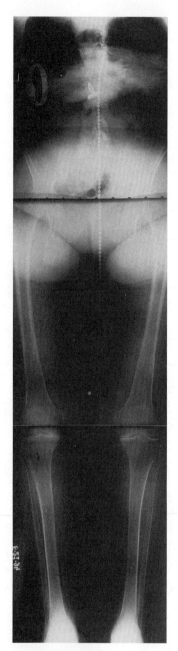

Figure 13-54 Alignment determined from standing views of the entire lower extremity. This weight-bearing view assists the surgeon preoperatively in determining the amount of varus or valgus deformity present secondary to the degenerative knee joint and in planning for the amount of surgical correction required. Various types of surgical procedures can correct knee joint deformities, including tibial osteotomy, in which a wedge of bone is removed from the proximal tibia to realign the leg and reduce and redistribute stresses over the largest possible articular surface; and total joint arthroplasty, which resects the involved articular surfaces and replaces them with artificial tibial, femoral, and patellar prostheses. Note that whatever procedure is chosen, it is likely that the leg length will be altered postoperatively. It is desirable in the patient's rehabilitation that this be compensated for in order to prevent further mechanical stresses in the other joints of the kinetic chain. This can be achieved simply by utilizing a heel lift in the shoe of the shorter leg.

The condition becomes most obvious when a child begins to ambulate. The etiology may be familial, related to hip or foot positioning, associated with trauma to the epiphyseal plate, fractures, or neurological deficits, or it may be idiopathic.

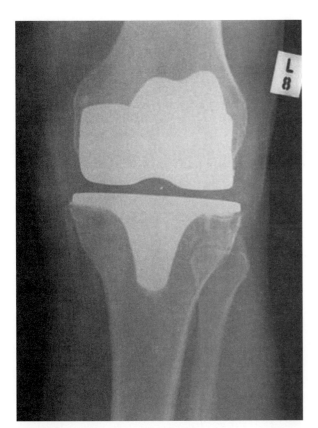

Figure 13-55 AP radiograph demonstrating a total knee replacement. *(Image courtesy of http://www.xray2000.co.uk.)*

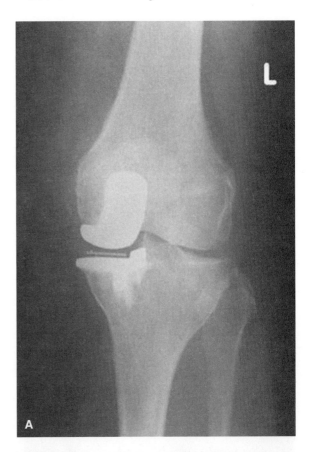

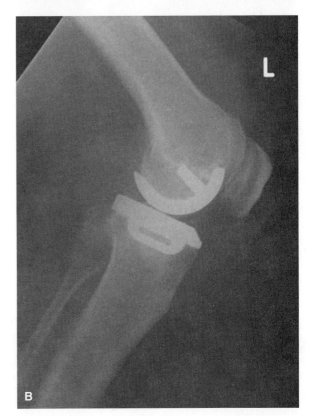

The AP radiograph of the entire lower extremity adequately demonstrates this deformity.

Treatment and prognosis depend on the etiologic factors and the severity of the angulation. Conservative treatment for mild cases consists of rehabilitation for orthotic correction of foot pronation and exercises to address flexibility and strength deficits. Surgery may be required in more severe cases to restore normal joint articulation.

Genu Varum

Genu varum is the angular deformity of the lower extremities commonly referred to as "bow legs." The knees are spaced widely apart when the ankle malleoli are in contact (Fig. 13-58A). It is common for a certain amount of apparent bowing to be present in infants and toddlers; this *physiological bowing* will be symmetrical and is usually outgrown during childhood, decreasing progressively as the child ages (Fig. 13-58B).

The etiology of genu varum may also be highly varied, related to renal or dietary rickets, epiphyseal injury, osteogenesis imperfecta, or osteochondritis, known as Blount's disease.

Radiologic Findings

Genu varum is assessed on AP radiographs of the entire lower extremity. Developmental physiological bowing of the

Figure 13-56 (A) AP radiograph demonstrating a unicompartmental knee replacement, which has resurfaced the medial joint compartment. **(B)** Lateral radiograph of the "half" knee replacement. *(Image courtesy of http://www.xray2000.co.uk.)*

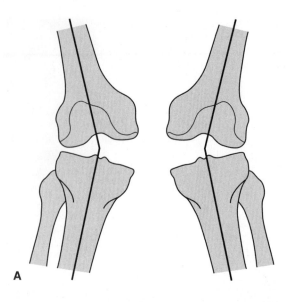

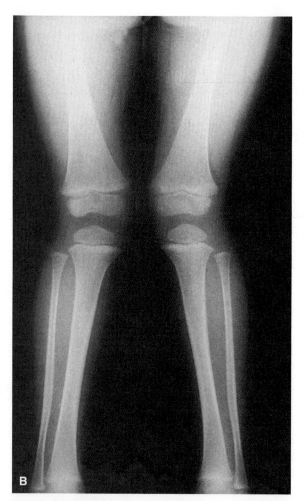

Figure 13-57 (A) Genu valgum, or "knock knees," is an angular deformity of the lower extremities in which the ankles are spaced widely apart when the knees are approximated. **(B)** This AP weight-bearing view of the lower extremities in a 3-year-old boy demonstartes bilateral genu valgum.

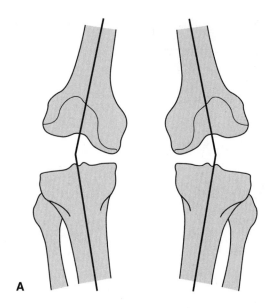

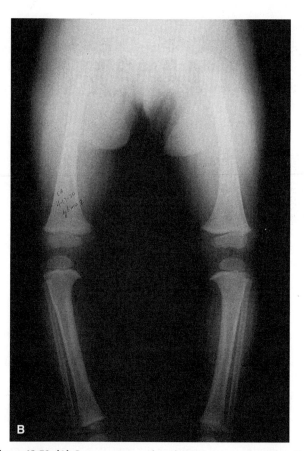

Figure 13-58 (A) Genu varum, or "bow legs," is an angular deformity of the lower extremities, whereby the knees are spaced widely apart when the ankles are in contact. **(B)** AP weight-bearing views of this 18-month-old girl demonstrate bilateral genu varum. This symmetrical apparent bowing is common in many toddlers and is usually outgrown in childhood.

extremities is distinguished from other disease processes by the normal appearance of cortical bone, epiphyses, plates, and metaphyses. Both the femoral and tibial medial and lateral cortical shafts will exhibit gentle bowing.

Genu Recurvatum

Genu recurvatum is excessive hyperextension of the knee (Fig. 13-59). Etiologies are varied and numerous and may be familial, idiopathic, or related to neurological and muscular deficits.

Treatment and prognosis are dependent on the etiological factors, but treatment is usually conservative, using bracing and exercise to restore alignment and muscular balance. The lateral radiograph demonstrates this deformity.

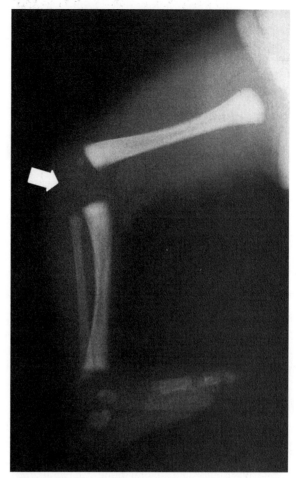

Figure 13-59 Genu recurvatum. This unusual example of genu recurvatum is seen in a radiograph of a 2-day-old infant. The arrow points to the *posterior* knee joint, which is in a position of extreme hyperextension.

Summary of Key Points

Routine Radiologic Evaluation

1. The routine radiographic evaluation of the knee includes four projections.
   - ➤ *AP*—demonstrates the femorotibial joint, distal femur, and proximal tibia. The patella is obscured because it is superimposed over the distal femur.
   - ➤ *Lateral*—demonstrates the patellofemoral joint in profile, the expanse of the quadriceps and patellar tendon, and the suprapatellar bursa.
   - ➤ *PA axial of the intercondylar fossa*—demonstrates the intercondylar fossa, the posterior aspect of the femoral condyles, and the intercondylar eminence of the tibial plateau.
   - ➤ *Tangential view of the patellofemoral joint*—demonstrates the patella and the articular relationship of the patellofemoral joint at one point in the range of motion.

Trauma at the Knee

2. *Radiographs* are sufficient for diagnosis and treament of most fractures at the knee. The ACR recommends radiographs as the *first initial study* for most traumatic and nontraumatic cases of knee pain.

3. *CT* with two- or three-dimensionally reconstructed images is valuable in the delineation of the degree of fragmentation or the depression of the articular surfaces as well as in preoperative planning.

4. *MRI* is essential in the evaluation of injuries to the articular cartilage, menisci, the cruciate and collateral ligaments, and the soft tissues.

5. *Bone scans* can identify occult or subtle fractures, stress fractures, and injury to the articular cartilage, with great sensitivity but inexact anatomic location.

Clinical Decision Rules

6. *Clinical decision rules* are guidelines that assist the practitioner in deciding if radiographs are needed to define a fracture. The clinical decision rules created in Ottawa and Pittsburgh are the best-known guidelines for the appropriate use of radiographs in acute knee injuries. These similar guides state that radiographs *should* be ordered

after trauma if any of the following is present: joint effusion after a direct blow or fall, inability to walk without limping, palpable tenderness over the patella or fibular head, or inability to flex the knee to 90 degrees. Radiographs *should not* be ordered if a patient had a twisting injury but is able to walk and no effusion is present.

Fractures at the Knee

7. Fractures of the *distal femur* are classified by anatomic location as supracondylar, intercondylar, or condylar fractures.

8. Fractures of the *proximal tibia* occur most frequently at the tibial plateaus, with the lateral plateau most often involved.

9. The *patella* is vulnerable to two types of injury: fracture sustained from a direct blow and avulsion fracture sustained from forceful contraction of the quadriceps.

Patellofemoral Subluxation

10. Chronic patellofemoral subluxation is evident by history or physical examination. Radiographs are necessary to determine whether osteochondral fragments or fractures are present and to provide information regarding the joint articular surfaces and joint congruity. Axial MRI and CT also provide information on joint congruity with the knee in extension.

Injuries to the Articular Cartilage

11. Three distinct conditions have similar terminology and should not be confused with each other:

    ➤ *Osteochondral fractures* are fractures at the articular cartilage and subchondral bone. *Chondral fractures* involve only the articular cartilage. The lateral femoral condyle is most often involved in this acute sports-related injury, and may be related to a transient patellar dislocation.

    ➤ *Osteochondritis dissecans* is a chronic osteochondral fracture, most often seen in adolescent athletes. The non–weight-bearing medial femoral condyle is most often involved.

    ➤ *Spontaneous osteonecrosis* involves the weight-bearing medial femoral condyle, and is seen most often in elderly females without a history of trauma.

Meniscal Tears

12. *Meniscal tears* are common sports-related injuries that present with intermittent clicking and locking of the knee joint. The medial meniscus is more frequently injured than the lateral meniscus. MRI is the standard modality for evaluating the menisci.

Injuries to the Ligaments

13. The *medial collateral ligament* is the more commonly injured collateral and in severe injury is associated with tears of the joint capsule, medial meniscus, and the anterior cruciate ligament, a combination of injuries known as *O'Donoghue's terrible* (or *unhappy*) *triad*. MRI is the study of choice with T2-weighted sequences the most revealing. Old tears may heal, ossify, and be evident on the AP radiograph as the characteristic *Pellegrini–Stieda* lesion.

14. Sports-related *anterior cruciate ligament* injuries occur at a rate of about 200,000 per year in the United States with females affected up to eight times more often than men participating in the same sports. Radiographs are required to evaluate possible avulsion fractures at the site of cruciate ligament attachments. Sagittal MR images are best to demonstrate the cruciates. An indirect sign of a tear of an anterior cruciate ligament on MRI is the *lateral femoral notch sign*, which represents the bone contusion that occurs from impaction of the lateral femoral condyle to the posterior tibial plateau.

15. *Sinding–Larsen–Johansson* disease and *Osgood–Schlatter* disease are mechanical traction disorders of the proximal and distal patellar ligament attachment sites, respectively. In chronic stages, the lateral radiograph will reveal bone fragmentation and calcification within the affected area of the patellar ligament.

Degenerative Joint Disease at the Knee

16. *Degenerative joint disease* at the knee is hallmarked radiographically by (a) decreased joint space, (b) sclerotic subchondral bone, (c) osteophyte formation at joint margins, (d) subchondral cyst formation, and (e) varus or valgus deformities.

Anomalies

17. Common congenital deformities of the knee and lower extremity include *genu valgum* or "knock-knees," *genu varum* or "bowlegs," and *genu recurvatum* or hyperextended knees. Valgus and varus deformities may also develop in adulthood secondary to altered joint congruity resulting from destructive joint processes such as DJD.

 Please refer to the text's enclosed CD-ROM for the American College of Radiology's current Musculoskeletal Appropriateness Criteria for the following topics: *Acute Trauma to the Knee, Nontraumatic Knee Pain, Imaging of Total Knee Arthroplasty.*

CASE STUDIES

CASE STUDY 1

Cancer Presenting as Knee Pain

The patient is a 60-year-old woman who self-referred to physical therapy because of the gradual onset of left knee pain.

Physical Therapy Examination

Patient Interview

The patient reported that her left knee pain had come on gradually over the past 6 weeks. As she had seen a physical therapist many years ago for a knee problem, she thought she would go directly to a physical therapist for evaluation.

She described the pain as a constant deep and boring pain that became sharper when standing and walking. She said that the knee pain had been keeping her awake at night over the previous 2 weeks, with little relief from over-the-counter pain medications.

The physical therapist questioned her carefully about her past medical history, discovering that she had been diagnosed with breast cancer 4 years previously and had been treated with lumpectomy, axillary dissection, and chemotherapy. Her checkups with the oncologist had all been fine, including the most recent appointment 6 months previously.

Physical Examination

The patient ambulated with an antalgic limp on the left. She was reluctant to bear her full weight through the left lower extremity. Screening examinations of the lumbar spine, hip, and ankle were unremarkable. Examination of the left knee was normal for range of motion and ligamentous integrity. Observation revealed no deformity or edema. Palpation about the knee was unremarkable, but the patient was very tender to palpation of the proximal tibia distal to the tibial tuberosity. Formal manual muscle testing was not performed because of the unusual nature of the patient's presentation and her medical history.

Intervention

The physical therapist provided crutches and gait training to the patient to promote safe ambulation and protect the painful knee. The physical therapist also immediately called the patient's oncologist and communicated concerns about an underlying serious pathology. Diagnostic imaging was ordered to rule out the primary concern: the possibility of a metastasis to bone.

Diagnostic Imaging

Anteroposterior (AP) and lateral radiographs of the knee and left lower leg were obtained as well as a whole-body bone scan. The radiographs demonstrated an osteolytic lesion in the proximal third of the tibia with a fracture extending through it (Fig. 13-60). The bone scan demonstrated metastases to multiple areas, including bilateral tibiae, bilateral ilia, left greater trochanter, lumbar spine, eighth rib, and skull (Fig. 13-61).

Outcome

The patient returned to her oncologist for treatment of the metastatic cancer. She was also referred to an orthopedic surgeon and had surgery to stabilize the left tibia prophylactically using an intramedullary nail. She returned to the physical therapist for rehabilitation following the surgery.

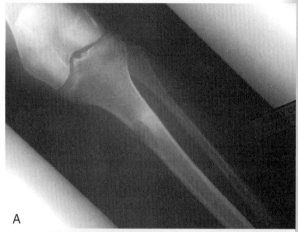
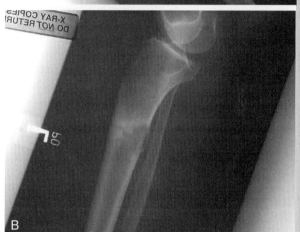

Figure 13-60 (A) AP and **(B)** lateral radiographs of the lower leg, demonstrating an osteolytic lesion with an incomplete, pathological fracture extending through it.

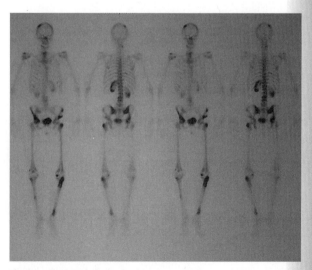

Figure 13-61 Whole-body bone scan, demonstrating multiple skeletal metastases.

Discussion

This case exemplifies the importance of a comprehensive patient interview, including a comprehensive medical history and an in-depth description of the pain pattern. This case also demonstrates the importance of understanding the indicators or "red flags" of serious pathology. The following factors were identified by the physical therapist as critical information:

1. A medical history positive for a cancer known to metastasize to bone

2. Constant pain, night pain, and pain unrelieved with rest or medication

3. Pain not reproducible with physical maneuvers of the knee

4. An area of pain remote from the knee joint, revealed by palpation

5. No traumatic incident or change of activities to explain the patient's onset of symptoms

The physical therapist acted correctly in limiting the physical examination (withholding muscle testing), protecting the affected limb (providing crutches), and contacting the appropriate professional (the oncologist) to get action taken as quickly as possible (appropriate diagnostic imaging ordered immediately).

The case is summarized in Figure 13-62.

CRITICAL THINKING POINT

Physical therapists who see patients in a direct-access role must be vigilant for nonmusculoskeletal sources of pain that may present as a musculoskeletal problem. Patients will often make incorrect assumptions about the source of their pain! They will not always readily report items from their history that they think are unrelated to the current problem. A comprehensive review of the patient's medical history is essential in the process of ruling out possible differential diagnoses that must include nonmusculoskeletal sources.

CASE STUDY 2

Discrepancy Between MRI Report and Surgical Report

The patient is a 40-year-old man referred to physical therapy for rehabilitation following arthroscopic knee surgery.

History of Trauma

The patient injured his right knee playing a game of pickup basketball with friends. He attempted to change directions quickly when he felt a painful sensation in the knee. He was unable to continue playing, and the knee swelled. Over the next few days, he experienced pain and locking in the knee and was unable to achieve full extension.

Initial Imaging

The patient was evaluated a few days later by an orthopedic surgeon. The surgeon aspirated the knee in the clinic and ordered a magnetic resonance imaging (MRI) scan. The radiologist's report stated the following: "There are signal changes in the body of the medial meniscus consistent with grade II degeneration. Evaluation of the lateral meniscus demonstrates a normal low-intensity signal and contour, without any findings to suggest a tear. Evaluation of the lateral tibiofemoral compartment

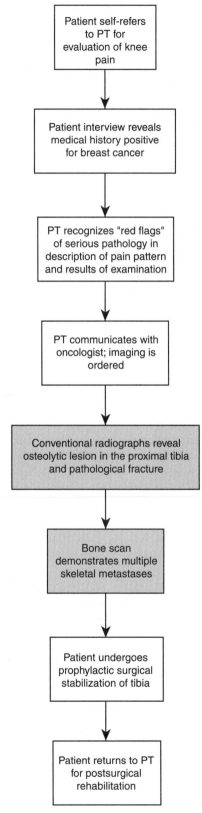

Figure 13-62 Pathway of case study events. Imaging is highlighted.

reveals an area of grade II to III chondromalacia of the posterior condyle. The anterior and posterior cruciate ligaments are without any evidence of disruption, distortion of their shape, or tears."

Intervention

The surgeon scheduled arthroscopic surgery for 1 week later. The operative report stated: "Intra-articular inspection reveals a 20-by-25-mm full-thickness chondral defect over the lateral aspect of the lateral femoral condyle. There is a small radial split in the lateral meniscus. The anterior cruciate ligament (ACL) is intact. The medial meniscus is intact."

The surgeon performed a partial meniscectomy of the *lateral* meniscus, débrided the articular defect, and created a microfracture of the underlying bone. The microfracture, which generated bleeding, was done to encourage healing of the femoral condyle's surface.

Physical Therapy Considerations

The physical therapist received both the initial MRI report and the surgical report with the patient's referral. The physical therapist was confused by the discrepancy between the MRI report and the surgical report. The MRI report did not mention a lateral meniscus tear, only degeneration of the medial meniscus. Furthermore, the MRI report spoke of chondromalacia of the femoral condyle but not a complete articular surface defect. When questioned by the therapist, the patient was unsure about the specifics of his procedure.

The therapist called the surgeon's office and was faxed the operative report, which explained the arthroscopic procedure in detail.

Discussion

This case exemplifies the inconsistencies that can sometimes exist between advanced imaging information and direct visualization. The physical therapist assumed, as do many clinicians, that MRI would show any and all pathology present in the patient's knee. Although this is usually true, direct observation inside the joint is still definitive.

This case is summarized in Figure 13-63.

CRITICAL THINKING POINTS

Any diagnostic imaging will have limitations in its sensitivity and specificity. Additionally, the chosen imaging planes, slice thicknesses, and selection of technical parameters—as well as interpreter skill—factor into the accuracy of the MRI report.

The clinician reading the report must remember that imaging is a technology that requires human interpretation and integration into treatment decisions.

Last, the physical therapist acted correctly in seeking out an answer prior to initiating treatment. *It is never a mistake not to touch something that is not understood.*

Case studies adapted by J. Bradley Barr, PT, DPT, OCS.

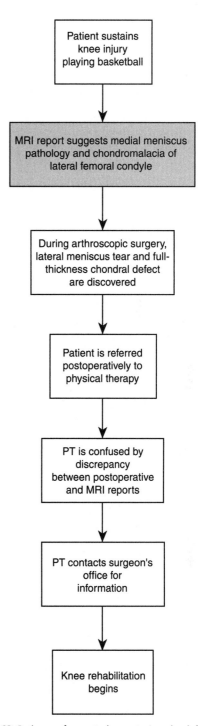

Figure 13-63 Pathway of case study events. Imaging is highlighted.

References

Normal Anatomy

1. Soderberg, GL: Kinesiology: Application to Pathological Motion. Williams & Wilkins, Baltimore, 1986.
2. Verna, A, et al: A screening method for knee trauma. Acad Radiol 8(5): 392, 2001.
3. Netter, FH: Atlas of Human Anatomy, ed. 4. WB Saunders, Philadelphia, 2006.
4. Nordin, M, and Frankel, VH: Basic Biomechanics of the Musculoskeletal System, ed. 3. Lippincott Williams & Wilkins, Philadelphia, 2001.
5. Whiting, W, and Zernicke, R: Biomechanics of Musculoskeletal Injury, ed. 2. Human Kinetics, Champaign, IL, 2008.
6. Norkin, CC, and Levangie, PK: Joint Structure and Function: A Comprehensive Analysis, ed. 2. FA Davis, Philadelphia, 1992.
7. Meschan, I: An Atlas of Radiographic Anatomy. WB Saunders, Philadelphia, 1960.
8. Weber, EC, Vilensky, JA, and Carmichael, SW: Netter's Concise Radiologic Anatomy. Saunders, Philadelphia, 2008.
9. Kelley, LL, and Peterson, CM: Sectional Anatomy for Imaging Professional, ed. 2. Mosby, St. Louis, MO, 2007.
10. Lazo, DL: Fundamentals of Sectional Anatomy: An Imaging Approach. Thomson Delmar Learning, Clifton Park, NY, 2005.

Routine Exam

11. American College of Radiology: Practice Guideline for the Performance of Radiography of the Extremities. 2006. Available at http://www.acr.org. Accessed July 22, 2008.
12. Weissman, B, and Sledge, C: Orthopedic Radiology. WB Saunders, Philadelphia, 1986.
13. Greenspan, A: Orthopedic Radiology: A Practical Approach, ed. 4. Lippincott Williams & Wilkins, Philadelphia, 2004.
14. Bontrager, KL: Textbook of Radiographic Positioning and Related Anatomy, ed. 6. Mosby, St. Louis, MO, 2005.
15. Fischer, HW: Radiographic Anatomy: A Working Atlas. McGraw-Hill, New York, 1988.
16. Wicke, L: Atlas of Radiographic Anatomy, ed. 5. Lea & Febiger, Malvern, PA, 1994.
17. Frank, E, Smith, B, and Long, B: Merrill's Atlas of Radiographic Positions and Radiologic Procedures, ed. 11. Elsevier Health Sciences, Philadelphia, 2007.
18. Squires, LF, and Novelline, RA: Fundamentals of Radiology, ed. 4. Harvard University Press, Cambridge, MA, 1988.
19. Chew, FS: Skeletal Radiology: The Bare Bones, ed. 2. Williams & Wilkins, Baltimore, 1997.
20. Weir, J, and Abrahams, P: An Atlas of Radiological Anatomy. Yearbook Medical, Chicago, 1978.
21. Krell, L (ed): Clark's Positioning in Radiology, Vol. 1, ed. 10. Yearbook Medical, Chicago, 1989.

Trauma

22. American College of Radiology: Appropriateness Criteria for Nontraumatic Knee Pain. 2005. Available at http://www.acr.org/SecondaryMainMenuCategories/quality_safety/app_criteria/pdf/ExpertPanelonMusculoskeletalImaging/NonTraumaticKneePainDoc15.aspx.
23. American College of Radiology: Appropriateness Criteria for Acute Trauma to the Knee. 2005. Available at http://www.acr.org/SecondaryMainMenuCategories/quality_safety/app_criteria/pdf/ExpertPanelonMusculoskeletalImaging/AcuteTraumatotheKneeDoc2.aspx.
24. Merchant, AC, et al: Roentgenographic analysis of patellofemoral congruence. J Bone Joint Surg 56A:1391, 1974.
25. Bucholz, RW, Heckman, J, and Court-Brown, C (eds): Rockwood and Green's Fractures in Adults, ed. 6. Lippincott Williams & Wilkins, Philadelphia, 2005.
26. Rockwood, CA, and Green, DP (eds): Fractures in Adults, ed. 5. Lippincott Williams & Wilkins, Philadelphia, 2002.
27. Beaty, J, and Kasar, J (eds): Rockwood and Wilkins' Fractures in Children, ed. 6. Lippincott Williams & Wilkins, Philadelphia, 2005.
28. Koval, KJ, and Zuckerman, JD: Handbook of Fractures, ed. 2. Lippincott Williams & Wilkins, Philadelphia, 2002.
29. Eiff, M, et al: Fracture Management for Primary Care. WB Saunders, Philadelphia, 2003.
30. Salter, RB: Textbook of Disorders and Injuries of the Musculoskeletal System, ed. 2. Williams & Wilkins, Baltimore, 1983.
31. Yochum, TR, and Rowe, LJ: Essentials of Skeletal Radiology, ed. 3. Williams & Wilkins, Baltimore, 2004.
32. Marchiori, DM: Clinical Imaging with Skeletal, Chest, and Abdomen Pattern Differentials. Mosby, St. Louis, MO, 1999.
33. Ip, D: Orthopedic Traumatology: A Resident's Guide. Springer, New York, 2006.
34. McConnell, J, Eyres, R, and Nightingale, J: Interpreting Trauma Radiographs. Blackwell, Malden, MA, 2005.
35. Berquist, TH: Imaging of Orthopedic Trauma, ed. 2. Raven Press, New York, 1989.
36. McCort, JJ, and Mindelzun, RE: Trauma Radiology. Churchill Livingstone, New York, 1990.
37. Drafke, MW, and Nakayama, H: Trauma and Mobile Radiography, ed. 2, FA Davis, Philadelphia, 2001.
38. Walsh, SJ, et al: Large osteochondral fractures of the lateral femoral condyle in the adolescent: Outcome of bioabsorbable pin fixation. J Bone Joint Surg Am 90(7):1473, 2008.
39. Akgun, I, et al: Arthroscopic microfracture treatment for osteonecrosis of the knee. Arthroscopy 21(7):834, 2005.
40. Langdown, AJ, et al: Oxford medial unicompartmental arthroplasty for focal spontaneous osteonecrosis of the knee. Acta Orthop 76(5):688, 2005.
41. Yates, PJ: Early MRI diagnosis and non-surgical management of spontaneous osteonecrosis of the knee. Knee 14(2):112, 2007.
42. Norman, A, and Baker, ND: Spontaneous osteonecrosis of the knee and medial meniscus tears. Radiology 129:653, 1978.
43. Kattapuram, TM, and Kattapuram, SV: Spontaneous osteonecrosis of the knee. Eur J Radiol 67(1):42, 2008.
44. Jacobs, B, et al: Knee osteochondritis dissecans. Emedicine, 2006. Available at http://www.emedicine.com/sports/TOPIC57.HTM. Accessed Sept 3, 2008.
45. Peterson, CS: Posterior cruciate ligament injury. Emedicine, 2006. Available at http://www.emedicine.com/sports/TOPIC105.HTM. Accessed Sept 3, 2008.
46. Souryal, T, et al: Anterior cruciate ligament injury. Emedicine, 2006. Available at http://www.emedicine.com/prm/topic3.HTM. Accessed Sept 3, 2008.
47. Parkkari, J, et al: The risk for cruciate ligament injury of the knee in adolescents and young adults: a population-based cohort study of 46,500 people with a 9-year follow-up. Br J Sports Med 42(6):422, 2008.
48. Granan, LP: Development of a national cruciate ligament surgery registry: the Norweigian National Knee Ligament Registry. Am J Sports Med 36(2):308, 2008.
49. McAllister, DR, and Petrigliano, FA: Diagnosis and treatment of posterior cruciate ligament injury. Curr Sports Med Rep 6(5):293, 2007.
50. Nagano, Y, et al: Gender differences in knee kinematics and muscle activity during single limb drop landing. Knee 14(3):218, 2007.
51. Hodler, J, von Schulthess, GK, and Zollikofer, CL: Musculoskeletal Disease: Diagnostic Imaging and Interventional Technology. Springer, Italy, 2005.
52. Daffner, RH: Clinical Radiology: The Essentials, ed. 3. Williams & Wilkins, Baltimore, 2007.
53. Bernstein, J (ed): Musculoskeletal Medicine. American Academy of Orthopedic Surgeons, Rosemont, IL, 2003.

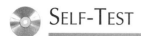

SELF-TEST

Radiographs A, B, and C

1. Identify each of the three *projections*, which belong to the same patient.

2. In film A, an arrow points to a small oval-shaped area of *increased density*. Would you guess that this object lies *inside* or *outside* of the joint capsule? What helps you determine this?

3. Name one possibility of what this object may represent.

4. Which *compartment(s)* of the knee show(s) *degenerative changes*?

5. Describe the *degenerative changes* that are present.

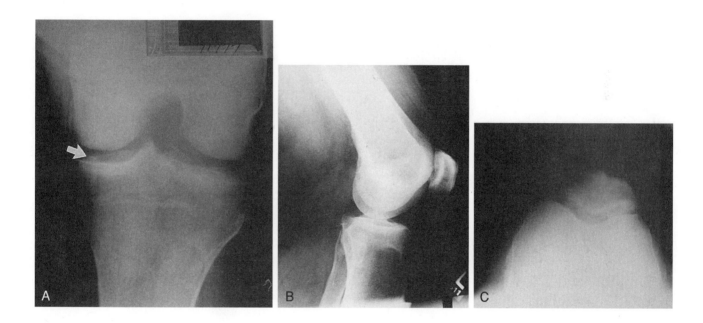

Chapter 14

RADIOLOGIC EVALUATION OF THE ANKLE AND FOOT

Injuries to the ankle and foot occur with great frequency. The ankle is considered the most commonly injured, major weight-bearing joint in the body. However, the true incidence of such injuries is unknown, because a variety of clinicians treat ankle injuries and their definitions are often imprecise. Most ankle injuries are straightforward ligamentous injuries. However, the clinical presentation of subtle ankle and foot fractures can be similar to that of ankle sprains, and these fractures can be missed on initial examination. Appropriate imaging can minimize delays in treatment that may result in long-term disability and surgery.

Review of Anatomy[1–8]

Osseous Anatomy

Ankle

The ankle joint is formed by the articulation of the distal tibia and fibula with the talus (Fig. 14-1). The distal end of the tibia is distinguished by a broad articular surface, the tibial plafond; an elongated medial process, the medial malleolus; an

expanded process at the anteromedial aspect, the anterior tubercle; and a posterior marginal rim, sometimes called the third malleolus or posterior malleolus. The distal end of the fibula, the lateral malleolus, is slightly posterior to and reaches below the level of the medial malleolus, extending alongside the talus. The inferior contours of the distal tibia and fibula combine to form a deep socket, or ankle mortise, into which the upper end of the talus fits. This articulation is the talocrural joint, or ankle joint proper.

Foot

The foot consists of 26 bones. There are 7 tarsals, 5 metatarsals, and 14 phalanges (Fig. 14-2).

Tarsals

The tarsals include the talus, calcaneus, cuboid, navicular, and three cuneiforms.

The talus is the second largest tarsal and is key in transmitting weight-bearing forces from the ankle to the foot. The *body* of the talus articulates in the talocrural joint. The superior surface of the body is referred to as the *talar dome*. The talar *neck* lies anterior to the body. The talar *head* articulates with the navicular anteriorly and the calcaneus inferiorly.

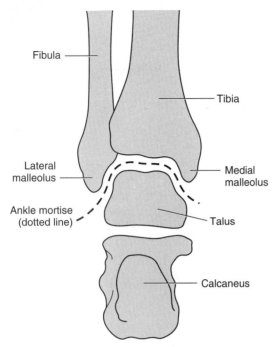

Figure 14-1 The talocrural or ankle joint.

The posterior articulation between the talus and calcaneus is the *subtalar joint.* The anterior articulation between the talus and calcaneus is part of the *talocalcaneonavicular joint,* the complex articulation, surrounded by one capsule, between the talus, navicular, and upper suface of the the *plantar calcaneonavicular ligament.*

The calcaneus is the largest tarsal bone. The posteroinferior aspect is the *tuberosity* or heel. A medial process and larger lateral process extend from either side of the tuberosity. The prominent *sustentaculum tali* is a process extending from the medial proximal aspect of the calcaneus. The calcaneus articulates with the talus and the cuboid. The superior articulation with the talus forms the subtalar joint. The anterior articulation with the cuboid forms the *calcaneocuboid joint.* A depression on the superior surface of the calcaneus, the calcaneal sulcus, corresponds with a groove on the inferior surface of the talus, the sulcus tali, to form the *tarsal sinus.*

The cuboid is located on the lateral aspect of the foot, articulating with the calcaneus posteriorly, the base of the fourth and fifth metatarsals anteriorly, and the third cuneiform medially. Occasionally the cuboid will also form an articulation with the navicular.

The navicular lies on the medial side of the foot, articulating with the talus posteriorly and the three cuneiforms anteriorly.

The cuneiforms are designated by number or by position. All three articulate with the navicular posteriorly and with each other adjacently. Anterior articulations with the metatarsals form the *tarsometatarsal joints.* The first, or medial cuneiform, articulates with the base of the first and second metatarsal; the second, or middle, cuneiform articulates with the base of the second metatarsal; the third, or lateral, cuneiform articulates with the second, third, and fourth metatarsals, and with the cuboid laterally.

Metatarsals

The metatarsals are numbered from 1 to 5, beginning on the medial side of the foot. Each metatarsal is composed of a small distal *head,* a *neck,* a long slender *shaft,* and a broad proximal *base.* The head of the first metatarsal articulates with two *sesamoid bones* on its inferior surface. The base of the fifth metatarsal supports a distally projecting *tuberosity.* Articulations between adjacent metatarsals form *intermetatarsal* joints. Articulations between the metatarsal heads and the proximal phalanges form the *metatarsophalangeal joints.*

Phalanges

The toes, or digits, are numbered from 1 to 5, beginning on the medial or great-toe side of the foot. The great toe is distinctive in that it is composed of only a *proximal* and a *distal phalanx.* The remaining toes each additionally possess a middle phalanx. The distal phalanges of the second through fifth digits are usually quite small and sometimes difficult to identify on radiograph. Middle and distal phalanges are not uncommonly fused.

Divisions of the Foot

The foot is often divided into three anatomic segments referred to as the *hindfoot, midfoot,* and *forefoot:*

- The hindfoot is composed of the talus and calcaneus.
- The midfoot is composed of the navicular, the cuboid, and the three cuneiforms.
- The forefoot is composed of the metatarsals and phalanges.

The hindfoot is separated from the midfoot by the *transverse tarsal joint* (consisting of the talonavicular and calcaneocuboid joints), commonly called *Chopart's joint.* The midfoot is separated from the forefoot by the *tarsometatarsal joint,* commonly called the *Lisfranc joint.*

Ligamentous Anatomy

Ligaments of the Ankle

Three principal sets of ligaments stabilize the ankle joint: the medial collateral ligament, the lateral collateral ligaments, and the distal tibiofibular syndesmotic complex (Fig. 14-3).

The medial collateral ligament, also known as the *deltoid ligament,* consists of a variable number of superficial and deep bands expanding in a fan-like shape from the medial malleolus to the talus, the navicular, and the sustentaculum tali of the calcaneus. This ligament possesses great tensile strength and is rarely injured in isolation.

The lateral collateral ligaments are three distinct ligamentous bands extending from the lateral malleolus to the talus and calcaneus: the *anterior talofibular, posterior talofibular,* and *calcaneofibular* ligaments. The lateral collateral ligaments are injured with much greater frequency than the medial collateral ligament.

The distal tibiofibular syndesmotic complex is considered to be among the most important stabilizing structures of the ankle, crucial in maintaining the width and stability of the ankle mortise. This complex is composed primarily of three structures: *the anterior tibiofibular ligament,* the *posterior*

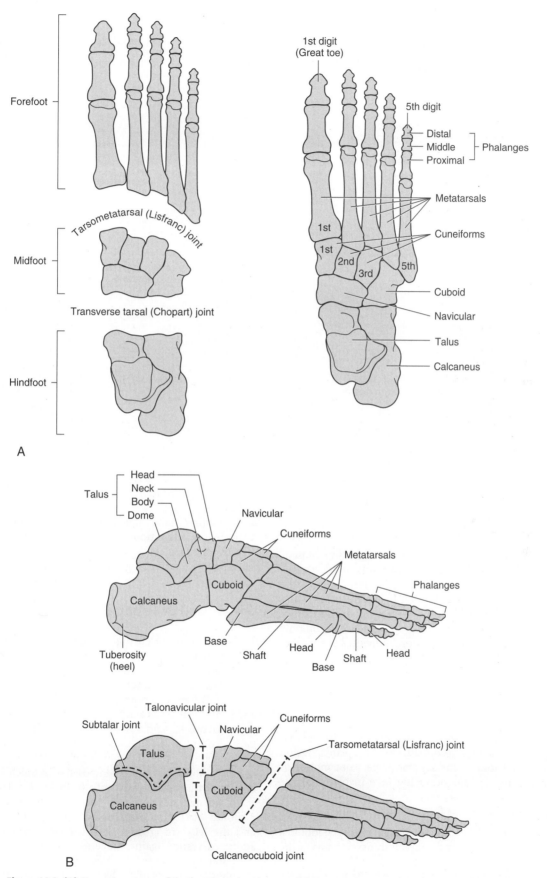

Figure 14-2 (A) Osseous anatomy of the foot from dorsal aspect. **(B)** Osseous anatomy of the foot from lateral aspect.

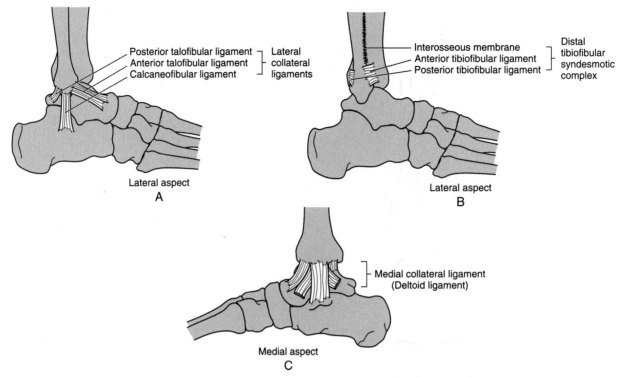

Figure 14-3 Three principal sets of ligaments stabilize the ankle joint: **(A)** the lateral collateral ligaments, **(B)** the distal tibiofibular syndesmotic complex, and **(C)** the medial collateral (deltoid) ligament.

tibiofibular ligament, and the *interosseous membrane,* which binds the fibular and tibial shafts together.

Ligaments of the Foot

The ligamentous support of the foot is fairly extensive. Muscular action, in concert with the ligaments, maintains the various arches of the foot and permits adaptive responses to the dynamic forces imposed on the foot by weight-bearing and ambulation. On plain radiographs, the individual ligaments of the foot are not readily identified and are not commonly affected by pathology. For this reason, individual description of the foot ligaments is not included here.

Joint Mobility

The ankle joint functions as a hinge joint. A transverse axis through the talus allows for dorsiflexion and plantarflexion of the talus and foot in the sagittal plane. Foot motion is complex, and movements occurring here involve multiple joints and planes.

The basic motions of the foot and ankle are the following:

- *Plantarflexion and dorsiflexion:* movement of the foot in a sagittal plane, occurring through a transverse axis at the ankle joint
- *Abduction and adduction:* movement of the forefoot away from or toward midline, occurring primarily at the transverse tarsal joints

- *Inversion and eversion:* elevation of the medial or lateral borders of the foot, occurring primarily at the subtalar joint
- *Supination and pronation:* Combined movements of inversion, adduction, and dorsiflexion, or the combined movements of eversion, abduction, and plantarflexion, respectively, occurring at multiple joints

Growth and Development

The foot is formed during the eighth week of gestation. At birth, only the calcaneus, talus, and occasionally the cuboid are ossified. The ossification centers for the diaphyses of the metatarsals and phalanges are also present at birth.

Ossification centers for the remaining tarsals, metatarsal and phalangeal heads and bases, and the distal tibia and fibula appear between 1 and 4 years of age (Figs. 14-4 and 14-5). The tarsals complete their development at adolescence, and the remainder of the foot and ankle is fully ossified at 18 to 20 years of age. Although the foot is composed of as much soft tissue as bone at birth, at skeletal maturity the foot is 90% bone.

In normal development the lower extremities of the 3-month-old fetus are flexed, the hips are externally rotated, and the legs are crossed with the feet plantarflexed and adducted, resting against the fetus's abdomen. By the second trimester the lower extremities uncross and "derotate," and the plantar surfaces of the feet come to rest on the mother's uterine wall. Failure of this postural change to occur may cause deformities of the feet to be present at birth.

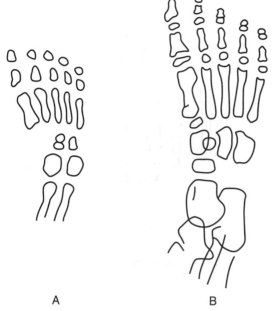

A   B

Figure 14-4 Radiographic tracings of the ossified portions of the foot **(A)** at birth and **(B)** at age 5. *(Adapted from Meschan,[5] p. 219.)*

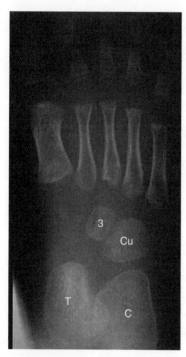

Figure 14-5 Normal radiographic appearance of a 2-year-old toddler. Visible are the ossified tarsals including the calcaneus (C), talus (T), and cuboid (Cu), and third cuneiform (3). The navicular and first and second cuneiforms are barely seen as small oval densities.

The feet of newborns will normally appear flat, owing to immature tarsal, muscular, and ligamentous development and the fat pad present on the sole of the foot. The longitudinal arch develops along with ambulatory skills, but persistence of pronated feet and genu valgum is not uncommon during early childhood and generally dissipates with further maturity.

Routine Radiologic Evaluation[7–21]

Practice Guidelines for Ankle and Foot Radiography in Children and Adults

The American College of Radiology (ACR), the principal professional organization of radiologists in the United States, defines the following practice guidelines as an educational tool to assist practitioners in providing appropriate radiologic care for patients.

Goals

The goal of the ankle or foot radiographic examination is to identify or exclude anatomic abnormalities or disease processes.

Indications

The indications for radiologic examination include but are not limited to trauma including suspected physical abuse of children; osseous changes secondary to metabolic disease, systemic disease, or nutritional deficiencies; neoplasms; primary nonneoplastic bone pathologies; infections; arthropathies; preoperative, postoperative, and follow-up studies; congenital syndromes and developmental disorders; vascular lesions; evaluation of soft tissue (such as a suspected foreign body); pain; and correlation of abnormal skeletal findings on other imaging studies.

Basic Projections and Radiologic Observations

The recommended projections at the ankle for a routine examination are *anteroposterior (AP), AP oblique (mortise),* and *lateral* views.

The recommended projections at the foot are the *AP, lateral,* and *oblique* views.

(Continued on page 432)

Routine Radiologic Evaluation of the Ankle

Anteroposterior

The AP view of the ankle demonstrates the distal tibia and fibula, including the medial and lateral malleoli and the dome of the talus.

Radiologic Observations[1,6–10]

The important observations are:

1. The lateral malleolus of the fibula extends below the medial malleolus. This anatomic feature provides joint stability (Fig. 14-6). Minimal shortening or displacement of the fibula after injury allows for abnormal talar tilt within the joint, which can lead to instability and degenerative joint disease.
2. The lateral malleolus is superimposed behind the lateral aspect of the tibia.
3. Only the upper and medial portions of the ankle mortise and its related joint space are visible.
4. The upper portion of the talar body, the dome, is visible as it articulates in the ankle mortise.
5. Medial or lateral shift or displacement of the talus within the mortise may indicate the presence of laxity, instability, or fracture at the ankle.
6. An abnormally wide joint space between the distal tibia and fibula indicates disruption of the distal tibiofibular syndesmotic complex.

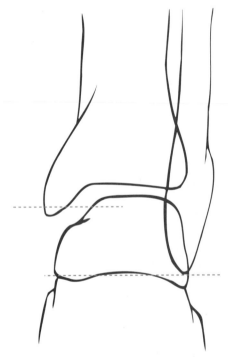

Figure 14-6 In the normal ankle, the fibular malleolus extends below the tibial malleolus.

Basic Projections

- **AP**
- AP oblique (mortise view)
- Lateral

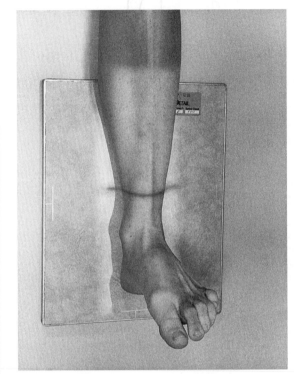

Setting up the Radiograph

Figure 14-7 Patient position for anteroposterior radiograph of the ankle.

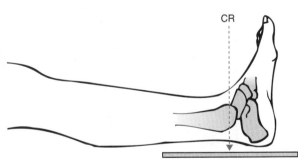

Figure 14-8 The central ray is directed vertically through the mid-point between the malleoli.

What Can You See?

Look at the radiograph (Fig. 14-9) and tracing (Fig. 14-10). Identify the following:

- Distal tibia
- Distal fibula
- Proximal talus or talar dome
- Ankle mortise

Try to identify these same osseous structures on the magnetic resonance (MR) image (Fig. 14-11). Can you also find the tendons of the posterior tibialis and peroneal muscles?

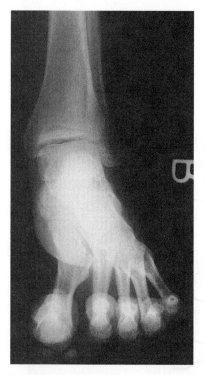

Figure 14-9 Anteroposterior radiograph of the ankle.

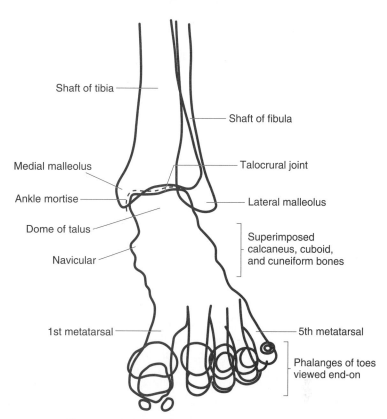

Shaft of tibia

Shaft of fibula

Medial malleolus

Talocrural joint

Ankle mortise

Lateral malleolus

Dome of talus

Superimposed
calcaneus, cuboid,
and cuneiform bones

Navicular

1st metatarsal

5th metatarsal

Phalanges of toes
viewed end-on

Figure 14-10 Tracing of anteroposterior radiograph of the ankle.

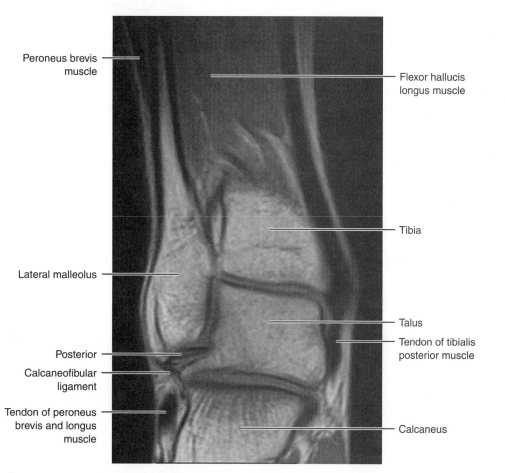

Peroneus brevis
muscle

Flexor hallucis
longus muscle

Tibia

Lateral malleolus

Talus

Tendon of tibialis
posterior muscle

Posterior

Calcaneofibular
ligament

Tendon of peroneus
brevis and longus
muscle

Calcaneus

Figure 14-11 Coronal T1-weighted MRI of the ankle. *(Image courtesy of http://www.medcyclopedia.com by GE Healthcare.)*

Routine Radiologic Evaluation of the Ankle

AP Oblique (Mortise View)

This view demonstrates the entire ankle mortise. This variation of the AP view is achieved by internally rotating the leg and foot 15 to 20 degrees to place both malleoli in the same plane, avoiding superimposition of the lateral aspect of the tibia over the fibula.

Radiologic Observations

The important observations are:

1. The entire radiographic joint space of the ankle proper, the ankle mortise, is visible (Fig. 14-12).
2. The mortise width is normally 3 to 4 mm over the entire surface of the talus; an extra 2 mm in widening is considered abnormal.
3. Abnormal widening of one side of the mortise or displacement of the talus indicates the presence of ligamentous laxity, injury, or fracture.
4. The tibiofibular joint articulation is not well demonstrated in this plane, because the lateral aspect of the tibia is slightly superimposed over the distal fibula. However, an abnormally wide space between the distal tibia and fibula suggests disruption of the distal tibiofibular syndesmotic complex.

Basic Projections

- AP
- **AP oblique (mortise view)**
- Lateral

Setting up the Radiograph

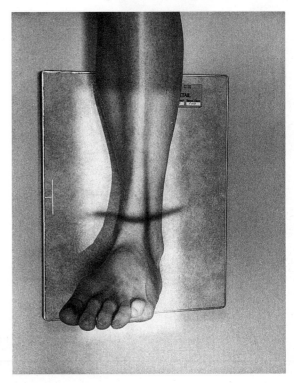

Figure 14-13 Patient position for AP oblique (mortise) view of the ankle.

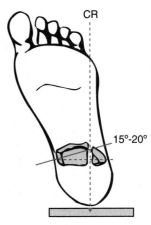

Figure 14-14 The leg is internally rotated 15 to 20 degrees until the intermalleolar plane is parallel with the image receptor. The central ray is directed at a midpoint between the malleoli.

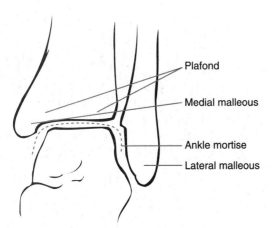

Figure 14-12 The space between the talar dome and the ankle mortise is usually 3 to 4 mm wide over the entire talar surface.

Plafond
Medial malleous
Ankle mortise
Lateral malleous

What Can You See?

Look at the radiograph (Fig. 14-15) and try to identify the radiographic anatomy. Trace the outlines of structures using a marker and transparency sheet. Compare results with the book tracing (Fig. 14-16). Can you identify the following:

- Distal tibia
- Distal fibula
- Proximal talus or talar dome
- Entire ankle mortise

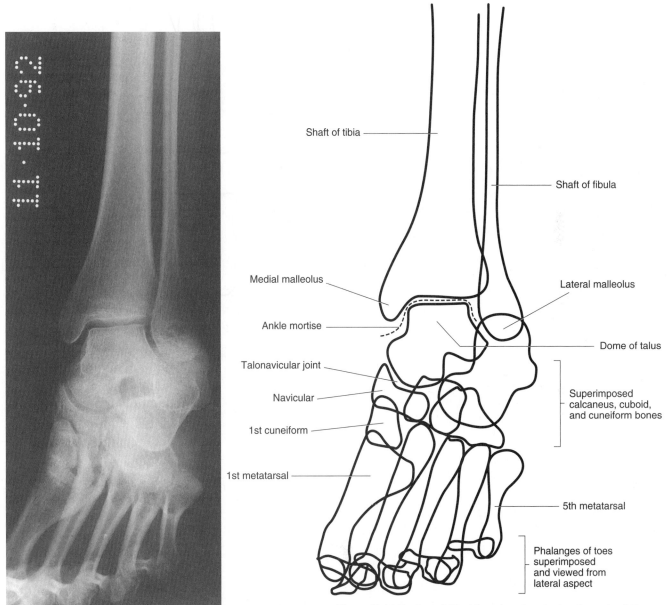

Figure 14-15 AP oblique (mortise view) radiograph of the ankle.

Figure 14-16 Tracing of AP oblique (mortise view) radiograph of the ankle.

Routine Radiologic Evaluation of the Ankle

Lateral

This view demonstrates the anterior and posterior aspects of the distal tibia, the lateral relationship of the tibiotalar and subtalar articulations, the talus, and the calcaneus.

Radiologic Observations

The important observations are:

1. The fibula is superimposed behind the posterior tibia and talus (Fig. 14-17).
2. The anterior tubercle and posterior rim (the so-called *third malleolus* or *posterior malleolus*) of the tibia are well demonstrated.
3. The subtalar joint is well demonstrated.
4. The talus and calcaneus are seen in their entirety, as well as their articulations with the navicular and cuboid bones.

What Can You See?

Look at the radiograph (Fig. 14-20) and try to identify the radiographic anatomy. Trace the outlines of structures using a marker and transparency sheet. Compare results with the book tracing (Fig. 14-21). Can you identify the following:

- Distal tibia, identifying the anterior tubercle and the posterior malleolus
- Distal fibula as it lies superimposed behind the tibia and talus
- Tarsal bones (identify the talus, calcaneus, navicular, and cuboid)
- Joints: tibiotalar, talocalcaneonavicular or subtalar, calcaneocuboid, and talonavicular

Basic Projections

- AP
- AP oblique (mortise view)
- **Lateral**

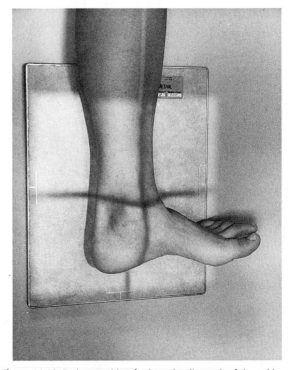

Setting up the Radiograph

Figure 14-18 Patient position for lateral radiograph of the ankle.

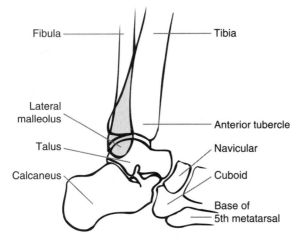

Figure 14-17 The fibula is superimposed behind the tibia and talus.

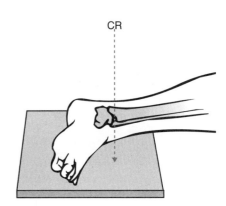

Figure 14-19 The central ray is directed vertically through the medial malleolus.

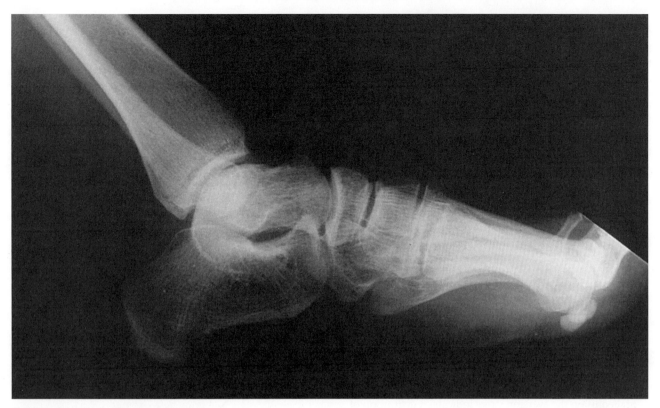

Figure 14-20 Lateral radiograph of the ankle.

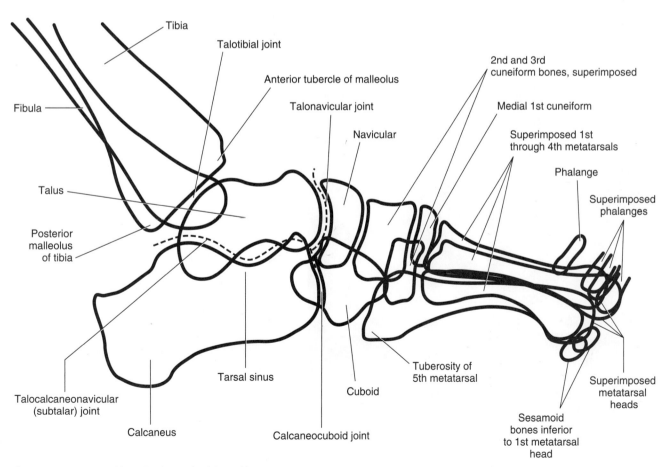

Figure 14-21 Tracing of lateral radiograph of the ankle.

Routine Radiologic Evaluation of the Ankle

Stress Views

Stress radiographic measurements have traditionally been used to assess the degree of joint instability. These measurements can play an important role in treatment decision making. Recent studies have questioned the value of stress radiographs in comparison with magnetic resonance imaging (MRI), as MRI offers the advantage of evaluating associated injuries related to the chronic instability. Stress views are presented here as they continue to be utilized in some settings and patient situations.

AP Inversion and Eversion Stress Views

Radiologic Observations

1. The leg and ankle are positioned in a true AP manner and the leg is firmly fixed by a mechanism or manually held in neutral. The plantar surface of the foot is turned medially for the inversion view (Fig. 14-22A) and laterally for the eversion view (Fig. 14-22B).
2. In a stable ankle with intact ligaments, the ankle mortise will remain relatively constant during the inversion and eversion maneuvers, as seen in Figure 14-22.
3. In an unstable ankle caused by ligamentous disruption, the ankle mortise will widen. An abnormally wide space between the medial border of the talus and the medial malleolus on the eversion stress indicates a disruption of the medial collateral ligament. An abnormally wide space between the lateral border of the talus and the lateral

malleolus indicates disruption of the lateral collateral ligament system (Fig. 14-23).
4. Displacement of the talus is referred to as "talar tilt." Talar tilt is measured as an angle determined by the intersection of lines drawn across the tibial plafond and the talar dome (Fig. 14-23). The contralateral ankle is measured to establish a baseline of normal for that individual. Normal values may range from less than 5 degrees to 15 degrees of tilt during forced inversion, and up to 10 degrees during forced eversion. Values significantly greater than this are pathological. Also, a difference of more than 5 degrees from the normal side to the injured side is considered significant.

Anterior Talar Drawer Stress View

Radiologic Observations

1. The leg and ankle are in a lateral position and the leg is fixed in place manually or with a mechanical device.
2. A stress is applied on the posterior aspect of the heel, resulting in anterior transposition of the talus on the tibia.
3. A measurement is taken from the posterior aspect of the tibia to the posterior aspect of the talus. Separation of 5 mm is considered normal, up to 10 mm may or may not be normal and requires comparison with the contralateral side, and greater than 10 mm indicates disruption of the anterior talofibular ligament (Fig. 14-24).

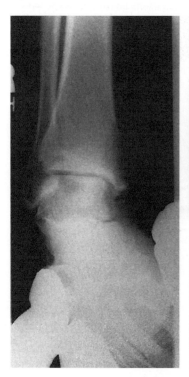
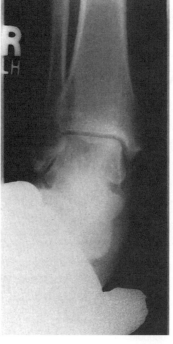

A   Inversion   B   Eversion

Figure 14-22 AP stress views: **(A)** inversion; **(B)** eversion. Because the ankle mortise joint space has remained relatively constant during both maneuvers, the ligaments are stable and intact. *(From Bontrager,[12] p. 228, Figs. 6-92 and 6-93, with permission.)*

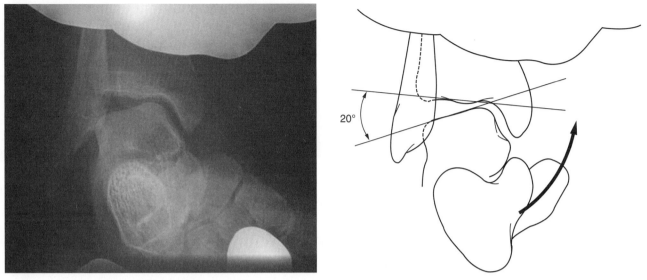

Figure 14-23 **(A)** AP stress radiograph and **(B)** tracing demonstrate 20 degrees of talar tilt upon passive inversion.

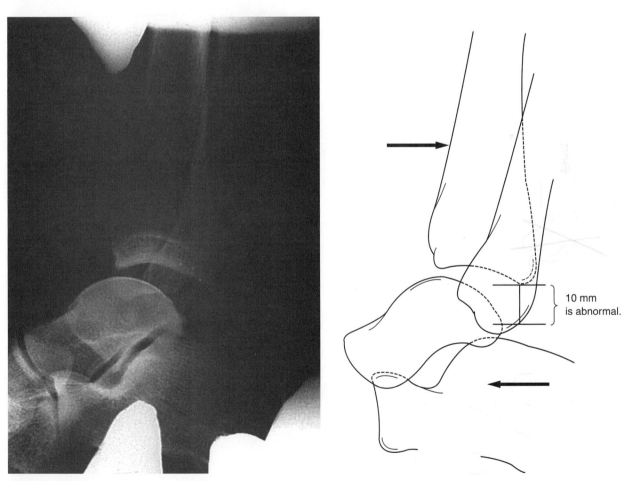

Figure 14-24 **(A)** Anterior drawer stress radiograph and **(B)** tracing demonstrating an abnormal anterior translation of the talus from the tibia greater than 10 mm.

Routine Radiologic Evaluation of the Foot

Anteroposterior

This dorsoplanar view demonstrates the phalanges, metatarsals, cuneiforms, cuboid, and navicular.

Radiologic Observations

The important observations are:

1. This view is made with the sole of the foot on the image receptor and the x-rays projected through the top of the foot in a dorsal to plantar direction.
2. All of the bones of the forefoot and midfoot are well demonstrated. The talus, calcaneus, and distal tibia are superimposed over one another and not well visualized.
3. Note any sesamoid bones, commonly present at the first and sometimes the second or third metatarsal heads.
4. The *first intermetatarsal angle* (Fig. 14-25) is an important anatomic feature formed by the intersection of the lines bisecting the first and second metatarsal shafts. This angle normally ranges from 5 to 15 degrees. The amount of angulation present in forefoot deformities can be quantified from this baseline.

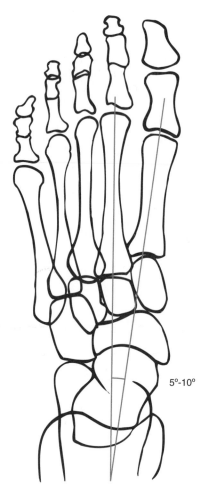

Figure 14-25 The first intermetatarsal angle is formed by the intersection of lines bisecting the first (*a*) and second (*b*) metatarsal shafts.

Basic Projections

- **AP**
- Lateral
- Oblique

Setting up the Radiograph

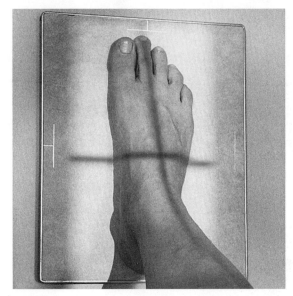

Figure 14-26 Patient position for anteroposterior radiograph of the foot.

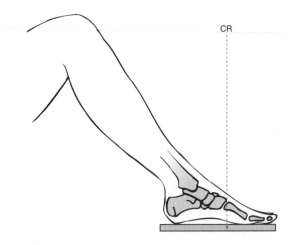

Figure 14-27 The central ray is directed toward the base of the third metatarsal.

What Can You See?

Look at the radiograph (Fig. 14-28) and try to identify the radiographic anatomy. Trace the outlines of structures using a marker and transparency sheet. Compare results with the book tracing (Fig. 14-29). Can you identify the following:

- Phalanges and their corresponding distal and proximal interphalangeal joints

- Metatarsals (identify head, shaft, and base of each)
- First intermetatarsal angle
- Sesamoid bones at the first metatarsal head
- Tarsals of the midfoot
- Transverse tarsal joint (Chopart joint) and the tarsometatarsal joint (Lisfranc joint)

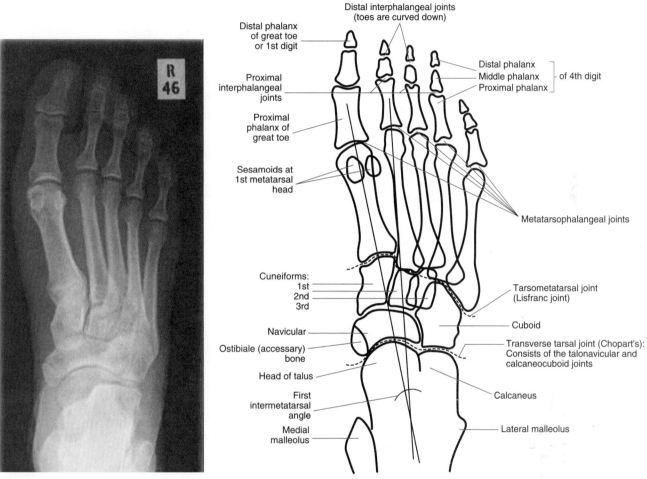

Figure 14-28 Anteroposterior radiograph of the foot.

Figure 14-29 Tracing of anteroposterior radiograph of the foot.

Routine Radiologic Evaluation of the Foot

Lateral

This view demonstrates the calcaneus and talus, the subtalar joint, and the talonavicular and calcaneocuboid articulations.

Radiologic Observations

The important observations are:

1. This lateral profile of the foot visualizes the hindfoot and midfoot, but the metatarsals and phalanges of the forefoot are obscured by superimposition.
2. The transverse tarsal (Chopart) and tarsometatarsal (Lisfranc) joints dividing the midfoot from the hindfoot and forefoot are well demonstrated.
3. Note the articular relationship of the talus to the calcaneus. The anterior and middle facets of the subtalar joint are separated from the posterior facet by the radiolucent oval representing the tarsal sinus.
4. The *Boehler angle* (Fig. 14-30A), also known as the *tuberosity* or *salient angle,* is frequently used to evaluate the angular relationship of the talus and the calcaneus in the presence of trauma. This angle is determined by the intersection of lines drawn: from the posterior aspect of the subtalar joint to the anterior process of the calcaneus (*a*) and across the posterior superior margin of the calcaneus (*b*). Normal values range from 25 to 40 degrees, and lesser values will be seen in the presence of calcaneal fractures.
5. *Calcaneal inclination* (or *calcaneal pitch,* Fig. 14-30B) is an angle described by the intersection of a line drawn along the plantar surface of the foot (*a*) and a line drawn tangentially to the inferior surface of the calcaneus (*b*). Normal values are 20 to 30 degrees. Higher values indicate a *pes cavus* deformity.

Basic Projections

- AP
- **Lateral**
- Oblique

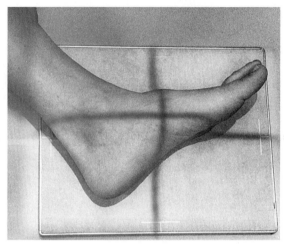

Setting up the Radiograph

Figure 14-31 Patient position for lateral radiograph of the foot.

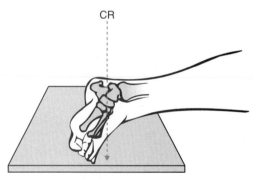

CR

Figure 14-32 The central ray is directed vertically through the base of the third metatarsal.

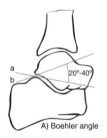

A) Boehler angle

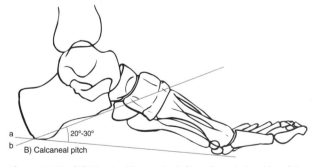

B) Calcaneal pitch

Figure 14-30 (A) The Boehler angle defines the relationship of the talus and calcaneus. **(B)** Calcaneal inclination or pitch describes the angular position of the calcaneus.

What Can You See?

Look at the radiograph (Fig. 14-33) and try to identify the radiographic anatomy. Trace the outlines of structures using a marker and transparency sheet. Compare results with the book tracing (Fig. 14-34). Can you identify the following:

- Tibia and fibula (note that the lateral malleolus is superimposed behind the talus)
- Transverse tarsal and tarsometatarsal joints
- Talus and calcaneus
- Tarsal sinus and the subtalar joint

Can you measure the following:

- Boehler angle
- The calcaneal inclination

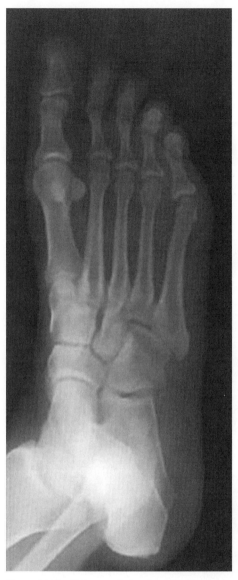

Figure 14-38 Oblique radiograph of the foot.

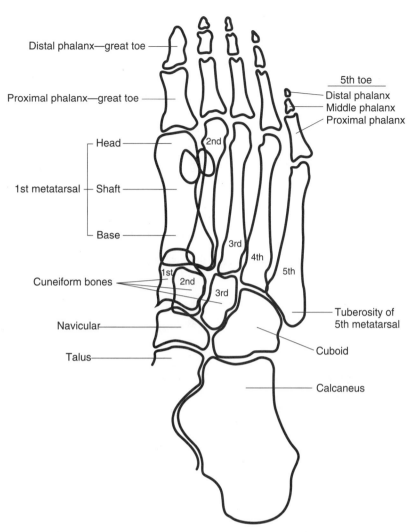

Figure 14-39 Tracing of oblique radiograph of the foot.

Magnetic Resonance Imaging of the Ankle and Foot

MRI is recommended as the most appropriate *next study* following radiography for the assessment of chronic ankle ankle/foot pain. Presented here are midsagittal and axial views of the ankle and foot.

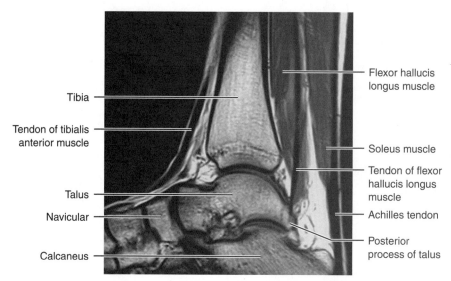

Tibia

Tendon of tibialis anterior muscle

Talus

Navicular

Calcaneus

Flexor hallucis longus muscle

Soleus muscle

Tendon of flexor hallucis longus muscle

Achilles tendon

Posterior process of talus

Figure 14-40 Sagittal T1-weighted MRI of the ankle. This slice is midsagittal at the long axis of the talus. *(Image courtesy of http://www.medcyclopedia.com by GE Healthcare.)*

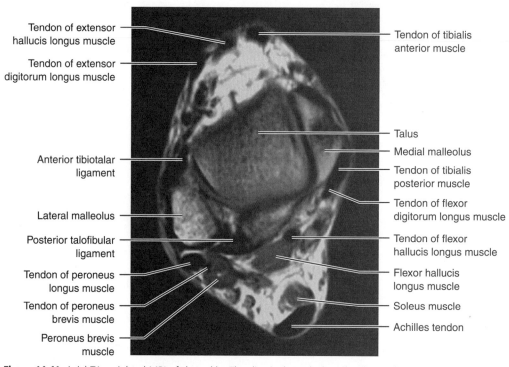

Tendon of extensor hallucis longus muscle

Tendon of extensor digitorum longus muscle

Anterior tibiotalar ligament

Lateral malleolus

Posterior talofibular ligament

Tendon of peroneus longus muscle

Tendon of peroneus brevis muscle

Peroneus brevis muscle

Tendon of tibialis anterior muscle

Talus

Medial malleolus

Tendon of tibialis posterior muscle

Tendon of flexor digitorum longus muscle

Tendon of flexor hallucis longus muscle

Flexor hallucis longus muscle

Soleus muscle

Achilles tendon

Figure 14-41 Axial T1-weighted MRI of the ankle. The slice is through the talar dome. *(Image courtesy of http://www.medcyclopedia.com by GE Healthcare.)*

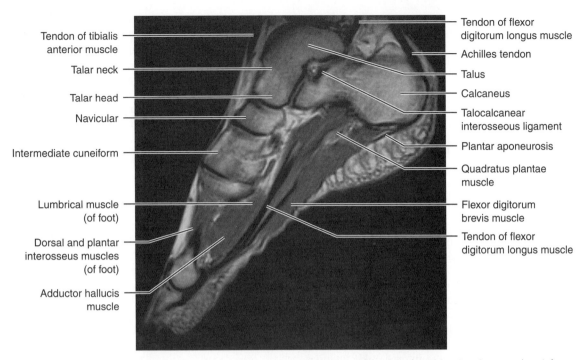

Tendon of tibialis anterior muscle
Talar neck
Talar head
Navicular
Intermediate cuneiform
Lumbrical muscle (of foot)
Dorsal and plantar interosseus muscles (of foot)
Adductor hallucis muscle

Tendon of flexor digitorum longus muscle
Achilles tendon
Talus
Calcaneus
Talocalcanear interosseous ligament
Plantar aponeurosis
Quadratus plantae muscle
Flexor digitorum brevis muscle
Tendon of flexor digitorum longus muscle

Figure 14-42 Sagittal T1-weighted MRI of the foot. This slice is through the middle of the foot, bisecting the second cunieform. *(Image courtesy of http://www.medcyclopedia.com by GE Healthcare.)*

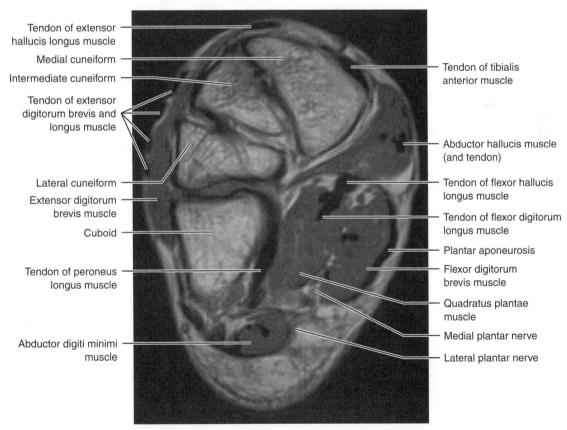

Tendon of extensor hallucis longus muscle
Medial cuneiform
Intermediate cuneiform
Tendon of extensor digitorum brevis and longus muscle
Lateral cuneiform
Extensor digitorum brevis muscle
Cuboid
Tendon of peroneus longus muscle
Abductor digiti minimi muscle

Tendon of tibialis anterior muscle
Abductor hallucis muscle (and tendon)
Tendon of flexor hallucis longus muscle
Tendon of flexor digitorum longus muscle
Plantar aponeurosis
Flexor digitorum brevis muscle
Quadratus plantae muscle
Medial plantar nerve
Lateral plantar nerve

Figure 14-43 Axial T1-weighted MRI of the foot at the level of the distal aspect of the cuboid. *(Image courtesy of http://www.medcyclopedia.com by GE Healthcare.)*

Trauma at the Ankle and Foot[11,22-61]

Diagnostic Imaging for Trauma of the Ankle and Foot

In adults the ankle is the most frequently injured major joint in the body. Consequently, ankle radiographs are among the most frequently ordered studies in the emergency department, exceeded in frequency only by chest and cervical spine radiographs. However, only a small percentage of these patients will have a fracture that requires definition by radiography.

To minimize unnecessary radiography and help the clinician decide when radiographs *are* and *are not* necessary, guidelines that are based on the patient's *clinical* presentation have been established. Commonly known as the Ottawa Ankle and Foot Rules, these guidelines state that radiographs should be ordered after ankle or foot trauma if the patient is unable to bear weight *and* has point tenderness in either the malleolar zone, midfoot zone, base of the fifth metatarsal, or at the navicular. Studies have shown this guideline to be 100% sensitive for detecting significant fractures. (See Chapter 18 for more on clinical decision rules.)

Radiographic examination of the injured ankle includes routine AP, lateral, and the mortise oblique views. The foot exam includes AP, lateral, and oblique views. Ankle and foot exams need *not* be performed if pain can be localized to one area or the other.

Advanced Imaging for Ankle and Foot Trauma

Radiographs are recommended by the ACR as the initial study for *all acute* conditions (meeting the Ottawa criteria) and *all chronic* pain conditions. Advanced imaging is used after the radiographic findings are either (1) insufficient to guide treatment or (2) after the radiographic findings are negative when further injury is suspected.

Computed tomography (CT) and MRI are often complementary studies in defining the characteristics of a pathology. Subtle fractures that are difficult to detect on radiographs are best seen with multidetector CT. CT is also used in evaluating intra-articular fractures, complex fractures, and the position of comminuted fragments. Stress fractures can be identified by MRI or radionuclide bone scans. MRI is best for identifying bone marrow edema, which can be interpreted as a biomechanical stress reaction of bone. Arthrography and MRI are used to evaluate ligamentous and cartilaginous injuries. If injury to the tendons is suspected, MRI is rated most appropriate, followed by diagnostic ultrasound.

Sprains at the Ankle

The precipitating force in ankle sprains is usually an inversion stress, accounting for 85% of all traumatic conditions at the ankle.[1] The degree of damage caused is dependent on the direction and magnitude of the applied force. Injuries may thus range in severity from minor overstretching of ligaments, effecting little functional loss, to ligamentous rupture or avulsion, creating ankle joint instability and significant functional impairment. The most severe injuries involve ligamentous disruption with associated fracture or fracture–dislocation.

Inversion Sprains

Sprains due to inversion stresses damage the lateral collateral ligaments (Fig. 14-44). The anterior talofibular and calcaneofibular ligaments are the most frequently injured components of the lateral collateral ligament system. Inversion sprains are the most common sprains; the resultant damage is usually ligamentous without bony involvement.

Eversion Sprains

Sprains due to eversion stresses damage the medial collateral ligament (Fig. 14-45). Forceful eversion stresses are generally associated with bony damage, because the medial collateral ligament has so much tensile strength that avulsion fractures and other fractures will often occur before the medial collateral ligament itself fails structurally and sustains damage.

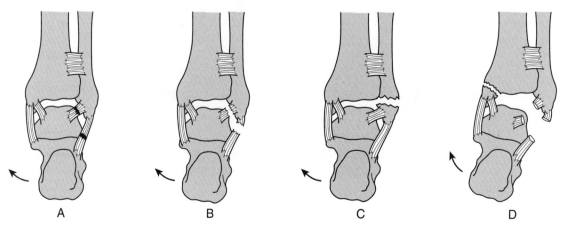

Figure 14-44 Spectrum of injuries resulting from inversion stresses: **(A)** sprain of lateral collateral ligament; **(B)** rupture or avulsion of lateral collateral ligament; **(C)** transverse fracture of lateral malleolus; **(D)** fracture of medial malleolus with rupture or avulsion of lateral collateral ligament.

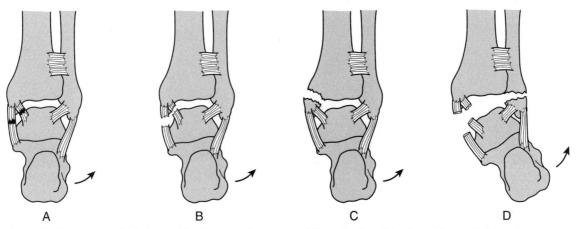

Figure 14-45 Spectrum of injuries resulting from eversion stresses: **(A)** sprain of medial collateral ligament; **(B)** rupture or avulsion of medial collateral ligament; **(C)** fracture of medial malleolus; **(D)** fracture of lateral malleolus with rupture or avulsion of medial collateral ligament.

Associated Injuries

Severe sprains disrupt other structures:

1. Avulsion fractures are due to the tensile pull of ligaments at their distal or proximal points of attachment.
2. Tearing of the distal tibiofibular syndesmotic complex is associated with either eversion or inversion stresses.
3. Instability from sprains is due to tearing of one or more of the three principal stabilizing ligaments, which consequently allows the ankle mortise to widen. Without this anatomic architecture intact, the talus is free to "tilt" within the mortise during foot movement. Chronic instability usually leads to further trauma and degenerative joint changes.

Radiologic Evaluation

Radiologic examination of severe ankle sprains is needed when an associated fracture is suspected. Joint instability can be revealed on routine radiographs or stress views by observing an abnormal position of the talus or increased width of the ankle mortise (Fig. 14-46). Ligamentous injury is further defined by MRI.

Treatment

Treatment to restore the stability of the ankle mortise may be conservative (cast immobilization) or surgical (screw fixation), followed by immobilization for several weeks. Rehabilitation after the immobilization phase is extensive and focuses on restoring joint arthrokinematics, osteokinematics, strength, and, if required, functional ambulation and athletic skills at the ankle and foot.

Fractures at the Ankle

Fractures and fracture–dislocations are common injuries at the ankle. The predisposing force mechanisms are often similar to those causing sprains, and fractures here are frequently seen to occur in combination with ligamentous ruptures, avulsions, and other fractures.

Mechanism of Injury

The mechanism of injury is generally axial or rotational loading. How the joint accepts these forces and the resultant injury pattern is dependent on many factors including chronicity of preexisting ankle instability, patient's age, bone density, comorbidity related to soft tissue conditions, position of the foot at the time of loading, and the magnitude, direction, and rate of loading.

Classification

Numerous classification systems exist to classify ankle fractures via injury mechanisms and structural damage. The purpose of classification systems is to aid treatment decisions and assess treatment outcomes. The most basic description in common usage describes the fracture site anatomically as one of the following (Fig. 14-47):

- A *unimalleolar fracture,* indicating fracture of either the lateral or the medial malleolus
- A *bimalleolar fracture,* indicating fracture of both the lateral and medial malleoli (Fig. 14-48)
- A *trimalleolar fracture,* indicating fracture of both malleoli and the posterior rim of the tibia, sometimes called the third malleolus

Other fractures involving the ankle joint include the following (Figs. 14-49, 14-50, and 14-51):

- *Shaft* fractures of the fibula and tibia
- *Comminuted* fractures of the distal tibia
- *Intra-articular* fractures of the tibial plafond or talar dome

Radiologic Evaluation

The routine radiographs demonstrate the characteristics of most ankle fractures sufficiently for treatment decisions. In viewing trauma radiographs, remember that positioning will not always be perfect, either because of inability to position the injured extremity precisely or because of the injury's resultant displacement of normal bone position. In Figure 14-48 the lateral view looks, at first glance, like an AP view, because of the displacement of the fibula. Remember that at least two views, made at right angles to each other, are necessary to evaluate three dimensions of anatomy.

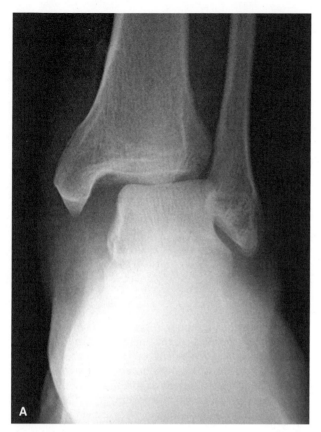
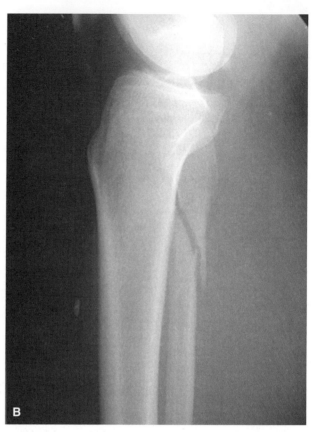

Figure 14-46 (A) The AP radiograph demonstrates instability of the ankle evidenced by the wide gap between the talus and medial malleoli; one may assume that the deltoid ligament is torn. This severe sprain also disrupted the interosseous membrane on the lateral side of the joint, and produced a spiral fracture at the proximal fibula seen on the lateral radiograph of the leg **(B)**. This combination of injuries is known as a Maisonneurve fracture. *(Image courtesy of John C. Hunter, MD, University of California, Davis School of Medicine.)*

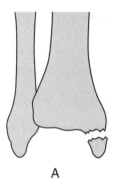
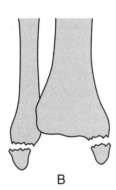
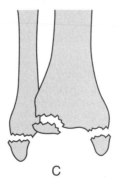

Figure 14-47 Basic classification of ankle fractures: **(A)** unimalleolar fracture, **(B)** bimalleolar fractures; **(C)** trimalleolar fracture (consisting of both malleoli and the posterior margin of the tibia).

Treatment

The goal of treatment is to stabilize fractures and reestablish the architecture of the ankle mortise.

Nonoperative treatment is indicated in stable fracture patterns with an intact distal tibiofibular syndesmosis. Long-leg casts are applied to control rotational components for 4 to 8 weeks. Radiologic evaluation is performed at 1- to 2-week intervals to monitor maintenance of reduction and progression of healing. Alternatively, short-leg casts or fracture braces may be sufficient if the fracture is very stable. Weight-bearing is restricted until fracture healing is evident radiographically.

Operative treatment is indicated when closed reduction is not possible, is not stable, or requires abnormal foot position to maintain the reduction. Operative treatment is also necessary when the fracture is unstable or results in talar tilt or

when the mortise is widened more than 2 mm over normal width. Plates, screws, and wires are used to achieve internal fixation, followed by short-leg casting. Weight-bearing is progressed based on the fracture pattern, stability of the fixation, and philosophy of the surgeon.

The amount of immobilization after reduction is usually lengthy if the mortise has been involved and extensive rehabilitation is necessary for recovery of function. Rehabilitation focuses on restoring normal joint arthrokinematics as well as normal range of motion, strength, and gait cycle.

Complications

The most common complications of ankle fractures are nonunion and degenerative joint changes associated with posttraumatic arthritis.

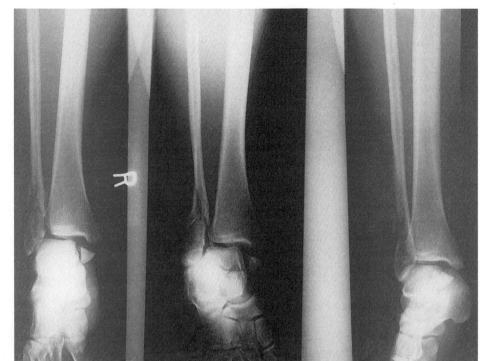

Figure 14-48 Bimalleolar fracture. A complete routine exam is shown. From left to right: an AP view, an oblique view, and a lateral view. This 29-year-old woman was injured after she stumbled catching her heel on an escalator step. There is a transverse fracture of the medial malleolus and a comminuted fracture of the lateral malleolus. Note the wide ankle mortise and wide interosseous membrane space on the AP and oblique views. On the lateral view, the dislocation and anterior displacement of the fibula is revealed.

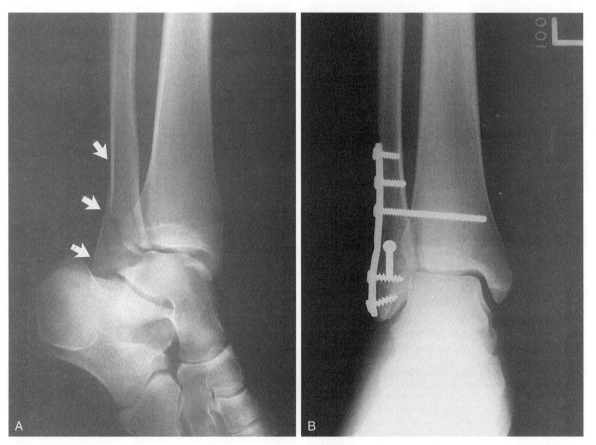

Figure 14-49 Comminuted fracture of the distal fibular shaft. This 24-year-old woman injured her ankle while skiing. **(A)** Lateral view of the ankle shows multiple fracture lines in the distal fibular shaft and lateral malleolus (white arrows). Note the posterior displacement of the entire fibula, evidenced by the abnormally wide interosseous space and the subluxation of the distal fibula out of the fibular notch of the tibia. **(B)** AP view of the ankle made postoperatively demonstrates the side plate and multiple-screw fixation device, which has restored normal alignment of the joint. Note that the long screw that enters the tibia has successfully restored the position of the fibula in the fibular notch of the tibia; consequently a normal ankle mortise has been re-established.

Fractures of the Foot

Foot fractures are generally described as being located at the hindfoot, midfoot, or forefoot. Fractures of the hindfoot (talus and calcaneus) are common, with the calcaneus being the most frequently fractured tarsal. With the exception of the navicular, which is noted to sustain stress fractures and also avulsion fractures of its tuberosity, isolated fractures of the midfoot tarsals are uncommon. Fractures of the forefoot metatarsals and phalanges are very common.

Hindfoot Fractures

Calcaneal Fractures

Mechanism of Injury Calcaneal fractures are often sustained during falls from a height in which the individual lands feet first. The injury is often bilateral and is frequently associated

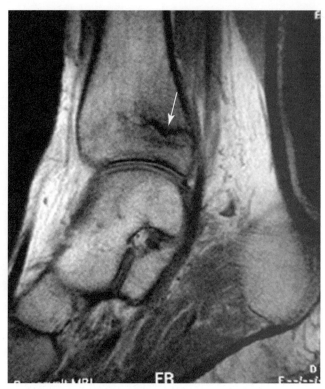

Figure 14-51 Sagittal T1-weighted MRI of the ankle. A *stress fracture* is seen as a low signal intensity line extending across the posterior distal tibia. This 48-year-old woman presented with ankle pain and swelling, negative radiographs, and a "hot" bone scan at the distal tibia. MRI is the modality of choice in defining stress fractures when radiographs are negative. *(Image courtesy of John C. Hunter, MD, University of California, Davis School of Medicine.)*

with a vertebral compression fracture in the thoracolumbar spine because of the transmitted axial forces.

Classification Calcaneal fractures are broadly classified as *intra-articular*, involving the subtalar joint, or *extra-articular*, sparing the subtalar joint (Fig. 14-52). Intra-articular fractures occur with three times greater frequency than extra-articular fractures (Figs. 14-53 and 14-54).

Radiologic Evaluation AP, lateral, and plantodorsal axial views of the calcaneus are obtained after an injury that results in hindfoot pain. Because calcaneal fractures are often bilateral, radiographs are often obtained of both feet. This is advantageous, because even if the other side was not injured, bilateral comparison is helpful in the measurements of normal anatomic angles such as the Boehler angle and the calcaneal pitch angle.

Treatment Nonoperative treatment is indicated for most extra-articular fractures or for severely comminuted fractures in osteopenic bone. Although some authors favor no cast immobilization but only protected weight bearing for 4 to 6 weeks, more common practice is short-leg casting—either weight-bearing or non–weight-bearing, depending on the site of fracture—for 4 to 8 weeks.

Operative treatment is indicated for intra-articular fractures when it is necessary to restore one or more of the following:

- The subtalar articulation
- The Boehler angle

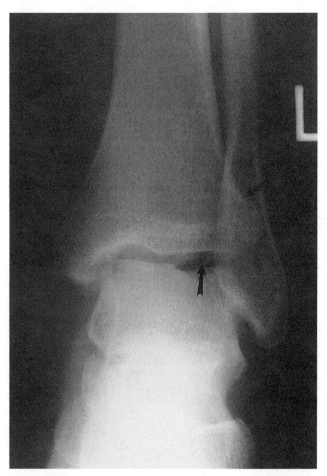

Figure 14-50 Impaction fracture of the tibial plafond and the talar dome. This 46-year-old man fell 20 feet out of a tree, where he had been hanging Christmas lights, and landed on his feet. The impaction at the ankle joint upon landing depressed the lateral aspect of the talar dome and impacted the lateral tibial plafond. A faint fracture line can be visualized extending from the articular surface of the tibia to the lateral distal tibial condyle (black arrows). This unfortunate man also sustained a burst fracture of the second lumbar vertebra as well as multiple rib fractures (see Figs. 9-39 and 11-38). This combination of injuries is not uncommon with this type of fall, because the axial force that is sustained at landing is readily transmitted through the extremities to the spine. For this reason, patients who present with this type of history are routinely screened at both the ankle and the spine regardless of what their primary complaint may be.

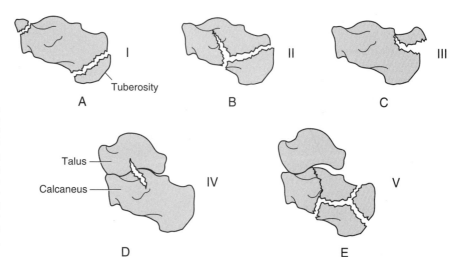

Figure 14-52 The *Rowe* classification of calcaneal fractures defines five injury patterns: **(A)** type I (incidence 21%): fractures of tuberosity, sustentaculum tali, or anterior process; **(B)** type II (incidence 3.8%), beak fractures and avulsion fractures of the Achilles' tendon insertion; **(C)** type III (incidence 19.5%), oblique fractures not extending into subtalar joint; **(D)** type IV (incidence 24.7%), fractures involving the subtalar joint; **(E)** type V (incidence 31%), fractures with central depression and comminution. *(Adapted from Greenspan,[11] p. 337.)*

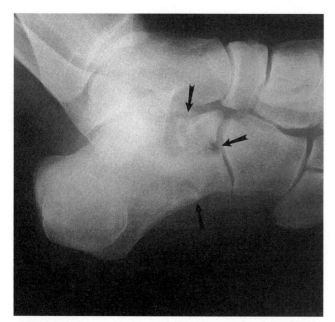

Figure 14-53 Fracture of the calcaneus. This 58-year-old woman was injured when she jumped down from a stepladder after losing her balance while washing windows. This *Rowe type V* fracture is comminuted with central depression and has intra-articular extensions into the subtalar joint and the calcaneocuboid joint (arrows).

- The normal width of the calcaneus
- The normal calcanealcuboid articulation
- Calcaneal height

Lag screws, plates, bone grafting are used to fixate and restore the calcaneus. More recent surgical procedures use percutaneous screw fixation and external fixators to minimize complications.

The patient does not bear weight for 8 to 12 weeks. Rehabilitation focuses on restoring normal joint arthrokinematics, strength, and normal gait cycle.

Complications Long-term complications usually result from malunion, including posttraumatic arthritis at the subtalar or calcaneocuboid joints and peroneal tendinitis from impingement of the tendons between the malpositioned calcaneus and the tip of the fibula.

Talar Fractures

Fractures of the talus occur second in frequency to calcaneal fractures.

Mechanism of Injury The injury mechanism is usually a large force applied through a dorsiflexed foot, as when a driver slams on the brakes in an auto collision.

Classification Because three-fifths of the talus is covered with articular cartilage, almost all talar fractures are considered to be intra-articular. Most classification schemes represent a continuum of fractures of the talar head, body, and neck (Fig. 14-55).

Radiologic Evaluation The routine radiologic evaluation of the foot demonstrates most talar fractures adequately. CT or MRI is used to further evaluate pain when radiographs are negative or to assist in preoperative planning (Figs. 14-56 and 14-57).

Treatment Nonoperative treatment is indicated in nondisplaced fractures and consists of immobilization in a short-leg cast for 8 to 12 weeks and avoidance of weight-bearing for the initial 6 weeks until radiographic evidence of healing is present (Fig. 14-58).

Operative treatment is required to treat displaced fractures in order to restore subtalar joint congruity (Fig. 14-59).

Complications Posttraumatic arthritis of the ankle and subtalar joints is a common long-term complication of talar fractures; it is related to the articular surface damage, the prolonged immobilization necessary for bony union, and the presence of any necrotic changes. Additionally, the blood supply to the talus is tenuous because no muscles attach to it and its cartilage-covered surface provides little area for vascular perforation. Thus the talus is predisposed to developing *avascular necrosis* after a fracture.

Midfoot Fractures

The relative immobility of the midfoot minimizes its susceptibility to isolated fractures. Fractures occurring in this region are often associated with other fracture or dislocation patterns. Sprains and fracture–subluxations or fracture–dislocations can occur at the transverse tarsal joint and tarsometatarsal joint, where the relatively rigid midfoot attaches to the more mobile

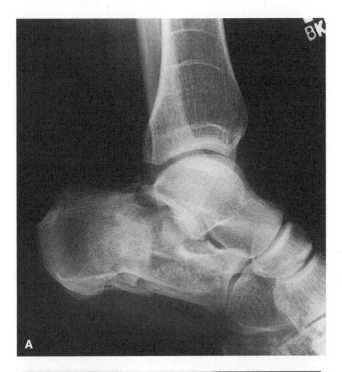

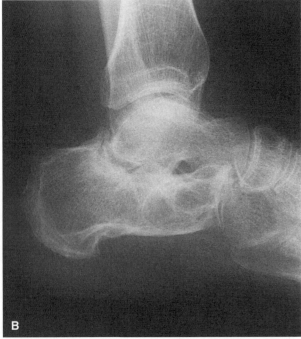

Figure 14-54 Fracture of the calcaneus. **(A)** This lateral view of the foot demonstrates a severely comminuted calcaneal fracture with central depression of the calcaneal body, which has disrupted the subtalar articulation (*Rowe type V*). This injury was sustained by a construction worker in a fall off a roof. **(B)** Follow-up film of the patient 1 year after open reduction and internal fixation with bone grafting shows fusion of the subtalar joint and the superior aspect of the calcaneocuboid joint. Functionally, these joints were stiff but painless, and motion at the talocrural joint was minimally limited. Note the Boehler angle and calcaneal pitch are both less than 20 degrees acutely and as a postoperative deformity. What do you anticipate will occur at the joints adjacent to the fused joint?

hindfoot and forefoot. In general, however, dislocations occur much less frequently than fractures.

A relatively rare fracture–dislocation at the tarsometatarsal (Lisfranc) joint is such an example (Fig. 14-60). The mechanism

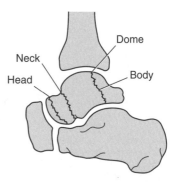

Figure 14-55 Fractures of the talus are described by their anatomic location at the body, dome, neck, or head. Because three-fifths of the talus is covered with articular cartilage, most fractures of the talus are considered to be intra-articular.

of injury of a fracture–dislocation is usually a high-energy trauma. Surgical reduction is often necessary to restore alignment and function.

Navicular Fractures

The navicular is one midfoot tarsal that is noted to sustain isolated injury. Four types of navicular fractures are known to occur:

- Dorsal avulsion fractures at the site of attachment of the deltoid ligament
- Tuberosity fractures
- Body fractures (Fig. 14-61)
- Stress fractures

Radiographs identify most fracture lines. Stress fractures are best defined by MRI when radiographs are negative. Treatment typically consists of non–weight-bearing immobilization in a short-leg cast for 4 to 6 weeks. Operative fixation is necessary for displaced fractures or large avulsed fragments. Lag screw fixation is most common, followed by partial weight-bearing short-leg cast immobilization.

Forefoot Fractures

Metatarsal Fractures

Mechanism of Injury Metatarsal fractures result most commonly from direct trauma, as when a heavy object is dropped on the foot. In these instances the fracture can occur at any location on the bone.

Classification An anatomic classification divides fractures into those occurring at the following:

1. First metatarsal, which requires excellent reduction and fixation because of its importance in weight-bearing function.
2. Second, third, and fourth metatarsals, which are injured from indirect twisting mechanisms and result in spiral fracture patterns. Stress fractures occur in the distal shafts of these bones.
3. Fifth metatarsal, due to direct trauma, to avulsion of the peroneus brevis, or to an inversion force (as is applied to a dancer's foot in descent from a demipointe position). Stress fractures occur in the proximal shaft of this bone at the metaphyseal–diaphyseal junction and can progress to displaced fractures (Fig. 14-62).

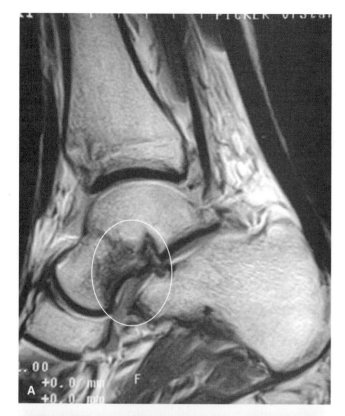

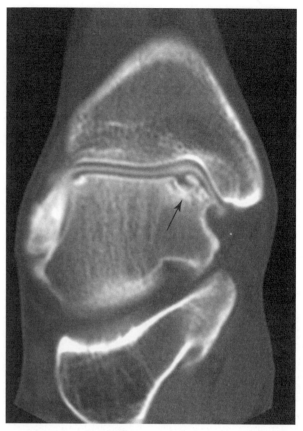

Figure 14-57 Coronal CT arthrogram of the ankle. The patient is a 33-year-old female who had had chronic ankle pain for 2 years. Radiographs were negative. An osteochondral defect was revealed by CT. The arthrogram was performed to assess the articular cartilage, which is now visible as intact. *(Image courtesy of John C. Hunter, MD, University of California, Davis School of Medicine.)*

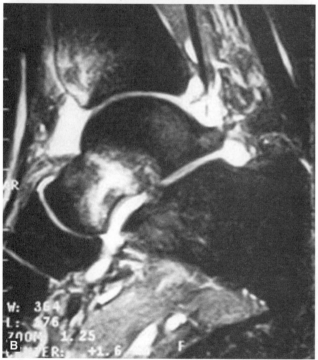

Figure 14-56 Occult fracture of the talar neck. The patient presented with chronic ankle pain. Radiographs were negative. **(A)** Sagittal T-1 weighted MRI shows a low intensity signal area (dark) at the neck, in circle. **(B)** Sagittal T-2 weighted MRI shows bone marrow edema at the neck as a high signal intensity (white). *(Image courtesy of John C. Hunter, MD, University of California, Davis School of Medicine.)*

Other classification schemes identify fracture patterns by the fracture pattern at the shaft or the amount of involvement of the articular ends of the bones.

Radiologic Findings AP, lateral, and oblique radiographs adequately demonstrate most metatarsal fractures. MRI is best in the identification of occult stress fractures.

Treatment Treatment of metatarsal fractures is dependent on the amount of displacement. Nondisplaced fractures are typically treated with short-leg weight-bearing cast immobilization for 2 to 4 weeks. Displaced fractures usually require open reduction and internal fixation (ORIF) to restore function; this is especially important at the first and fifth metatarsals, which provide stability and protection to the interposed metatarsals. Cast immobilization usually follows for 6 weeks.

Rehabilitation focuses on restoring joint arthrokinematics at the ankle and foot as well as function strength, range of motion, and normal gait cycle.

Complications Nonunion, delayed union, and posttraumatic arthritis are the most common complications associated with metatarsal fractures.

Phalangeal Fractures

Mechanism of Injury Phalangeal fractures result most commonly from objects being dropped on the toes or from "stubbing" injuries. The first and fifth toes are most often injured because of their exposed location.

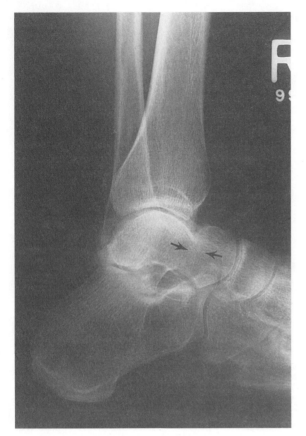

Figure 14-58 Nondisplaced fracture of the talar neck. The most common mechanism of talar neck fracture is hyperdorsiflexion of the foot on the leg; the posterior capsular ligaments of the subtalar joint rupture and the neck of the talus hits the leading anterior edge of the distal tibia.

Radiologic Findings Phalangeal fractures are usually identifiable on routine radiographs of the foot, although isolation of the digit of interest for the lateral view aids in diagnosis.

Treatment Treatment generally consists of manual reduction, splinting or "buddy" taping to the adjacent digit, and protected weight-bearing with a hard-sole shoe orthosis for 3 to 4 weeks. Injuries to the great toe are treated more aggressively to ensure anatomic reduction sufficient for weight-bearing function; they may require internal fixation with lag screws or wires.

Rehabilitation after immobilization is important to re-establish normal dorsiflexion of the first metatarsophalangeal joint, which allows for a normal gait cycle.

Complications Hallux limitus (partial loss of motion at the great toe) and hallux rigidus (complete loss of motion at the great toe) describe the severity of the chronic posttraumatic degenerative changes at the first metatarsophalangeal joint, which can seriously impair function.

Deformities of the Foot[11,62–81]

Abnormal foot positions may be congenital or developmental or may result from traumatic conditions or neuromuscular impairment. The entire foot may exhibit structural or anatomic deformity, or the deformity may be confined to a segment of the foot, such as the forefoot, midfoot, or hindfoot.

Radiologic Evaluation

The evaluation and description of foot deformities are derived from lines and angles drawn on the AP and lateral conventional radiographs. These measurements are used to describe anatomic deviations from the norm.

Although lateral films are routinely taken in a non–weight-bearing position, additional weight-bearing lateral films provide further information regarding the flexibility, rigidity, or adaptability of a deformity to weight-bearing function.

Examples of some commonly seen foot deformities follow.

Hallux Valgus

Hallux valgus is a deformity of the forefoot in which the first metatarsal is deviated medially and the great toe is deviated laterally (Fig. 14-63). The etiology is varied, and associations have been made with biomechanical dysfunction, improper footwear, and predisposing congenital factors such as a wide first intermetatarsal angle and pes planus. Females are affected with much greater frequency than males.

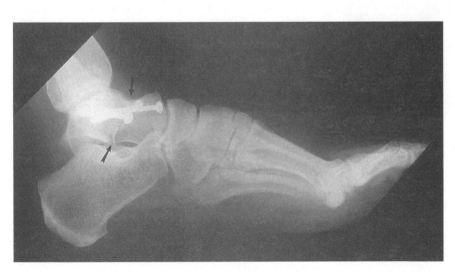

Figure 14-59 Displaced fracture of the talar neck. Displaced talar fractures such as this may be treated with closed reduction and immobilization, but they often require open reduction and internal fixation to achieve adequate anatomic reduction of the fracture and to preserve subtalar joint junction. The arrows mark the extent of the fracture line; the multiaxis compression screws appear to have achieved satisfactory reduction.

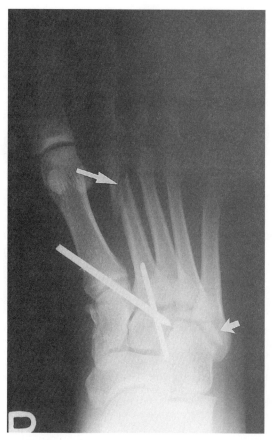

Figure 14-60 Tarsometatarsal (Lisfranc) dislocation with associated fractures. This 37-year-old man was injured when he fell off his horse and his foot remained caught in the stirrup. The forefoot was forcefully twisted and abducted laterally, resulting in a spiral fracture of the second metatarsal neck (long arrow), a shear fracture of the cuboid (small arrow), and a dislocation of the tarsometatarsal joint. This AP view of the foot shows the tarsometatarsal dislocation reduced and stabilized with two Steinmann pins.

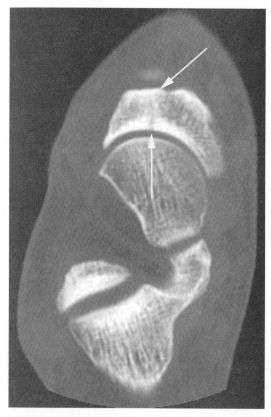

Figure 14-61 Axial CT showing a stress fracture in the navicular. The patient is an 18-year-old female dancer with a 6-month history of pain in the navicular and midfoot. Initial MRI and bone scans were positive for edema and increased tracer activity (respectively) in the navicular bone. After 6 months of limited improvement despite immobilization and other conservative treatment, the physician elected to do a CT when radiographs remained unremarkable. Why was a CT chosen instead of a repeat of MRI and/or bone scan? Since the other diagnostic consideration was osteoid osteoma, it was felt that detecting a fracture line would answer all questions and avoid the need to biopsy; additionally CT is superior to MRI in defining osteoid osteoma. *(Image courtesy of John C. Hunter, MD, University of California, Davis School of Medicine.)*

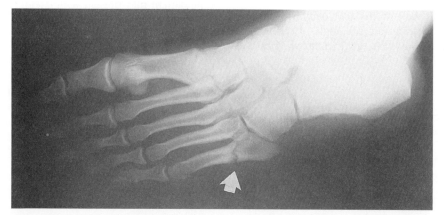

Figure 14-62 Fracture of the base of the fifth metatarsal. All fractures in this region have generally been referred to as "Jones fractures" after the original description put forth in 1902 by Sir Robert Jones, who personally sustained this fracture while dancing. Unfortunately, the persistence of this eponym has resulted in significant confusion in the management of these fractures, because at least two distinct fracture patterns occur at the base of the fifth metatarsal: avulsion fracture of the tuberosity at the attachment of the peroneus brevis and transverse fracture of the proximal diaphysis, as seen here (arrow). The management of these two types of fractures is distinctly different, because the healing potential of the diaphyseal fracture is diminished and the rate of fibrous union or subsequent "refracture" is high. Inadequate initial treatment may contribute to nonunion or delayed union of the diaphyseal fracture; thus this fracture must be distinguished from the less complicated, more proximal avulsion fracture.

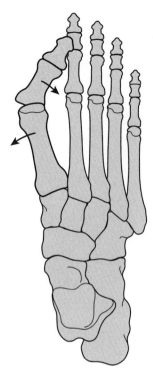

Figure 14-63 Hallux valgus is a deformity of the forefoot in which the first metatarsal is deviated medially and the great toe is deviated laterally.

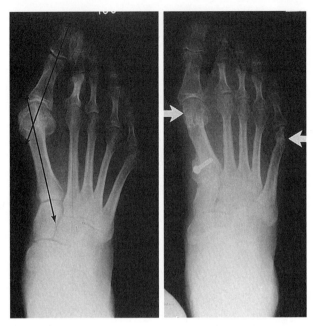

Figure 14-64 Hallux valgus. The AP view of the foot on the left is a preoperative film of a 58-year-old woman. Note the medial deviation of the first metatarsal and the lateral deviation of the great toe. Bunions have formed at the medial side of the first metatarsal head and the lateral side of the fifth metatarsal head. The AP film on the right is a postoperative film demonstrating an osteotomy with screw stabilization at the base of the first metatarsal and bunionectomies at the first and fifth metatarsal heads (white arrows).

Clinical Presentation

Clinically, the first metatarsophalangeal joint undergoes friction and stress in this deformity, and bunion formation on the medial side of the joint is a common occurrence. Although some patients may be asymptomatic, the more severe cases of hallux valgus significantly alter function and cause pain, especially if degenerative joint changes progress.

Radiologic Evaluation

Radiologically, the AP view of the foot demonstrates this deformity; the first intermetatarsal angle describes the degree of medial deviation of the first metatarsal, known as *metatarsus primus varus.*

Treatment

Treatment may consist of corrective orthoses, bunionectomy, arthrodesis, or resection arthroplasty (Fig. 14-64). Rehabilitation focuses on restoring joint arthrokinematics and sufficient dorsiflexion at the joint to permit normal toe-off in the gait cycle.

Pes Cavus

In *pes cavus,* sometimes called "claw foot," the medial longitudinal arch is abnormally high (Fig. 14-65).

Etiology

The etiology of pes cavus is known in approximately 80% of patients. Conditions include malunion of calcaneal or talar fractures, sequelae of burns or compartment syndromes,

residual talipes equinovarus, or neurological disorders such as Charcot–Marie–Tooth disease, muscular dystrophy, poliomyelitis, syringomyelia, Friedreich's ataxia, cerebral palsy, and spinal cord tumors. The other 20% of cases are idiopathic and usually nonprogressive.

Clinical Presentation

The patient may present with lateral foot pain secondary to excessive weight-bearing, metatarsalgia, plantar keratosis, and ankle instability.

Radiologic Evaluation

Weight-bearing radiographs are essential for inspection of degenerative joint changes, calcaneal position, and forefoot alignment. A calcaneal pitch over 30 degrees is indicative of pes cavus. The talometatarsal angle, as seen on the lateral view (Fig. 14-66), gives a value for the height of the arch in the sagittal plane.

Treatment

The goal of treatment is to allow the patient to ambulate without pain. This usually involves producing a plantigrade foot that allows for even distribution of weight-bearing loads.

Conservative treatment includes stretching, strengthening, and the use of orthotics. Extra deep shoes are needed to offload bony prominences. Lateral wedges may be applied to the outside sole to shift weight off the lateral foot. Bracing may be helpful for flexible deformities or foot-drop.

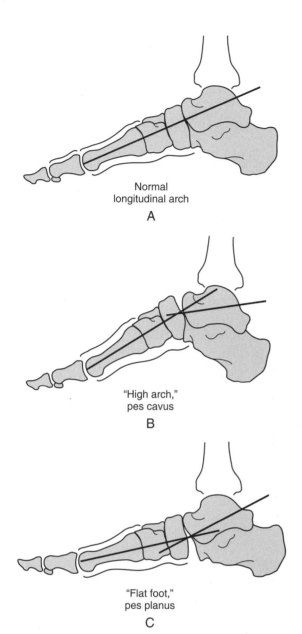

Normal
longitudinal arch

A

"High arch,"
pes cavus

B

"Flat foot,"
pes planus

C

Figure 14-65 The talometatarsal angle is formed by the intersection of a line drawn along the midshaft of the first metatarsal and a line bisecting the talus on the lateral view of the foot. Normally zero **(A)**, this angle has been used to define **(B)** pes cavus and **(C)** pes planus. The determination of flexible versus rigid arches requires comparison of weight-bearing and non–weight-bearing views. *(Adapted from Richardson and Iglarsh,[62] p. 536.)*

Surgical treatment involves both soft tissue and bony procedures. Examples include tendon transfers, osteotomies, plantar fascia releases, and joint arthrodeses.

Pes Planus

Classification

Pes planus, or "flat foot," is categorized as being either rigid (pathological) or flexible (physiological). A flexible flat foot demonstrates a low arch on weight-bearing and a return to a more normal arch when non–weight-bearing. A rigid flat foot demonstrates a low arch whether weight-bearing or non–weight-bearing (Fig. 14-67).

Flat Feet in Children

A flexible flat foot is considered normal in young children and usually resolves with growth and maturity. Unfortunately some children do not outgrow flat feet, and the deformity persists lifelong. Early intervention in the treatment of flexible pes planus is highly controversial. Some practitioners recommend no treatment for a painless flat foot. Others who treat the damaging effects of excessive pronation in adults argue that much pathology can be curbed if the condition is addressed in childhood.

Etiology

Etiological factors of flexible flat foot are widely varied and include torsional abnormalities, muscular imbalance, ligamentous laxity, neuropathy, obesity, agenesis of the sustentaculum tali, calcaneovalgus, equinus, varus or valgus tibia, limb length discrepancy, compensated forefoot varus, and an external tibial ossicle. Biomechanically, the condition is primarily one of peritalar subluxation that occurs secondary to excessive pronation of the subtalar joint. Etiology of rigid flat foot includes *tarsal coalition* and *congenital vertical talus.*

Clinical Presentation

Flexible flat feet in adults may or may not be painful. Rigid flat feet with tarsal coalition are seen to become symptomatic in the second decade of life, when the foot ossifies and greater stresses are put on the tarsals owing to increased body weight and the increased activity of sports or work.

Radiologic Evaluation

Lateral radiographs may show deviations in calcaneal inclination, talar *declination* producing a negative talometatarsal angle, or a *medial column sag* at the talonavicular or naviculocuneiform joints. A *talar beak* is a secondary change due to limitations of subtalar joint motion (Fig. 14-68). The AP radiograph may show altered talonavicular congruity and cuboid adduction.

Tarsal coalition is the bony or fibrocartilaginous connection between two or more tarsal bones. *Talonavicular* and *calcaneonavicular* coalitions are the most common and are bilateral in over 50% of known cases. Coalitions are usually identified on radiograph, although CT or MRI allows for the more precise determination of articular involvement (Fig. 14-69). MRI is advantageous in identifying nonosseous fibrous and cartilaginous coalitions.

Congenital vertical talus is the most serious pathological flat foot and may occur in association with other congenital anomalies such as myelomeningocele, arthrogryposis, and developmental hip dyplasias. At birth the foot is dorsiflexed and the arch is convex. Radiographs confirm the diagnosis (Fig. 14-70).

Treatment

Conservative treatment includes the use of orthotic heel stabilizers from the time a child begins walking until a normal supinatus is developed in the forefoot-to hindfoot relationship near age 6. At this time, a functional orthosis can be effective. Functional foot orthoses place the subtalar joint in neutral via rigid control of the rearfoot at the stance phase of the gait cycle. Another option is an ankle–foot orthosis that functions in the stance phase as well as the swing phase by exerting control over the ankle and tibia.

Surgical treatment for painful flat foot after failure of conservative treatment is varied. Subtalar joint *arthroereisis* is implantation of a disk the size of a pencil eraser in the sinus tarsi to block pronation of the subtalar joint. The implant is outside the joint and is easily removed at maturity or if the patient does not tolerate it. Subtalar arthroereisis is utilized alone or in combination with heel cord lengthening, medial arch stabilization, or both. Surgical intervention for coalition includes resection of the bridge and interposition of fat, tendon, or muscle at the coalition site.

Rehabilitation is involved to help correct the dynamic factors that influence the kinetic chain of the limbs, including joint mobilization, muscle balancing, flexibility, functional limb length modifications, and orthotic fabrication.

Talipes Equinovarus

The most common congenital deformity of the lower extremity is *talipes equinovarus,* commonly known as *clubfoot* (Fig. 14-71). (*Talipes* is a term designating deformities of the ankle and foot.)

Etiology

The etiology of clubfoot during fetal development appears to be multifactorial. Both genetic and environmental factors are implicated. The less severe forms of the deformity, known as

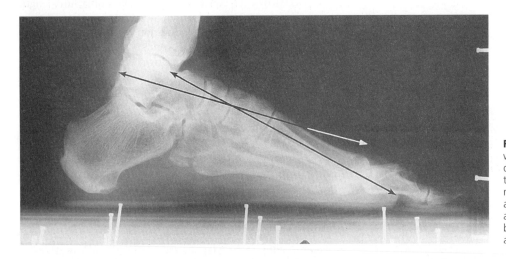

Figure 14-66 Pes cavus. This lateral weight-bearing view of the foot demonstrates a "high" medial longitudinal arch. One radiographic measurement used to quantify this arch is the talometatarsal angle, arrived at by the intersection of lines bisecting the first metatarsal shaft and the body of the talus.

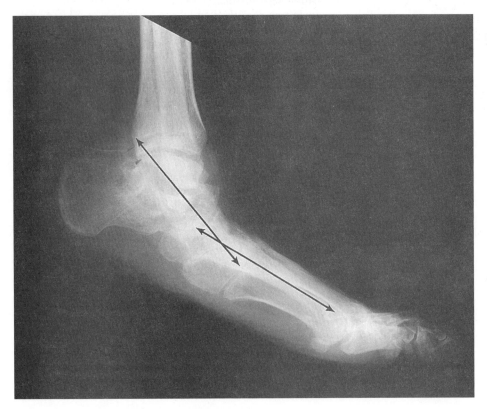

Figure 14-67 Rigid pes planus. The "low" medial longitudinal arch of the foot is quantified on this lateral view by measuring the talometatarsal angle, an intersection of the lines inscribed across the body of the talus and through the midshaft of the first metatarsal. This radiograph shows persistence of the deformity when non–weight-bearing, which determines that the deformity is rigid rather than flexible.

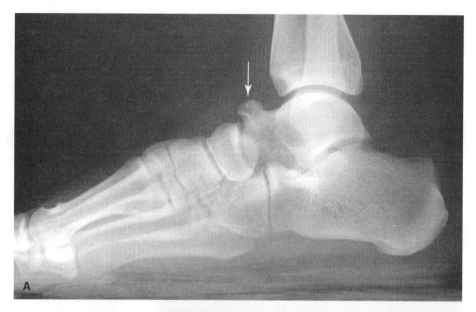

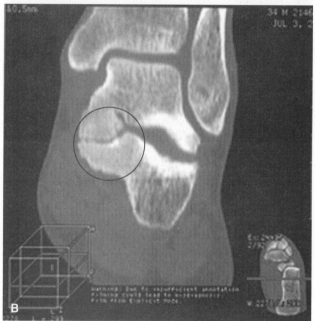

Figure 14-68 The patient is a 34-year-old male with chronic foot pain. **(A)** The lateral radiograph is unremarkable except for the large osteophyte at the talar head, known as a *talar beak* (arrow). The talar beak is commonly associated with talocalcaneal coalition and occurs because of subtalar joint limitation and subsequent dorsal subluxation of the navicular. **(B)** Coronal CT shows the talocalcaneal coalition (circled). This coalition is nonosseous, as a dark line is present through the coalition. MRI would further define cartilaginous or fibrous coalition. *(Image courtesy of John C. Hunter, MD, University of California, Davis School of Medicine.)*

postural clubfoot, are associated with abnormal intrauterine positioning.

Risk factors include a family history of the condition. Boys are predominantly affected. The incidence is 1 in 800 live births.

Clinical Presentation

There is bilateral involvement in up to 50% of cases. The deformity may range from mild and flexible to severe and rigid. The hallmarks of this deformity include the following:

1. An equinus or plantarflexed position of the heel
2. Inversion of the subtalar joint with a varus position of the hindfoot

3. Metatarsal adduction with varus position of the forefoot
4. In the most severe cases, subluxation or dislocation of the subtalar or talocalcaneonavicular joint (this element cannot be evaluated on radiograph before the navicular ossifies by age 2 or 3).

Radiologic Evaluation

Radiographs are of limited value in assessing talipes equinovarus at birth because the bones are minimally ossified. Radiographic assessment is significant later in monitoring osseous growth and development and assessing surgical outcome.

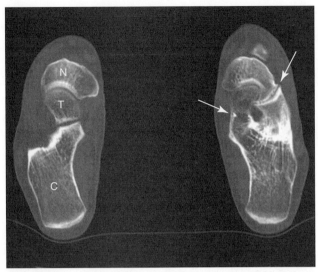

Figure 14-69 The patient is a 28-year-old male with chronic pain in the left foot. Prior radiographs demonstrated a narrowing of the subtalar joint. Coronal CT of both feet on the same exam allows for comparison. The right foot is normal and the bones are identified: N = navicular, T = talus, C = calcaneus; the left shows an *osseous talocalcaneal coalition* (white arrow) and a *fibrous calcaneonavicular coalition* (black arrow). *(Image courtesy of John C. Hunter, MD, University of California, Davis School of Medicine.)*

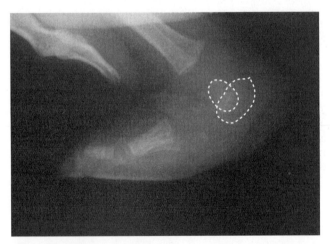

Figure 14-70 Lateral radiograph of a 2-month old child, with the foot held in maximum dorsiflexion, shows no change in the vertical orientation of the talus relative to the calcaneus, as compared to the plantarflexed radiograph (not shown). Both bones are outlined to show the abnormal perpendicular relationship of the talus to the calcaneus. *(Image courtesy of R. E. Christopher Rose, MBBS, FRCSC, University of the West Indies.)*

Treatment

Conservative treatment begins immediately after birth to take advantage of adaptable flexibility. The foot is manipulated into a more normal position and then casted. Recasting and repositioning continues at intervals; this is usually complete after 3 months. After the foot is so realigned, normal position is maintained through stretching exercises, night splints, and orthopedic shoes for up to several years as needed. Surgical treatment is required when conservative measures fail or to correct contractures or irreducible joint subluxations.

Rehabilitation is involved extensively to restore strength, flexibility, and function as well as to facilitate normal developmental motor skills.

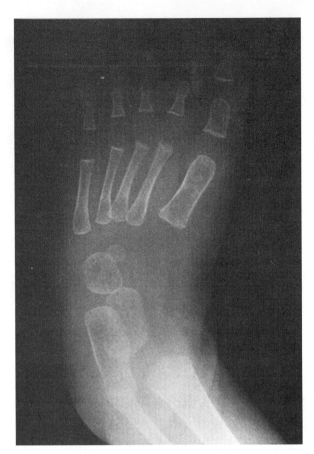

Figure 14-71 AP radiograph of a 2-year-old with talipes equinovarus. The forefoot is in adduction relative the the hindfoot. Compare with the normal anatomy in Figure 14-5.

The prognosis is generally good for a functional foot and pain-free ambulation.

Foot Anomalies

Accessory Bones[11]

Accessory bones are anomalous bones that usually form because of a failure of one or more ossification centers to unite with the main mass of bone. Accessory bones appear with some frequency at the foot. Studies have reported an incidence as high as 30% in adults. Accessory bones may be seen radiographically at various locations in the foot; the locations and names of these are presented in Figure 14-72. The most commonly occurring accessory bones of the foot are the *os trigonum,* the *os intermetatarseum,* and the *os tibiale* or accessory navicular (see Figs. 14-29 and 14-73).

Accessory bones can complicate the evaluation of foot injuries if they are present in the area of a suspected fracture. Comparison films are not always helpful because accessory and sesamoid bones are not always bilaterally symmetrical. In general, accessory bones are differentiated from acute fractures by the presence of an intact, smooth cortical shell with an underlying line of increased density. In contrast, acute fractures will have an irregular cortical surface and no appearance of increased density beneath the surface.

Figure 14-72 Names and locations of accessory bones seen in the foot. The asterisk * indicates those that occur with frequency: (1) talotibial ossicle (os talotibiale); (2) supratalar ossicle (os supratalare); (3) supranavicular ossicle (os supranaviculare); (4)* intermetatarsal ossicle (os intermetatarsale); (5) secondary cuboid (cuboides secundarium); (6) secondary calcaneus (calcaneus secundarius); (7)* external tibial ossicle (os tibiale externum); (8)* trigone ossicle (os trigonum); (9) peroneal ossicle (os peronaeum); (10) vesalian ossicle (os vesalianum); (11) accessory talus (talus accessorius); (12) secondary talus (talus secundarius). *(Adapted from Greenspan,⁸ p. 309.)*

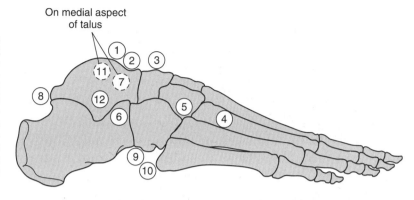

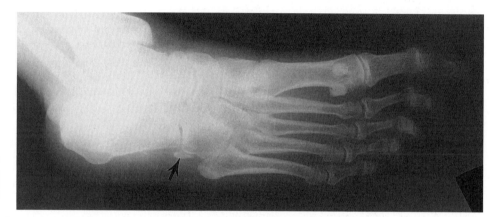

Figure 14-73 Os peroneum, accessory bone. On the oblique view of this foot, a large os peroneum is visible (arrow) embedded within the tendon of the peroneus brevis muscle.

Summary of Key Points

Routine Radiologic Evaluation of the Ankle

1. The routine radiographic evaluation of the ankle includes three projections:

   ➤ *AP view*—demonstrates the distal tibia and fibula and dome of the talus.

   ➤ *AP oblique (mortise view)*—demonstrates the entire joint space of the ankle mortise.

   ➤ *Lateral*—demonstrates the anterior and posterior aspects of the tibia, the tibiotalar joint, and the subtalar joint.

Routine Radiologic Evaluation of the Foot

2. The routine evaluation of the foot includes three projections:

   ➤ *Anteroposterior*—demonstrates all the bones of the forefoot and midfoot and their associated articulations; the first intertarsal angle is measured on this view.

   ➤ *Lateral*—demonstrates the bones of the hindfoot and midfoot and their associated articulations (the Boehler angle and calcaneal inclination are measured on this view).

   ➤ *Oblique*—demonstrates the shafts of the metatarsal bones and the intermetatarsal joints.

Trauma Radiography

3. The ACR recommends radiographic examination as the *initial study* for all acute injuries meeting Ottawa criteria; and for assessment of all chronic ankle/foot pain.

4. Advanced imaging is used when radiographs are (a) insufficient to guide treatment, or (b) after the radiographic findings are negative when further injury is suspected.

   ➤ CT or MRI is recommended for the evaluation of complex and cartilaginous fractures.

   ➤ MRI, tenography, and ultrasound are recommended for the evaluation of soft tissue injuries.

   ➤ MRI or bone scans are recommended for the identification of stress fractures.

Ankle Sprains

5. The ankle is the most frequently sprained joint in the body. The majority of injuries are precipitated by an inversion force. Damage may range in severity from minor sprains to ligamentous rupture, bony avulsions, and joint instability.

6. Radiologic signs of ankle instability following severe sprains are seen on the AP view as an abnormal position of the talus and increased width of the ankle mortise joint space.

Fractures at the Ankle

7. The basic classification system to describe ankle fractures groups them into *unimalleolar fractures, bimalleolar fractures,* and *trimalleolar fractures.*

8. The goal of treatment is to stabilize the fracture site and reestablish the architecture of the ankle mortise. Without sufficient reduction of the ankle mortise, the ankle will be vulnerable to instability and posttraumatic arthritis.

Fractures at the Foot

9. Fractures of the foot are generally described by anatomic location as fractures of the hindfoot, midfoot, or forefoot.

10. At the hindfoot, the calcaneus is the most frequently fractured bone; a fracture of it is often associated with a vertebral compression fracture in the thoracolumbar spine.

11. Most fractures of the talus are considered to be intraarticular. Complications of talar fractures include posttraumatic arthritis of the ankle and subtalar joints as well as avascular necrosis.

12. At the midfoot, fractures are usually seen in combination with sprains and dislocations at the transverse tarsal and tarsometatarsal joints; an exception is stress fractures of the navicular.

13. At the forefoot, fractures of the metatarsals and phalanges are usually caused by direct trauma or "stubbing" injuries. Stress fractures are also common injuries in the forefoot, usually appearing at the distal shafts of the second through fourth metatarsals and the proximal shaft of the fifth metatarsal.

Deformities of the Foot

14. Deformities of the foot are described and evaluated radiologically by the measurements of lines and angles drawn on the AP and lateral radiographs of the foot.

15. *Hallux valgus* is a deformity of the forefoot in which the first metatarsal is deviated medially and the great toe is deviated laterally.

16. *Pes cavus* is an abnormally high medial longitudinal arch of the foot, with a calcaneal inclination greater than 30 degrees as measured on the lateral view.

17. *Pes planus* is an abnormally low medial longitudinal arch of the foot, biomechanically resulting from peritalar subluxation or congenital deformities such as tarsal coalition.

18. *Talipes equinovarus* or *clubfoot* is the most common congenital deformity of the lower extremity. Radiographs are of limited value at birth because of the minimal ossification present at that time. Radiographic assessment is significant later in monitoring osseous growth and assessing treatment outcomes.

 Please refer to the text's enclosed CD-ROM for the American College of Radiology's current Musculoskeletal Appropriateness Criteria for the following topics: *Chronic Ankle Pain, Suspected Ankle Fractures, Chronic Foot Pain.*

CASE STUDIES

The following two case studies involve fractures of the proximal fifth-metatarsal shaft, commonly known as *Jones fractures,* after Sir Robert Jones (1857–1933), who described his own case in 1902 (and who also reported the first clinical use of x-rays in 1897).[21] The contrast in treatment decisions and outcomes illustrates how the "same" fracture can present entirely different challenges to the physician and physical therapist.

Case Study 1

Fifth-Metatarsal Shaft Fracture, Uncomplicated

The patient is a 16-year-old boy referred to physical therapy following surgical fixation of a fifth-metatarsal shaft fracture.

History of Trauma

The patient reported that the initial injury occurred during a soccer game. While his foot was planted, he was slide-tackled and the foot was forced to twist. He was held out of the remainder of the game and was sent to the emergency room for conventional radiographs.

Initial Imaging

Anteroposterior (AP) and lateral radiographs (Fig. 14-74) of the left foot revealed an incomplete transverse fracture of the fifth metatarsal shaft at the diaphyseal–metaphyseal junction. Some bony sclerosis was evident at the fracture site, suggesting that a pre-existing stress fracture had progressed to become a displaced fracture.

Intervention

The patient was treated via open reduction and internal fixation with a lag screw 2 days after the injury and was immobilized for 4 weeks in cast. Radiographs demonstrated evidence of good bony union at the fracture site. He was referred to outpatient physical therapy for rehabilitation (Fig. 14-75).

Outcome

The patient underwent comprehensive rehabilitation in physical therapy and returned to soccer 12 weeks after injury without complications or complaints of pain.

Discussion

This case outlines a successful surgical management and rehabilitation of a fifth-metatarsal fracture. This type of fracture, also known as a Jones fracture, is relatively common in athletes who perform quick running and cutting maneuvers. The repetitive forces involved in these movements can lead to a stress fracture that eventually displaces or becomes complete with a single inversion-type injury, as appeared to have taken place in this patient's case.

The case is summarized in Figure 14-76.

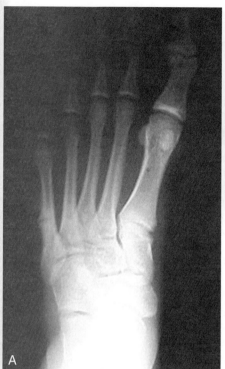

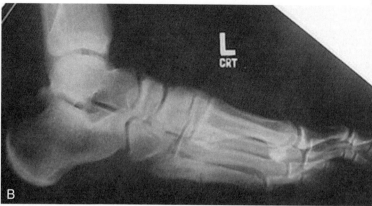

Figure 14-74 (A) AP view of the foot demonstrating an incomplete proximal fifth-metatarsal fracture. **(B)** Lateral view of the foot. Note the area of increased density at the fracture site. This represents a pre-existing stress fracture.

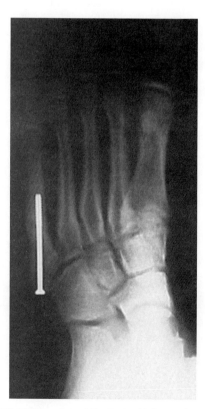

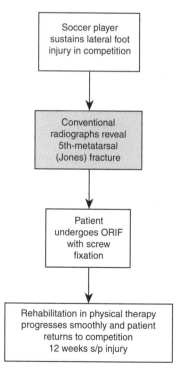

Figure 14-75 Oblique view of the foot with internal screw fixation of the fracture site.

Soccer player
sustains lateral foot
injury in competition

Conventional
radiographs reveal
5th-metatarsal
(Jones) fracture

Patient
undergoes ORIF
with screw
fixation

Rehabilitation in physical therapy
progresses smoothly and patient
returns to competition
12 weeks s/p injury

Figure 14-76 Pathway of case study events. Imaging is highlighted.

CRITICAL THINKING POINTS

The fracture was incomplete and undisplaced. Usually this dictates conservative treatment at any fracture site. Why did the surgeon choose open reduction and internal fixation?

Probably one reason is the evidence that a stress fracture had pre-existed for some time. The acute injury was simply the "last straw," or final imposed force, that caused the bone to fail and fracture. Therefore the surrounding bone at the fracture site was already in structural failure. Treating by cast immobilization alone had some potential for delayed union or nonunion.

Another factor may have been the patient's age and activity level. If the surgeon treated conservatively with cast immobilization, would the patient be absolutely compliant with the non–weight-bearing requirements? Inability to ensure compliance may have presented another risk factor for delayed union or nonunion.

Last, how important was it to the patient to return as quickly as possible to the game of soccer? Were concerns regarding eligibility and scholarship factored into the decision to operate immediately? Could the patient afford the time required to start with conservative treatment and then start again with surgical treatment in the event that conservative treatment failed?

Although classification systems of fracture configurations exist for the surgeon to use as guidelines for treatment decisions, each case is still individual, and treatment decisions are based on that surgeon's perception of the critical factors in the patient's case.

CASE STUDY 2

Fifth-Metatarsal Shaft Fracture, Complicated

The patient is an 18-year-old male basketball player referred to physical therapy for rehabilitation following surgical fixation of the fracture of a fifth-metatarsal shaft.

History of Trauma

The patient sustained the initial injury during a basketball game and was immediately assessed by an athletic trainer. The trainer suspected that he had sprained his ankle and treated accordingly with ice, compression, and elevation. He was also given crutches, an ankle brace, and instructions to bear weight as tolerated. A few days later, the patient returned to the trainer with complaints of persistent lateral foot pain with every step. The trainer then referred the patient to an orthopedic surgeon.

Initial Imaging

The surgeon ordered radiographs of the foot. AP and lateral radiographs demonstrated a complete fracture of the proximal fifth metatarsal at the diaphyseal-metaphyseal junction.

Intervention

This patient was initially treated conservatively with cast immobilization for 4 weeks. Follow-up radiographs demonstrated nonunion at the fracture site. The patient then underwent open reduction and internal screw fixation across the fracture site and was immobilized in a short-leg cast for 4 weeks.

Outcome

After successful union was radiographically evident, the patient was referred to physical therapy and began rehabilitation. During the initial weeks of rehabilitation the patient progressed steadily. After 8 weeks of rehabilitation, during the final phase of rehabilitation, the patient began to experience pain with full eversion and during running.

The physical therapist reviewed the patient's most recent radiographs, taken 4 weeks after surgery (Fig. 14-77). The position of the screw head appeared to be encroaching on the joint space between the fifth-metatarsal base and the cuboid bone. This would be consistent with the patient's complaints of a "pinching" pain with forced eversion.

The physical therapist contacted the surgeon and discussed the possibility of the screw as a source of pain. The surgeon determined that bone healing was adequate at this point and removed the screw. The patient completed rehabilitation and returned to playing basketball without complaints of pain.

Discussion

This patient's fracture was complete, yet the surgeon elected to treat conservatively. The eventual nonunion at the fracture site necessitated open reduction and internal fixation. The decision to treat conservatively is in contrast to the treatment decision made in Case Study 1. Why did this patient's complete fracture not receive immediate internal fixation?

Possible reasons are:

- The fracture was nondisplaced and had a good chance of healing with conservative treatment.

- The patient was older and was willing to be compliant with the non–weight-bearing status required for several weeks.

- Time was not a factor in the event that conservative treatment failed and surgery would be required (as happened).

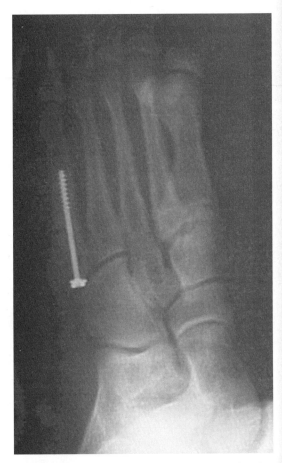

Figure 14-77 Oblique view of the foot demonstrating internal screw fixation after failed conservative treatment and nonunion.

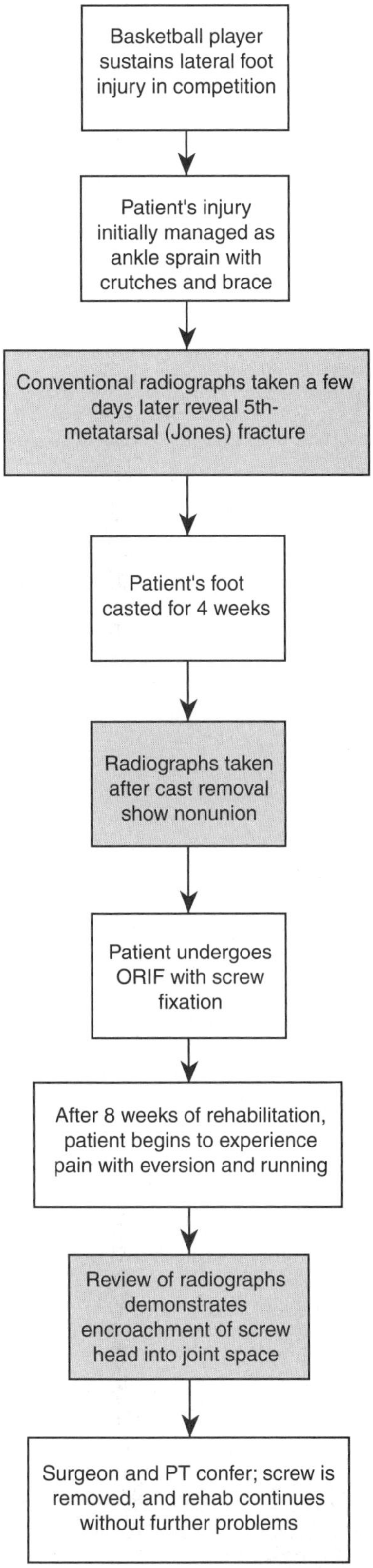

```
┌─────────────────────┐
│  Basketball player  │
│  sustains lateral   │
│  foot injury in     │
│  competition        │
└─────────────────────┘
          │
          ▼
┌─────────────────────┐
│  Patient's injury   │
│  initially managed  │
│  as ankle sprain    │
│  with crutches and  │
│  brace              │
└─────────────────────┘
          │
          ▼
┌─────────────────────┐
│  Conventional       │
│  radiographs taken  │
│  a few days later   │
│  reveal 5th-        │
│  metatarsal (Jones) │
│  fracture           │
└─────────────────────┘
          │
          ▼
┌─────────────────────┐
│  Patient's foot     │
│  casted for 4 weeks │
└─────────────────────┘
          │
          ▼
┌─────────────────────┐
│  Radiographs taken  │
│  after cast removal │
│  show nonunion      │
└─────────────────────┘
          │
          ▼
┌─────────────────────┐
│  Patient undergoes  │
│  ORIF with screw    │
│  fixation           │
└─────────────────────┘
          │
          ▼
┌─────────────────────┐
│  After 8 weeks of   │
│  rehabilitation,    │
│  patient begins to  │
│  experience pain    │
│  with eversion and  │
│  running            │
└─────────────────────┘
          │
          ▼
┌─────────────────────┐
│  Review of          │
│  radiographs        │
│  demonstrates       │
│  encroachment of    │
│  screw head into    │
│  joint space        │
└─────────────────────┘
          │
          ▼
┌─────────────────────┐
│  Surgeon and PT     │
│  confer; screw is   │
│  removed, and rehab │
│  continues without  │
│  further problems   │
└─────────────────────┘
```

Figure 14-78 Pathway of case study events. Imaging is highlighted.

As discussed in the previous case study, the surgeon's decisions are based on the individual patient and may not always seem to be in accordance with what is anticipated based on general guidelines for fracture treatment.

The case is summarized in Figure 14-78.

CRITICAL THINKING POINTS

1. Visualizing the placement of surgical hardware can be important to physical therapists during rehabilitation of a patient following open reduction and internal fixation (ORIF). This visual information may help the physical therapist to make decisions regarding interventions such as range of motion, weight bearing, and joint mobilization. In this case, the surgical hardware was identified as a likely source of pain.

2. Surgical hardware can sometimes become problematic because of its placement or potential to shift or migrate. Radiographs identify these potential problems.

3. Remember that at least two radiographic views, made at right angles to each other, are required to determine the position of surgical hardware (or any other object appearing on the radiograph).

4. Physical therapists must communicate clearly and accurately with the surgeon if surgical hardware may be related to problems that arise during a patient's rehabilitation.

Case studies adapted by J. Bradley Barr, PT, DPT, OCS.

References

Normal Anatomy

1. Netter, FH: Atlas of Human Anatomy, ed. 4. WB Saunders, Philadelphia, 2006.
2. Nordin, M, and Frankel, VH: Basic Biomechanics of the Musculoskeletal System, ed. 3. Lippincott Williams & Wilkins, Philadelphia, 2001.
3. Whiting, W, and Zernicke, R: Biomechanics of Musculoskeletal Injury, ed. 2. Human Kinetics, Champaign, IL, 2008.
4. Norkin, CC, and Levangie, PK: Joint Structure and Function: A Comprehensive Analysis, ed. 2. FA Davis, Philadelphia, 1992.
5. Meschan, I: An Atlas of Radiographic Anatomy. WB Saunders, Philadelphia, 1960.
6. Weber, EC, Vilensky, JA, and Carmichael, SW: Netter's Concise Radiological Anatomy. WB Saunders, Philadelphia, 2008.
7. Kelley, LL, and Peterson, CM: Sectional Anatomy for Imaging Professional, ed. 2. Mosby, St. Louis, MO, 2007.
8. Lazo, DL: Fundamentals of Sectional Anatomy: An Imaging Approach. Thomson Delmar Learning, Clifton Park, NY, 2005.

Routine Exam

9. American College of Radiology: Practice Guideline for the Performance of Radiography of the Extremities. 2006. Available at http://www.acr.org. Accessed July 22, 2008.
10. Weissman, B, and Sledge, C: Orthopedic Radiology. WB Saunders, Philadelphia, 1986.
11. Greenspan, A: Orthopedic Radiology: A Practical Approach, ed. 4. Lippincott Williams & Wilkins, Philadelphia, 2004.
12. Bontrager, KL: Textbook of Radiographic Positioning and Related Anatomy, ed. 6. Mosby, St. Louis, MO, 2005.
13. Fischer, HW: Radiographic Anatomy: A Working Atlas. McGraw-Hill, New York, 1988.
14. Wicke, L: Atlas of Radiographic Anatomy, ed. 5. Lea & Febiger, Malvern, PA, 1994.
15. Frank, E, Smith, B, and Long, B: Merrill's Atlas of Radiographic Positions and Radiologic Procedures, ed. 11. Elsevier Health Sciences, Philadelphia, 2007.
16. Squires, LF, and Novelline, RA: Fundamentals of Radiology, ed. 4. Harvard University Press, Cambridge, MA, 1988.
17. Chew, FS: Skeletal Radiology: The Bare Bones, ed. 2. Williams & Wilkins, Baltimore, 1997.
18. Weir, J, and Abrahams, P: An Atlas of Radiological Anatomy. Yearbook Medical, Chicago, 1978.
19. Krell, L (ed): Clark's Positioning in Radiology, Vol 1, ed. 10. Yearbook Medical, Chicago, 1989.
20. Nyska, M, et al: Radiological assessment of a modified anterior drawer test of the ankle. Foot Ankle 13(7):400, 1992.
21. Lohrer, H, et al: Observer reliability in ankle and calcaneocuboid stress radiography. Am J Sports Med 36(6):1143, 2008.

Trauma

22. American College of Radiology: Appropriateness Criteria for Suspected Ankle Fracture. 2005. Available at http://www.acr.org/SecondaryMain MenuCategories/quality_safety/app_criteria/pdf/ExpertPanelonMusculoskele talImaging/SuspectedAnkleFracturesDoc21.aspx.
23. American College of Radiology: Appropriateness Criteria for Chronic AnklPain. 2005. Available at http://www.acr.org/SecondaryMainMenuCate gories/quality_safety/app_criteria/pdf/ExpertPanelonMusculoskeletalImag ing/ChronicAnklePainDoc5.aspx.
24. Bucholz, RW, Heckman, J, and Court-Brown, C (eds): Rockwood and Green's: Fractures in Adults, ed. 6. Lippincott Williams & Wilkins, Philadelphia, 2005.
25. Rockwood, CA, and Green, DP (eds): Fractures in Adults, ed. 5. Lippincott Williams & Wilkins, Philadelphia, 2002.
26. Beaty, J, and Kasar, J (eds): Rockwood and Wilkins' Fractures in Children, ed. 6. Lippincott Williams & Wilkins, Philadelphia, 2005.
27. Koval, KJ, and Zuckerman, JD: Handbook of Fractures, ed. 2. Lippincott Williams & Wilkins, Philadelphia, 2002.
28. Eiff, M, et al: Fracture Management for Primary Care. WB Saunders, Philadelphia, 2003.
29. Yochum, TR, and Rowe, LJ: Essentials of Skeletal Radiology, ed. 3. Williams & Wilkins, Baltimore, 2004.
30. Marchiori, DM: Clinical Imaging with Skeletal, Chest, and Abdomen Pattern Differentials. Mosby, St. Louis, 1999.
31. Ip, D: Orthopedic Traumatology: A Resident's Guide. Springer, New York, 2006.
32. McConnell, J, Eyres, R, and Nightingale, J: Interpreting Trauma Radiographs. Blackwell, Malden, MA, 2005.
33. Berquist, TH: Imaging of Orthopedic Trauma, ed. 2. Raven Press, New York, 1989.
34. McCort, JJ, and Mindelzun, RE: Trauma Radiology. Churchill Livingston, New York, 1990.
35. Drafke, MW, and Nakayama, H: Trauma and Mobile Radiography, ed. 2. FA Davis, Philadelphia, 2001.
36. Hodler, J, von Schulthess, GK, and Zollikofer, CL: Musculoskeletal Disease: Diagnostic Imaging and Interventional Technology. Springer, Italy, 2005.
37. Daffner, RH: Clinical Radiology: The Essentials, ed. 3. Williams & Wilkins, Baltimore, 2007.
38. Bernstein, J (ed): Musculoskeletal Medicine. American Academy of Orthopedic Surgeons, Rosemont, IL, 2003.
39. Ardizzone, R, and Valmassy, RL: Continuing education: How to diagnose lateral ankle injuries. Podiatry Today 18(10), 2005. Availalable at http://www.podiatrytoday.com/article/4627.
40. Wyblier, M, et al: Musculoskeletal radiology: Ankle and foot in adults. J Radiol 89(5 Pt 2):711, 2008.
41. Elias, I, et al: Bone stress injury of the ankle in professional ballet dancers seen on MRI. BMC Musculoskel Disord 28;9:39, 2008.
42. Ting, AY, et al: MR imaging of midfoot injury. Magn Reson Imaging Clin North Am 16(1):105, 2008.
43. Collins, MS: Imaging evaluation of chronic ankle and hindfoot pain in athletes. Magn Reson Imaging Clin North Am 16(1):39, 2008.
44. Haverstock, BD: Foot and ankle imaging in the athlete. Clin Podiatr Med Surg 25(2):249, 2008.
45. Marin, LE: Percutaneous reduction and external fixation for foot and ankle fractures. Clin Podiatr Med Surg 25(4):721, 2008.
46. Borowski, LA, et al: The epidemiology of U.S. high school basketball injuries 2005-2007. Am J Sports Med 36:2328, 2008.
47. Porter, DA: Functional outcome after operative treatment for ankle fractures in young athletes: A retrospective case series. Foot Ankle Int 29(9):887, 2008.
48. Raikin, SM, et al: The association of varus hindfoot and fracture of the fifth metatarsal metaphyseal–diaphyseal junction: The Jones fracture. Am J Sports Med 36(7):1367, 2008.
49. Wukich, DK, and Kline, AJ: The management of ankle fractures in patients with diabetes. J Bone Joint Surg Am 90(7):1570, 2008.
50. Kierzynka, G, and Grala, P: Compartment syndrome of the foot after calcaneal fractures. Ortop Traumatol Rehabil 10(4):372, 2008.
51. Abbassian, A, and Thomas, R: Ankle ligament injuries. Br J Hosp Med 69(6):339, 2008.
52. Schepers, T, et al: Percutaneous reduction and fixation of calcaneal fractures. Oper Orthop Traumatol 20(2):168, 2008.
53. Can, U, et al: Safety and efficiency of the Ottawa Ankle Rule in a Swiss population with ankle sprains. Swiss Med Wkly 138(19–20):292, 2008.
54. Gupta, RT, et al: Lisfranc injury:imaging findings for this important but often-missed diagnosis. Curr Probl Diagn Radiol 37(3):115, 2008.
55. Cottom, JM, et al: Treatment of Lisfranc fracture dislocations with an intrerosseous suture button technique: A review of 3 cases. J Foot Ankle Surg 47(3):250, 2008.
56. Rammelt, S, and Zwipp, H: Talar neck and body fractures. Injury 40(2):120, 2009.
57. Dodson, NB, et al: Imaging strategies for diagnosing calcaneal and cuboid stress fractures. Clin Podiatr Med Surg 25(2):183, 2008.
58. Budny, AM, and Young, BA: Analysis of radiographic classifications for rotational ankle fractures. Clin Podiatr Med Surg 25(2):139, 2008.
59. Goulart, M, et al: Foot and ankle fractures in dancers. Clin Sports Med 27(2):295, 2008.
60. Singer, G, et al: A study of metatarsal fractures in children. J Bone Joint Surg 90(4):772, 2008.
61. Hunter, TB, et al: Musculoskeletal eponyms: Who are those guys? Radiographics 20:819, 2000.

Deformities of the Foot

62. Richardson, J, and Iglarsh, A: Clinical Orthopaedic Physical Therapy. WB Saunders, Philadelphia, 1994.
63. Kennedy, JG, and Collumbier, JA: Bunions in dancers. Clin Sports Med 27(2):321, 2008.
64. Oh, IS, et al: Clinical and radiological results after distal metatarsal osteotomy for hallux vallgus. Foot Ankle Int 29(5):473, 2008.
65. Chhaya, SA, et al: Understanding hallux valgus deformity: What the surgeon wants to know from conventional radiographs. Curr Probl Diagn Radiol 37(3):127, 2008.

66. Deenik, AR, et al: Hallux valgus angle as main predictor for correction of hallux valgus. BMC Musculoskel Disord 9:70, 2008.

67. Roddy, E, et al: Prevalence and associations of hallux valgus in a primary care population. Arthritis Rheum 59(6):857, 2008.

68. Lipscombe, S, et al: Scarf osteotomy for the correction of hallux valgus: Midterm clinical outcome. J Foot Ankle Surg 47(4):273, 2008.

69. Okuda, R, et al: Proximal metatarsal osteotomy for hallux valgus: Comparison of outcome for moderate and severe deformities. Foot Ankle Int 29(7):664, 2008.

70. Berg, RP, et al: Scarf osteotomy in hallux valgus: A review of 72 cases. Acta Orthop Belg 73(2):219, 2007.

71. Pollard, JD, and Schuberth, JM: Posterior bone block distraction arthrodesis of the subtalar joint: A review of 22 cases. J Foot Ankle Surg 47(3):191, 2008.

72. Hattori, T, et al: Radiological study of joint destruction patterns in rheumatoid flatfoot. Clin Rheumatol 27(6):733, 2008.

73. Pehlivan, O, et al: Radiographic correlation of symptomatic and asymptomatic flexible flatfoot in young male adults. Int Orthop 33(2):447, 2009.

74. Hardy, MA, and Logan, DB: Principles of arthrodesis and advances in fixation for the adult acquired flatfoot. Clin Podiatr Med Surg 24(4):789, 2007.

75. Maskill, MP, et al: Triple arthrodesis for the adult-acquired flatfoot deformity. Clin Podiatr Med Surg 24(4):765, 2007.

76. Rose, RE: Flat feet in children: When should they be treated? Internet J Orthop Surg 6(1), 2007.

77. Chang, TJ, and Lee, J: Subtalar joint arthroereisis in adult-acquired flatfoot and posterior tibial tendon dysfunction. Clin Podiatr Med Surg 24(4):687, 2007.

78. Ochman, S, et al: Calcaneonavicular coalition fracture: A rare differential diagnosis of post-traumatic ankle pain. Unfallchirurgie 111(11):944, 2008.

79. Nalaboff, KM, and Schweitzer, ME: MRI of tarsal coalition: Frequency, distribution, and innovative signs. Bull NYU Hosp Jt Dis 66(1):14, 2008.

80. Staser, J, et al: Radiographic diagnosis of posterior facet talocalcaneal coalition. Pediatr Radiol 37(1):7, 2007.

81. Wang, E, et al: Tarsal coalition. Emedicine, 2008. Available at: http://www.emedicine.com/Radio/topic673.htm.

Self-Test

Radiograph A

1. Identify this *projection*.

2. Name the *deformity* at the first digit.

3. Describe the *bony changes* seen at the *medial side* of the *first metatarsal head*.

4. Describe the *positional* relationship of the *first* and *second toes* to each other.

Radiograph B

5. Identify this *projection*.

6. Describe the *joint positions* of the *ankles* and *feet* as much as possible from this one projection.

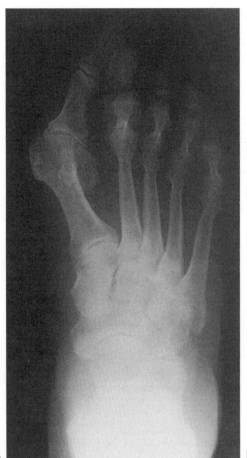

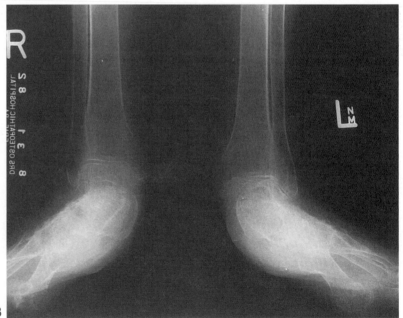

A

B

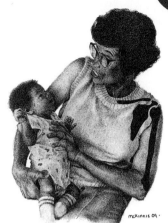

RADIOLOGIC EVALUATION OF THE SHOULDER

The glenohumeral joint is sometimes referred to as the *true* shoulder joint, but it is only one of four articulations that constitute what is commonly called the *shoulder, shoulder girdle,* or *shoulder joint complex.* The combined and coordinated movements of the glenohumeral, acromioclavicular, and sternoclavicular joints plus the scapulothoracic articulation permit the arm to be positioned in space for efficient use of the hand. Impairment of a single articulation will inhibit normal functioning of the collective. To provide a comprehensive radiographic look at the entire shoulder joint complex, radiographs of the acromioclavicular and scapulothoracic articulations are included herein. Radiographs of the sternoclavicular joints are presented in Chapter 9.

Review of Anatomy[1–8]

Osseous Anatomy

The bones of the *shoulder* are the *proximal humerus,* the *scapula,* and the *clavicle.* The articulation between the humerus and the scapula is the *glenohumeral joint,* and the articulation between the scapula and the clavicle is the *acromioclavicular joint.*

Humerus

The most proximal part of the humerus is the humeral head, which articulates in the scapular glenoid fossa (Fig. 15-1). The humeral anatomic neck is the slightly constricted region that lies just below the head. Inferior to the anatomic neck is the laterally projecting greater tuberosity and the anteriorly projecting lesser tuberosity. The tuberosities are separated by the intertubercular or bicipital groove. The narrowed region distal to the tuberosities is the surgical neck. Below the surgical neck is the humeral *shaft.*

Scapula

The scapula is a flat, triangular bone with three borders, three angles, two surfaces, and prominent processes. The borders are identified as the *medial* or *vertebral border,* the *lateral* or *axillary border,* and the *superior border.* The angles or corners of the triangular scapula are named the *superior, inferior,* and *lateral angles.* The superior and inferior angles are at the ends of the medial border. The lateral angle and border give rise to the prominent process of the scapula and

455

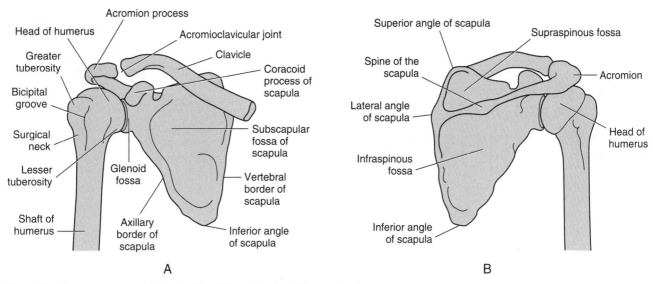

Figure 15-1 Osseous anatomy of the shoulder: **(A)** anterior view; **(B)** posterior view.

thus compose the greatest mass and weight of the scapula. The broadened end of the lateral angle supports the shallow glenoid fossa, which is deepened by the attachment of the fibrocartilaginous glenoid labrum and receives the humeral head. Medial to the glenoid fossa is the coracoid process, which projects superiorly and anteriorly.

The body of the scapula is thin and somewhat curved for greater strength. The *costal surface* of the scapular body lies in close approximation to the thoracic ribs, and this bone–muscle–bone articulation is referred to as the *scapu-lothoracic joint.* The costal surface of the body presents a shallow concave cavity, the *subscapular fossa.* The convex *dorsal surface* is divided into the *supraspinous fossa* and the *infraspinous fossa,* separated by a bony ridge, the spine of the scapula. The spine of the scapula begins at the medial border and extends across most of the body of the scapula, forming at its end the large curving projection, the *acromion.*

Clavicle

The clavicle, also discussed in Chapter 9, is a long bone with two curvatures. The lateral end of the clavicle articulates with the acromion, forming the acromioclavicular joint. The medial end of the clavicle articulates with the sternal manubrium, forming the sternoclavicular joint. The elongated portion of bone between the two ends is termed the body or shaft of the clavicle. In general, the

clavicle in males is noted to be thicker and more curved than that in females.

Ligamentous Anatomy

Glenohumeral Joint

The glenohumeral joint is supported by various muscles, ligaments, and tendons that reinforce the joint capsule. The joint capsule attaches to the scapula at the glenoid fossa and to the humerus at the anatomic neck. The joint capsule is reinforced anteriorly by the glenohumeral ligaments and superiorly by the coracohumeral ligament. The rotator cuff muscles also reinforce the joint capsule (Fig. 15-2). These muscles are the subscapularis, supraspinatus, infraspinatus, and teres minor, located anteriorly, superiorly, posterosupe-riorly, and posteriorly, respectively, enveloping the gleno-humeral joint. The inferior aspect of the joint is the weakest structural area, because it is not directly reinforced by capsular ligaments or muscles.

Acromioclavicular Joint

The acromioclavicular joint is stabilized principally by the coracoclavicular ligament located medially to the joint, attaching the clavicle to the scapula via the coracoid process. The acromioclavicular joint capsule itself is rather

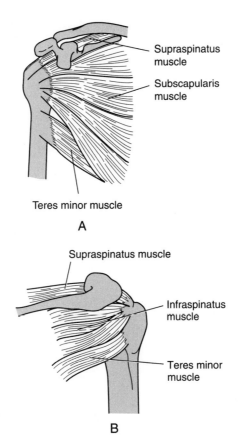

Figure 15-2 Rotator cuff muscles: **(A)** anterior view; **(B)** posterior view.

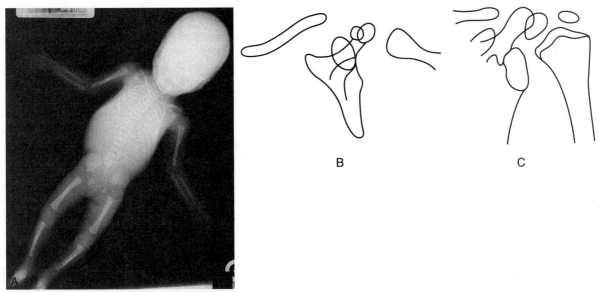

Figure 15-3 (A) Normal radiographic appearance of a healthy 6-month-old infant. **(B)** Radiographic tracings of the ossified portions at the shoulder girdle at birth; **(C)** at age 2 years. *(Adapted from Meschan,[3] p. 65.)*

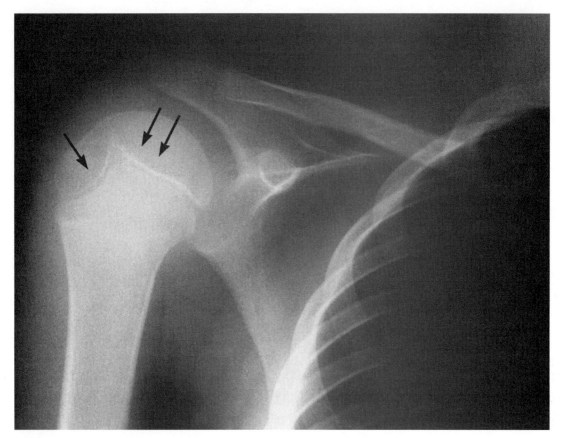

Figure 15-4 Normal radiographic appearance of the shoulder of a healthy 8-year-old. By this age, the greater (single arrow) and lesser (double arrow) tuberosities of the humerus have coalesced and formed one epiphysis.

weak and is reinforced by strong superior and inferior acromioclavicular ligaments.

Joint Mobility

Four articulations are involved in shoulder joint mobility. The glenohumeral, acromioclavicular, sternoclavicular, and scapulothoracic joints work in concert to afford the shoulder the greatest sum of functional mobility available at any single articulation in the body.

Arm elevation is possible in both the sagittal and frontal planes to 180 degrees or greater. Internal and external rotation are each accomplished to approximately 90 degrees, varying somewhat with the starting position of shoulder elevation. Backward extension in the sagittal plane is possible to 60 degrees. About 180 degrees of movement is possible in the horizontal plane. Other motions available at the shoulder include adduction and abduction. Circumduction, a combination of movement through these elemental planes, is freely available at the shoulder. Gliding of the articular surfaces occurs as components move during all motions.

Growth and Development

The clavicle, scapular body, and humeral shaft begin ossification at the seventh to eighth week of fetal life. The ossification center for the proximal humeral head appears at 36 weeks of fetal development. At birth only these structures are ossified and are readily visible on radiograph (Fig. 15-3).

Secondary centers for the greater and lesser tuberosities of the humerus appear between 3 and 5 years of age and coalesce at about 6 years of age, forming one epiphysis. In many individuals, the greater tuberosity may remain separated until it fuses with the humeral shaft at about age 16 (Fig. 15-4).

The remainder of the scapula—including the acromion, coracoid process, glenoid fossa, vertebral border, and inferior angle—is largely cartilaginous at birth. Secondary centers of ossification appear at the coracoid process at about 1 year of age and in most of the other structures of the scapula at puberty, fusing with the main body of the scapula at 18 to 25 years of age.

Routine Radiologic Evaluation[7-19]

Practice Guidelines for Shoulder Radiography in Children and Adults[9]

The American College of Radiology (ACR), the principal professional organization of radiologists in the United States, defines the following practice guidelines as an educational tool to assist practitioners in providing appropriate radiologic care for patients.

Goals

The goal of the radiographic examination at the shoulder joint complex is to identify or exclude anatomic abnormalities or disease processes.

Indications

The indications for radiologic examination include but are not limited to trauma, including suspected physical abuse; osseous changes secondary to metabolic disease, systemic disease, or nutritional deficiencies; neoplasms; infections; primary nonneoplastic bone pathologies; arthropathies; preoperative, postoperative, and follow-up studies; congenital syndromes and developmental disorders; vascular lesions; evaluation of soft tissue (as for suspected foreign body); pain; and correlation of abnormal skeletal findings on other imaging studies.

Basic Projections and Radiologic Observations

The minimum recommended projections are as follows:

- Shoulder: *anteroposterior (AP)* views, ideally an *internal rotation* view and an *AP external rotation view.* The purpose of performing these two variations on the AP projection is to allow greater visualization of the humeral head and proximal third of the humeral shaft. In the presence of suspected fracture or dislocation, only one AP projection is made with the upper extremity positioned in *neutral.*
- Acromioclavicular joint: an *upright AP* view. The stability of the acromioclavicular joints is evaluated by performing *two* upright AP radiographs, one without weights and one with weights tied to the wrists. The purpose of the weights is to place a longitudinal pull through the arms that will stress the acromioclavicular joints.
- Scapula: an *AP* view and a *lateral* view. A certain portion of the scapula is well demonstrated on the shoulder AP radiograph, but much of the scapular body is superimposed by the ribs. If the scapula is the area of interest, it will be filmed with special positioning to free it from as much superimposition as possible.

Trauma at the Shoulder[11,20-65]

Diagnostic Imaging for Trauma of the Shoulder

The shoulder area possesses less mechanical protection and less bony stability than any other large joint in the body, rendering it susceptible to a variety of fractures, joint dislocations, and soft-tissue and cartilage injuries.

The ACR Appropriateness Criteria[20] recommends AP and axillary or scapular Y radiographs *as the initial study for all trauma cases to rule out fracture or dislocation.* MRI is recommended for acute and subacute shoulder pain *if initial radiographs are normal* and if *rotator cuff pathology, instability,* or *labral tears* are suspected. As an alternative, computed tomography (CT) arthrography is recommended if MRI is unavailable or contraindicated. Diagnostic ultrasound, "with appropriate expertise," is also recommended in the evaluation of soft tissue pathology.

Fractures of the Proximal Humerus

Fractures of the proximal humerus constitute about 5% of all fractures. An increased incidence is noted with increased age, thought to be related to osteoporosis.

Mechanism of Injury

The most common mechanism of injury is a fall on an outstretched hand. This is especially common in elderly women with osteoporosis. Younger adults are more often injured in high-energy trauma, such as motor vehicle accidents. These injuries are often complicated by associated fractures, dislocations, and soft tissue disruption.

(Continued on page 474)

Routine Radiologic Evaluation of the Shoulder

Anteroposterior External Rotation Projection

This view is taken in the true AP *anatomic* position, which places the shoulder and arm in *external rotation*. This view demonstrates the *proximal third of the humerus,* the *lateral two-thirds of the clavicle,* the *acromioclavicular joint,* and the *upper and lateral portion of the scapula.*

Radiologic Observations

The important observations are:

1. The greater tuberosity is visualized in profile at the most lateral aspect of the humeral head.
2. The lesser tuberosity is superimposed at the midarea of the humeral head.
3. The medial portion of the humeral head is partially superimposed in the glenoid fossa. Thus, the glenohumeral joint space is not visualized as completely "open."
4. The average width of the glenohumeral joint can be observed by drawing lines across the joint surfaces (Fig. 15-5). This distance, *x*, averages 5 mm. Distances greater than this can be suggestive of joint effusion, acromegaly, or posterior humeral dislocation. Distances narrower than this can suggest degenerative joint disease or rheumatoid arthritis.
5. The crest of the spine of the scapula can be seen extending across the scapula and broadening into the acromion.
6. The vertebral and lateral borders of the scapula are superimposed behind the rib cage.
7. The coracoid process is visualized end-on.
8. The acromioclavicular joint is seen superior to the glenohumeral joint.
9. Any *calcium deposits* present in the muscles, tendons, or bursae of the shoulder may also be demonstrated.

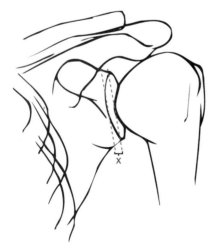

Figure 15-5 On the AP view of the shoulder, the distance *x* from the glenoid fossa to the humeral head averages 5 mm.

Basic Projections

- **AP external rotation projection**
- AP internal rotation projection

Setting up the Radiograph

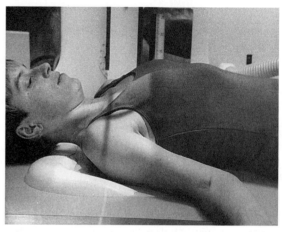

Figure 15-6 Patient position for AP external rotation radiograph of the shoulder.

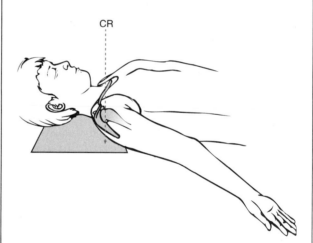

CR

Figure 15-7 The central ray is directed perpendicular to a point 1 inch inferior to the coracoid process.

What Can You See?

Look at the radiograph (Fig. 15-8) and try to identify the radiographic anatomy. Trace the outlines of structures using a marker and transparency sheet. Compare results with the tracing (Fig. 15-9). Can you identify the following:

- Proximal humerus (identify the greater and lesser tuberosities)
- Anatomic neck and surgical neck of the humerus
- Borders of the scapula (identify the crest of the spine of the scapula, coracoid process, glenoid fossa, and acromion)
- Clavicle (identify the acromioclavicular joint)

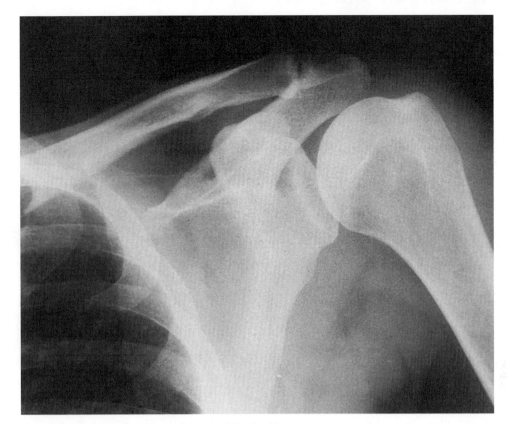

Figure 15-8 AP external rotation radiograph of the shoulder.

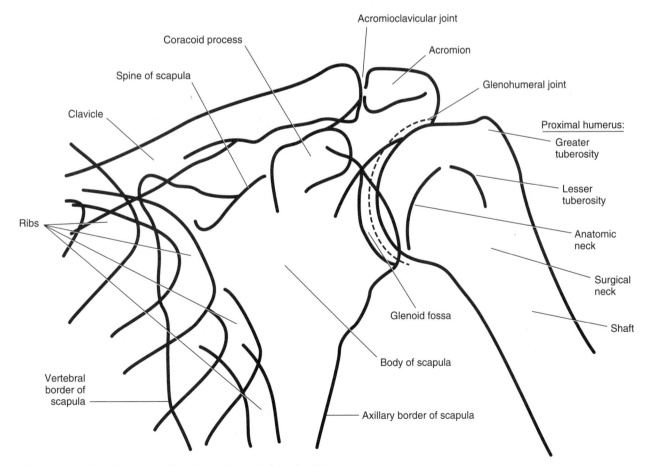

Figure 15-9 Tracing of AP external rotation radiograph of the shoulder.

Routine Radiologic Evaluation of the Shoulder

Anteroposterior Internal Rotation Projection

This view is taken with the arm and shoulder positioned in internal rotation. This view demonstrates the proximal third of the humerus, lateral two-thirds of the clavicle, acromioclavicular joint, and upper and lateral portion of the scapula.

Radiologic Observations

The important observations are:

1. The greater tuberosity is now superimposed over the mid-area of the humeral head.
2. The lesser tuberosity is now seen in profile on the medial aspect of the humeral head (Fig. 15-10).
3. The medial portion of the humeral head is partially superimposed on the glenoid fossa. Thus the glenohumeral joint space is not visualized as an "open" joint space.
4. The crest of the spinous process of the scapula can be seen extending across the scapula and broadening into the acromion.
5. The vertebral and lateral borders of the scapula are superimposed behind the rib cage.
6. The coracoid process is visualized end-on.
7. The acromioclavicular joint is seen superior to the glenohumeral joint.
8. Any *calcium deposits* present in muscles, tendons, or bursae of the shoulder may also be demonstrated.

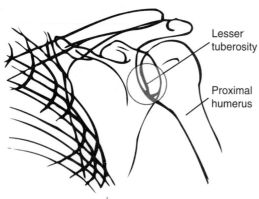

Figure 15-10 Internal rotation of the arm results in the ability to see the lesser tuberosity in profile at the medial aspect of the humeral head.

Basic Projections

- AP external rotation projection
- **AP internal rotation projection**

Setting up the Radiograph

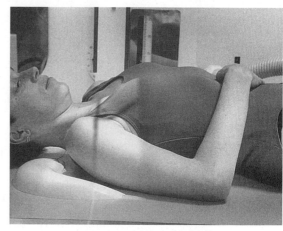

Figure 15-11 Patient position for AP internal rotation radiograph of the shoulder.

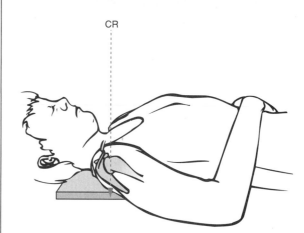

Figure 15-12 The central ray is directed perpendicular to a point 1 inch inferior to the coracoid process.

What Can You See?

Look at the radiograph (Fig. 15-13) and try to identify the radiographic anatomy. Trace the outlines of structures using a marker and transparency sheet. Compare results with the tracing (Fig. 15-14). Can you identify the following:

- Proximal humerus (identify the greater and lesser tuberosities)
- Anatomic neck and surgical neck of the humerus
- Borders of the scapula (identify the crest of the spinous process, coracoid process, glenoid fossa, and acromion)
- Clavicle (identify the acromioclavicular joint)

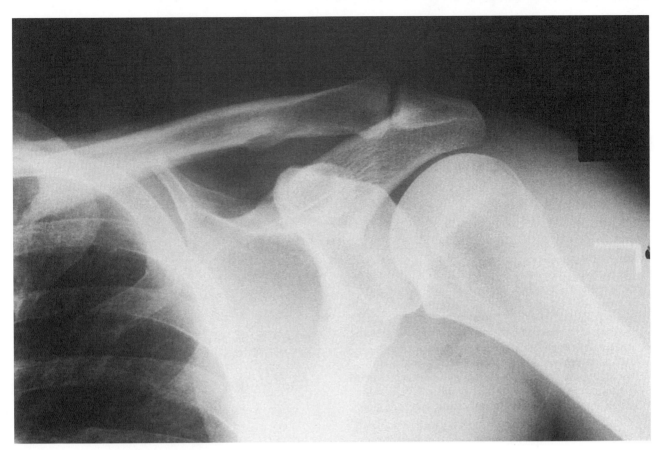

Figure 15-13 AP internal rotation radiograph of the shoulder.

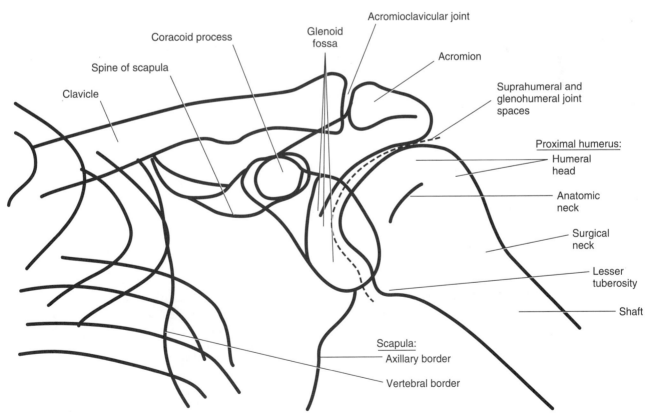

Figure 15-14 Tracing of AP internal rotation radiograph of the shoulder.

Routine Radiologic Evaluation of the Acromioclavicular Joint

AP Bilateral With and Without Weights

These two views demonstrate both acromioclavicular (AC) joints at once for comparison purposes. After the first radiograph is made without weights, a second radiograph is made with a minimum of 10 to 15 lb (5 to 7 kg) of weight hanging from each wrist. This second radiograph is considered a stress view, done to determine possible AC joint instability. Other structures visible on either radiograph are the entire length of the clavicles, both sternoclavicular joints, and both shoulders as described in the AP views.

Radiologic Observations

The important observations are:

1. This AP radiograph is made with the the patient standing, arms at the sides.
2. The AC joint is evaluated by examining the relationship of the acromion to the clavicle (Fig. 15-15). The normal joint space distance at this articulation ranges from 0.3 to 0.8 cm. Additionally, the relationship of the coracoid process to the clavicle is also examined. The normal distance between the inferior aspect of the clavicle and the coracoid process, the *coracoclavicular distance*, ranges from 1.0 to 1.3 cm. The amount of abnormal increases in these distances helps determine the severity of the ligamentous injury. Grading of AC separation can thus be quantified using these distances:

   - *Grade I, mild sprain.* Minimal widening of the acromioclavicular joint space with the coracoclavicular distance still within normal range: AC ligaments are sprained.
   - *Grade II, moderate sprain.* Widening of the AC joint space to 1.0 to 1.5 cm with a 25% to 50% increase in the coracoclavicular distance: AC ligaments are torn, coracoclavicular ligaments are sprained.
   - *Grade III, severe sprain.* Widening of the acromioclavicular joint space 1.5 cm or greater with a 50% or more increase in the coracoclavicular distance: Both the AC and coracoclavicular ligaments are torn. The AC joint is dislocated, and the clavicle appears to be displaced superiorly.

What Can You See?

Look at the radiograph (Fig. 15-19) and try to identify the radiographic anatomy. Trace the outlines of structures using a marker and transparency sheet. Compare results with the tracing (Fig. 15-20). Can you identify the following:

- Sternum, as it lies superimposed over the thoracic spine
- Clavicles

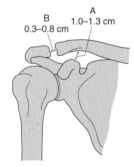

Figure 15-15 The AC joint is evaluated by measuring **(A)** the coracoclavicular distance and **(B)** the AC joint space distance. Normal value range is given. *(Adapted from Greenspan,[5] pp. 5 and 23.)*

A 1.0–1.3 cm
B 0.3–0.8 cm

Basic Projections

- AP, bilateral, without weights
- **AP, bilateral, with weights**

Setting up the Radiograph

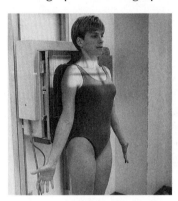

Figure 15-16 Patient position for bilateral AP view of acromioclavicular joints without weights.

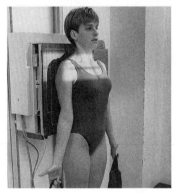

Figure 15-17 Patient position for bilateral AP view of acromioclavicular joints with weights (in handbags).

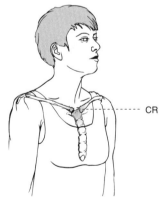

CR

Figure 15-18 The central ray is directed perpendicular to the midline of the body at the level of the acromioclavicular joints.

- Acromion process
- Coracoid process
- Acromioclavicular joint distance
- Coracoclavicular distance

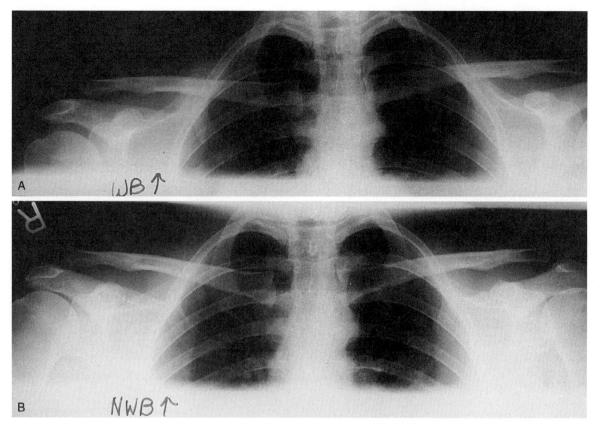

Figure 15-19 AP radiograph of bilateral acromioclavicular joints **(A)** with weights (WB, weight-bearing) and **(B)** without weights (NWB, non–weight-bearing).

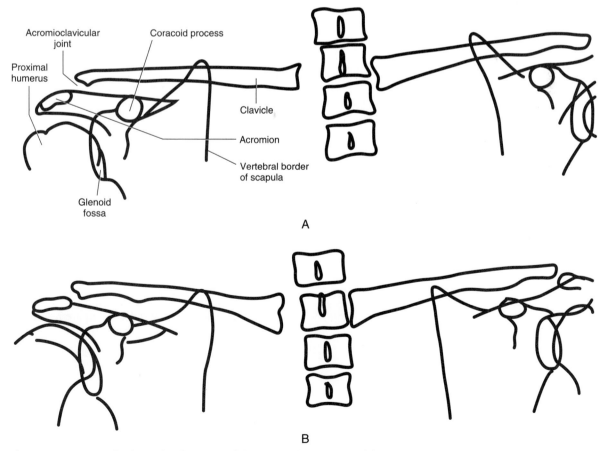

Figure 15-20 Tracing of radiographs of AP views of the acromioclavicular joints **(A)** with weights and **(B)** without weights.

Routine Radiologic Evaluation of the Scapula

Anteroposterior

This view demonstrates the entire *scapula*. The lateral half of the scapula is seen free of superimposition of the ribs and lungs. These structures are superimposed on the medial half of the scapula.

Radiologic Observations

The important observations are:

1. The patient's arm is abducted and externally rotated. This position allows the scapula to abduct and rotate upward so that the lateral half is now cleared of the rib cage and can be evaluated in more detail.
2. All three borders and angles of the scapula are usually visible.

Basic Projections

- **AP**
- Lateral

Setting up the Radiograph

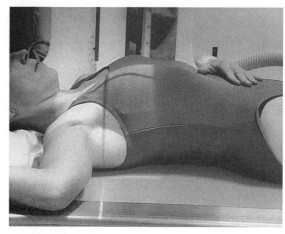

Figure 15-21 Patient position for AP radiograph of the scapula.

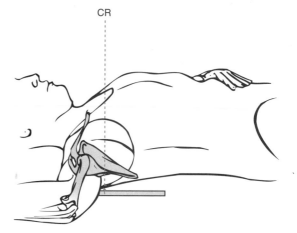

Figure 15-22 The central ray is directed perpendicular to the mid-scapular area at a point 2 inches inferior to the coracoid process.

What Can You See?

Look at the radiograph (Fig. 15-23) and try to identify the radiographic anatomy. Trace the outlines of structures using a marker and transparency sheet. Compare results with the tracing (Fig. 15-24). Can you identify the following:

- Body of the scapula (identify the vertebral, axillary, and superior borders and the superior, inferior, and lateral angles)
- Coracoid process
- Acromion
- Spinous process
- Glenoid fossa

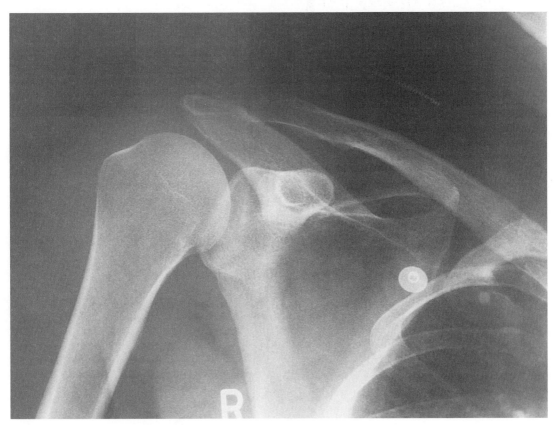

Figure 15-23 AP radiograph of the scapula. Note that the radiograph does not match the positioning photo in Figure 15-21 because the radiographed patient was unable to abduct the arm fully.

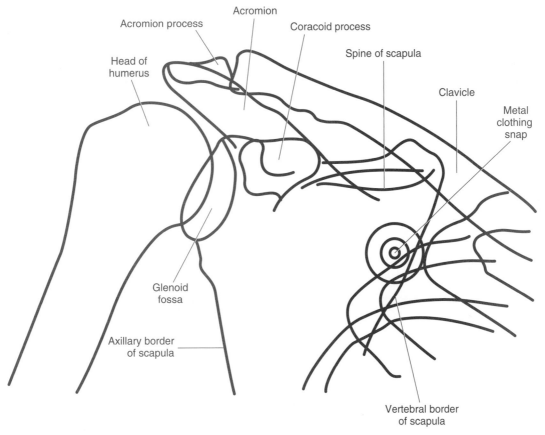

Figure 15-24 Tracing of AP radiograph of the scapula.

Routine Radiologic Evaluation of the Scapula

Lateral

This view demonstrates the scapula from a lateral aspect. The scapula is projected clear of the rib cage. The *body* of the scapula is best evaluated in this radiograph.

Radiologic Observations

The important observations are:

1. The patient's arm is positioned across the front of his or her chest to free the body of the scapula from superimposition of the humeral shaft, or the patient's arm may be positioned behind his or her back to free the acromion and coracoid process from superimposition of the humeral head.
2. The profile of the scapular body is clearly seen. Fractures of the scapular body are readily visible on this view.

Basic Projections

- AP
- **Lateral**

Setting up the Radiograph

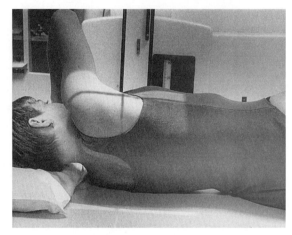

Figure 15-25 Patient position for lateral view of the scapula.

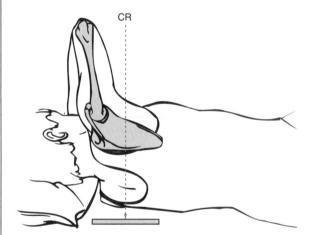

CR

Figure 15-26 The central ray is directed perpendicular to the midlateral border of the scapula.

What Can You See?

Look at the radiograph (Fig. 15-27) and try to identify the radiographic anatomy. Trace the outlines of structures using a marker and transparency sheet. Compare results with the tracing (Fig. 15-28). Can you identify the following:

- Proximal humerus superimposed behind the scapula
- Body of the scapula
- Acromion
- Coracoid process
- Glenoid fossa

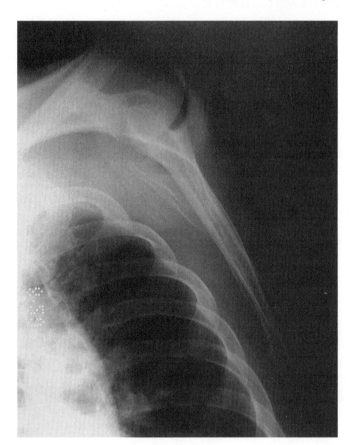

Figure 15-27 Lateral radiograph of the scapula.

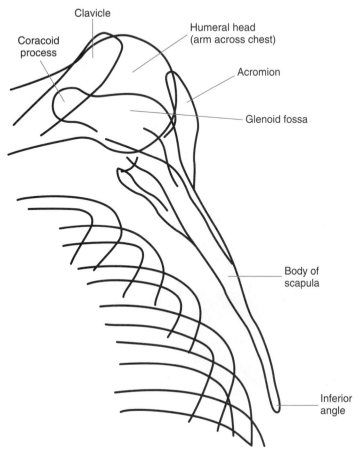

Figure 15-28 Tracing of lateral radiograph of the scapula.

Routine Radiologic Evaluation

Additional Views

- Axillary view of the glenohumeral joint
- Scapular "Y" lateral view

The shoulder joint can be radiographically evaluated by many special projections designed to demonstrate specific anatomy or abnormal conditions. The literature defines many variations of oblique, tangential, and axial projections that may be used to demonstrate, for example, different aspects of the glenoid fossa, the glenohumeral joint, the intertubercular groove, the subacromial joint space, and the insertion sites for individual rotator cuff muscles as well as different aspects of the clavicle, scapula, and acromioclavicular joint.

Examples of two common additional views used to evaluate the injured shoulder are the axillary view and the *scapular "Y" lateral view.*

Axillary View of the Glenohumeral Joint

One of the more essential special projections is an *inferosuperior axial projection* of the glenohumeral joint (Figs. 15-29, 15-30, and 15-31). This projection is also commonly known as an *axillary view.* One variation on this projection is the *West Point* view, made with the patient prone. In any variation of this projection the central ray is directed through the shoulder joint in an inferosuperior direction, and the images are somewhat similar. The inferosuperior axial projection is helpful in determining the exact relationship of the humeral head to the glenoid fossa in the evaluation of glenohumeral dislocations. The rims of the glenoid fossa and the coracoid process are also well demonstrated.

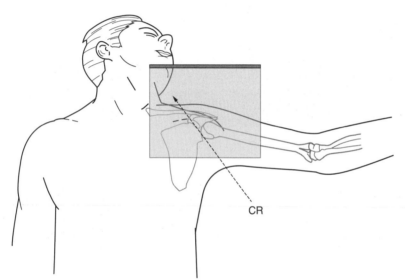

CR

Figure 15-29 The inferosuperior axial projection of the glenohumeral joint. The central ray is directed horizontally through the axilla toward the acromioclavicular joint.

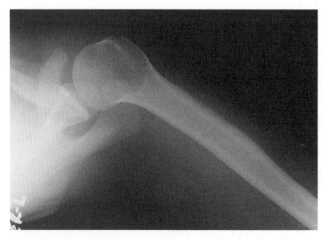

Figure 15-30 Radiograph of an axillary view of the glenohumeral joint.

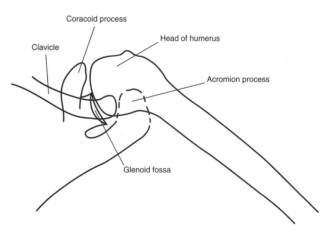

Coracoid process
Clavicle
Head of humerus
Acromion process
Glenoid fossa

Figure 15-31 Tracing of axillary view radiograph.

Anterior Oblique: The Scapular Y Lateral View

An essential special projection often utilized for the evaluation of a traumatized shoulder is the *anterior oblique* view of the shoulder, more commonly known as the *scapular Y lateral* view. The patient's upper extremity remains in neutral at the patient's side and does not have to undergo any movement for positioning purposes (Figs. 15-32, 15-33, and 15-34).

This view got its name from the characteristic appearance of the scapula as seen from this perspective. The acromion and the coracoid process form the upper portion of the Y, and the scapular body forms the vertical portion of the Y.

This projection is most frequently used in the assessment of fractures or dislocations of the proximal humerus and scapula.

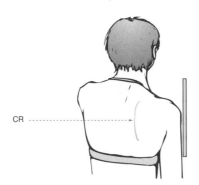

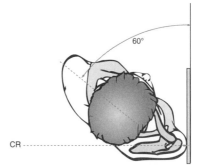

Figure 15-32 For a scapular "Y" lateral projection, the patient is in a 60-degree anterior oblique position, and the central ray is directed through the glenohumeral joint, perpendicular to the image receptor.

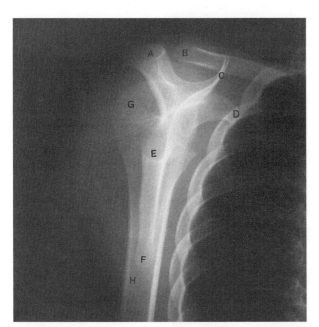

Figure 15-33 Radiograph of scapular "Y" view. This oblique view of the shoulder demonstrates the relationship of the humeral head to the glenoid cavity and also demonstrates the parts of the scapula projected clear of the rib cage. *A*, acromion; *B*, distal end of the clavicle; *C*, superior border of the scapula; *D*, coracoid process; *E*, body of scapula; *F*, inferior angle of the scapula; *G*, humeral head; *H*, humeral shaft.

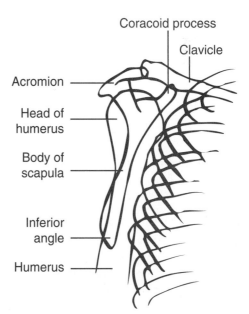

Figure 15-34 Tracing of scapular Y lateral radiograph.

Magnetic Resonance Imaging of the Shoulder

Examples of normal anatomy as seen on proton-density-sequence magnetic resonance imaging (MRI) are presented in Figures 15-35 through 15-38.

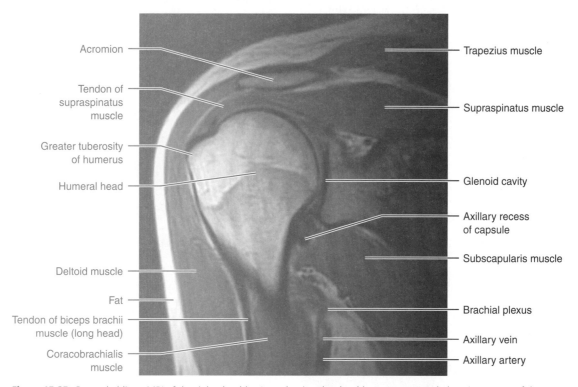

Acromion

Tendon of supraspinatus muscle

Greater tuberosity of humerus

Humeral head

Deltoid muscle

Fat

Tendon of biceps brachii muscle (long head)

Coracobrachialis muscle

Trapezius muscle

Supraspinatus muscle

Glenoid cavity

Axillary recess of capsule

Subscapularis muscle

Brachial plexus

Axillary vein

Axillary artery

Figure 15-35 Coronal oblique MRI of the right shoulder. In evaluating the shoulder, a true coronal plane is not as useful as one that is somewhat oblique. MRI can construct practical views that allow us to see tissues in a plane easy to follow from our understanding of the anatomy. The coronal oblique is parallel to the course of the supraspinatus muscle and tendon.

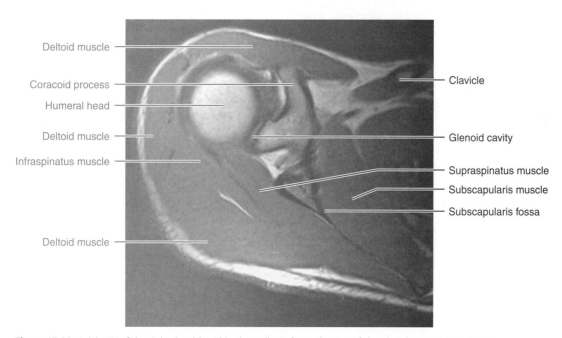

Deltoid muscle

Coracoid process

Humeral head

Deltoid muscle

Infraspinatus muscle

Deltoid muscle

Clavicle

Glenoid cavity

Supraspinatus muscle

Subscapularis muscle

Subscapularis fossa

Figure 15-36 Axial MRI of the right shoulder. This plane allows for evaluation of the glenohumeral articulation.

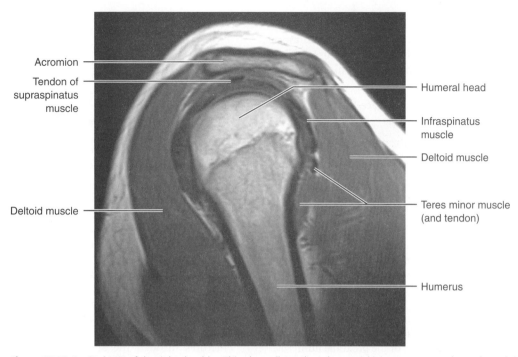

Acromion
Tendon of supraspinatus muscle
Deltoid muscle

Humeral head
Infraspinatus muscle
Deltoid muscle
Teres minor muscle (and tendon)
Humerus

Figure 15-37 Sagittal MRI of the right shoulder. This plane allows the subacromial joint structures to be evaluated.

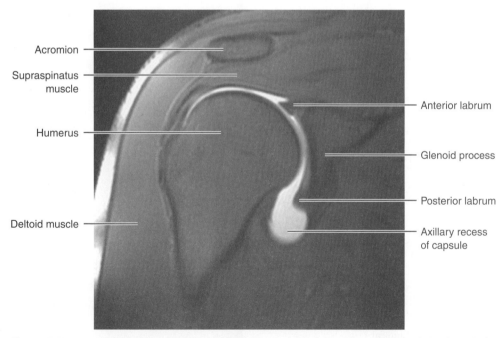

Acromion
Supraspinatus muscle
Humerus
Deltoid muscle

Anterior labrum
Glenoid process
Posterior labrum
Axillary recess of capsule

Figure 15-38 MR arthrography, coronal oblique view. The contrast media outlines tissues and also distends the joint. This distention is useful in the evaluation of structures that are often too crowded to see adequately, such as the labrum, glenohumeral ligaments, and biceps anchor. *(Image courtesy of Alex Freitas, MD.)*

Classification

The Neer four-part classification system is used most widely to describe proximal humerus fractures. This system is based on the four major anatomic segments (Fig. 15-39):

1. The head, from the articular surface to the anatomic neck
2. The greater tuberosity
3. The lesser tuberosity
4. The shaft, at the level of the surgical neck

Fractures are then identified as *nondisplaced* or *displaced*. A fracture is displaced if 1 cm or more separates the fragments or if 45 degrees or more of angulation is present.

Nondisplaced fractures are considered *one-part fractures*, regardless of how many fracture lines exist, because the fragments are in continuity as one unit, held together by soft tissue. The majority of proximal humeral fractures are nondisplaced.

Displaced fractures are further classified as *two-part, three-part,* or *four-part* fractures, with the division lines corresponding to the gross anatomic divisions of the proximal humerus. When one fragment displaces, a two-part fracture exists. When two fragments displace, a three-part fracture exists. When three fragments displace, a four-part fracture exists.

Fractures of the Greater Tuberosity

Fractures of the greater tuberosity in middle-aged and older adults usually result from a fall directly on the point of the shoulder. These fractures are often undisplaced and treated conservatively with several weeks of sling immobilization.

Avulsion fractures of the greater tuberosity are more common in younger adults and usually occur by indirect injury, such as a fall with the arm adducted, combined with forceful contraction of the rotator cuff muscles attempting to limit excursion of the arm. Thus on the clinical exam, these fractures can be difficult to distinguish from rotator cuff tears. In treatment, immobilization in an abduction splint or shoulder spica cast for several weeks is required to prevent the rotator cuff muscles from pulling on the avulsed fracture site (Fig. 15-40).

Fractures of the Lesser Tuberosity

Fractures of the lesser tuberosity are rare and are usually caused by avulsion forces resulting from forceful contraction of the subscapularis muscle.

Fractures of the Humeral Head

Fractures of the humeral head are rare and, when present, are often associated with dislocation. During the dislocation, a portion of humeral head may be sheared off against the glenoid labrum. This type of fracture may be considered an *osteochondral fracture* because the fracture fragment would be partly composed of articular cartilage.

Fractures through the anatomic neck, the constricted region just below the humeral head, are also rarely seen in isolation, more often present in combination with other fractures. These usually require surgical treatment and are associated with a high risk of avascular necrosis.

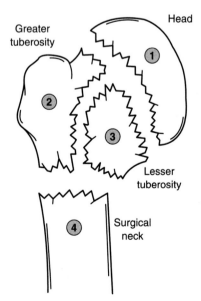

Figure 15-39 In the Neer classification of proximal humerus fractures, the proximal humerus is divided into four anatomic segments.

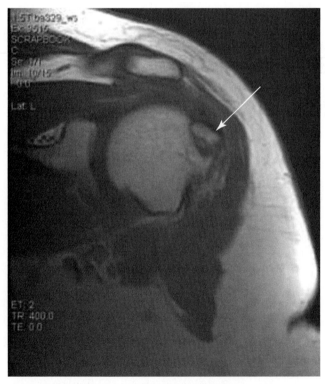

Figure 15-40 Sagittal T1-weighted MRI of the shoulder demonstrating an occult fracture of the greater tuberosity of the humerus. This young woman was injured while skiing. Initial radiographs were normal. The MRI was ordered to rule out rotator cuff pathology, and the fracture was discovered. Clinically, this type of injury can be difficult to distinguish from a cuff tear.

Fractures of the Surgical Neck

Fractures of the surgical neck of the humerus are common (Fig. 15-41). Fractures occurring here resulting from direct blows tend to be transverse and somewhat comminuted. Fractures resulting from an indirect injury, such as a fall on an outstretched hand whereby forces are transmitted up the arm, are more likely to produce a spiral fracture line and may extend to involve the tuberosities or anatomic neck.

Impacted fractures at the surgical neck are common in the elderly, especially in osteoporotic women, often resulting from a relatively minor fall. Impacted fractures are treated conservatively with sling immobilization. The more severely displaced surgical neck fractures may require open reduction. The thick periosteum of the humeral shaft, related to the great amount of muscle surrounding the humerus, aids in rapid healing of fractures in this area.

Pathological Fractures

The proximal humerus is a frequent site for pathological fractures, usually presenting in the region of the surgical neck. Pathological fractures occur through bone that has been abnormally weakened by either localized, disseminated, or generalized disease processes. These fractures are often the result of benign or malignant primary bone tumors, metastatic lesions, or related to radiation therapy. The proximal humerus is also a common site of fracture in patients with generalized osteoporosis (see Fig. 2-48); the weakened architecture of osteoporotic bone is vulnerable to fracture from relatively minor trauma.

Radiologic Evaluation

A neutral AP and a scapular Y lateral is sufficient for evaluating simple proximal humerus fractures. Complex fractures may require CT to evaluate position of fragments, articular involvement, and glenoid rim fractures.

Treatment

Generally, minimally displaced fractures are treated nonsurgically with sling immobilization. Rehabilitation for early shoulder mobilization may be instituted at 7 to 10 days after injury, if the fracture is stable or impacted. Pendulum-type exercises are taught to the patient. Sling immobilization continues for 4 to 6 weeks.

Displaced fractures can be difficult to maintain via closed reduction, because of opposing muscle forces. Displaced and irreducible fractures generally require surgical fixation. Older patients may benefit from primary prosthetic replacement (hemiarthroplasty).

Rehabilitation is extensive because of the necessary length of immobilization. Adhesions that restrict joint motion are a usual sequela and require aggressive joint mobilization to restore normal joint arthrokinematics and normal scapulohumeral rhythm necessary for normal active movements of the upper extremity.

Complications

A complication of displaced proximal humeral fractures is avascular necrosis. A high risk is involved in up to a third of four-part fractures as well as a significant amount of three-part fractures or anatomic neck fractures.

Loss of joint motion secondary to adhesions may require open lysis if rehabilitation fails to restore normal joint arthrokinematics.

Vascular injuries are infrequent, compromising about 5% of proximal humeral fractures. The axillary artery is most often involved, and the elderly are at higher risk secondary to atherosclerosis and loss of vessel wall elasticity. The presence of an intact radial pulse does not guarantee the integrity of the axillary artery because of the collateral contribution of the radial artery.

Neural injury to the brachial plexus or axillary nerve is also infrequently seen, with an incidence of 6%.

Fractures of the Clavicle

Mechanism of Injury

Falls onto an outstretched hand or directly onto the shoulder account for the majority of fractures of the clavicle. About three-fourths of these fractures occur in children younger than age 13 and are known to heal well. The clavicle may also be fractured during childbirth trauma. Palpation of the newborn's clavicles is essential, especially more so after difficult deliveries. A fracture is revealed by crepitus or movement at the fracture site. Stress fractures have been associated with athletes who use overhead throwing.

Classification

Fractures of the clavicle are designated by their location at the proximal, middle, or distal third of the bone (Fig. 15-42). Most fractures (80%) occur in the middle third (Fig. 15-43). The lateral third is the next most common site. Relatively rare proximal-third fractures need to be differentiated from epiphyseal injuries, if the sternal ossification center is not yet fused, and from sternoclavicular dislocation injuries.

Radiologic Evaluation

An AP view as well as a 45-degree caudal tilt view are usually sufficient to demonstrate the injury. The caudal tilt view is a variation on the AP view in which the central ray is angled to project the clavicle above the ribs and scapula, so it can be seen free of superimposition.

Fractures of the distal third may be compromised by ligamentous injury, and joint stability is assessed via the AP weighted and unweighted acromioclavicular views.

CT may be needed in fractures of the proximal third, to differentiate epiphyseal or sternoclavicular injury, or in fractures of the distal third, to identify articular involvement.

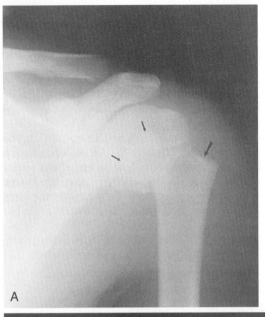

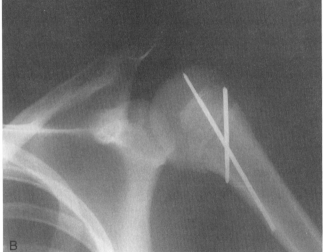

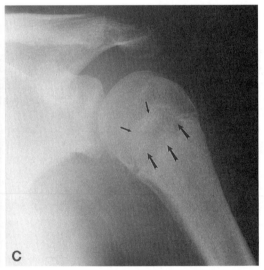

Figure 15-41 Fracture of the surgical neck of the humerus. This 15-year-old boy injured his shoulder in a car accident. **(A)** This AP view of the left shoulder demonstrates a severely displaced surgical neck fracture. The distal fragment has displaced laterally and superiorly. The fracture line is transverse (large arrow). Note the epiphyseal plate of the humeral head (small arrows), which is distinguished from the fracture by smoothly rounded margins and increased density on the border of the epiphysis. **(B)** Follow-up films made 1 month after surgical pin fixation. Note good alignment and positioning at the fracture site and evidence of callus formation bridging the fracture gap. **(C)** 4½ months after injury. The pins had been removed a few weeks prior. Large arrows point to the barely visible remnant of the fracture line, which is undergoing progressive remodeling. Small arrows point to the epiphyseal growth plate, which has also changed in appearance because of maturity after this length of time.

Treatment

Most clavicular fractures in children or adults are successfully treated with figure-eight bandage splinting of the shoulder girdles. This treatment restricts shoulder motion to less than 30 degrees of abduction, flexion, or extension. Slings may also be used, alone or in combination with the figure-eight bandage. Immobilization continues for 4 to 8 weeks until no crepitus or tenderness is present at the fracture site.

Treatment of the newborn infant involves minimizing movement of the affected extremity during dressing, feeding, bathing, and handling. Pinning the sleeve of the affected side to the chest with the elbow at 90 degrees may also help. When the symptoms of pain resolve, the infant will start using the arm normally.

Surgical treatment is required in open fractures, fractures with neurovascular injury, and fractures of the distal third of the clavicle that are rendered unstable by associated rupture of the coracoclavicular ligaments. Surgery can be elective for cosmetic reasons, such as an uncontrolled deformity due to malunion.

Complications

Serious complications from fractures of the middle third are uncommon. When complications of fractures of the middle third do arise, they are most often due to malunion resulting in angulation, shortening, or poor cosmetic appearance. Nonunion is rare. A late complication, secondary to hypertrophic callus formation at the fracture site, is a compression neuropathy of the brachial plexus.

Fractures of the Scapula

Mechanism of Injury

Fractures of the body of the scapula are relatively rare and, when present, are usually the result of a direct blow or violent trauma (Fig. 15-44). Motor vehicle accidents account for over

half of scapular fractures, and the high incidence of other associated serious injuries reflects the great force required to fracture the scapula.

Other fracture patterns are seen at the scapula. Fractures of the glenoid are associated with shoulder dislocations. Acromion fractures result from direct downward blows.

Classification

A basic classification of scapular fractures divides the bone as follows:

- *Type I:* fractures of the scapular body
- *Type II:* apophyseal fractures, including the acromion and coracoid process
- *Type III:* fractures of the superolateral angle, including the glenoid neck and fossa

Radiologic Evaluation

Most fractures of the scapula are demonstrated on the AP, axillary, and scapular Y lateral views. CT scanning is often needed in the evaluation of glenoid fractures to assess the congruity of the joint and assist in treatment decisions.

An acromial fracture should not be confused with an *os acromiale*, an unfused apophysis at the epiphyseal level, present in approximately 3% of the population.

Treatment

Fractures to the scapular body and spinous process are usually minimally displaced because of the protection of the surrounding muscles. These heal well in 4 to 6 weeks

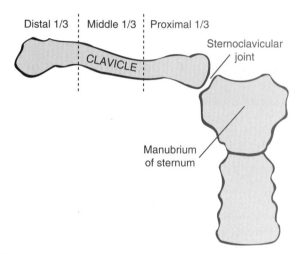

Figure 15-42 The location of trauma to the clavicle is designated by dividing the length of the clavicle into thirds.

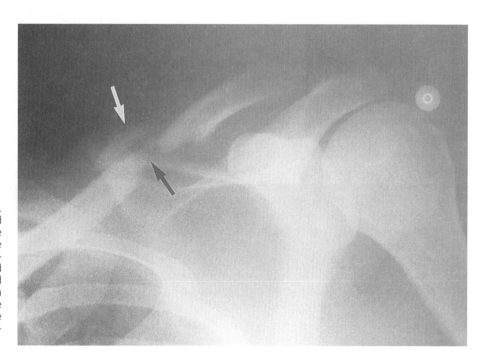

Figure 15-43 Fracture of the clavicle. Because the clavicle is an S-shaped bone, mechanical forces from the side cause a shearing effect on its middle third, where the majority of clavicle fractures such as this occur. This 24-year-old man was injured as he fell to his side and was tackled during a game of touch football. The AP view demonstrates the fracture site (black arrow) and the large wedge-shaped fragment that has displaced superiorly (white arrow).

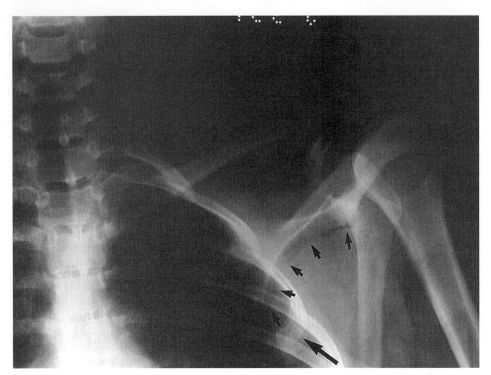

Figure 15-44 Fracture of the body of the scapula. This 33-year-old woman was injured when she neglected to duck and was struck by the swinging boom on a sailboat. This AP view of the scapula demonstrates the transverse and minimally displaced fracture line through the body of the scapula (small arrows). Note an associated fracture of the rib (large arrow) sustained when the scapula impacted on the rib cage.

without any type of immobilization. Nondisplaced acromion fractures heal well in 2 to 3 weeks with sling immobilization. Fractures at the lateral angle, glenoid neck, or glenoid may heal well with conservative treatment if they are undisplaced and do not disrupt the glenohumeral articular relationship.

Surgical treatment is usually necessary with significantly displaced fractures that disrupt the articular surface.

Complications

The most serious complications are from associated injuries caused by the high-energy trauma: rib fractures, pneumothorax, pulmonary contusion, brachial plexus and vascular avulsions, and spinal column injuries.

Suprascapular nerve injuries are associated with fracture of the coracoid as well as other fractures at the scapular neck or body.

Dislocations of the Glenohumeral Joint

The glenohumeral joint is susceptible to subluxation and dislocation because of the relative lack of bony stability and the large, redundant articular capsule. Displacement of the humeral head from its normal articulation to the glenoid fossa is the most common of all joint dislocations and may occur with or without associated fractures. It occurs most often in young adults, less often in the elderly, and rarely in children.

Mechanism of Injury

The mechanism of anterior dislocation is usually forceful external rotation and extension while the arm is abducted. The greater tuberosity is levered against the acromion, and the humeral head is forced out of the glenoid fossa and through the restraint of the anterior ligaments and anterior capsule (Fig. 15-45).

Posterior dislocations are usually caused by a direct blow to the front of the shoulder.

Recurrent instability related to acquired laxity may occur with minor trauma or by volitional mechanisms.

Classification

Classification of glenohumeral dislocations is by the direction that the humeral head displaced in relationship to the glenoid fossa: anterior, posterior, superior, or inferior.

The vast majority of dislocations are anterior (over 90%). The humeral head comes to rest under the coracoid process or under the anterior aspect of the glenoid fossa. These may be referred to as subcoracoid or subglenoid dislocations, respectively.

Posterior dislocations are the second most common glenohumeral dislocation. Inferior and superior dislocations are rare.

Associated Fractures

Associated fractures include a compression fracture of the posterolateral aspect of the humeral head, known as the

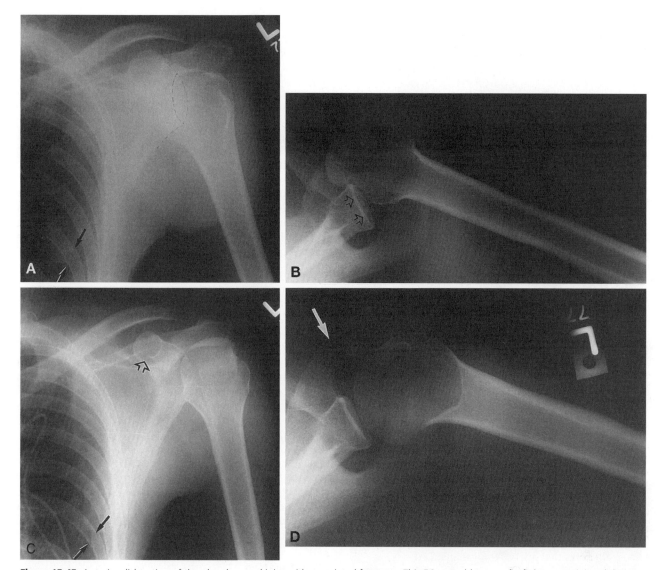

Figure 15-45 Anterior dislocation of the glenohumeral joint with associated fractures. This 56-year-old man, a firefighter, was injured during a rescue when the flooring in the second story of a house collapsed underneath him. **(A)** AP view of the shoulder demonstrates the displacement of the humeral head from the glenoid fossa (dotted line). Note the rib fracture (arrows). **(B)** Axillary view of the glenohumeral joint clearly demonstrates that the humeral head has displaced anteriorly from the glenoid fossa (fossa marked by open arrows). **(C)** AP film of the shoulder made after reduction. Note the fracture of the coracoid process now visible (open arrow). **(D)** Axillary view after reduction shows normal relationship of the humeral head to the glenoid fossa. The coracoid process fracture is more clearly demonstrated on this view and is now identified as a complete, transverse fracture of the tip of the coracoid process (white arrow).

Hill–Sachs lesion. The humeral head sustains an impact as it strikes the glenoid rim during the dislocation (Fig. 15-46).

Other associated fractures may occur at the greater tuberosity, surgical neck, or glenoid rim. A fracture of the anteroinferior rim of the glenoid, also described as a bony avulsion of the labrum from the rim, is known as a *Bankart fracture.* If the pathology is within the fibrocartilaginous labrum without osseous damage, it is known as a *Bankart lesion* (Fig. 15-47).

Radiologic Evaluation

A trauma series is usually obtained, including AP, axillary, and scapular Y lateral views. The axillary and scapular Y lateral views are essential for determining the exact relationship of the humeral head to the glenoid fossa. Posterior dislocations, for example, are problematic in diagnosing on the AP views. The abnormal position of the humeral head posterior to the glenoid fossa may be overlooked as normal superimposition.

CT is useful in defining humeral head or glenoid impaction fractures, loose bodies, and anterior labral bony avulsions. MRI is recommended to assess injury to the rotator cuff, capsule, or labrum.

Treatment

Treatment after an initial dislocation is generally nonsurgical and consists of reduction followed by immobilization,

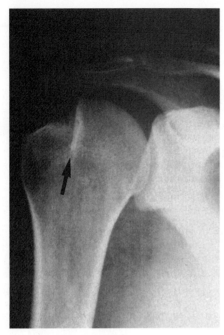

Figure 15-46 Hill–Sachs deformity associated with anterior humeral dislocation. The impact of the angular surface of the interior glenoid rim produces the compression deformity of the articular surface, which has also been referred to as the "hatchet deformity" (arrow). *(From Yochum and Rowe,[18] p. 494, with permission.)*

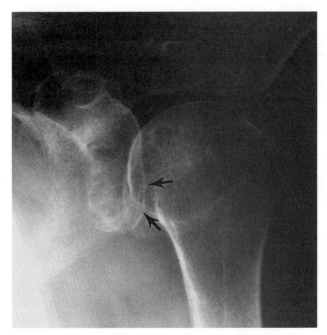

Figure 15-47 Bankart fracture of the glenoid rim. This 69-year-old woman presented with a chronic history of anterior glenohumeral instability, initiated by a traumatic anterior dislocation 10 years prior. This AP view of the shoulder demonstrates a fracture of the anteroinferior rim of the glenoid, represented by the radiolucent line paralleling the margins of the fossa (arrows). The osteoarthritic changes in the joint, including sclerosis, spurring of the inferior joint surfaces, superior migration of the humeral head, and joint space narrowing, are likely to be secondary osteoarthritic changes related to the chronic instability of the joint.

allowing enough time for the anterior capsule to heal. Rehabilitation focuses on strengthening and gradual return to full function.

Surgical treatment is indicated in the presence of large fracture fragments or selectively in a distinct patient population, such as young athletes.

Complications

Recurrent anterior subluxation or dislocation and chronic joint instability are common problems. The incidence of recurrent dislocation is estimated at up to 90% in athletes at age 20, up to 60% at age 30, and 15% at age 40. Most recurrences happen within the first 2 years after the initial dislocation. Surgical repair is necessary to establish stability and full function in the joint.

Acromioclavicular Joint Separation

Acromioclavicular joint separation, also commonly called *shoulder separation,* refers to various degrees of ligamentous sprain or rupture at the joint. This injury may happen in isolation or be complicated by associated clavicle, acromion, or coracoid fractures (Fig. 15-48).

Mechanism of Injury

The mechanism of injury is typically a downward force applied to the acromion process from either a fall on the point of the shoulder or a direct blow. Various other forces may disrupt the joint, such as traction on the arm, a fall on an outstretched hand, or a fall on a flexed elbow.

Classification

The stability of this joint is achieved primarily by the coracoclavicular ligament and additionally by the acromioclavicular ligament and joint capsule (Fig. 15-49). Sprains are graded as mild, moderate, and severe in reference to the degree of disruption of these structures.

Radiologic Evaluation

The trauma series is usually obtained after acute injury. In addition, bilateral AP views of the acromioclavicular joints, with and without weights, is used to assess ligamentous injury. Refer to "Routine Radiologic Evaluation of the Acromioclavicular Joint" above, for radiologic assessment.

Treatment

Treatment is controversial; management of all grades of sprain may be treated conservatively with varying lengths of immobilization, or surgical repair may be instituted in moderate and severe sprains. Several types of surgical repair exist, including wire or pin fixation of the acromioclavicular

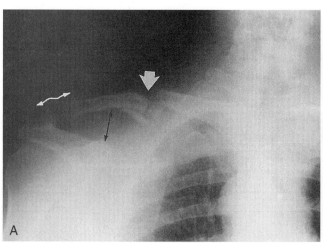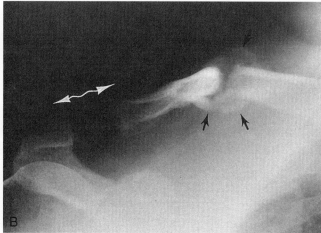

Figure 15-48 AC joint separation with clavicle fracture. **(A)** This 55-year-old man, a farmer, was injured when several sacks of grain fell down on him from the loft in his barn. This AP view of the AC joint demonstrates marked widening of both the acromioclavicular joint (white wavy arrow) and the coracoclavicular distance (black arrow), indicating a moderate to severe sprain of the AC joint. There is an associated comminuted fracture of the midshaft of the clavicle (large white arrow). **(B)** Management of this patient was complicated by the extremely slow union of the clavicular fracture. This AP film of the AC joint made 11 months later shows some callus (black arrows) uniting the fracture fragments, but the fracture is not united, as evidenced by the wide radiolucent gap at the fracture site. The disruption of the AC joint remains unchanged.

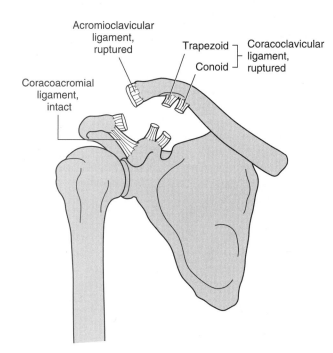

Figure 15-49 The stability of the acromioclavicular joint is achieved primarily by the coracoclavicular ligaments. Severe sprains or ruptures of these ligaments result in acromioclavicular joint separation.

joint; reconstruction, repair, or fixation of the coracoclavicular ligament; excision of the distal clavicle; or dynamic muscle transfers.

Rehabilitation focuses on restoring shoulder range of motion and strength for function.

Complications

Complications identifiable on radiograph include arthritic changes in the joint, chronic subluxation, soft tissue calcification, distal clavicle osteolysis associated with chronic dull pain and weakness, and loosening or migration of metal fixation devices.

Rotator Cuff Tears

The four muscles of the rotator cuff are the subscapularis, supraspinatus, infraspinatus, and teres minor. The tendons of these muscles converge and fuse with the fibrous capsule of the glenohumeral joint, inserting into the anatomic neck and tuberosities of the humerus. Underlying the rotator cuff is the synovial lining and joint space. Above the rotator cuff lies the subacromial bursa and its extension, the subdeltoid bursa.

Mechanism of Injury

Rotator cuff tears may result from an acute traumatic episode, as during a glenohumeral dislocation, a fall on an outstretched hand, or a forceful abduction movement of the arm. Rotator cuff tears may also result from the progressive tendon irritation caused by repetitive overhead movements or impingement. Degenerative changes in the hypovascular region of the cuff, seen most commonly in patients over 50 years of age, predispose the structure to rupture from relatively minor trauma.

Classification

The most common tear involves the hypovascular *critical zone* in the supraspinatus tendon 1 cm above its insertion on the greater tuberosity. Tears are either incomplete (partial) or complete (full thickness).

Radiologic Evaluation

In the past, the radiologic evaluation of suspected rotator cuff tears was accomplished with arthrography. An intact rotator cuff would confine the contrast medium to the joint capsule and the structures that normally communicate with the capsule—the sheath of the biceps tendon inferiorly and the subscapular bursa anteriorly. A complete tear of the cuff would allow the contrast medium to travel up through the tear and fill the subacromial–subdeltoid bursa, causing the bursa to be radiopaque (Fig. 15-50). Incomplete tears were identified by a collection of contrast medium at the tear site.

Today, arthrography is recommended only if the patient cannot have MRI and ultrasound expertise is not available. The advantage of MRI is that it is noninvasive and can provide the surgeon with specific information regarding the tendons involved, including the location, size, quality of the torn edges, and the amount of muscle atrophy and tendon retraction present (Fig. 15-51A,B).

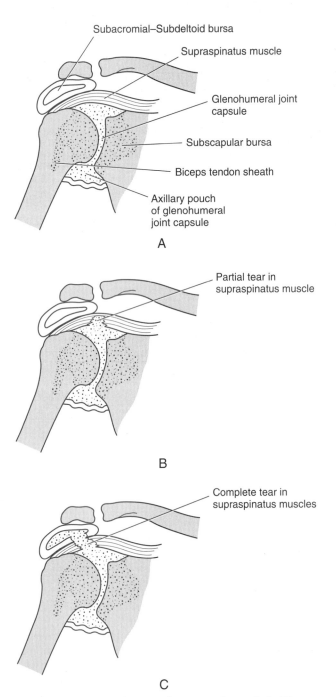

A

B

C

Figure 15-50 Schematic diagrams of contrast arthrography in **(A)** a normal glenohumeral joint, where contrast medium is confined to the joint capsule and communicating structures (biceps tendon and subscapular bursa); **(B)** a partial rotator cuff tear, where contrast medium leaks into the tear site; and **(C)** a complete rotator cuff tear, where contrast medium travels up through the tear and fills the subacromial–subdeltoid bursa.

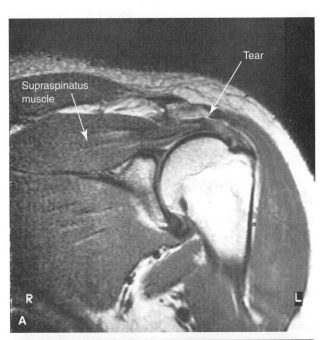

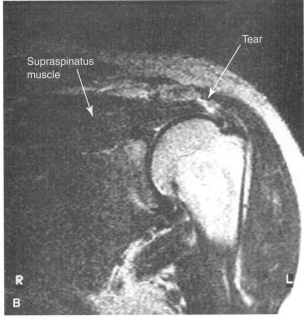

Figure 15-51 Supraspinatus tendon tear demonstrated on different MRI sequences. **(A)** Proton density coronal oblique image shows the tear as a loss of continuity of the supraspinatus tendon (dark, irregular area) in the critical zone, just proximal to its insertion at the greater tuberosity. **(B)** T2-weighted coronal oblique image demonstrates the tear as a high-signal-intensity (white) focal lesion at the critical zone.

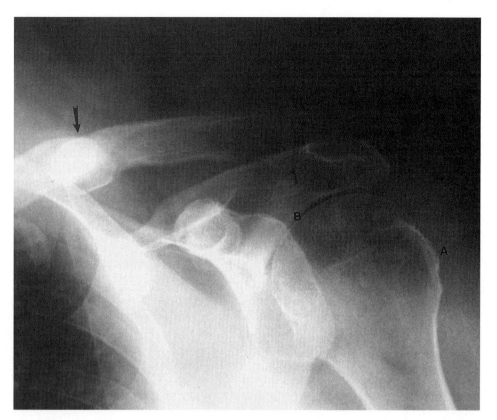

Figure 15-52 Rotator cuff tear, radiographic findings. This 64-year-old man presents with complaints of progressive weakness in the muscles of his left shoulder. There was a history of trauma 2 years prior when he fractured his clavicle in a fall off his bicycle. This AP view of his shoulder demonstrates the classic plain film findings associated with chronic tears of the rotator cuff: (a) irregularity of the greater tuberosity; (b) narrowing of the distance between the acromion and the humeral head; (c) erosion or loss of bone in the inferior aspect of the acromion. The small arrow indicates early osteoarthritic changes present at the AC joint, and the large arrow indicates the site of the healed clavicle fracture.

Chronic rotator cuff tears are evident on radiographs by the secondary changes that subsequently occur. These include the following (Fig. 15-52):

1. *Irregularity of the greater tuberosity:* The tuberosity may appear flattened, atrophied, or sclerotic because of rupture of the supraspinatus tendon and lack of traction stress at the insertion site.
2. *Narrowing of the distance between the acromion and the humeral head:* This space is normally occupied by the bursa and cuff muscles. Atrophy of the cuff muscles will decrease the thickness of the cuff, decreasing the space. Additionally, weak rotator cuff muscles will not oppose the pull of the deltoid muscle, and the humeral head will be pulled proximally, further decreasing the space.
3. *Erosion of the inferior aspect of the acromion:* The upward migration of the humeral head may cause changes at the acromion, including sclerosis, subchondral cyst formation, and loss of bone.

Treatment

Minor tears are treated conservatively with rest, nonsteroidal anti-inflammatory drugs, and perhaps cortisone injections. Most tears, however, do not heal well with time and require surgical repair. The rehabilitation is extensive, beginning in the acute phase with controlled motion and culminating with return to full function in 4 to 6 months.

Complications

Most complications of rotator cuff tears are related to the degenerative changes at the glenohumeral and acromioclavicular joints, as noted in the radiographic findings just described.

Failure to regain full range of motion and strength following surgery can lead to impaired scapulohumeral rhythm and chronic tendon irritation and inflammation as well as poor function.

Glenoid Labrum Tears

The labrum has two basic functions in the joint: to deepen the glenoid fossa so the humeral head stays in place, and to serve as an attachment site for the capsular ligaments and the biceps tendon. Symptoms of a labral tear may include pain that is worse with overhead movements, clicking or catching, and a sense of instability.

Mechanism of Injury

The labrum can be injured acutely in association with a dislocation, a forceful lifting manuever, or a fall on an outstretched hand. The labrum can also be injured from repetitive movements of the arm. The overhead athlete (e.g., baseball, swimming, tennis) is susceptible to biceps tendon stress at the superior labral attachement as well as repetitve impingement of the posterior humeral head against the rotator cuff and labrum.

Also, muscle imbalances that decentralize the position of the humeral head within the fossa can trigger a cascade of abnormal shoulder biomechanics that result in a pathological laxity and abnormal shear forces at the labrum.

Classification

Labral tears are highly varied. A simple way to categorize tears is to divide them into three groups:

- The first group involves avulsions of the labrum off the glenoid rim. This is most often seen in acute trauma.
- The second group involves tearing within the substance of the labrum. This type of tearing may or may not be symptomatic and is seen frequently in adults over age 40.
- The third group of tears is in relation to the biceps tendon as it blends into the superior labrum to attach to the glenoid tubercle. These lesions are well-documented in the literature, described with the acronym *SLAP*. This stands for a tear at the *superior labrum, anterior and posterior* (to the biceps tendon). Depending on the author, four or five SLAP subtypes exist.

Table 15-1 contains many acronyms used to describe a variety of labral tears and associated lesions.

Radiologic Evaluation

MR arthrography is the most appropriate procedure to assess suspected instability and labral tears. The advantage of direct MR arthrography is that the contrast distends the joint, permittting better visualization of the labrum, capsular structures, and the underside of the rotator cuff. Routine MRI is appropriate with high resolution and appropriate expertise, and CT arthrography is the second procedure of choice if MRI is contraindicated or not available. Figures 15-53 and 15-54 are examples of labral tears diagnosed using MR arthrography.

Treatment

Many tears heal with conservative care because of the rich blood supply of the labrum. Other tears require surgical intervention to restore joint function and stability. Avulsions are reattached to the glenoid rim with sutures and anchors. The

---

TABLE 15-1 ● *Acronyms and MRI Terminology of Glenohumeral and Labral Lesions*[a]

Acronym	Definition	Clinical Comments
ALPSA	Anterior labral periosteal sleeve avulsion	Associated with prior anterior dislocation
Bankart fracture	Avulsion of labrum off the anteroinferior glenoid rim	Associated with prior anterior dislocation
Bankhart lesion	Tear of anteroinferior labrum	Associated with prior anterior dislocation
Bennett lesion	Mineralization of the posterior band of the inferior glenohumeral ligament	Common in major league pitchers and overhead athletes; may be asymptomatic
BHAGL	Bony humeral avulsion glenohumeral ligament	Associated with dislocation and tear of the subscapularis tendon
Buford complex	A cord-like middle glenohumeral ligament with absence of the anterosuperior labrum	Normal variant
GARD	Glenoid rim articular divot	Not associated with instability
GIRD	Glenohumeral internal rotation deficit	Common in swimmers and overhead athletes; at risk to develop SLAP
GLAD	Glenolabral articular disruption involving anteroinferior labrum and adjacent humeral articular cartilage	Spectrum of injury varies from cartilaginous flap to osteochondral fracture
GLOM	Glenoid labrum ovoid mass	Represents an anterosuperior tear and retraction of the labrum or middle glenohumeral ligament
HAGL	Humeral avulsion glenohumeral ligament	Avulsion of the capsule and inferior glenohumeral ligament from the neck of the humerus
Hill–Sachs lesion	Impaction fracture of the posterolateral surface of the humeral head	Associated with prior anterior dislocation
McLaughlin sign	Impaction fracture of the anterior humeral head (also called a reverse Hill–Sachs)	Associated with prior posterior dislocation
MDI or AMDI	A traumatic multidirectional instability of the glenohumeral joint	Labrum and rotator cuff interval are potential sites of pathology
OCD	Osteochondritis dissecans	Osteochondral lesion of the glenoid cavity secondary to impaction forces
Paralabral ganglion cyst	Ganglion cyst adjacent to the labrum	Associated with labral tear
Perthes lesion	Incomplete avulsion of the capsulolabral complex from the scapular neck	Similar to ALPSA except that the periosteum is intact and the labral avulsion is incomplete
POLPSA	Posterior labral periosteal sleeve avulsion	Associated with prior posterior dislocation
SLAP	Superior labral anterior to posterior, anterior and posterior are in reference to the biceps tendon	Seen in overhead athletes, often involves the biceps anchor. Divided into four or five types
Trough lesion	Fracture of the medial humeral head	Associated with prior posterior dislocation
TUBS	Traumatic instability. T = traumatic event, U = unidirectional instability in the anteroinferior direction, B = Bankart lesion usually present, and S = surgical repair required to restore function	Usually due to a fall on an outstretched hand during athletic activity

[a] As with any acronym, definitions in the literature may vary and be anatomically inexact.

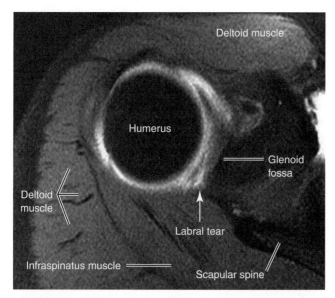

Figure 15-53 SLAP lesion. T1-weighted axial MR arthrography of the right shoulder demonstrates fraying of the posterior superior labrum with an irregular collection of contrast between the posterior superior labrum and the posterior aspect of the glenoid (arrow). The patient is a collegiate baseball player with pain in the follow-through phase of throwing.

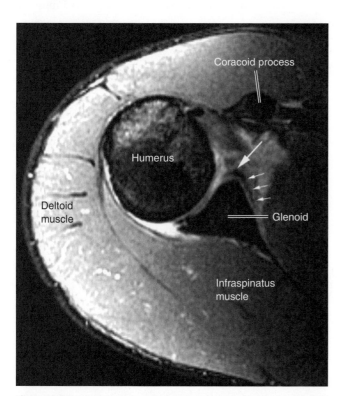

Figure 15-54 ALPSA (anterior labral periosteal sleeve avulsion) lesion. MR arthrography demonstrates a detached anterior labrum (large arrow) which has remained attached to the periosteum of the scapular margin (small arrows). The patient had a history of prior anterior dislocations. *(Image courtesy of John C. Hunter, MD.)*

torn edges of minor tears are debrided; large tears require suture repair. *Biceps tenodesis* is most often performed in patients over age 40 with associated biceps tendon tears. This procedure cuts the biceps from where it attaches to the labrum and reinserts it in another area.

Rehabilitation after repair or tenodesis is delayed 4 to 6 weeks to allow full healing at the repair site. Overhead athletes with SLAP repairs can expect about 6 months to return to full throwing velocity. Physical therapy is essential to restore strength and flexibility, and address the biomechanical factors that may have contributed to the labral injury.

Abnormal Conditions at the Shoulder[11,35–65]

Impingement Syndrome

Two types of *impingement syndrome* are described. *External* impingement is the compression of the rotator cuff tendons as they are entrapped in the *supraspinatus outlet*—the space between the humeral head inferiorly and the coracoacromial ligament and acromion superiorly—when the arm is elevated. *Internal impingement* compresses the posterior capsule and rotator cuff between the humeral head and glenoid when the arm is elevated and rotated. This is most commonly seen in overhead athletes. Both types of impingement are associated with tendinitis, bursitis, rotator cuff lesions, muscle imbalances, and labral tears. Note that although we study all these conditions separately, biomechanically they are linked and thus each has the potential to predispose the development of the other.

Radiologic Evaluation

The history and physical exam are diagnostic for impingement syndromes. MRI can indentify the various associated soft tissue pathologies including bursitis, tendinitis, and tears of the rotator cuff and labrum (Fig. 15-55).

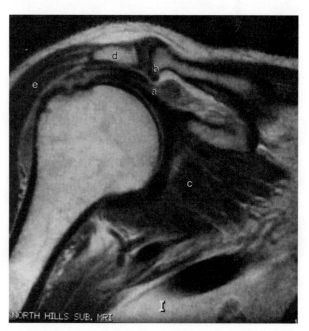

Figure 15-55 Impingement syndrome, MRI findings. This coronal MR image of the shoulder demonstrates the supraspinatus muscle (a) impinged by a large osteophyte (b) on the inferior aspect of the distal clavicle. Other structures noted are: (c) subscapularis muscle, (d) acromion, (e) deltoid muscle.

Radiographic evidence of impingement syndrome in the later stages includes subacromial proliferation of bone, osteophyte formation on the inferior surfaces of the acromion or acromioclavicular joint, and cysts or sclerosis of the greater tuberosity at the insertion of the rotator cuff tendons (Fig. 15-56).

Treatment

Treatment in the earlier stages may be successful with conservative measures, including rehabilitation to address muscle imbalances and modalities to control inflammation. Surgical intervention designed to decompress the subacromial space and alleviate impingement of the soft tissues may be indicated when conservative treatment has failed. Resection of the coracoacromial ligament, anterior acromion, or distal clavicle and excision of acromioclavicular joint osteophytes are examples of such procedures.

Adhesive Capsulitis

Adhesive capsulitis, commonly known as a "frozen shoulder," is defined as chronic inflammation and fibrosis of the glenohumeral joint capsule. The condition is characterized by pain and global restriction of motion at the glenohumeral joint.

Classification

The etiology of adhesive capsulitis is unknown. Two categories are clinically apparent, however: primary (idiopathic) and secondary.

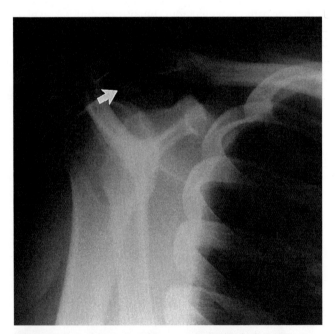

Figure 15-56 Impingement syndrome, radiographic findings. This anterior oblique view of the shoulder (scapular Y position) is obtained by rotating the patient 30 degrees from a true lateral position. Structures best shown include an oblique lateral view of the proximal humerus superimposed over a lateral view of the scapula. The relationship of the humeral head to the glenoid cavity is well demonstrated. Additionally, the subacromial space is well visualized. Note that in the subacromial region of this shoulder of a 40-year-old man, a large calcification is seen in the (tendon of the rotator cuff arrow). This may represent a calcification of a partial rotator cuff tear, or fibrosis and calcification of frictioned tendons.

Primary adhesive capsulitis appears spontaneously without identifiable stimulus. It affects 2% to 3% of the population and tends to occur most commonly after age 50. Women are affected more often than men.

Secondary adhesive capsulitis is associated with a pre-existing trauma to the shoulder or some other painful condition originating elsewhere in the body that results in prolonged voluntary or involuntary immobilization of the shoulder. Some systemic diseases and conditions are associated with secondary adhesive capsulitis, including diabetes, hyperthyroidism, rheumatoid arthritis, myocardial infarction, hemiplegia, scleroderma, lung cancer, cervical radiculitis, and mastectomy.

Clinical Presentation

Both categories exhibit similar clinical manifestations and histologic changes in the joint capsule. The natural clinical course of adhesive capsulitis is divided into three stages:

1. An acute, painful stage, characterized by increasing pain at movement or at rest and at night, lasting 3 to 8 months.
2. An adhesive stage, marked by increasing stiffness and decreasing pain, lasting 4 to 6 months.
3. A recovery stage, characterized by minimal pain and severe restriction of movement, lasting 1 to 3 months.

The last stage is self-limiting, with a gradual and spontaneous increase in range of motion.

Radiologic Evaluation

Conventional radiographs may reveal only localized osteoporosis at the shoulder owing to disuse atrophy. Radiographic examination is important, however, to assess underlying possible causes of secondary adhesive capsulitis, such as fracture, avascular necrosis, osteoarthritis, crystalline arthropathy, calcific tendinitis, and neoplasm.

Contrast arthrography, although invasive, is useful to document decreased joint volume. An unaffected glenohumeral joint will accommodate 20 to 30 mL of contrast material, whereas an affected joint will hold only 5 to 10 mL. Restrictions in the capsule will also prohibit the normal filling of the axillary and subscapular recesses of the capsule (Fig. 15-57). Additionally, some studies have shown that 10% to 30% of patients are found to have a rotator cuff tear revealed on the arthrogram.

The usefulness of MRI has also been evaluated. MRI can demonstrate capsular thickening, but a decrease in joint fluid is not demonstrated.

Treatment

Adhesive capsulitis tends to be self-limiting and usually resolves spontaneously in several months. However, pain and functional disability usually require earlier active intervention. Significant disability can be minimized with early therapeutic intervention in those patients who are at a known risk for developing adhesive capsulitis. Analgesics and physical therapy represent the treatment approach of choice.

Complications

Approximately 7% to 15% of patients permanently lose full range of motion.

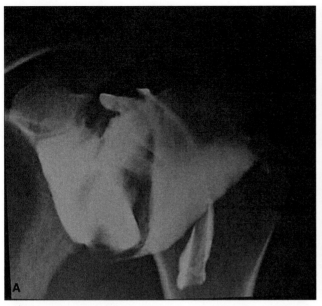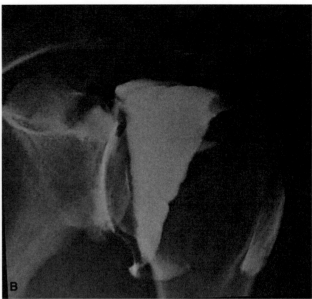

Figure 15-57 Arthrography of the glenohumeral joint, normal and abnormal findings. **(A)** AP radiograph of the shoulder after injection of contrast shows normal filling of the glenohumeral joint capsule. The contrast material extends into the subscapular recess, axillary recess, and biceps tendon sheath. **(B)** AP radiograph after injection of contrast demonstrates characteristic findings of adhesive capsulitis. The capacity of the axillary pouch is markedly decreased, and the subscapularis recess and biceps tendon sheath remain unopacified. *(Source of images: http://www.xray2000.co.uk.)*

Summary of Key Points

Routine Radiologic Evaluation of the Shoulder

1. The routine radiographic evaluation of the shoulder includes two AP projections demonstrating different aspects of the proximal humerus as well as part of the clavicle and scapula.
   - ➤ *AP view with the arm externally rotated*—the greater tuberosity is in profile
   - ➤ *AP view with the arm internally rotated*—the lesser tuberosity is in profile

Routine Radiologic Evaluation of the Acromioclavicular Joints

2. The routine radiographic evaluation of the acromioclavicular joints includes two projections: *bilateral AP without weights* and *bilateral AP with weights*. These provide traction through the patient's arms for a *stress view* to evaluate the stability of the acromioclavicular joints.

Routine Radiologic Evaluation of the Scapula

3. The routine radiographic evaluation of the scapula includes two projections:
   - ➤ *AP*—demonstrates the lateral half of the scapula while the ribs and lung are superimposed on the medial half
   - ➤ *Lateral*—evaluates the body of the scapula in profile

Trauma Series

4. The trauma series includes an AP with the arm in neutral and special projections indicated by clinical presentation, such as:

   - ➤ *Axillary view of the glenohumeral joint*—demonstrates the exact relationship of the humeral head to the glenoid fossa
   - ➤ *Anterior oblique (scapular Y lateral view)*—demonstrates a lateral view of the humeral head and scapula without having to move the arm from a neutral position

5. MRI is recommended for acute and subacute shoulder pain if *initial radiographs are normal*, and if *rotator cuff pathology*, *instability*, or *labral tears* are suspected. As an alternative, CT arthrography is recommended if MRI is unavailable or contraindicated. Diagnostic ultrasound, "with appropriate expertise," is also recommended in the evaluation of soft tissue pathology.

Fractures of the Proximal Humerus

6. Fractures of the proximal humerus are commonly classified by the *Neer four-part system*. Fractures are described by how many parts the proximal humerus has separated into: one-part (nondisplaced), two-part, three-part, or four-part.

7. The surgical neck of the proximal humerus is a frequent site of *pathological fracture.*

Fractures of the Clavicle

8. Fractures of the clavicle are designated by their location at the proximal, middle, or distal thirds of the bone. The *middle third* is the most frequent site of fracture. AP and angled AP radiographs are diagnostic.

Fractures of the Scapula

9. Fractures of the scapula are divided into fractures of the *body, apophysis,* and *superolateral* fractures. AP and lateral radiograph are diagnostic.

10. Fractures of the rim of the *glenoid fossa* are associated with glenohumeral dislocation.

Dislocations at the Glenohumeral Joint

11. More than 90% of glenohumeral dislocations are *anterior* dislocations. The AP, axillary, and scapular Y views are diagnostic.

12. The *Hill–Sachs lesion* is a compression fracture of the posterolateral aspect of the humeral head sustained during dislocation.

13. The *Bankart lesion* is a detachment of the labrum from the anterior inferior glenoid rim, indicative of recurrent dislocations. If a bony avulsion of the rim is involved, it is visible on radiographs and known as a *Bankart fracture.*

Acromioclavicular Joint Separations

14. Acromioclavicular joint separations are ligamentous sprain or rupture at the acromioclavicular joint. They are graded as *mild, moderate,* or *severe,* in reference to the degree of instability. Radiographs evaluate the coracoclavicular distance and the acromioclavicular distance in AP stress films.

Rotator Cuff Tears

15. The most common rotator cuff tear involves the hypovascular *critical zone* of the supraspinatus tendon, 1 cm proximal to its insertion on the greater tuberosity.

16. Diagnosis is by MRI. Radiographic findings are evident in chronic cases.

Impingement Syndrome

17. Two types of *impingement* occur when the arm is overhead: *external impingement* compresses the rotator cuff in the supraspinatus outlet; *internal impingement* compresses the posterior capsule and rotator cuff between the humeral head and glenoid.

18. History and physical exam are diagnostic. MRI can define associated soft tissue pathologies commonly associated with impingement, such as rotator cuff tears, labral tears, and tendinitis.

Adhesive Capsulitis

19. Adhesive capsulitis, or "frozen shoulder," is a chronic inflammation and fibrosis of the glenohumeral joint capsule. Contrast arthrography can demonstrate decreased capsular volume. Radiographs can evaluate possible underlying pathology.

 Please refer to the text's enclosed CD-ROM for the American College of Radiology's current Musculoskeletal Appropriateness Criteria for the following topic: *Shoulder Trauma.*

CASE STUDIES

Case Study 1
Rotator Cuff Tear

The patient, a 45-year-old man, was referred to outpatient physical therapy by his primary care physician for the evaluation and treatment of left shoulder pain.

History of Trauma

The patient fell approximately 15 feet off of a ladder at work, hitting the ground on his left side. He experienced left hip and shoulder pain immediately and was taken to the local emergency department. There the attending physician ordered conventional radiographs of the left hip and pelvis and the left shoulder. The physician also cleared him of any head or spine injury by physical examination.

Initial Imaging

Conventional radiographs of the hip and pelvis were taken and read by the radiologist. No bony abnormalities were identified. Radiographs of the left shoulder revealed no fractures or dislocations.

Intervention

The patient was released from the emergency department. He was sent home ambulating independently, using a cane in his right hand. He was also given a sling for his left shoulder, to wear as needed for comfort. The patient was instructed to follow up with his primary care physician to determine whether any further treatment was necessary for his hip or shoulder.

The patient saw his physician one week after the injury. His hip pain had nearly resolved by this time, and he was ambulating without an assistive device, but he continued to experience left shoulder pain. The primary care physician sent him to physical therapy with a referral stating, "Evaluate and treat for left shoulder pain."

Physical Therapy Examination

Patient Complaint

At the initial physical therapy appointment 1½ weeks after the injury, the patient complained of left shoulder pain extending down the lateral arm from the acromion to the elbow. He was not experiencing any neck pain or symptoms below the elbow. The patient brought the radiologist's report from his emergency department radiographs to the first appointment.

Physical Examination

The physical therapist completed screening examinations for the cervical spine and elbow. These were both within normal limits. Examination of the left shoulder revealed a number of significant findings. The patient was reluctant to move the left shoulder and reported pain with any attempt to elevate actively above 45 degrees, but the therapist could achieve full passive shoulder flexion and abduction with mild discomfort. Manual muscle testing of the shoulder revealed weakness with external rotation, flexion, and abduction. The patient had difficulty slowly lowering his arm to his side during the drop arm test.

Considering a working hypothesis of partial or complete rotator cuff tear, the physical therapist contacted the patient's primary care physician. The therapist described his findings and recommended magnetic resonance imaging (MRI) of the patient's shoulder. The physician agreed to order the imaging study.

Additional Imaging

The MR image of the patient's shoulder (Fig. 15-58) showed a complete tear of the rotator cuff and some degenerative spurring on the undersurface of the acromioclavicular joint.

Outcome

The patient was referred to an orthopedic surgeon for surgical repair of the rotator cuff. Following the surgery, the physical therapist followed the patient through rehabilitation.

Discussion

In many cases physical therapists receive referrals to examine and plan interventions for patients who have not been given a definite diagnosis. This patient's shoulder pain had not been diagnosed prior to the physical therapist's first appointment. It then becomes the therapist's responsibility to determine whether physical therapy intervention was appropriate at that time.

Should the Physical Therapist Have Recommended the MRI Right Away?

The therapist in this case might have tried a period of conservative management, perhaps 1 or 2 weeks, before contacting the physician to recommend further investigation with diagnostic imaging. In fact, the patient's primary care physician might have been considering MRI but wanted to try a course of physical therapy before ordering this expensive test.

The answer depends upon the relative advantages and disadvantages of waiting a few weeks if a rotator cuff tear does exist. The significant amount of pain experienced by this patient so recently after the injury clouded the physical examination somewhat. Muscle testing is less reliable in the presence of significant pain. A period of time to reduce his pain level through symptomatic intervention might have helped to clear the clinical picture.

The physical therapist should consider the following:

1. How definitive the examination findings are

2. Whether there are any detrimental (or beneficial) effects of delaying surgical repair

3. The comparative costs of 2 weeks of physical therapy versus MRI

4. The patient's wishes

Each case must be considered individually to determine the optimal course of action. This case is summarized in Figure 15-59.

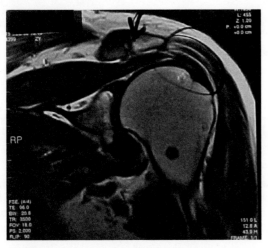

Figure 15-58 Coronal MR image of the left shoulder showing a complete rotator cuff tear and degenerative spurring of the acromioclavicular joint.

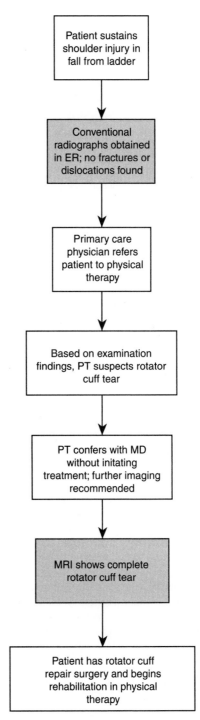

Figure 15-59 Pathway of case study events. Imaging is highlighted.

CRITICAL THINKING POINTS

1. It is always the physical therapist's responsibility to determine the appropriateness of physical therapy for a patient.

2. Good examination skills, knowledge of the characteristics of differential diagnoses, and past experience assist the physical therapist in judging when physical therapy is necessary or when diagnostic imaging needs to be employed to make this decision.

3. Good communication between the physical therapist and the referring physician is necessary to make good diagnostic imaging recommendations.

CASE STUDY 2

Shoulder Hemiarthroplasty

The patient, a 75-year-old woman, is referred to physical therapy following shoulder hemiarthroplasty surgery.

History

The patient reported a long history, beginning 15 years earlier, of left shoulder pain and dysfunction. She had been told that she had chronic tendinitis and bursitis. Five years ago she stumbled while descending some stairs, catching herself by pushing against the wall alongside the staircase. She had diagnostic imaging at that time and was told she had torn her rotator cuff. She elected not to have a surgical repair done at that time because it was her nondominant upper extremity and she did not want to complete a long course of rehabilitation.

Her shoulder pain gradually worsened over time until she told her primary care physician that she wanted something done. The physician referred her to an orthopedic surgeon, who recommended a shoulder hemiarthroplasty, based on the results of physical examination and diagnostic imaging.

Diagnostic Imaging

Conventional radiographs of the left shoulder (Fig. 15-60) demonstrated severe osteoarthritis affecting the glenohumeral joint. The joint surfaces and inferior surface of the acromion showed marked erosion, sclerosis, and significant spurs encroaching on the glenohumeral and subacromial joint space. The humeral head had migrated superiorly in the joint.

MRI was ordered at the same time; it confirmed a large rotator cuff tear with retraction of the supraspinatus and infraspinatus tendons away from their attachment sites on the humerus.

Intervention

The patient underwent hemiarthroplasty surgery, which included replacement of the humeral head and smoothing of the acromion's inferior surface. The surgeon was unable to reattach the supraspinatus and infraspinatus tendons because of the amount of retraction and degeneration of these tendons. Radiographs taken following the surgery (Fig. 15-61) showed the new humeral head component and significant improvement of the

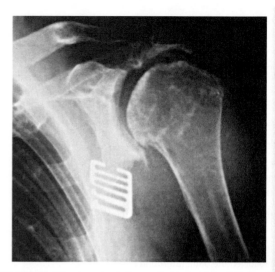

Figure 15-60 AP external rotation radiograph of the left shoulder, showing severe degenerative changes of the humeral head and acromion.

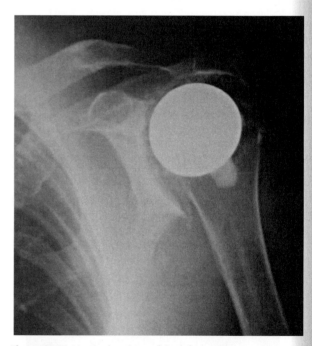

Figure 15-61 Hemiarthroplasty of the left shoulder.

acromion's appearance. The humeral head continued to show superior positioning on the glenoid fossa due to the absence of the supraspinatus and infraspinatus tendons.

Outcome

The patient completed a course of rehabilitation. Upon discharge from physical therapy, she reported no left shoulder pain. Her functional use of the left upper extremity was limited to activities in very close proximity to her trunk and near waist level. She continued to

```
┌─────────────────────┐
│   Patient with chronic   │
│ left shoulder pain and  │
│   dysfunction sees      │
│       physician         │
└─────────────────────┘
           │
           ▼
┌─────────────────────┐
│  Radiographs and MRI   │
│  show severe OA and    │
│   rotator cuff tear with  │
│  retraction of tendons   │
└─────────────────────┘
           │
           ▼
┌─────────────────────┐
│   Patient has shoulder   │
│     hemiarthroplasty     │
│         surgery          │
└─────────────────────┘
           │
           ▼
┌─────────────────────┐
│    Patient referred to    │
│     physical therapy     │
│    for post-surgical      │
│     rehabilitation        │
└─────────────────────┘
           │
           ▼
┌─────────────────────┐
│  PT uses diagnostic      │
│ imaging to make prognosis │
│ and educate patient about │
│    expected functional    │
│         outcome           │
└─────────────────────┘
           │
           ▼
┌─────────────────────┐
│  Patient discharged      │
│ with limited left upper   │
│   extremity function      │
│  but pain-free shoulder   │
└─────────────────────┘
```

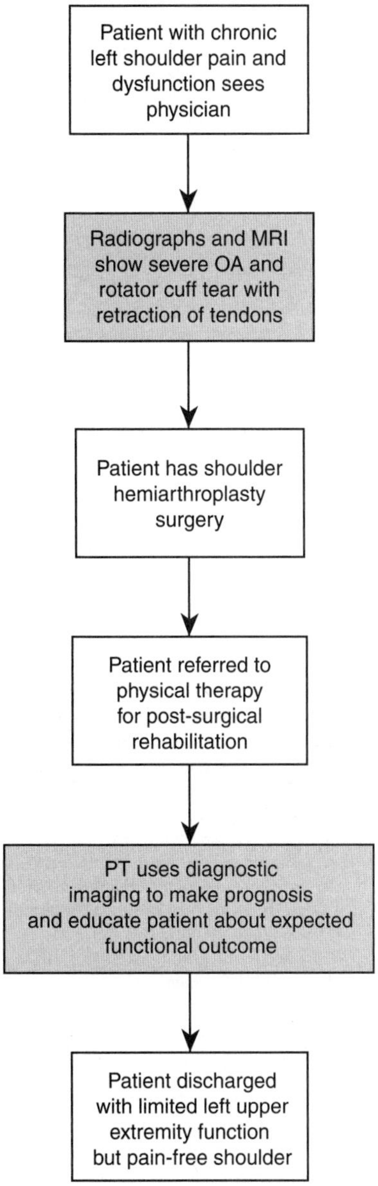

Figure 15-62 Pathway of case study events. Imaging is highlighted.

have significant limitations in left shoulder active range of motion secondary to the loss of the muscular force couple normally provided by an intact rotator cuff.

Discussion

Diagnostic imaging was helpful to the physical therapist elucidating the poor pre-existing and chronic degenerative condition of the patient's shoulder. A more accurate, realistic postsurgical prognosis was possible using this visual information. The patient could be informed of what she might expect to gain in rehabilitation. The patient and the therapist were able to set reasonable goals and achieve the most successful outcome possible.

This case is summarized in Figure 15-62.

CRITICAL THINKING POINTS

Even when the physical therapist has no role in suggesting diagnostic imaging, the information can still be very important in terms of intervention planning, goal setting, and making an accurate prognosis. Setting realistic goals with the patient's input is important to the ultimate success of any patient's rehabilitation.

When function is expected to be less than optimal, educating the patient becomes even more critical. In many cases, diagnostic imaging is an excellent tool for helping to make prognoses and for educating patients about their expected functional return.

Case studies adapted by J. Bradley Barr, PT, DPT, OCS.

References

Normal Anatomy

1. Netter, FH: Atlas of Human Anatomy, ed. 4. WB Saunders, Philadelphia, 2006.
2. Nordin, M, and Frankel, VH: Basic Biomechanics of the Musculoskeletal System, ed. 3. Lippincott Williams & Wilkins, Philadelphia, 2001.
3. Whiting, W, and Zernicke, R: Biomechanics of Musculoskeletal Injury, ed. 2. Human Kinetics, Champaign, IL, 2008.
4. Norkin, CC, and Levangie, PK: Joint Structure and Function, A Comprehensive Analysis, ed. 2. FA Davis, Philadelphia, 1992.
5. Meschan, I: An Atlas of Radiographic Anatomy. WB Saunders, Philadelphia, 1960.
6. Weber, EC, Vilensky, JA, and Carmichael, SW: Netter's Concise Radiologic Anatomy. Saunders, 2008.
7. Kelley, LL, and Peterson, CM: Sectional Anatomy for Imaging Professional, ed. 2. Mosby, St. Louis, MO, 2007.
8. Lazo, DL: Fundamentals of Sectional Anatomy: An Imaging Approach. Thomson Delmar Learning, Clifton Park, NY, 2005.

Routine Exam

9. American College of Radiology: Practice Guideline for the Performance of Radiography of the Extremities, 2006. Available at http://www.acr.org. Accessed October 8, 2008.
10. Weissman, B, and Sledge, C: Orthopedic Radiology. WB Saunders, Philadelphia, 1986.
11. Greenspan, A: Orthopedic Radiology: A Practical Approach, ed. 4. Lippincott Williams & Wilkins, Philadelphia, 2004.
12. Bontrager, KL: Textbook of Radiographic Positioning and Related Anatomy, ed. 6. Mosby, St. Louis, MO, 2005.
13. Fischer, HW: Radiographic Anatomy: A Working Atlas. McGraw-Hill, New York, 1988.
14. Wicke, L: Atlas of Radiographic Anatomy, ed. 5. Lea & Febiger, Malvern, PA, 1994.
15. Frank, E, Smith, B, and Long, B: Merrill's Atlas of Radiographic Positions and Radiologic Procedures, ed. 11. Elsevier Health Sciences, Philadelphia, 2007.
16. Squires, LF, and Novelline, RA: Fundamentals of Radiology, ed. 4. Harvard University Press, Cambridge, MA, 1988.
17. Chew, FS: Skeletal Radiology: The Bare Bones, ed. 2. Williams & Wilkins, Baltimore, 1997.
18. Weir, J, and Abrahams, P: An Atlas of Radiological Anatomy. Yearbook Medical, Chicago, 1978.
19. Krell, L (ed): Clark's Positioning in Radiology, vol 1, ed. 10. Yearbook Medical, Chicago, 1989.

Trauma/Abnormal Conditions

20. American College of Radiology: Appropriateness Criteria for Shoulder Trauma. Available at http://www.acr.org/SecondaryMainMenuCategories/quality_safety/app_criteria/pdf/ExpertPanelonMusculoskeletalImaging/ShoulderTraumaDoc18.aspx.
21. Bucholz, RW, Heckman, J, and Court-Brown, C (eds): Rockwood and Green's Fractures in Adults, ed. 6. Lippincott Williams & Wilkins, Philadelphia, 2005.
22. Rockwood, CA, and Green, DP (eds): Fractures in Adults, ed. 5. Lippincott Williams & Wilkins, Philadelphia, 2002.
23. Beaty, J, and Kasar, J (eds): Rockwood and Wilkins' Fractures in Children, ed. 6. Lippincott Williams & Wilkins, Philadelphia, 2005.
24. Koval, KJ, and Zuckerman, JD: Handbook of Fractures, ed. 2. Lippincott Williams & Wilkins, Philadelphia, 2002.
25. Eiff, M, et al: Fracture Management for Primary Care. WB Saunders, Philadelphia, 2003.
26. Yochum, TR, and Rowe, LJ: Essentials of Skeletal Radiology, ed. 3. Williams & Wilkins, Baltimore, 2004.
27. Marchiori, DM: Clinical Imaging with Skeletal, Chest, and Abdomen Pattern Differentials. Mosby, St. Louis, 1999.
28. Ip, D: Orthopedic Traumatology: A Resident's Guide. Springer, New York, 2006.
29. McConnell, J, Eyres, R, and Nightingale, J: Interpreting Trauma Radiographs. Blackwell, Malden, MA, 2005.
30. Drafke, MW, and Nakayama, H: Trauma and Mobile Radiography, ed. 2. FA Davis, Philadelphia, 2001.
31. Hodler, J, von Schulthess, GK, and Zollikofer, CL: Musculoskeletal Disease: Diagnostic Imaging and Interventional Technology. Springer, Italy, 2005.
32. Daffner, RH: Clinical Radiology: The Essentials, ed. 3. Williams & Wilkins, Baltimore, 2007.
33. Bernstein, J (ed): Musculoskeletal Medicine. American Academy of Orthopedic Surgeons, Rosemont, IL, 2003.
34. Shahabpour, M, et al: The effectiveness of diagnostic imaging methods for the assessment of soft tissue and articular disorders of the shoulder and elbow. Eur J Radiol 65(2):194, 2008.
35. Rudez, J, and Zanetti, M: Normal anatomy, variants, and pitfalls on shoulder MRI. Eur J Radiol 68(1):25, 2008.
36. Fotiadou, AN, et al: Ultrasonography of symptomatic rotator cuff tears compared with MR imaging and surgery. Eur J Radiol 68(1):174, 2008.
37. Lecouvet, FE, et al: Multidetector spiral CT arthrography of the shoulder. Clinical applications and limits, with MR arthrography and arthroscopic correlation. Eur J Radiol 68(1):120, 2008.
38. Goud, A, et al: Radiographic evaluation of the shoulder. Eur J Radiol 68(1):2, 2008.
39. Van Grinsven, S, et al: MR arthrography of traumatic anterior shoulder lesions showed modest reproducibility and accuracy when evaluated under clinical circumstances. Arch Orthop Trauma Surg 127(1):11, 2007.
40. Opsha, O, et al: MRI of the rotator cuff and internal derangement. Eur J Radiol 68(1):36, 2008.
41. De Filippo, M, et al: Multidetector CT arthrography of the shoulder: Diagnostic accuracy and indications. Acta Radiol 49(5):540, 2008.
42. Emery, KH: Imaging of sports injuries of the upper extremity in children. Clin Sports Med 25(3):543, 2006.
43. Chaipat, L, and Palmer, WE: Shoulder magnetic resonance imaging. Clin Sports Med 25(3):371, 2006.
44. Trieb, K, et al: A rare reason for the end of a career in competitive tennis. J Sports Med Phys Fitness 48(1):120, 2008.
45. Birks, M, et al: Stress fracture of the clavicle in a patient with no obvious risk factors. Ann R Coll Surg Engl 87(1):W5, 2005.
46. Edelson, G, et al: Natural history of complex fractures of the proximal humerus using a three-dimensional classification system. J Shoulder Elbow Surg 17(3):399, 2008.
47. Curtis, C, et al: Delayed union of a scapular fracture—An unusual cause of persistent shoulder pain. Med Sci Sports Exerc 39(12):2095, 2007.
48. Gallo, RA, et al: Defining the relationship between rotator cuff injury and proximal humerus fractures. Clin Orthop Relat Res 458:70, 2007.
49. Saupe, N, et al: Acute traumatic posterior shoulder dislocations: MR findings. Radiology 248(1):185, 2008.
50. Probyn, LJ, et al: Recurrent symptoms after shoulder instability repair: Direct MR arthrographic assessment—Correlation with second look surgical evaluation. Radiology 245(3):814, 2007.
51. Antonio, GE, et al: First-time shoulder dislocation: High prevalence of labral injury and age-related differences revealed by MR arthrography. J Magn Reson Imaging 26(4):983, 2007.
52. Al-Shawi, A, et al: The detection of full thickness rotator cuff tears using ultrasound. J Bone Joint Surg Br 90(7):889, 2008.
53. Guerini, H, et al: Harmonic sonography of rotator cuff tendons: Are cleavage tears visible at last? J Radiol 89(3 pt 1):333, 2008.
54. Hedtmann, A, and Heers, G: Imaging in evaluating rotator cuff tears. Orthopade 36(9):796, 2007.
55. Vanhoenacker, FM, et al: MR arthrography of the rotator cuff. JBR-BTR 90(5):338, 2007.
56. Andrews, J, et al: Glenoid labrum tears related to the long head of the biceps. Am J Sports Med 13:337, 1985.
57. Neer, CS II: Impingement lesions. Clin Orthop 173:70, 1983.
58. Chang, D, et al: SLAP lesions: Anatomy, clinical presentation, MR imaging diagnosis and characterization. Eur J Radiol, 68(1):72, 2008.
59. Kendall, CB, et al: SLAP tear associated with a minimally displaced proximal humerus fracture. Arthroscopy 23(12):1362.e1, 2007.
60. Wright, R, and Paletta, G: Prevalence of the Bennett lesion of the shoulder in major league pitchers. Am J Sports Med 32:121, 2004.
61. Silva, L, et al: Accuracy of physical examination in subacromial impingement syndrome. Rheumatology (Oxford) 47(5):679, 2008.
62. Grainger, AJ: Internal impingement syndromes of the shoulder. Semin Musculoskel Radiol 12(2):127, 2008.
63. DeBerardino, T, and Chang, W: Shoulder impingement syndrome. Emedicine, 2006. Accessed October 15, 2008 at http://www.emedicine.com/sports/topic119.htm.
64. Sofka, CM, et al: Magnetic resonance imaging of adhesive capsulitis: Correlation with clinical staging. HSS J 4(2):164, 2008.

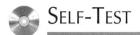

SELF-TEST

Radiograph A

1. Identify the *projection.*

2. Identify three findings that suggest an *advanced pathological state.* (*Hint:* Look at gross bony architecture, soft tissue shadows, and density changes.)

Radiograph B

3. Identify the *projection.*

4. What *joint* is being stabilized by the *internal fixation device?*

Radiograph C

5. Identify the *projection.*

6. The large number of internal fixation devices required to regain anatomic position leads you to believe that what *type of fracture pattern* existed?

7. What would you guess was the *mechanism* of this injury?

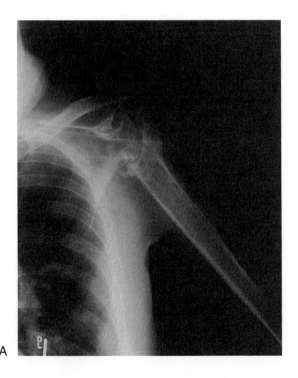

A

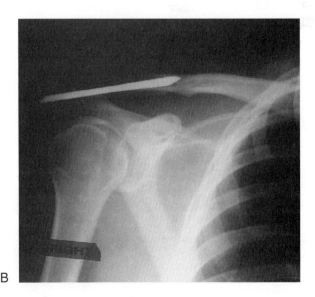

B

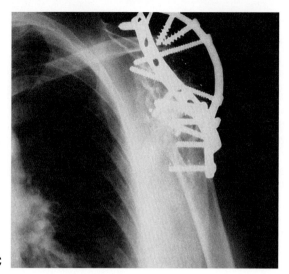

C

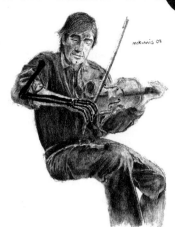

RADIOLOGIC EVALUATION OF THE ELBOW

The elbow is the anatomic junction between the arm and forearm. Whereas the shoulder functions to place the upper extremity anywhere within the wide sphere of its range of motion, the elbow functions to adjust the extremity's height and length and the functional position of the hand to accomplish prehensile tasks efficiently. The elbow's three separate synovial articulations housed within one joint capsule present unique challenges to clinicians involved in treating trauma and dysfunction at this joint.

Review of Anatomy[1–8]

Osseous Anatomy

Elbow Joint

The bones of the elbow are the distal humerus, the proximal ulna, and the proximal radius (Fig. 16-1). The articulation between the humerus and ulna is the humeroulnar joint. The articulation between the humerus and radius is the humeroradial joint. The articulation between the proximal portions of the ulna and radius is the proximal radioulnar joint. These three separate articulations are within a common joint capsule and together make up the *elbow joint.*

Distal Humerus

The humeral shaft expands at its distal end into medial and lateral humeral condyles. The articular portions of these condyles are the trochlea and capitulum. The spool-shaped trochlea is divided by a semicircular groove or trochlear sulcus. The trochlea is on the medial aspect of the distal humerus and articulates with the ulna. The rounded capitulum, also called the capitellum, is on the lateral aspect and articulates with the radius. The medial and lateral epicondyles are projections located proximally to the trochlea and capitulum, respectively. The distal humerus is marked by three depressions or fossae. Anteriorly, the coronoid fossa and radial fossa receive the ulnar coronoid process and radial head at full elbow flexion. Posteriorly, the olecranon fossa receives the ulnar olecranon process at elbow extension.

Proximal Ulna

The proximal ulna has two beak-like processes: the large olecranon process at its tip and the coronoid process on its anterior surface. Between these two processes lies the articular concave trochlear notch, which receives the trochlea. The shallow radial notch on the lateral side of the ulna articulates with the radial head.

Proximal Radius

The proximal radius is distinguished by a head, a neck, and a tuberosity. The radial head is disk-like and cupped on its upper end, articulating with the capitulum above and the ulna medially. The neck is the constricted area below the head, and the tuberosity is an oval prominence distal to the neck.

Forearm

The radial and ulnar bones together are referred to as the bones of the forearm. These bones are articulated with each other proximally, as just noted: through their shafts via the strong interosseous membrane and distally at the distal radioulnar joint, a pivot joint formed between the head of the ulna and ulnar notch of the radius. The forearm articulates to the wrist at the radiocarpal joint, formed by the distal radius, the articular disk of the distal radioulnar joint, and the proximal row of carpal bones.

Ligamentous Anatomy

Approximately half of the elbow's stability is provided by the bony configuration of the joint, and the remainder of its stability results primarily from the joint capsule and its medial and lateral ligamentous reinforcements (Fig. 16-2). The *ulnar (medial) collateral ligament* attaches to the medial humeral epicondyle and extends in a broad triangular expanse to the olecranon. The *radial (lateral) collateral ligament* attaches to the lateral humeral epicondyle and extends to the annular ligament and radial notch of the ulna.

The *annular ligament* of the radius is an oval band enclosing the head of the radius and attaching to the anterior and posterior margins of the radial notch of the ulna. The radial head is able to rotate within this ligamentous sling, which provides its articular stability to the ulna.

The main muscles acting on the elbow joint are the triceps, biceps, and brachialis. They also are potentially important factors in joint stability.

Joint Mobility

The humeroulnar and humeroradial joints of the elbow function as hinge joints, permitting extension and flexion through a range from 0 to 135 degrees or greater. The proximal radioulnar joint is a trochoid joint, allowing approximately 90 degrees each of forearm pronation and supination.

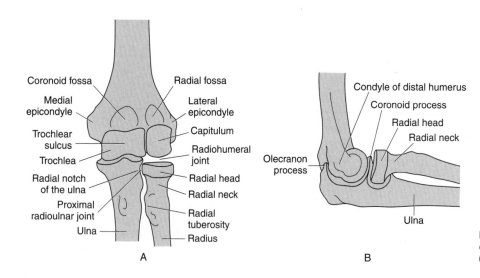

Figure 16-1 Osseous anatomy of the elbow: **(A)** anterior aspect (left elbow), **(B)** lateral aspect (right elbow).

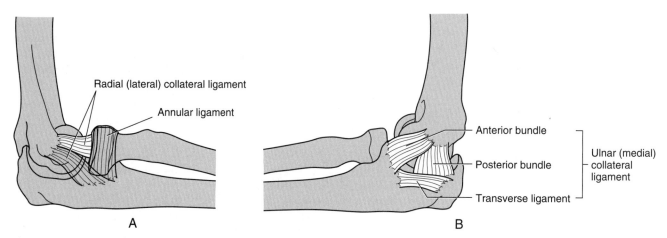

Figure 16-2 Ligaments of the elbow joint, from **(A)** the lateral aspect and **(B)** the medial aspect.

Growth and Development

Ossification of the elbow begins in the shafts of the humerus, ulna, and radius in the eighth week of fetal life. At birth only these structures are ossified and visible on radiograph (Fig. 16-3). The elbow joint is entirely cartilaginous at birth.

The remaining architecture of the elbow is formed by seven secondary ossification centers. Four secondary ossification centers belong to the humerus:

- The center for the capitulum and the lateral portion of the trochlea appears in infancy.
- The center for the medial epicondyle appears after age 5 (Fig. 16-4A).
- The center for the medial trochlea appears around age 10.
- The center for the lateral epicondyle appears around age 14.

The capitulum and trochlea coalesce to form one epiphysis by puberty (Fig. 16-4B).

Three secondary ossification centers belong to the forearm:

- The center for the radial head appears around age 5.
- The center for the proximal ulna appears around age 11.
- Occasionally a separate center for the radial tuberosity appears around puberty.

All of these secondary centers complete fusion in the mid-to-late teenage years, with girls showing earlier bone maturation than boys.

Routine Radiologic Evaluation[9–19]

Practice Guidelines for Radiography of the Elbow in Children and Adults[9]

The American College of Radiology (ACR), the principal professional organization of radiologists, defines practice guidelines to assist practitioners in providing appropriate radiologic care for patients. These guidelines exist as an educational tool to direct a reasonable course of action.

Goals

The goal of the radiographic examination at the elbow is to identify or exclude anatomic abnormalities or disease processes.

Indications

The indications for radiologic examination include but are not limited to trauma, including suspected physical abuse; osseous changes secondary to metabolic disease, systemic disease, or nutritional deficiencies; neoplasms; infections; primary non-neoplastic bone pathologies; arthropathies; preoperative, postoperative, and follow-up studies; congenital syndromes and developmental disorders; vascular lesions; evaluation of soft tissue (as for suspected foreign body); pain; and correlation of abnormal skeletal findings on other imaging studies.

Basic Projections, Radiologic Observations, and MRI Anatomy

The minimum recommended projections for the elbow are *anteroposterior (AP)* and *lateral* views. *Oblique* views of the elbow are sometimes included in a facility's protocol or are requested depending on clinical indications.

As with any complex joint, numerous special projections exist to demonstrate different perspectives sought on specific structures. For most screening purposes and typical complaints, however, these standard views suffice.

The radiographic evaluation of trauma at the elbow necessitates the additional evaluation of the forearm. Fracture or dislocation at the proximal radius and ulna is sometimes accompanied by associated trauma at the distal aspects or distal articulations of these bones. Thus, in evaluating trauma cases, the radiographic evaluation of the elbow is not complete without evaluation of the entire forearm. Recommended projections for the forearem include AP and lateral views.

ACR Appropriateness Criteria[20] recommends magnetic resonance imaging (MRI) evaluation for chronic elbow pain if radiographs are nondiagnostic. Normal MRI anatomy is presented in axial, coronal, and sagittal scanning planes.

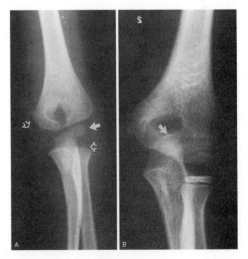

Figure 16-4 (A) Normal radiographic appearance of the elbow in a 5-year-old boy. At this stage of maturity, the secondary ossification center for the capitulum is easily visible (solid arrow). The secondary ossification centers for the medial epicondyle of the humerus and the radial head are just beginning to ossify and are difficult to identify (open arrows). **(B)** Normal radiographic appearance of the elbow in a healthy 11-year-old boy. At this stage of development, the capitulum and the trochlea have coalesced to form one epiphysis. The epiphysis of the radial head and medial epicondyle are also visible. The secondary ossification center for the proximal ulna (arrow) has just begun to ossify and is visible superimposed in the olecranon fossa.

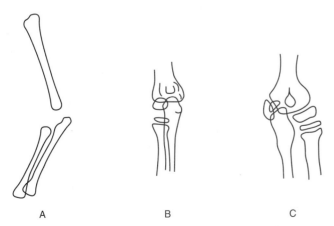

Figure 16-3 Radiographic tracings of the ossified portions of the elbow **(A)** at birth, **(B)** at age 5 years, and **(C)** at age 11 years.

Routine Radiologic Evaluation of the Elbow

Anteroposterior

This view demonstrates the *distal humerus* and *proximal radius* and *ulna* seen in the anatomic position. The visible structures of the distal humerus include the lower third of the *shaft*, the *medial* and *lateral epicondyles*, the *olecranon fossa*, the *capitulum* and the *trochlea*. The *humeroradial joint space* is visible, as is the *humeroulnar joint space*, superimposed by the *olecranon process*.

Radiologic Observations

The important observations are:

1. The patient's arm is in anatomic position, fully extended and externally rotated. The *carrying angle* of the elbow is revealed on this view (Fig. 16-5). Normally the long axis of the forearm forms a valgus angle with the long axis of the humerus. Values for this angle are usually stated as being larger in women, although some researchers have noted no sex difference. Average normal values range from approximately 5 to 15 degrees. Abnormal increases or decreases in this angle may be a sign of fracture or posttraumatic deformity.
2. The olecranon process is articulated in the olecranon fossa in this position of elbow extension. The olecranon process can be visualized superimposed behind the trochlea of the humerus.
3. A portion of the radial head, neck, and tuberosity is superimposed on the ulna.
4. The humeroradial and humeroulnar joint spaces are well demonstrated.

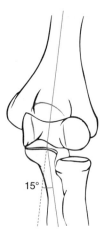

Figure 16-5 The angle formed by the longitudinal axes of the distal humerus and the proximal ulna constitutes the carrying angle of the forearm.

Basic Projections

- **AP**
- Lateral
- Obliques

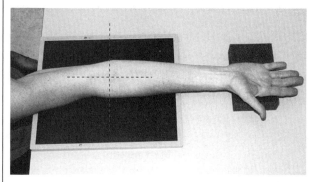

Setting up the Radiograph

Figure 16-6 Patient position for AP radiograph of the right elbow.

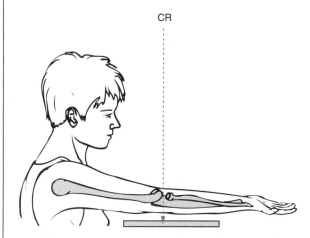

Figure 16-7 The central ray is perpendicular to the elbow joint.

What Can You See?

Look at the radiograph (Fig. 16-8) and try to identify the radiographic anatomy. Trace the outlines of structures using a marker and transparency sheet. Compare results with the book tracing (Fig. 16-9). Can you identify the following:

- Distal humerus (identify the medial and lateral epicondyles, the capitulum, and the trochlea)
- Ulna (identify the olecranon process and shaft)
- Radius (identify the radial head, neck, and tuberosity)
- Humeroulnar and humeroradial joint spaces
- Carrying angle of the elbow (measure by noting the angle of intersection between a line connecting midpoints in the distal humeral shaft and a line connecting midpoints in the proximal ulnar shaft)

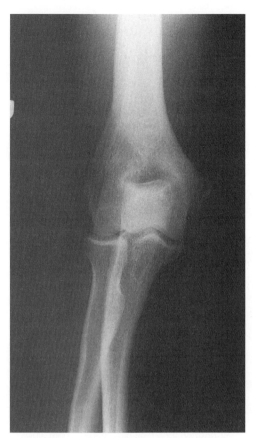

Figure 16-8 AP radiograph of the right elbow.

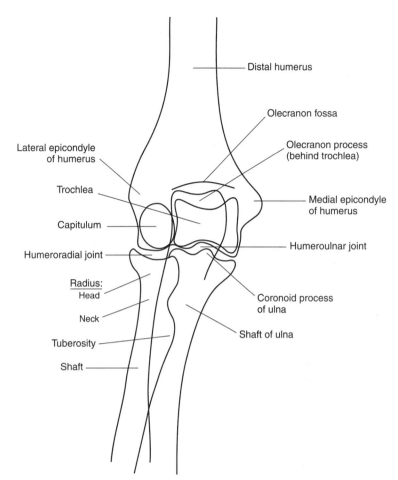

Figure 16-9 Tracing of AP radiograph of right elbow.

Routine Radiologic Evaluation of the Elbow

Lateral

The lateral view, taken with the elbow flexed to 90 degrees, demonstrates the *distal humerus* and *proximal radius* and *ulna*. Visible structures include the *olecranon process*, the anterior portion of the *radial head*, and the *humeroradial joint*.

Radiologic Observations

The important observations are:

1. The olecranon process is seen in profile articulating in the olecranon fossa.
2. The coronoid process of the olecranon is superimposed on the posterior portion of the radial head.
3. Only the anterior portion of the radial head is viewed free of superimposition.
4. In adults, this true lateral projection superimposes structures of the distal humerus, causing distinct images to appear. The directly superimposed medial and lateral epicondyles form a large teardrop-shaped image. Below this image is a radiodense circular image, partially surrounded by concentric arcs. The circular image is produced by the trochlear sulcus. The inner concentric arcs are formed by the rims of the capitulum and trochlea. The outermost arc is formed by the trochlear notch.
5. In children, the normal position of the capitulum relative to the distal humerus and the proximal radius can be found by the intersection of two lines (Fig. 16-10). A line drawn along the longitudinal axis of the proximal radius (*a* in the figure) normally passes through the center of the capitulum, and a line drawn along the anterior border of the humerus (*b* in the figure) normally intersects the middle third of the capitulum. Disruptions in this relationship are an indication of fracture or other abnormality.
6. The *fat pads* of the coronoid and radial fossae are normally visualized superimposed together as a thin triangular lucency just anterior to the distal humerus. In the presence of joint effusion, the fat pads will displace further anteriorly.

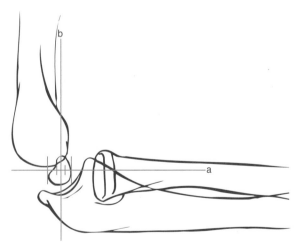

Figure 16-10 The normal position of the capitellum is relative to the distal humerus and proximal radius. Line *a* is drawn along the longitudinal axis of the proximal radius and normally passes through the center of the capitellum. Line *b* is drawn along the anterior border of the humerus and normally intersects the middle third of the capitellum.

Basic Projections

- AP
- **Lateral**
- Obliques

Setting up the Radiograph

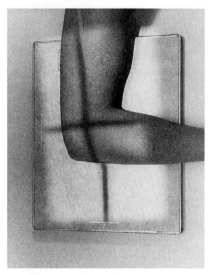

Figure 16-11 Patient position for lateral radiograph of right elbow.

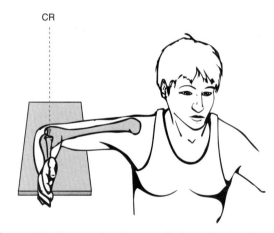

Figure 16-12 The central ray is perpendicular to the elbow joint.

What Can You See?

Look at the radiograph (Fig. 16-13) and try to identify the radiographic anatomy. Trace the outlines of structures using a marker and transparency sheet. Compare results with the book tracing (Fig. 16-14). Can you identify the following:

- Olecranon (identify the olecranon process and the coronoid process)
- Radius (identify the radial head, neck, and tuberosity)
- Distal humerus (identify the epicondyles and the concentric images of the trochlear sulcus, capitulum, trochlear rims, and trochlear notch)
- Radiolucent image representing the anterior fat pads

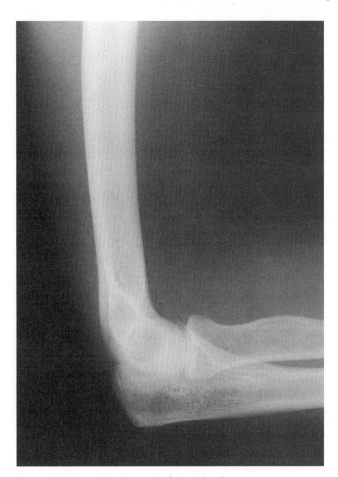

Figure 16-13 Lateral radiograph of the right elbow.

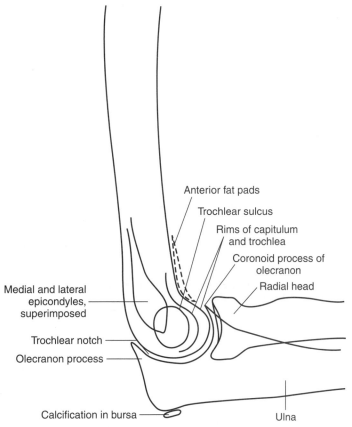

Anterior fat pads

Trochlear sulcus

Rims of capitulum and trochlea

Coronoid process of olecranon

Radial head

Medial and lateral epicondyles, superimposed

Trochlear notch

Olecranon process

Calcification in bursa

Ulna

Figure 16-14 Tracing of lateral radiograph of the elbow.

Routine Radiologic Evaluation of the Elbow

Obliques

Oblique views of the elbow may be obtained with the patient's arm in internal or external rotation. The choice is determined by the specific area of interest. The elbow is in full extension for either projection.

Oblique: Internal Rotation

The internal oblique view is obtained with the patient's extended arm and forearm internally rotated 90 degrees from the anatomic position, or *pronated*. This position crosses the proximal radius over the ulna, superimposing most of these structures. The *coronoid process*, however, is visible without superimposition and is best demonstrated on this view.

Radiologic Observations

The important observations are:

1. The coronoid process is visualized free of superimposition.
2. The olecranon process is articulated in the olecranon fossa.
3. The joint space between the trochlear notch and trochlea is visible.

Basic Projections

- AP
- Lateral
- **Oblique, internal rotation**

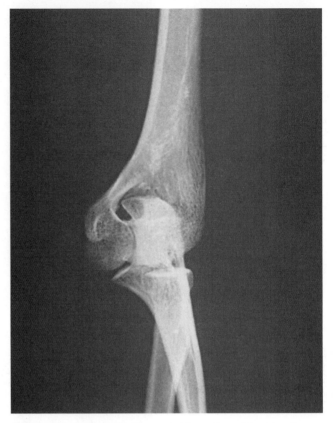

Figure 16-16 Radiograph of internal oblique view of the right elbow.

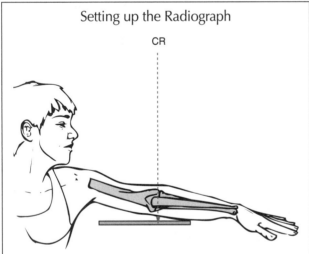

Setting up the Radiograph

CR

Figure 16-15 Patient position for external oblique view of the elbow. The central ray is perpendicular to the arm and enters at the elbow joint.

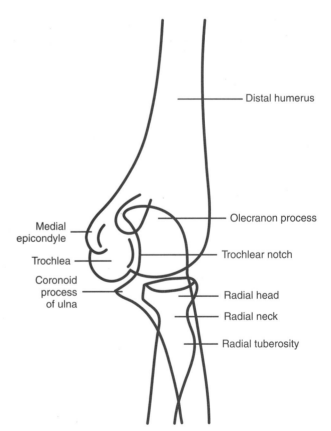

Distal humerus

Olecranon process

Medial epicondyle

Trochlear notch

Trochlea

Coronoid process of ulna

Radial head

Radial neck

Radial tuberosity

Figure 16-17 Tracing of radiograph of internal oblique view of the right elbow.

Routine Radiologic Evaluation of the Elbow

Oblique: External Rotation

The external oblique view is obtained with the patient's extended arm and forearm externally rotated 45 degrees from the anatomic position, or fully *supinated*. This position best demonstrates the *radial head, neck, and tuberosity* viewed free of any superimposition.

Radiologic Observations

The important observations are:

1. The radial head, neck, and tuberosity are visualized free of superimposition.
2. The capitulum and lateral epicondyle are viewed in profile.
3. The humeroulnar and humeroradial joint spaces are visible.

Basic Projections

- AP
- Lateral
- **Oblique, external rotation**

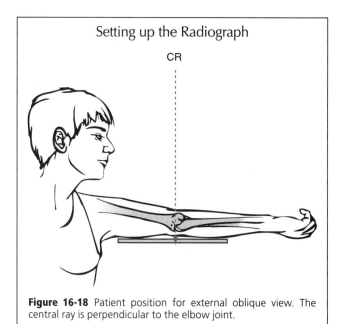

Setting up the Radiograph

CR

Figure 16-18 Patient position for external oblique view. The central ray is perpendicular to the elbow joint.

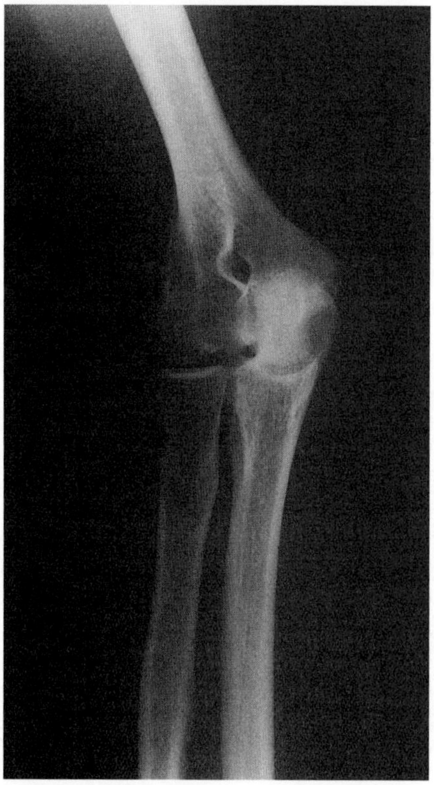

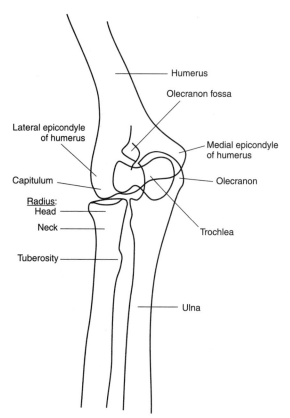

Figure 16-19 Radiograph of external oblique view of the right elbow.

Labels (Figure 16-20): Humerus; Olecranon fossa; Lateral epicondyle of humerus; Medial epicondyle of humerus; Capitulum; Olecranon; Radius: Head; Neck; Trochlea; Tuberosity; Ulna

Figure 16-20 Tracing of radiograph of external oblique view of the right elbow.

Routine Radiologic Evaluation of the Forearm

Anteroposterior

This view demonstrates the elbow, the entire radius and ulna, and the wrist.

Radiologic Observations

The important observations are:

1. The patient's elbow is extended and the forearm is in the anatomic position.
2. The entire length of the radius and ulna is visible. Note the normal bowing and contour of the shafts.
3. The olecranon is articulated in the olecranon fossa and is superimposed on the trochlea.
4. Both the proximal and distal articulations of the forearm are visible. Elbow and wrist joint spaces will appear only partially open because of x-ray beam divergence over the length of the film. (Note that some facilities may include only the wrist articulation if the elbow has already been demonstrated on AP elbow projection.)

Basic Projections

- **AP**
- Lateral

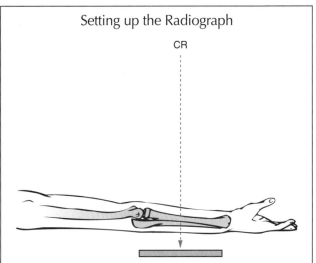

Setting up the Radiograph

CR

Figure 16-21 Patient position for AP view of the right forearm. The central ray is perpendicular to the forearm and enters the forearm at its midpoint.

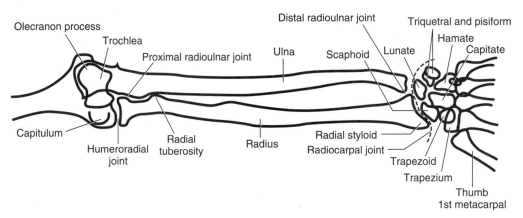

Figure 16-22 Radiograph of AP view of the right forearm.

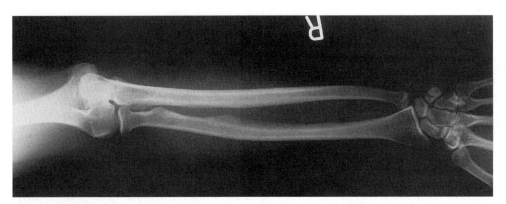

Figure 16-23 Tracing of AP view of the right forearm.

Routine Radiologic Evaluation of the Forearm

Lateral

This view demonstrates the *elbow,* the entire length of the *radius* and *ulna,* and the *wrist,* seen in profile.

Radiologic Observations

The important observations are:

1. The patient's elbow is flexed, and the forearm is resting on its ulnar border, supinated approximately 45 degrees.
2. Much of the radius and ulna are superimposed over each other. Note the normal bowing and contour of the shafts.
3. Elbow structures are as described on the lateral view of the elbow.
4. The radial head is superimposed on the coronoid process.
5. Both the proximal and distal articulations of the forearm are visible. Elbow and wrist joint spaces appear only partially open because of beam divergence.

Basic Projections

- AP
- **Lateral**

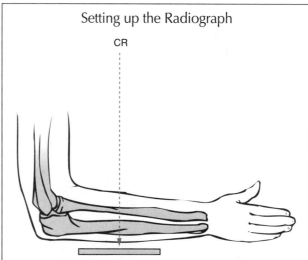

Setting up the Radiograph

CR

Figure 16-24 Patient position for lateral view of the right forearm. The central ray is perpendicular to the forearm and enters at the midpoint.

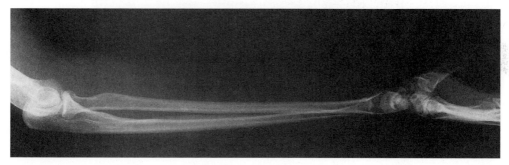

Figure 16-25 Lateral radiograph of the right forearm.

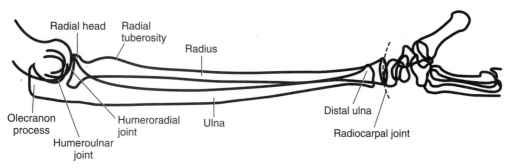

Radial head   Radial tuberosity   Radius

Olecranon process   Humeroradial joint   Ulna   Distal ulna   Radiocarpal joint

Humeroulnar joint

Figure 16-26 Tracing of lateral radiograph of the right forearm.

Magnetic Resonance Imaging of the Elbow

Chronic elbow pain can be caused by a variety of bony or soft tissue abnormalities. Radiographs may reveal the cause of the problem and be sufficient to direct conservative treatment. However, when radiographs are nondiagnostic and conservative treatment has failed, MRI is recommended for most clinical conditions. Normal MRI anatomy displayed in T1-weighted images follows.

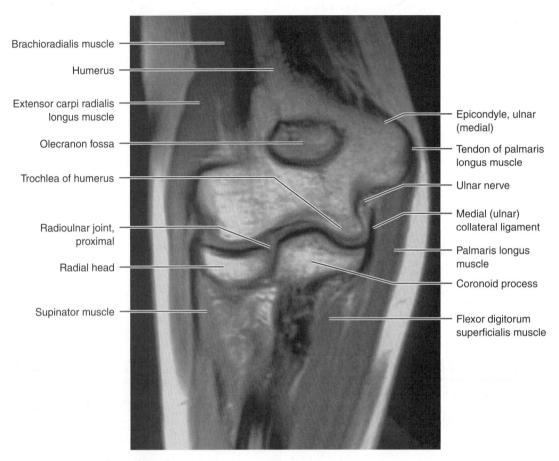

Brachioradialis muscle

Humerus

Extensor carpi radialis longus muscle

Olecranon fossa

Trochlea of humerus

Radioulnar joint, proximal

Radial head

Supinator muscle

Epicondyle, ulnar (medial)

Tendon of palmaris longus muscle

Ulnar nerve

Medial (ulnar) collateral ligament

Palmaris longus muscle

Coronoid process

Flexor digitorum superficialis muscle

Figure 16-27 Coronal MRI of the elbow.

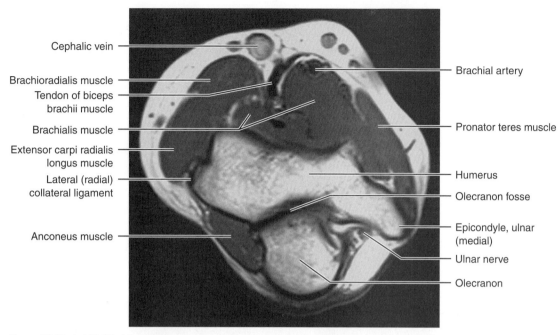

Cephalic vein

Brachioradialis muscle

Tendon of biceps brachii muscle

Brachialis muscle

Extensor carpi radialis longus muscle

Lateral (radial) collateral ligament

Anconeus muscle

Brachial artery

Pronator teres muscle

Humerus

Olecranon fosse

Epicondyle, ulnar (medial)

Ulnar nerve

Olecranon

Figure 16-28 Axial MRI of the elbow at the level of the humeral epicondyles.

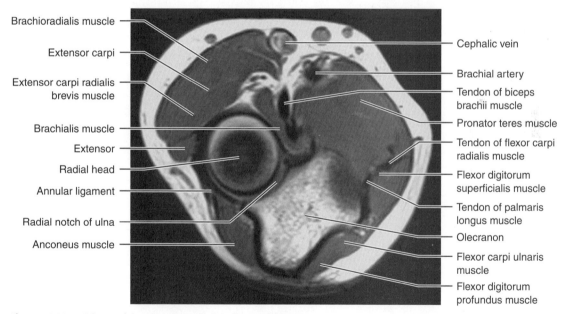

Brachioradialis muscle

Extensor carpi

Extensor carpi radialis brevis muscle

Brachialis muscle

Extensor

Radial head

Annular ligament

Radial notch of ulna

Anconeus muscle

Cephalic vein

Brachial artery

Tendon of biceps brachii muscle

Pronator teres muscle

Tendon of flexor carpi radialis muscle

Flexor digitorum superficialis muscle

Tendon of palmaris longus muscle

Olecranon

Flexor carpi ulnaris muscle

Flexor digitorum profundus muscle

Figure 16-29 Axial MRI of the elbow at the level of the radial head.

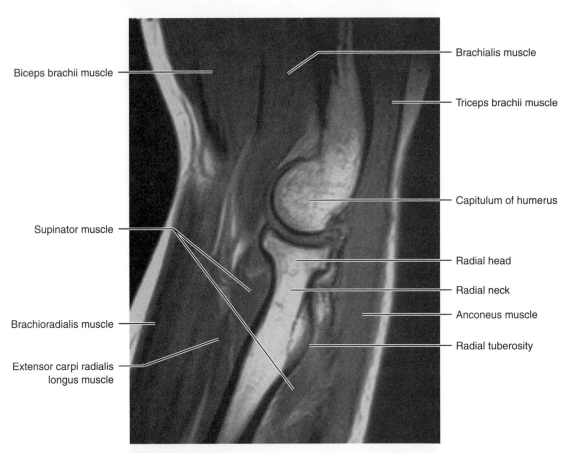

Biceps brachii muscle

Brachialis muscle

Triceps brachii muscle

Capitulum of humerus

Supinator muscle

Radial head

Radial neck

Anconeus muscle

Brachioradialis muscle

Radial tuberosity

Extensor carpi radialis longus muscle

Figure 16-30 Sagittal MRI of the elbow through the humeroradial joint.

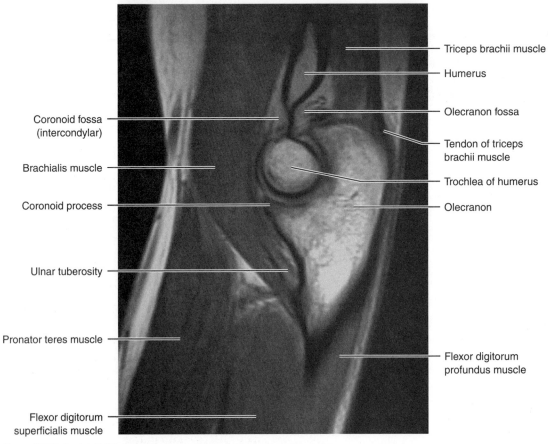

Triceps brachii muscle

Humerus

Coronoid fossa (intercondylar)

Olecranon fossa

Tendon of triceps brachii muscle

Brachialis muscle

Trochlea of humerus

Coronoid process

Olecranon

Ulnar tuberosity

Pronator teres muscle

Flexor digitorum profundus muscle

Flexor digitorum superficialis muscle

Figure 16-31 Sagittal MRI of the elbow joint through the humeroulnar joint.

Trauma at the Elbow[20–80]

Trauma to the elbow is common in all age groups. The mechanism of injury is often a fall on an outstretched hand. Athletic activities also provide occasions for direct trauma as well as repetitive microtrauma and overuse conditions seen in adolescents and young adults.

In general, trauma to the elbow joint is often poorly tolerated in adults. Residual pain, deformity, loss of motion, and posttraumatic arthritic joint changes are not uncommon following elbow fractures, dislocations, or subluxations. Children usually fare better than adults because of greater remodeling capacity. The surgical and postsurgical rehabilitation needs are often challenging to the orthopedist and the therapist, both of whom strive to restore the functional abilities of the joint.

A paradox is observed to exist in the functional potential of the posttraumatic elbow and the radiologic findings of the posttraumatic elbow. Weissman[10] notes that after fracture healing, the final clinical result may not coincide with the final radiographic appearance. That is, "excellent function may coexist with distorted anatomy, and poor function may be present in spite of optimal radiographic appearances."

Diagnostic Imaging for Trauma of the Elbow

The diagnostic imaging evaluation for elbow trauma always begins with routine radiographs of the elbow and forearm. Most fractures, dislocations, and subluxations are adequately demonstrated on these projections. Advanced imaging is warranted if radiographs are negative but the suspicion for fracture is high, or if soft tissue abnormalities need to be evaluated.

Subtle or osteochondral fractures may be diagnosed with either MRI or with computed tomography (CT) if MRI is not available or contraindicated. In some cases of complex fractures, three-dimensionally reformatted CT is used to further characterize the fracture configuration to assist the surgeon in preoperative planning (Fig. 16-32).

Soft tissue injuries or abnormalities of the tendons, ligaments, capsule, cartilage, or synovium may be evaluated by the use of MRI, MR arthrography, or ultrasound. The utility of ultrasound for elbow trauma has been shown to be excellent in the evaluation of medial and lateral epicondylitis, collateral ligament tears, tendon ruptures, bursitis, intra-articular bodies, nerve entrapments, and even occult fractures. Although the use of diagnostic ultrasound at the elbow is increasing, it remains underutilized owing to the limited availability of ultrasonographers with musculoskeletal expertise.

The ACR Appropriateness Guidelines[20] for evaluation of nine variants of chronic elbow pain can be accessed on the text's DavisPlus website at http://www.fadavis.com.

Radiographic Soft Tissue Signs of Trauma

Some subtle fractures may not be easy to see on radiograph. However, the *joint effusion* that *any* fracture produces is much easier to see. At the elbow, this joint effusion creates two abnormal soft tissue signs that are highly associated with fracture. The *positive fat pad sign* and the *abnormal supinator line* are radiographic soft tissue clues to underlying fracture.

Positive Fat Pad Sign

Fat pads are located anteriorly and posteriorly at the fossae of the distal humerus, overlying the joint capsule. Normally, the anterior fat pads of the coronoid and radial fossae are visualized on the lateral radiograph superimposed together as a thin, triangular lucency just anterior to the distal humerus. The posterior fat pad lies deep in the olecranon fossa and is not visible on the lateral radiograph. A positive fat pad sign is produced when an effusion distends the capsule enough to displace the fat pads from their normal position—rendering them visible as radiolucent images within the gray soft tissues. See Figure 2-24 for examples.

Note that although the positive fat pad sign is most often associated with fracture, any condition that produces enough joint effusion will also displace the fat pads. Examples include hemophilia, inflammatory arthritis, infection, intra-articular masses, and osteochondritis dissecans.

Abnormal Supinator Line

The fat plane overlying the supinator muscle, sometimes referred to as the *supinator line*, is normally seen on the lateral radiograph as a thin, lucent line parallel to the anterior aspect of the proximal third of the radius approximately 1 cm from the anterior margin of the radius. In virtually all cases of acute radial head fracture, this line may become elevated, widened, or blurred. Conditions other than trauma causing this abnormal soft tissue sign include infection and inflammatory diseases.

Fractures and Dislocations[11,20–33]

Mechanism of Injury

Most fractures and dislocations at the elbow result from falls on an outstretched hand with or without an abduction or adduction component, or a force applied through a flexed elbow. Fractures of the radial and ulnar shafts are more often caused by direct trauma, often associated with violent blows, motor vehicle accidents, or falls from heights.

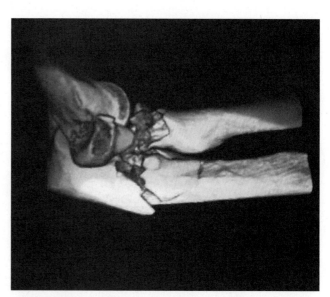

Figure 16-32 Three-dimensional CT reformation of the elbow. A displaced fracture of the proximal ulna and proximal radius is shown. (*Image courtesy of Amy Rasely.*)

Fractures of the Distal Humerus

Fractures of the distal humerus are classified anatomically as (Fig. 16-33):

1. *Supracondylar,* occurring above the condyles
2. *Transcondylar,* occurring across the condyles at the level of the olecranon fossa
3. *Intercondylar,* splitting the condyles apart in a Y or T shape or comminuted configuration
4. *Condylar,* involving either the medial or the lateral condyle
5. *Articular,* involving the trochlea or capitulum
6. *Epicondylar,* occurring at the medial or lateral epicondyle

Supracondylar fractures are the second most common of all extremity fractures in children, following fractures of the forearm. Supracondylar fractures are divided into *extension* and *flexion* types. The infrequently seen flexion-type injury displaces the distal fragment anterior to the humeral shaft. The frequently seen extension-type displaces the distal fragment posterior to the humeral shaft and is more likely to be associated with neurovascular damage in the antecubital region (Fig. 16-34). Complications include malunion with resultant *cubitus varus* or *gunstock* deformity, peripheral nerve injury, and Volkmann's ischemia, a form of compartment syndrome due to occlusion of the brachial artery (Fig. 16-35).

Transcondylar fractures occur more often in falls of elderly persons who are compromised by osteoporosis. (Fig. 16-36). *Intercondylar fractures* are the most common distal humeral fracture in adults and result from a direct force that causes the wedgelike olecranon to be driven into the distal humeral articular surface, splitting the condyles.

Condylar fractures are uncommon in adults but are seen with some frequency in children. The oblique fracture line extends through both nonarticular and articular portions of the condyle. Fractures of the lateral condyle are most common, generally thought to occur as a result of a varus force avulsing the condyle.

Articular fractures include fractures of the capitulum and trochlea and are rare in all age groups. When present, the fracture line is usually in the coronal plane, parallel to the anterior surface of the humerus. Because the fracture fragments are largely cartilaginous, radiographs may not always reveal their true size.

Epicondylar fractures are uncommon in adults and, when present, are usually the result of a direct blow, with the prominent medial epicondyle more likely to be involved. In children and adolescents, the medial epicondyle is more commonly injured from avulsion forces sustained through the physeal growth plate (*Little Leaguer's elbow*) or in association with elbow dislocations (see Fig. 3-15).

Radiologic Evaluation

Routine radiographs demonstrate most fractures of the distal humerus sufficiently. At times, MRI or CT is required to delineate patterns of comminution or identify fragments that may be partially cartilaginous.

Treatment

Treatment of all distal humeral fractures is aimed at restoring joint surfaces and articular congruity to achieve functional joint motion.

Nonoperative treatment is the choice in patients with nondisplaced or minimally displaced fragments, or in elderly patients with severe comminution and severe osteopenia.

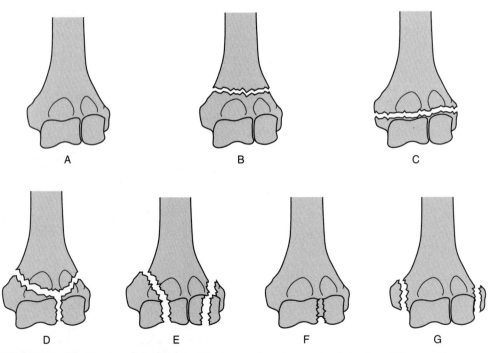

Figure 16-33 Classification of distal humeral fractures as based on anatomic location: **(A)** normal humerus; **(B)** supracondylar fracture; **(C)** transcondylar fracture; **(D)** intercondylar fracture, T- or Y-shaped; **(E)** condylar fracture; **(F)** articular fracture; **(G)** epicondylar fracture. *(Adapted from Greenspan,[6] p. 5.33.)*

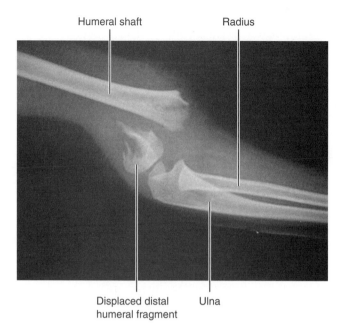

Humeral shaft   Radius

Displaced distal   Ulna
humeral fragment

Figure 16-34 Extension-type supracondylar fracture of the distal humerus. The distal humeral fragment is posterior to the shaft.

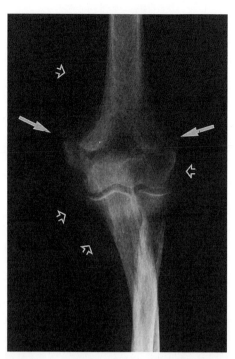

Figure 16-36 Transcondylar fracture of the distal humerus. This 82-year-old man was injured during a fall on his outstretched hand. The fracture is complete, extending transversely through both cortices at the transcondylar level (arrows). Note the excessive amount of joint effusion seen, confined by the extent of the joint capsule (open arrows).

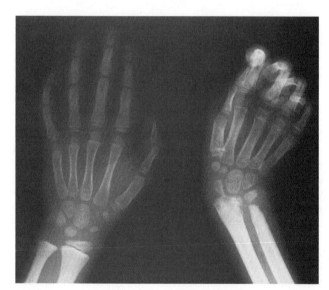

Figure 16-35 Volkmann's ischemia. This is a posteroanterior (PA) view of the hands of a 6-year-old boy. The left hand is normal. The child suffered a supracondylar fracture on the right at the age of 2½. Healing was complicated by occlusion of the brachial artery and infection, which obliterated the biceps muscle, median nerve, and ulnar nerve. The hand is nonfunctional. Note the shortening of the forearm bones, deformity of the distal radius and ulna, diminished size of the carpals and metacarpal bones, contractures of the fingers, and diffuse muscle wasting.

open reduction with plate-and-screw fixation, to resection arthroplasty and prosthetic joint replacement. Fragments may also have to be resected, and ligaments may have to be reattached.

Rehabilitation involves restoration of optimal range of motion and strength at the elbow, forearm, and wrist.

Complications

Loss of motion is the most frequently encountered complication of distal humerus fractures due to malunion deformity, excessive callus formation within the capsule, or arrested growth or overgrowth. Up to a 20-degree loss of condylar-shaft angle may be tolerated because of the compensatory motion of the shoulder. Posttraumatic arthritis can result from direct articular injury or poor joint congruity from malunion deformities. Other complications include the presence of intraarticular loose bodies, myositis ossificans, and associated ulnar nerve injury.

Fractures of the Radial Head

Fractures of the radial head are common in adults, comprising about one-third of all fractures about the elbow. Radial head fractures are divided into four types by the Mason classification system (Figs. 16-37 and 16-38):

- *Type I:* undisplaced fractures, typically treated with immobilization
- *Type II:* displaced fractures with separation, depression, or angulation of the fracture fragment, treated conservatively or by radial head excision if the articular surface is significantly displaced

General practice is to support the extremity in a long-arm posterior splint with 90 degrees of elbow flexion for at least 6 weeks or until adequate callus formation is present. The exception is flexion-type supracondylar fractures, which are supported in relative elbow extension.

Operative treatment is indicated for open fractures, displaced fractures, or associated vascular injury. Repair may range from closed reduction with percutaneous pinning, to

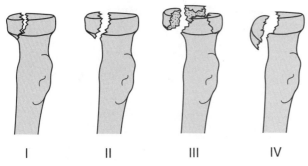

Figure 16-37 The Mason classification of radial head fractures identifies three types of injury patterns: type I, undisplaced fractures; type II, marginal fractures with displacement; and type III, comminuted fractures. Type IV fractures were later suggested to encompass radial head fractures associated with dislocation. *(Adapted from Greenspan,[6] p. 5.37.)*

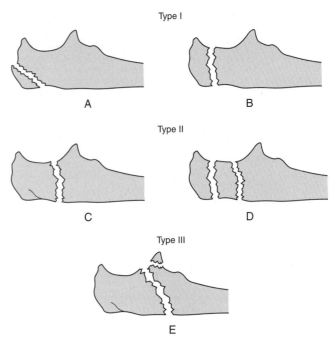

Figure 16-39 Classification of olecranon fractures. Type I are fractures of the proximal third of the olecranon, subdivided into **(A)** extra-articular and **(B)** intra-articular groups. Type II are fractures of the middle third, subdivided into **(C)** one or **(D)** two fracture lines. Type III are fractures of the distal third **(E)**. The most common is type II. *(Adapted from Greenspan,[6] p. 5.40.)*

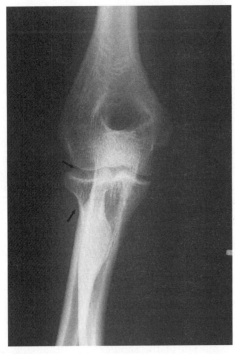

Figure 16-38 Radial head fracture. The arrows mark the ends of the fracture line, which extends longitudinally through the articular surface of the radial head. The fracture fragment shows minimal depression and displacement. This fracture is probably classified as a type I fracture in the Mason classification system.

Treatment

Nonoperative treatment for minimally displaced fractures consists of sling immobilization and early range-of-motion exercises. Operative treatment for severe displacement or comminution includes radial head is excision just proximal to the annular ligament or prosthetic replacement of the radial head to prevent proximal migration. If this migration causes significant pain or impaired function, radioulnar synostosis may be necessary.

Complications

Some complications associated with radial head fractures are related to initially unrecognized associated injuries, including wrist pain secondary to interosseous ligament, complex tears of the triangular fibrocartilage, and capitular osteochondral injuries. Prolonged pain or swelling may be an indication of an underlying pathology. Posttraumatic arthritis may occur, especially if free osteochondral fragments are present or if joint congruity is disrupted.

Fractures of the Proximal Ulna

Fractures of the proximal ulna that disrupt the trochlear notch have the potential to impair both flexion–extension mobility and mediolateral stability at the elbow. Olecranon fractures are generally classified as undisplaced, displaced, or comminuted. The fracture line may be extra-articular, confined to the olecranon tip, or intra-articular, extending to the articular surface (Fig. 16-39).

- *Type III:* comminuted fractures, generally treated by radial head resection
- *Type IV:* radial head fractures associated with elbow dislocations, treated after reduction based on the amount of displacement or comminution present[5,17]

Radiologic Evaluation

These fractures are adequately demonstrated radiographically on the AP, lateral, and oblique views.

Radiologic Evaluation

Fractures of the olecranon are well demonstrated on routine AP and lateral radiographs (Fig. 16-40). The internal oblique view demonstrates the coronoid process free of superimposition.

Treatment

Nonoperative treatment for undisplaced fractures includes immobilization in a posterior splint or long-arm cast with the elbow flexed; range-of-motion exercises are initiated at 2 weeks after injury. Displaced fractures are most often treated operatively with open reduction and internal fixation via plate-and-screw fixation.

Complications

Limited motion complicates up to half of proximal ulnar fractures. Stable internal fixation and early motion is thought to minimize loss of motion. Loose bodies and posttraumatic arthritis can complicate intra-articular fractures. Ulnar nerve symptoms may be secondary to the original injury or after surgical fixation, but often resolve spontaneously without definitive treatment. Triceps strength may be decreased secondary to the elongation of the muscle in the immobilization position. An unrecognized coronoid process fracture that goes untreated may fail to unite, leading to chronic instability in the joint.

Fractures of the Forearm

Fractures of both the radial and the ulnar shaft are usually displaced fractures, due to the severity of force necessary to injure both bones (Fig. 16-41).

Fractures of the radial shaft alone usually occur in the distal third of the shaft; the proximal third is rarely fractured due to the protection of surrounding muscle. Fractures in the distal third of the radial shaft are often associated with subluxation or dislocation of the distal radioulnar joint. This fracture–dislocation pattern is known as *Galeazzi's fracture* (Fig. 16-42). The injury sustained at the distal radioulnar joint injury may be purely ligamentous tearing or may be avulsion of the ligament at the ulnar styloid. In children, fractures of the distal third radial shaft are the most common of all fractures in the body. The relative weakness of the metaphyseal region that has not yet remodeled is probably accountable for the susceptibility of this area to fracture.

Fractures of the ulnar shaft alone are fairly common. The mechanism of injury is most often a direct blow to a defensive maneuver, earning this fracture the name *nightstick*

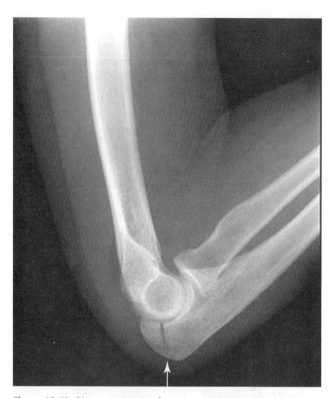

Figure 16-40 Olecranon process fracture, type I, intra-articular. On this lateral radiograph, the fracture line is vertical and extends into the trochlear notch (arrow).

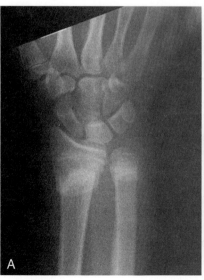
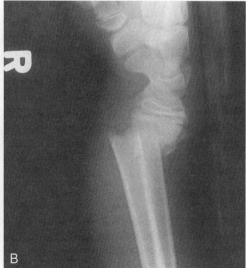

Figure 16-41 Fractures of the radial and ulnar shafts. This 14-year-old boy was injured when he was thrown from a dirt bike. **(A)** This PA view of the wrist demonstrates complete, transverse, displaced fractures at the level of the metaphyses of both the radius and ulna. **(B)** This lateral view of the wrist demonstrates the great amount of displacement and overriding of the fracture fragments, not appreciated on the PA view. Note the soft tissue outline paralleling the deformity. Despite the great amount of displacement, this fracture was successfully treated with closed reduction and cast immobilization. There was no residual deformity.

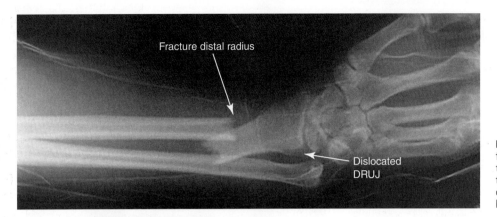

Fracture distal radius

Dislocated DRUJ

Figure 16-42 AP radiograph of the forearm demonstrates the combination of fracture at the distal third of the radial shaft and dislocation of the distal radioulnar joint, commonly known as *Galeazzi's fracture*.

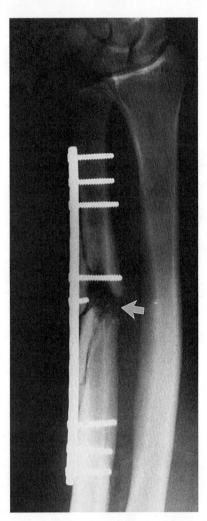

Figure 16-43 Fracture of the ulnar shaft. This 35-year-old man was injured when he was accidentally struck with a baseball bat. This severely comminuted midshaft fracture also demonstrates a segment of bone loss (arrow). This postoperative AP film of the forearm demonstrates a combination of side plate and screw fixation, which has successfully reduced the fragments and preserved the distal radioulnar joint.

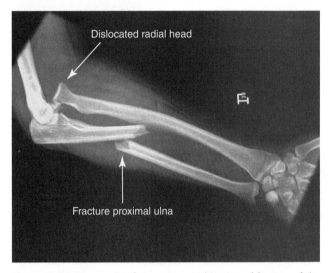

Dislocated radial head

Fracture proximal ulna

Figure 16-44 *Monteggia's fracture* is a combination of fracture of the proximal third of the ulna with dislocation of the radial head. *(Source of image: www.xray2000.co.uk.)*

Radiologic Evaluation

The imaging evaluation of forearm fractures begins with routine radiographs of both the elbow and forearm, including the wrist. The additional projections are necessary because the anatomic relationships of the radius and ulna form a ring-like configuration, and fracture at one site may disrupt an adjacent articulation. Also, associated fractures may simultaneously occur at the wrist or distal humerus.

Treatment

Fractures of both the radius and ulnar shafts often require open reduction and internal fixation to correct angular and rotational deformities in order to regain normal supination and pronation mobility.

Most fractures of the radial shaft alone are treated nonoperatively with cast immobilization. Undisplaced fractures occurring *proximal* to the level of insertion of the pronator teres are treated by immobilization with the forearm in nearly full supination to prevent the unopposed pull of the supinator brevis and biceps brachii from subsequently displacing the proximal fracture fragment. Fractures occurring *distal* to the insertion of the pronator teres do not require immobilization in this manner, because the pronator teres balances the pull of the supinators.

fracture (Fig. 16-43). A common fracture–dislocation injury involving the ulnar shaft is known by the eponym *Monteggia's fracture* (Fig. 16-44). This eponym refers to a fracture of the proximal third of the ulna combined with dislocation of the radial head.

Fracture–dislocations usually require operative treatment to restore supination–pronation mobility and avoid posttraumatic arthritis at the distal radioulnar joint.

Ulnar shaft fractures are treated with immobilization if undisplaced, but displaced fractures generally require open reduction and internal fixation.

Complications

The common complications of forearm fractures include distal radioulnar dysfunction, loss of motion, and arthritic changes at the wrist. Malunion can be caused by improper positioning in the cast or failure to perform cast changes as needed.

In children, the incidence of radial shaft refracture is as high as 12%, and refracture may occur up to 1 year after injury. Precautions are advised against return to active sports for at least 1 month after cast removal. Overgrowth is not uncommon for the 6- to 8-month period after injury. The average amount is 6 to 7 mm and is considered functionally insignificant.

Monteggia's fracture–dislocation may be compromised by radial head instability and nonunion. Damage to the radial and medial nerves is associated with this injury.

Dislocations of the Elbow

Elbow dislocations are most often due to a fall on an outstretched hand that levers the olecranon away from the trochlea. Dislocations of the elbow joint are described by the direction that the radius and ulna have displaced in relation to the distal humerus (Fig. 16-45). Three types of elbow dislocations are those involving:

1. Only the radius
2. Only the ulna
3. Both the radius and ulna together

The most common type, accounting for 80% to 90% of all elbow dislocations, involves both the radius and the ulna, displaced in a posterior or posterolateral direction (see Fig. 3-16).

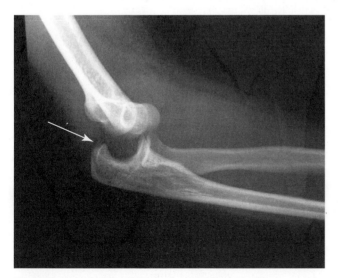

Figure 16-45 Dislocations of the elbow are named in reference to the direction in which the radius and ulna have displaced in relationship to the distal humerus. Posterior, or posterolateral, dislocations, shown here, are the most common.

Imaging Evaluation

Dislocations are readily diagnosed on routine AP and lateral radiographs. The presence of dislocation signals the possibility of associated injury to the forearm or wrist; therefore radiographs of the forearm, including the wrist, are obtained to complete the evaluation.

Treatment

Conservative treatment consists of closed reduction under sedation and analgesia, followed by short-term sling immobilization with early active elbow range-of motion-exercise. Recovery of motion and strength may require 3 to 6 months' time.

Operative treatment is required for cases in which bony or soft tissue entrapment prevents successful closed reduction or in which a large displaced coronoid fragment is present, which may contribute to joint instability.

Complications

Complications include loss of motion with prolonged immobilization, calcification of the collateral ligaments and capsule, development of myositis ossificans, typically seen in an extensively damaged brachialis muscle, and ulnar or median nerve injury.

Abnormal Conditions at the Elbow[11,34–80]

Epicondylitis[34–52]

Medial epicondylitis (golfer's elbow) and *lateral epicondylitis (tennis elbow)* are overuse injuries characterized in the acute stage by tendinitis (Fig. 16-46A,B). Chronically, a tendinosis develops due to the repetitive stress, which prevents the tendon from healing normally.

Medial epicondylitis affects the flexor muscle group at the musculotendinous junction and its origin on the medial epicondyle. It is the most common cause of medial elbow pain. Lateral epicondylitis is seen with much greater frequency and involves the musculotendinous junction of the extensor carpi radialis brevis muscle at the lateral epicondyle. The underlying collateral ligamentous complex and joint capsule also have been implicated.

Imaging Evaluation

Radiographs are used to rule out associated disorders such as intra-articular loose bodies, bony avulsions, osteoarthritis, or calcification in the tendons. MRI is recommended in patients whose radiographs are nondiagnostic and whose pain does not respond to conservative treatment. MRI can rule out associated disorders, assess the collateral ligaments, and identify degenerative tissue. Ultrasound, if available, is recommended as an alternative to MRI.

Treatment

The mainstay of treatment is nonsurgical. Many treatments are discussed in the literature, including physical therapy exercises; thermal modalities; low-level laser therapy; Cyriax protocol manipulation; supportive bracing; and injections of corticosteroids, blood, or botulinum toxin. For recalcitrant tendinosis, many traditional open, arthroscopic, and percutaneous surgical procedures have been described, including débridement of tissue, tendon release, decortication of the epicondyle, and radiofrequency microtenotomy. No single intervention, nonsurgical or surgical, has been proven to be most efficient.

Osteochondritis Dissecans[53-80]

Osteochondritis dissecans (OCD) is a localized joint injury that involves a separation of a segment of cartilage and subchondral bone from the articular surface (Fig. 16-47A,B). Over 75% of cases occur at the knee, but the elbow, ankle, and wrist are also susceptible. In the elbow joint, the most common site of OCD is in the anterolateral aspect of the capitellum. It is theorized that repeated valgus stress, a tenuous blood supply within the capitellum, and disparity in

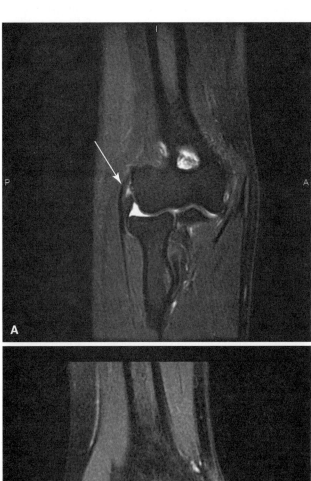

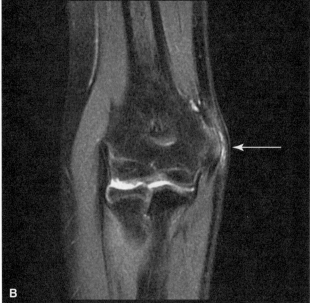

Figure 16-46 T2-weighted coronal MRIs demonstrating epicondylitis. **(A)** *Lateral epicondylitis* is characterized by high signal intensity in the origin of the common extensor tendon which involves the lateral collateral ligament (arrow). **(B)** *Medial epicondylitis* is characterized by marrow edema at the medial epicondyle, increased signal at the origin of the common flexor tendon, and subcutaneous edema of the soft tissues (arrow).

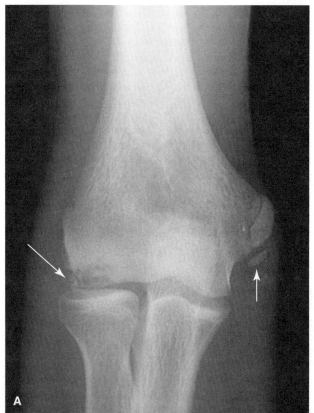

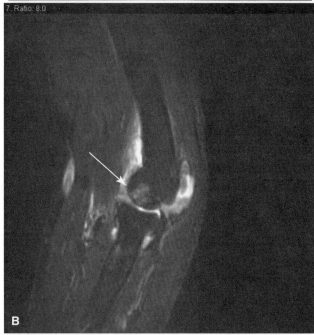

Figure 16-47 Osteochondritis dissecans of the capitellum. **(A)** AP radiograph demonstrates the defect as a radiolucent lesion with irregular ossification (large arrow). An intra-articular loose body has migrated to the medial side of the joint (small arrow). Note the open growth plate at the medial epicondyle in this teenage patient. *(Image courtesy of John Hunter, MD, University of California, Davis School of Medicine.)* **(B)** T2-weighted sagittal MRI demonstrates OCD as a localized area of high signal intensity (arrow).

the mechanical properties of the radial head and lateral capitellum factor into the localization of OCD at the capitellum.

OCD typically presents in the young adolescent athlete with open growth plates. Repetitive microtrauma activities such as throwing creates valgus compressive forces in the radiocapitellar joint; a similar mechanism is noted in the upper extremity weight-bearing skills of gymnasts. The pain is usually dull, poorly localized, aggravated with use, and improved with rest.

Imaging Evaluation

Routine radiographs are the first imaging study obtained in the evaluation of OCD. Early in the course of OCD, radiographs may appear without abnormalities. The first radiographic signs include a sclerotic rim of subchondral bone adjacent to the articular surface, irregular ossification, radiolucency due to hyperemia, and a bony defect adjacent to the articular surface. Lateral radiographs may show flattening of the capitellum. Later, the radiographic appearance is based on whether separation of osteochondral fragments occurs. With separation, loose bodies may be visualized within the joint. Note that loose bodies may exist without being evident on radiograph. Without separation, the central sclerotic fragment becomes less distinctive, the rarefaction area ossifies, and the lesion slowly heals. In the late stages of OCD, degenerative changes leading to incongruity between the articulation of the radial head and the capitellum become evident.

MRI is useful for early detection of OCD, and assists in determining the size and extent of the lesion and the vascular supply to the area. On T2-weighted images, separated fragments are noted to have pockets of high signal (fluid) surrounding them.

Ultrasound can demonstrate localized capitellar bony flattening, useful in early detection. Nondisplaced fragments appear as highly echogenic areas in the capitellar subchondral bone. Displaced fragments appear as highly echogenic loose bodies overlying intact subchondral bone.

Treatment

Nonoperative treatment is appropriate for patients who are skeletally immature with an intact lesion and no loose bodies. Activity modification and immobilization are key to the promotion of healing in the subchondral bone and prevention of chondral collapse, subsequent fracture, and crater formation.

Surgical options for the treatment of persistently symptomatic OCD lesions include arthroscopic removal of loose bodies, débridement, microfracture techniques, and osteochondral autografting.

Summary of Key Points

Routine Radiologic Evaluation

1. The routine radiologic evaluation of the elbow includes three projections demonstrating the distal humerus, proximal ulna, proximal radius, and their associated articulations:

   ➤ *Anteroposterior*—The elbow is demonstrated in anatomic position.

   ➤ *Lateral*—The elbow is flexed 90 degrees and the forearm is in neutral.

   ➤ *Oblique*—The elbow is extended and the forearm is either fully pronated (internal oblique) or supinated (external oblique).

2. The routine radiologic evaluation of the forearm includes AP and lateral projections of the entire length of the forearm as well as the articular ends.

Trauma Radiography

3. The radiographic evaluation in trauma cases includes the routine projections plus additional AP and lateral views of the forearm including the wrist. Trauma at the elbow is often associated with fracture or dislocation at these structures.

4. Two abnormal soft issue signs indicative of joint trauma are visible on radiographs:

   ➤ *Fat pad sign*—Fat pads become displaced out of their fossae in response to increased capsular volume from effusion.

   ➤ *Abnormal supinator line*—An elevation or blurring of the outline of the supinator muscle is seen in association with radial head fractures.

5. Advanced imaging is warranted if radiographs are nondiagnostic. Subtle or osteochondral fractures may be diagnosed with either MRI or with CT if MRI is not available or contraindicated. Soft tissue injuries or abnormalities of the tendons, ligaments, capsule, cartilage, or synovium may be evaluated by the use of MRI, MR arthrography, or ultrasound.

Fractures at the Elbow

6. Fractures of the distal humerus are classified by location as supracondylar, transcondylar, intercondylar, articular, or epicondylar. The supracondylar type is the most common elbow fracture in children. The intercondylar type is most common in adults.

7. Fractures of the radial head comprise about one-third of all elbow fractures in adults.

8. Fractures of the proximal ulna that disrupt the trochlear notch have the potential to impair the stability and function of the elbow joint.

9. In children, fractures of the distal radial shaft are the most common of all fractures in the body.

Dislocations at the Elbow

10. Elbow dislocations are described by the direction in which the radius and ulna have displaced in relationship to the distal humerus. The majority of elbow dislocations involve both the radius and ulna displaced in a posterior or posterolateral direction.

Epicondylitis

11. *Medial epicondylitis (golfer's elbow)* and *lateral epicondylitis (tennis elbow)* are overuse injuries characterized by tendinitis that can progress to tendinosis. Radiographs rule out associated disorders; MRI or ultrasound can demonstrate tissue inflammation and tendon degeneration.

Osteochondritis Dissecans of the Capitellum

12. OCD is a localized joint injury that involves a separation of a segment of cartilage and subchondral bone from the articular surface. It typically presents in adolescent athletes. Initial radiographs may be normal. MRI or ultrasound can be used to diagnosis the earliest stages of OCD.

 Please refer to the text's enclosed CD-ROM for the American College of Radiology's current Musculoskeletal Appropriateness Criteria for the following topic: *Chronic Elbow Pain.*

CASE STUDIES

Case Study 1

Distal Humeral Fracture

The patient is an 8-year-old boy evaluated for elbow pain by a physical therapist in an emergency room setting.

History of Trauma

The boy fell off of his skateboard onto an outstretched right hand. His parents took him to the emergency room, where he complained of elbow pain. This emergency room uses physical therapists as screeners for musculoskeletal problems, so a physical therapist was the first professional to examine the patient.

Physical Therapy Examination

Patient Complaint

The patient could not identify a specific location of pain, but complained of generalized elbow pain. He did not experience any numbness or tingling or any other areas of pain.

Physical Examination

The therapist examined the patient and noted diffuse edema about the elbow and tenderness to palpation all around the joint. There was no obvious deformity about the elbow. The patient was very reluctant to move the extremity. Active range of motion was restricted to approximately 30 to 90 degrees, limited by pain. No muscle testing was completed. The radial pulse, capillary refill, and distal sensation were all normal.

Initial Imaging

The physical therapist recommended anteroposterior (AP) and lateral radiographs of the elbow to test the hypothesis of an elbow fracture. The AP radiograph appeared normal, but there were significant findings on the lateral view (Fig. 16-48). Following the posterior cortical margin of the humerus, the therapist noticed a break in the normally smooth contour near the elbow joint (A), indicating a fracture. Assessment of the soft tissues revealed radiolucent shadows both anterior and posterior to the distal humerus (B), suggesting displacement of the fat pads due to joint effusion.

Intervention

The therapist referred the patient to the pediatric orthopedist on call, who confirmed the diagnosis and managed the fracture from that point. Because the fracture was nondisplaced, the

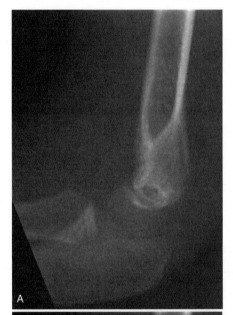
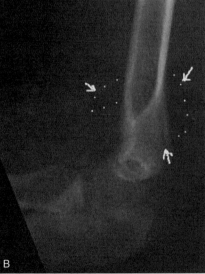

Figure 16-48 (A and B) These are the same lateral radiograph of the elbow. There is a fracture of the posterior border of the distal humerus. **(B)** This view outlines the anterior and posterior fat pads, which have been displaced by the traumatic effusion and are visible within the soft tissues.

orthopedist treated conservatively with immobilization in a long-arm cast. After 3 weeks, the patient's cast was removed and he began rehabilitation.

Discussion

Even though no deformity of the elbow joint was clinically obvious, the therapist had enough evidence (history of trauma, generalized joint edema, unwillingness to move) to support a hypothesis of fracture. Conventional radiographs were the logical choice to confirm this hypothesis. Using the ABCs (alignment, bone density, cartilage, soft tissues) search pattern, the therapist was able to manage the patient efficiently through referral to the appropriate practitioner.

The case is summarized in Figure 16-49.

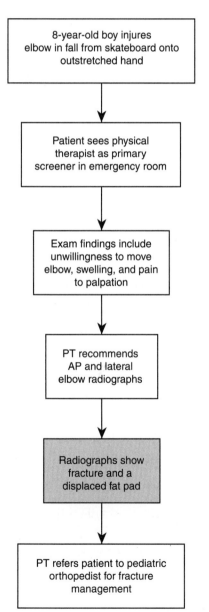

Figure 16-49 Pathway of case study events. Imaging is highlighted.

CRITICAL THINKING POINTS

1. Soft tissue findings on conventional radiographs, such as positive fat pad signs, can serve as reliable clues to underlying pathology.

2. Physical therapists functioning as first-contact musculoskeletal providers should be familiar with the routine radiographic views required to screen a given joint adequately.

3. Physical therapists should be able to assess a radiograph with a basic search pattern and recognize obvious abnormalities.

CASE STUDY 2

Little Leaguer's Elbow

The patient is a 15-year-old male baseball player referred by his primary care physician to physical therapy for examination and treatment of elbow pain.

History

The patient reported gradual onset of right elbow pain over the course of his summer baseball league season. He began to notice an increase in pain after a weekend tournament during which he had pitched a large number of innings. He saw his family physician the following week and was referred to physical therapy. No diagnostic imaging was initially obtained.

Physical Therapy Examination

Patient Complaint

The patient reported pain along the medial aspect of his elbow. All throwing activities aggravated the pain, including easy tossing. The patient stated his elbow was now bothering him even at rest. He had been held out of practice since the weekend tournament.

Physical Examination

Key findings during the physical examination included moderate edema at the medial aspect of the right elbow and tenderness to palpation of the medial epicondyle. Elbow active range of motion was full with minimal discomfort. Resisted tests of the elbow flexors and extensors were also minimally uncomfortable. Resisted wrist flexion was more painful. Valgus stress testing of the elbow was very painful, but no gross instability was noted. Neurovascular examination was normal.

Intervention

The physical therapist decided to proceed with conservative management for 2 weeks and then reexamine the patient. He advised the patient to continue to rest the elbow by avoiding all throwing and upper extremity resistance exercise. His edema was managed by compression and ice.

After 2 weeks, much of the edema had resolved and the patient reported no pain at rest. However, the patient was unable to perform any throwing without severe medial elbow pain. Palpation of the medial epicondyle and valgus stress testing continued to be very painful. The physical therapist discussed the situation with the patient's primary care physician and requested radiographic examination prior to continuing any further physical therapy.

Diagnostic Imaging

The physician ordered conventional radiographs of the patient's elbow. AP and lateral radiographs (Fig. 16-50) were positive for an avulsion fracture of the patient's right medial epicondyle.

Outcome

The primary care physician referred the patient to an orthopedic surgeon with a sports emphasis practice. The surgeon recommended continued conservative management, with no throwing for the next 12 weeks. He planned to reexamine the athlete at that time to decide whether a gradual return to throwing would be possible.

Discussion

The medial epicondyle is a traction apophysis for the medial collateral ligament and the flexor muscles of the wrist. The forces across this physis are tensile rather than compressive. Ossification begins at approximately age 5, but this ossification center fuses with the metaphysis at approximately age 15. Chronic medial epicondylar apophyseal injuries are related to overuse injuries from repetitive throwing, as seen in the skeletally immature baseball player.

Little Leaguer's elbow is the eponym that describes this injury. Valgus extension overload on the elbow produces a traction apophysitis on the medial epicondyle and compression of the lateral side of the joint at the radial head and capitulum. This excessive tension and compression can result not only in avulsion of the apophysis but also in loose bodies, osteochondritis dissecans, and osteoathritis in adulthood.

Radiographic examination can sometimes be challenging. The posteromedial position of the ossification center may be difficult to visualize on the AP view. The medial epicondylar apophysis is sometimes incorrectly identified as a fracture because of the occasionally fragmented appearance of the ossification center and the superimposition of the distal medial metaphysis. Radiologists can request slightly obliqued lateral views to promote better visualization. Complete absence of the apophysis on routine elbow views requires comparison views and a search for the displaced fragment. Fat pad

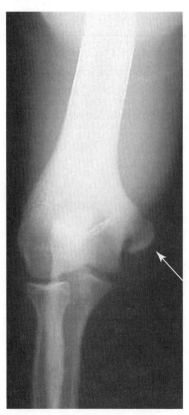

Figure 16-50 AP radiograph demonstrates avulsion of the medial epicondyle.

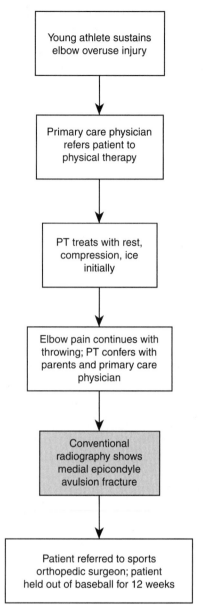

Figure 16-51 Pathway of case study events. Imaging is highlighted.

signs are unreliable because the epicondyles are extra-articular and outside the joint capsule in older children.

The case is summarized in Figure 16-51.

CRITICAL THINKING POINTS

1. A trial of conservative treatment for an unknown injury is always appropriate in the absence of neurovascular compromise. The physical therapist did not prolong the trial of conservative treatment but initiated diagnostic imaging to help make a definitive diagnosis.

2. Prevention is the key to management of Little Leaguer's elbow. Sensible guidelines that limit pitching in practice and games protect young players from overuse injuries. Proper pitching techniques that prevent excessive valgus stress may also reduce injury. Patient and parent education is essential.

Case studies adapted by J. Bradley Barr, PT, DPT, OCS.

References

Normal Anatomy

1. Netter, FH: Atlas of Human Anatomy, ed. 4. WB Saunders, Philadelphia, 2006.
2. Nordin, M, and Frankel, VH: Basic Biomechanics of the Musculoskeletal System, ed. 3. Lippincott Williams & Wilkins, Philadelphia, 2001.
3. Whiting, W, and Zernicke, R: Biomechanics of Musculoskeletal Injury, ed. 2. Human Kinetics, Champaign, IL, 2008.
4. Norkin, CC, and Levangie, PK: Joint Structure and Function: A Comprehensive Analysis, ed. 2. FA Davis, Philadelphia, 1992.
5. Meschan, I: An Atlas of Radiographic Anatomy. WB Saunders, Philadelphia, 1960.
6. Weber, EC, Vilensky, JA, and Carmichael, SW: Netter's Concise Radiologic Anatomy. WB Saunders, Philadelphia, 2008.
7. Kelley, LL, and Peterson, CM: Sectional Anatomy for Imaging Professional, ed. 2. Mosby, St. Louis, MO, 2007.
8. Lazo, DL: Fundamentals of Sectional Anatomy: An Imaging Approach. Thomson Delmar Learning, Clifton Park, NY, 2005.

Routine Exam

9. American College of Radiology: Practice Guideline for the Performance of Radiography of the Extremities. Amended 2006. Accessed October 19, at http://www.acr.org.
10. Weissman, B, and Sledge, C: Orthopedic Radiology. WB Saunders, Philadelphia, 1986.
11. Greenspan, A: Orthopedic Radiology: A Practical Approach, ed. 4. Lippincott Williams & Wilkins, Philadelphia, 2004.
12. Bontrager, KL: Textbook of Radiographic Positioning and Related Anatomy, ed. 6. Mosby, St. Louis, MO, 2005.
13. Fischer, HW: Radiographic Anatomy: A Working Atlas. McGraw-Hill, New York, 1988.
14. Wicke, L: Atlas of Radiographic Anatomy, ed. 5. Lea & Febiger, Malvern, PA, 1994.
15. Frank, E, Smith, B, and Long, B: Merrill's Atlas of Radiographic Positions and Radiologic Procedures, ed. 11. Elsevier Health Sciences, Philadelphia, 2007.
16. Squires, LF, and Novelline, RA: Fundamentals of Radiology, ed. 4. Harvard University Press, Cambridge, MA, 1988.
17. Chew, FS: Skeletal Radiology: The Bare Bones, ed. 2. Williams & Wilkins, Baltimore, 1997.
18. Weir, J, and Abrahams, P: An Atlas of Radiological Anatomy. Yearbook Medical, Chicago, 1978.
19. Krell, L (ed): Clark's Positioning in Radiology, vol. 1, ed. 10. Yearbook Medical, Chicago, 1989.

Trauma/Abnormal Conditions

20. American College of Radiology: Appropriateness Criteria for Chronic Elbow Pain. Reviewed 2008. Available at http://www.acr.org/Secondary MainMenuCategories/quality_safety/app_criteria/pdf/ExpertPanelonMus culoskeletalImaging/ChronicElbowPainDoc6.aspx.
21. Bucholz, RW, Heckman, J, and Court-Brown, C (eds): Rockwood and Green's Fractures in Adults, ed. 6. Lippincott Williams & Wilkins, Philadelphia, 2005.
22. Rockwood, CA, and Green, DP (eds): Fractures in Adults, ed. 5. Lippincott Williams & Wilkins, Philadelphia, 2002.
23. Beaty, J, and Kasar, J (eds): Rockwood and Wilkins' Fractures in Children, ed. 6. Lippincott Williams & Wilkins, Philadelphia, 2005.
24. Koval, KJ, and Zuckerman, JD: Handbook of Fractures, ed. 2. Lippincott Williams & Wilkins, Philadelphia, 2002.
25. Eiff, M, et al: Fracture Management for Primary Care. WB Saunders, Philadelphia, 2003.
26. Yochum, TR, and Rowe, LJ: Essentials of Skeletal Radiology, ed. 3. Williams & Wilkins, Baltimore, 2004.
27. Marchiori, DM: Clinical Imaging with Skeletal, Chest, and Abdomen Pattern Differentials. Mosby, St. Louis, MO, 1999.
28. Ip, D: Orthopedic Traumatology: A Resident's Guide. Springer, New York, 2006.
29. McConnell, J, Eyres, R, and Nightingale, J: Interpreting Trauma Radiographs. Blackwell, Malden, MA, 2005.
30. Drafke, MW, and Nakayama, H: Trauma and Mobile Radiography, ed. 2. FA Davis, Philadelphia, 2001.
31. Hodler, J, von Schulthess, GK, and Zollikofer, CL: Musculoskeletal Disease: Diagnostic Imaging and Interventional Technology. Springer, Italy, 2005.
32. Daffner, RH: Clinical Radiology: The Essentials, ed. 3. Williams & Wilkins, Baltimore, 2007.
33. Bernstein, J (ed): Musculoskeletal Medicine. American Academy of Orthopedic Surgeons, Rosemont, IL, 2003.
34. Dodson, CC, et al: Elbow arthroscopy. J Am Acad Orthop Surg 16(10):574, 2008.
35. Savoie, FH: Guidelines to becoming an expert elbow arthroscopist. Arthroscopy 23(11):1237, 2007.
36. Steinmann, SP: Elbow arthroscopy: Where are we now? Arthroscopy 23(11)1231, 2007.
37. Brunton, LM, et al: MRI of the elbow: Update on current techniques and indications. J Hand Surg (Am) 31(6):1001, 2006.
38. Harada, M, et al: Using sonography for the early detection of elbow injuries among young baseball players. AJR Am J Roentgenol 187(6):1436, 2006.
39. Zhu, J, et al: Ultrasound-guided, minimally invasive, percutaneous needle puncture treatment for tennis elbow. Adv Ther 25(10):1031, 2008.
40. Kraus, R, et al: Efficient imaging of elbow injuries in children and adolescents. Klin Padiatr 219(5):282, 2007.
41. McCartney, CJ, et al: Ultrasound examination of peripheral nerves in the forearm. Reg Anesth Pain Med 32(5):434, 2007.
42. Tran, N, and Chow, K: Ultrasonography of the elbow. Semin Musculoskelet Radiol 11(2):105, 2007.
43. Lew, HL, et al: Introduction to musculoskeletal diagnostic ultrasound: Examination of the upper limb. Am J Phys Med Rehabil 86(4):310, 2007.
44. Khoury, V, and Cardinal, E: "Tenomalacia": A new sonographic sign of tendinopathy? Eur Radiol 19(1):144, 2009.
45. Zuazo, I, et al: Acute elbow trauma in children: Role of ultrasonography. Pediatric Radiol 38(9):982, 2008.
46. Zhang, JD, and Chen, H: Ultrasonography for non-displaced and mini-displaced humeral lateral condyle fracture in children. Chin J Traumatol 11(5):297, 2008.
47. Sans, N, and Railhac, JJ: Elbow: Plain radiographs. J Radiol 89(5 pt 2):633, 2008.
48. Rosenberg, ZS, et al: MRI features of posterior capitellar impaction injuries. AJR Am J Roentgenol 190(2):435, 2008.
49. Sutcliffe, J, et al: Magnetic resonance findings of golf-related injuries. Curr Probl Diagn Radiol 37(5):231, 2008.
50. Shahabpour, M, et al: The effectiveness of diagnostic imaging methods for the assessment of soft tissue and articular disorders of the shoulder and elbow. Eur J Radiol 65(2):194, 2008.
51. Worthing, AB, and Cupps, TR: The rheumatic causes of elbow instability. Hand Clin 24(1):79, 2008.
52. Ouellette, H, et al: MR imaging of the elbow in baseball pitchers. Skel Radiol 37(2):115, 2008.
53. Lindenhovius, AL, and Jupiter, JB: The posttraumatic stiff elbow: A review of the literature. J Hand Surg (Am) 32(10):1605, 2007.
54. Wright, RW, et al: Radiographic findings in the shoulder and elbow of major league baseball pitchers. Am J Sports Med 35(11):1839, 2007.
55. Ring, D: Apparent capitellar fractures. Hand Clin 23(4):471, 2007.
56. Lattanza, LL, and Keese, G: Elbow instability in children. Hand Clin 24(1):139, 2008.
57. Ring, D, and King, G: Radial head arthroplasty with a modular metal spacer to treat acute traumatic elbow instability. J Bone Joint Surg Am 90(Suppl 2 Pt 1):63, 2008.
58. Park, GY, et al: Diagnostic value of ultrasonography for clinical medial epicondylitis. Arch Phys Med Rehabil 89(4):738, 2008.
59. Faro, F, and Wolf, JM: Lateral epicondylitis: Review and current concepts. J Hand Surg (Am) 32(8):1271, 2007.
60. Karkhanis, S, Frost, A, and Maffulli, N: Operative mangement of tennis elbow: A quantitative review. Br Med Bull 88(1):171, 2008.
61. Meknas, K, et al: Radiofrequency microtenotomy: A promising method for treatment of recalcitrant lateral epicondylitis. Am J Sports Med 36(10):1960, 2008.
62. Kohia, M, et al: Effectiveness of physical therapy treatments on lateral epicondylitis. J Sports Rehabil 17(2):119, 2008.
63. Tsai, P, and Steinberg, DR: Median and radial nerve compression about the elbow. Instr Course Lect 57:177, 2008.
64. Altan, L, and Kanat, E: Conservative treatment of lateral epicondylitis: Comparison of two different orthotic devices. Clin Rheumatol 27(8):1015, 2008.
65. Oken, O, et al: The short-term efficacy of laser, brace, and ultrasound treatment in lateral epicondylitis: A prospective, randomized, controlled trial. J Hand Ther 21(1):63, 2008.
66. Calfee, RP, et al: Management of lateral epicondylitis: Current concepts. J Am Acad Orthop 16(1):19, 2008.
67. Bunata, RE, et al: Anatomic factors related to the cause of tennis elbow. J Bone Joint Surg Am 89(9):1955, 2007.
68. Wahegaonkar, AL, et al: Technique of osteochondral autograft transplantation mosaicplasty for capitellar osteochondritis dissecans. J Hand Surg (Am) 32(9):1454, 2007.

69. Miyamoto, W, et al: Oblique osteochondral plug transplantation technique for osteochondritis dissecans of the elbow joint. Knee Surg Sports Traumatol Arthros 2008 (Epub ahead of print).

70. Takahara, M, et al: Classification, treatment, and outcome of osteochondritis dissecans of the humeral capitellum. J Bone Joint Surg Am 90(Suppl 2 Pt 1):47, 2008.

71. Krabak, BJ, et al: Shoulder and elbow injuries in the adolescent athlete. Phys Med Rehabil Clin North Am 19(2):271, 2008.

72. Nobuta, S, et al: Clinical outcome of fragment fixation for osteochondral dissecans of the elbow. Ups J Med Sci 113(2):201, 2008.

73. Rahusen, FT, et al: Results of arthroscopic debridement for osteochondritis dissecans of the elbow. Br J Sports Med 40(12):966, 2006.

74. Kusumi, T, et al: Osteochondritis dissecans of the elbow: Histopathological assessment of the articular cartilage and subchondral bone with emphasis on their damage and repair. Pathol Int 56(10):604, 2006.

75. Yamamoto, Y, et al: Osteochondral autograft transplantation for osteochondritis dissecans of the elbow in juvenile baseball players: Minimum 2-year follow-up. Am J Sports Med 34(5):714, 2006.

76. Bojanic, I, et al: Arthroscopy and microfracture technique in the treatment of osteochondritis dissecans of the humeral capitellum: A report of three adolescent gymnasts. Knee Surg Sports Traumatol Arthrosc 14(5):491, 2006.

77. Brownlow, HC, et al: Arthroscopic treatment of osteochondritis dissecans of the capitellum. Knee Surg Sports Traumatol Arthrosc 14(2):198, 2006.

78. Kijowski, R, and De Smet, AA: MRI findings of osteochondritis dissecans of the capitellum with surgical correlation. AJR Am J Roentgenol 185(6):1453, 2005.

79. Debeer, P, and Brys, P: Osteochondritis dissecans of the humeral head: Clinical and radiological findings. Acta Orthop Belg 71(4):484, 2005.

80. Kijowski, R, and DeSmet, A: Radiography of the elbow for evaluation of patients with osteochondritis dissecans of the capitellum. Skel Radiol 34(5):266, 2005.

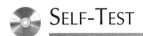

SELF-TEST

Radiographs A, B, and C

1. Identify the *projections.*

2. All three films represent *normal findings* for different age groups. Identify which film belongs to the 5-year-old girl, the 10-year-old boy, and the 30-year-old man.

3. What *anatomic features* helped you determine the ages of the patients?

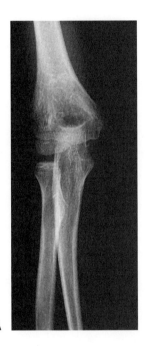

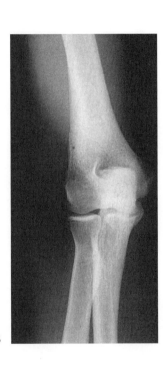

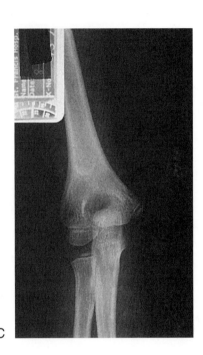

A   B   C

Chapter 17

RADIOLOGIC EVALUATION OF THE HAND AND WRIST

With contributions by Corlia van Rooyen, MPT, RHT

The hand and wrist are among the most often radiographed areas of the skeleton in any age group. The high frequency of traumatic fractures as well as the painful degenerative conditions from repetitive microtrauma or arthritic deformities account for this. The clinicians involved in treatment of the hand and wrist rely on imaging to assist in accurate diagnosis to minimize delays in providing appropriate treatment—delays that may result in long-term disability and surgery.

Review of Anatomy[1–10]

Osseous Anatomy

The 27 bones that make up one hand and wrist are divided into three groups: the phalanges, the metacarpals, and the carpals (Fig. 17-1).

The *phalanges* are the fingers and thumb, or digits, of the hand. They number 14, with a *proximal, middle,* and *distal phalanx* forming each finger and a *proximal* and *distal*

phalanx forming the thumb. Each phalanx is a miniature long bone characterized by the presence of a *base,* a *shaft,* and, most distal, a *head.* The thumb is designated as the first digit, and the fingers are consecutively numbered as digits 2 through 5.

Five *metacarpals* form the palm of the hand. They are numbered in the same manner as the digits, with the first metacarpal at the thumb and the fifth metacarpal at the little finger side of the hand. The metacarpals are also miniature long bones, each possessing a base, shaft, and head.

Eight *carpals* make up the wrist. They are divided into proximal and distal rows for ease of learning their positions. The proximal row from the thumb side consists of the *scaphoid, lunate, triquetrum,* and *pisiform* bones. The distal row, from the thumb side, consists of the *trapezium, trapezoid, capitate,* and *hamate* bones.

The distal *radius* has two articular facets separated by a ridge for articulation with the scaphoid and lunate. The *sigmoid notch* of the distal radius articulates with the distal *ulna.*

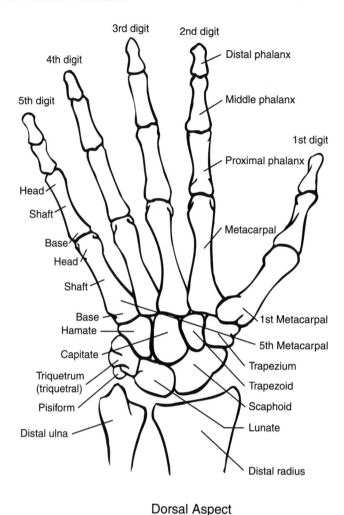

Dorsal Aspect

Figure 17-1 Osseous anatomy of the hand, dorsal aspect.

Joints and Ligaments of the Hand and Wrist

Interphalangeal Joints

The interphalangeal (IP) joints are located between the segments of each phalanx (Fig. 17-2). In the fingers they are designated as the distal interphalangeal joints and the proximal interphalangeal joints. The thumb possesses only one interphalangeal joint. Each joint is supported by an articular capsule and palmar (volar) and collateral ligaments. The dorsal aspect is reinforced by expansion of the extensor tendon sheath.

Metacarpophalangeal Joints

The metacarpophalangeal (MCP) joints are located between the bases of the proximal phalanges and the metacarpal heads. They are also each supported by articular capsules, volar and collateral ligaments, and expansions of the extensor tendons on their dorsal aspects. Sesamoid bones, small ossicles located within the tendons, are commonly present at these joints.

Intermetacarpal Joints

These joints are located between the adjacent bases of the four metacarpal bones of the fingers. Dorsal and palmar ligaments, as well as interosseous ligaments, support the intermetacarpal joints.

Carpometacarpal Joints

These joints are located between the metacarpal bases and the distal row of carpal bones. The first carpometacarpal joint at the thumb is an independent articulation between the first metacarpal base and the trapezium, housed in its own strong articular capsule. The remaining carpometacarpal joints of the hand share the intercarpal synovial cavity. Dorsal and palmar carpometacarpal ligaments and interosseous ligaments support these articulations.

The distal row of carpals (trapezium, trapezoid, capitate, hamate) are connected to one another and to the bases of the metacarpals by strong ligaments, making the distal row relatively immobile.

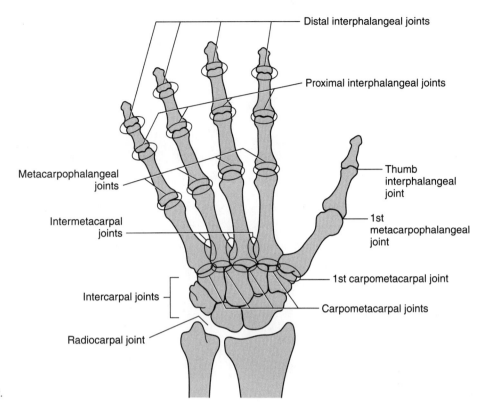

Figure 17-2 Joints of the hand and wrist.

Intercarpal Joints

These joints are the articulations between the carpals themselves, contained within the intercarpal synovial cavity. This cavity also includes the intermetacarpal and second through fifth carpometacarpal joints. Dorsal and palmar intercarpal ligaments support the capsule, and within the capsule interosseous ligaments unite the individual carpal bones.

Radiocarpal Joint

Referred to as the wrist joint, this joint is formed by the proximal row of carpal bones and their interosseous ligaments articulating with the distal radius and articular disk of the distal radioulnar joint (DRUJ). The articular capsule encloses the joint and is strengthened by the dorsal and palmar radiocarpal ligaments and the radial and ulnar collateral ligaments.

In general, the dorsal ligaments are weaker than the palmar ligaments. The important palmar ligaments of the wrist are the *radioscaphocapitate* (which guides scaphoid kinematics), *radioscapholunate* (which stabilizes the scapholunate articulation), *radiolunate*, and *radiolunotriquetral* (which supports the proximal row and stabilizes the radiolunate and lunotriquetral joints).

The *space of Poirier* is a ligament-free area in the capitolunate space, rendering it an area of potential weakness.

The *triangular fibrocartilage complex* (*TFCC*) is a major stabilizer of the ulnar carpus and distal radioulnar joint,

absorbing 20% of the axial load across the wrist joint. The components of the TFCC include the *radiotriquetral ligament*, the fibrocartilage *articular disk*, the *extensor carpi ulnaris tendon sheath, palmar and dorsal radioulnar ligaments*, and the *ulnocarpal ligament* (consisting of *ulnotriquetral, ulnolunate,* and *ulnocapitate ligaments*) and *ulnocarpal meniscus (meniscal homolog)*.

Joint Mobility

The varying articular surface shapes of the small joints of the hand permit many differences in range of motion between the individual fingers and the thumb. Amounts of range of motion can also greatly differ among individual persons, often relating to the amount of ligamentous laxity present. In general, the hand is extremely mobile and can coordinate between its components an infinite variety of movement.

The *interphalangeal joints* function as hinge joints permitting full extension or hyperextension and a great amount of flexion, ranging from 90 to 110 degrees or more. The *metacarpophalangeal joints* of the fingers are condyloid, allowing multiplanar motion and approximately 90 degrees of flexion. The *first metacarpophalangeal joint* at the thumb is a saddle joint allowing full extension or hyperextension and as much as 90 degrees of flexion. The *carpometacarpal joints* of the hand are gliding joints,

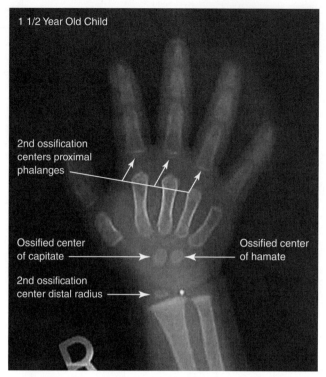

1 1/2 Year Old Child

2nd ossification centers proximal phalanges

Ossified center of capitate

Ossified center of hamate

2nd ossification center distal radius

Figure 17-3 Normal radiographic appearance of the hand of an 18-month-old child. The secondary centers of ossification visible on radiograph at this age are labeled.

permitting enough flexion and extension to allow cupping of the palm. The *first carpometacarpal joint* of the thumb is a saddle joint allowing a wide range of motion through a conical space, the most important of which is opposition to the fingers.

Motions at the *wrist joint complex*, consisting of the intercarpal joints, the radiocarpal joint, and the distal radioulnar joint, are intricately integrated, permitting motion in two planes and in combinations of those planes. The major motions are flexion-extension and abduction-adduction, also called radial and ulnar deviation. Varying widely among individuals, approximately 90 degrees of flexion, 80 degrees of extension, 20 degrees of radial deviation, and 30 degrees of ulnar deviation are possible. Forearm pronation and supination result from motion arising at the proximal and distal radioulnar joints, permitting the hand to rotate axially approximately 150 degrees.

Growth and Development

The hand and wrist are often used as indicators of skeletal age in children. The timing of the appearances of ossification centers and configuration of the epiphyses has been radiographically demonstrated in large group studies of children and is referenced in the Greulich and Pyle atlas.[4]

Ossification of the shafts of the metacarpals and phalanges begins at 8 weeks of fetal life. At birth these structures are fairly well formed. The carpals are ordinarily cartilaginous at birth and are not visible on radiographs. Ossification at the carpals takes place from a single center in each bone.

First to appear on radiograph are the centers for the capitate and hamate, usually by 6 months of age (Fig. 17-3). The center for the triquetrum appears after age 2, followed by the centers for the lunate, trapezium, trapezoid, and scaphoid in yearly intervals to age 6. The pisiform begins ossification much later, after age 11 (Fig. 17-4). Ossification is usually complete at the carpals by ages 14 to 16, with girls maturing 1 or 2 years earlier than boys.

At the metacarpals, secondary ossification centers appear in the distal epiphyses at age 2. Fusion of the metacarpals is complete by 16 to 18 years of age.

At the phalanges, secondary ossification centers appear in the proximal epiphyses at age 2, and their development parallels that of the metacarpals.

The radial and ulnar shafts begin ossification in the eighth week of fetal life and are well formed at birth. The secondary center of ossification for the distal radial epiphysis appears at the end of the first year and for the distal ulnar epiphysis at 5 or 6 years of age. These epiphyses complete fusion to their respective shafts at 18 to 20 years of age.

Routine Radiologic Evaluation[11–21]

Practice Guidelines for Extremity Radiography in Children and Adults

The American College of Radiology (ACR), the principal professional organization of radiologists, defines practice guidelines to assist practitioners in providing appropriate radiologic care for patients.

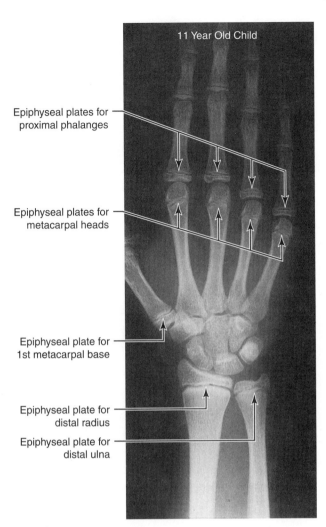

11 Year Old Child

Epiphyseal plates for proximal phalanges

Epiphyseal plates for metacarpal heads

Epiphyseal plate for 1st metacarpal base

Epiphyseal plate for distal radius

Epiphyseal plate for distal ulna

Figure 17-4 Normal radiographic appearance of the hand in an 11-year-old child. At this stage of development all the carpals are ossified, and the epiphyses of the radius, ulna, metacarpals, and phalanges are almost completely ossified. The epiphyseal plates appear "open" as radiolucent lines parallel to the ends of the epiphyses.

Goals

The goal of hand or wrist radiographic examination is to identify or exclude anatomic abnormalities or disease processes.

Indications

The indications for radiologic examination include but are not limited to trauma; suspected physical abuse in young children; osseous changes secondary to metabolic disease, systemic disease, or nutritional deficiences; neoplasms; infections; arthropathy; preoperative, postoperative, and follow-up studies; congenital syndromes and developmental disorders; vascular lesions; evaluation of soft tissue (as for suspected foreign body); pain; and correlation of abnormal skeletal findings on other imaging studies.

Basic Projections and Radiologic Observations

The hand and wrist have separate radiographic examinations. Also, if an individual finger is the area of interest, a separate radiographic examination of the finger is performed. The

recommended projections for either the hand, wrist, or finger are the *posteroanterior (PA)*, *lateral*, and *oblique* views.

Radiographic positioning for the three basic projections of the hand, wrist, or finger are essentially the same, the difference being where the x-ray beam is centered and how it is *collimated* or "coned down" for a closeup view of the anatomy.

For evaluation of individual carpals, many optional projections are available to visualize specific anatomic sites. Two common optional projections, the ulnar and radial deviation views of the wrist, are presented.

Radiographs of the hand and wrist are examined with the fingers pointing up. Consistent with this custom is the fact that metacarpal and phalangeal *heads* are then positioned *superiorly*, and their *bases inferiorly*, when viewed.

Trauma at the Hand and Wrist[22–48]

Fractures of the hand are common, comprising 10% of all fractures. The distal phalanges, being the most exposed portion of the hand, account for more than half of all hand fractures in adults. Over 50% of hand fractures are work-related.

The distal radius is the most commonly injured bone at the wrist, followed by the scaphoid. The true incidence of fractures at the wrist is unknown, because carpal injuries are often not recognized in the presence of more obvious associated injuries (such as forearm or metacarpal fractures). These fractures at the wrist are often dismissed as sprains. The mechanism for the majority of wrist fractures is a fall on an outstretched hand.

In children, the most frequently fractured bone anywhere in the skeleton is the distal radius. In adults, the incidence of distal radial fractures in the elderly correlates with osteopenia and rises in incidence with age, nearly in parallel with the increased incidence of hip fractures.

Diagnostic Imaging for Trauma of the Hand and Wrist

The ACR Appropriateness Guidelines

The ACR Appropriateness Guidelines[22,23] identify 12 variants of *acute* hand and wrist pain and 11 variants of *chronic* wrist pain. In all cases, routine radiographic evaluation is recommended as the first imaging study to perform. Generally speaking, advanced imaging is recommended next only if initial radiographs are normal or nondiagnostic.

For the follow-up of known fractures, radiographic intervals are generally 7 to 10 days after immobilization to check the position of fragments and confirm initiation of healing processes. Unless a fracture is at high risk for development of complications or if the patient presents with persistent pain, radiographs are usually not necessary until near the end of the healing time frame. Radiographs at this point serve to:

- Confirm radiographic evidence of union
- Justify removal of external fixation
- Permit rehabilitation to proceed

Routine Radiologic Evaluation of the Hand

Posteroanterior

This view demonstrates the *hand*, *wrist*, and *distal forearm*. Structures best shown are the *phalanges*, *metacarpals*, *carpals*, and all *joints* of the hand.

Radiologic Observations

The important observations are:

1. The patient's palm and fingers are positioned flat on the film cassette. This results in a true PA view of the hand but an *oblique* view of the thumb.
2. Note the *symmetrical* appearance of the concave sides of the shafts of each phalanx and metacarpal. The oblique perspective of the thumb is the exception.
3. Note the normal *tufted* appearance of the terminal ends of the distal phalanges.
4. Normally the long axis of the second metacarpal is in line with the long axis of the radius (*a* in Fig. 17-5).
5. Normally there is slight ulnar deviation of the proximal phalanges of the fingers in respect to the metacarpals (*b* in Fig. 17-5).
6. Normally a line drawn along the distal articular surfaces of the fourth and fifth metacarpals should also extend along the distal articular surface of the third metacarpal. If the line intersects the third metacarpal at a more proximal point, the fourth metacarpal may be abnormally short (as in fracture or Turner's syndrome). This is known as the *metacarpal sign* (*c* in Fig. 17-5).
7. The interphalangeal and metacarpophalangeal joint spaces are visible.
8. Sesamoid bones are a frequent occurrence at the metacarpophangeal and interphalangeal joints of the thumb and at the metacarpophalangeal joint of the fifth finger.
9. The bases of the second through fifth metacarpals partially overlap.
10. At the wrist there is overlap of the trapezium and the trapezoid as well as of the pisiform and the triquetrum.

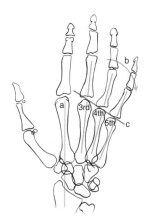

Figure 17-5 Radiographic spatial relationships, PA view of the hand.

Basic Projections

- **PA**
- Lateral
- Oblique

Setting up the Radiograph

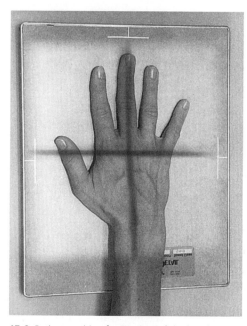

Figure 17-6 Patient position for PA view of the hand.

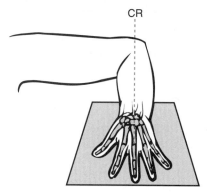

Figure 17-7 The central ray is perpendicular to the hand at the third metacarpophalangeal joint.

What Can You See?

Look at the radiograph (Fig. 17-8) and try to identify the radiographic anatomy. Trace the outlines of the structures using a marker and transparency sheet. Compare results with the book tracing (Fig. 17-9). Can you see the following:

- Phalanges (identify proximal, middle, and distal segments and the base, shaft, and head of a single phalanx)
- Metacarpals (identify the base, shaft, and head of one metacarpal)

- Sesamoid bones at the first metacarpophalangeal joint
- Carpal bones (identify the proximal row of carpals—scaphoid, lunate, triquetrum, and pisiform—and the distal row of carpals—trapezium, trapezoid, capitate, and hamate)
- Joints of the hand (identify the distal and proximal interphalangeal joints, the metacarpophalangeal joints, and the carpometacarpal joints)

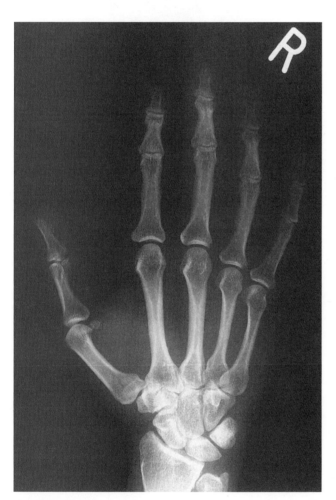

Figure 17-8 PA radiograph of the hand.

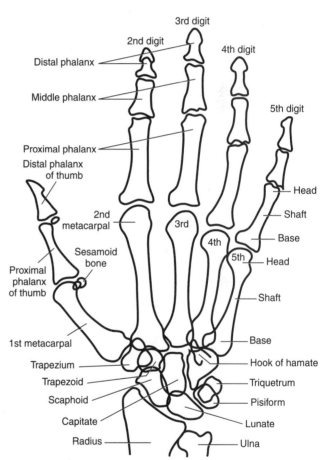

Figure 17-9 Tracing of PA radiograph of the hand.

Routine Radiologic Evaluation of the Hand

Oblique

This view demonstrates the *phalanges, metacarpals, carpals,* and all *joints* of the hand in an oblique view.

Radiologic Observations

The important observations are:

1. The patient's hand and wrist have been placed flat on the film as for a PA projection, and then the thumb side of the hand is lifted, rotating the hand and wrist 45 degrees from the PA position.
2. Some routine oblique views use a foam wedge to support the hand at 45 degrees (Fig. 17-10). This prevents foreshortening of the phalanges and obscuring of the interphalangeal joints. This position is used more often if the phalanges are the area of interest.
3. The phalanges and metacarpals are demonstrated without superimposition. This lack of overlap of the long bones of the hand makes the *oblique view* advantageous over the direct *lateral view*, which superimposes many structures. The lateral view is necessary, however, to determine the exact amounts of any displacements that may be present.
4. The interphalangeal and metacarpophalangeal joint spaces are visible.

Basic Projections

- PA
- Lateral
- **Oblique**

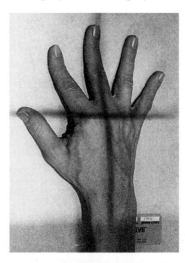

Setting up the Radiograph

Figure 17-11 Patient position for oblique view of the hand.

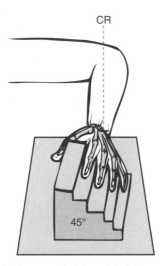

Figure 17-10 A 45-degree angled foam block is used to position the hand for an oblique radiograph. The elevation of the fingers opens MCP and IP joint spaces. The block is used when the phalanges are a primary area of interest.

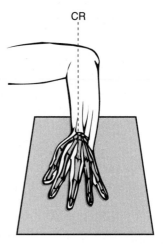

Figure 17-12 The central ray passes through the third metacarpophalangeal joint.

What Can You See?

Look at the radiograph (Fig. 17-8) and try to identify the radiographic anatomy. Trace the outlines of the structures using a marker and transparency sheet. Compare results with the book tracing (Fig. 17-9). Can you see the following:

- Phalanges (identify proximal, middle, and distal segments and the base, shaft, and head of a single phalanx)
- Metacarpals (identify the base, shaft, and head of one metacarpal)

- Sesamoid bones at the first metacarpophalangeal joint
- Carpal bones (identify the proximal row of carpals—scaphoid, lunate, triquetrum, and pisiform—and the distal row of carpals—trapezium, trapezoid, capitate, and hamate)
- Joints of the hand (identify the distal and proximal interphalangeal joints, the metacarpophalangeal joints, and the carpometacarpal joints)

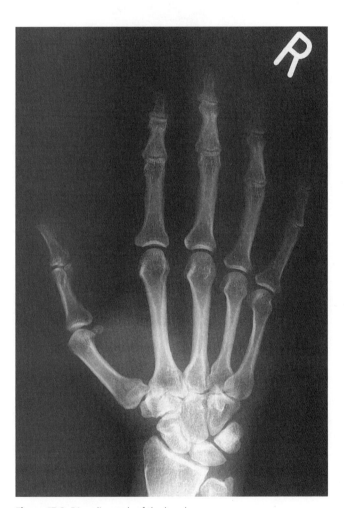

Figure 17-8 PA radiograph of the hand.

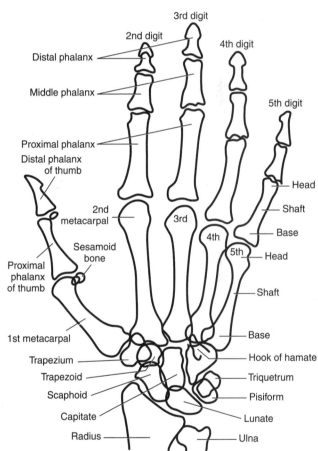

Figure 17-9 Tracing of PA radiograph of the hand.

Routine Radiologic Evaluation of the Hand

Oblique

This view demonstrates the *phalanges, metacarpals, carpals,* and all *joints* of the hand in an oblique view.

Radiologic Observations

The important observations are:

1. The patient's hand and wrist have been placed flat on the film as for a PA projection, and then the thumb side of the hand is lifted, rotating the hand and wrist 45 degrees from the PA position.
2. Some routine oblique views use a foam wedge to support the hand at 45 degrees (Fig. 17-10). This prevents foreshortening of the phalanges and obscuring of the interphalangeal joints. This position is used more often if the phalanges are the area of interest.
3. The phalanges and metacarpals are demonstrated without superimposition. This lack of overlap of the long bones of the hand makes the *oblique view* advantageous over the direct *lateral view*, which superimposes many structures. The lateral view is necessary, however, to determine the exact amounts of any displacements that may be present.
4. The interphalangeal and metacarpophalangeal joint spaces are visible.

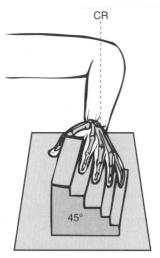

Figure 17-10 A 45-degree angled foam block is used to position the hand for an oblique radiograph. The elevation of the fingers opens MCP and IP joint spaces. The block is used when the phalanges are a primary area of interest.

Basic Projections

- PA
- Lateral
- **Oblique**

Setting up the Radiograph

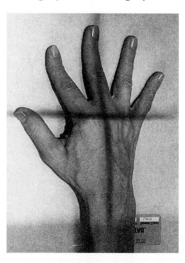

Figure 17-11 Patient position for oblique view of the hand.

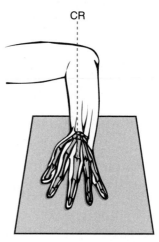

Figure 17-12 The central ray passes through the third metacarpophalangeal joint.

What Can You See?

Look at the radiograph (Fig. 17-13) and try to identify the radiographic anatomy. Trace the outlines of the structures using a marker and transparency sheet. Compare results with the book tracing (Fig. 17-14). Can you see the following:

- Phalanges (identify proximal, middle, and distal segments and the base, shaft, and head of a single phalanx)
- Metacarpals (identify the base, shaft, and head of one metacarpal)
- Joints of the hand: the distal and proximal interphalangeal joints, the metacarpophalangeal joints, and the carpometacarpal joints
- Sesamoid bones at the first metacarpophalangeal joint

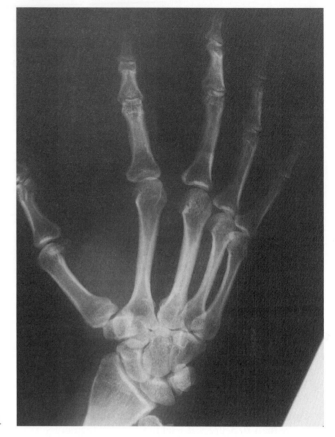

Figure 17-13 Oblique radiograph of the hand.

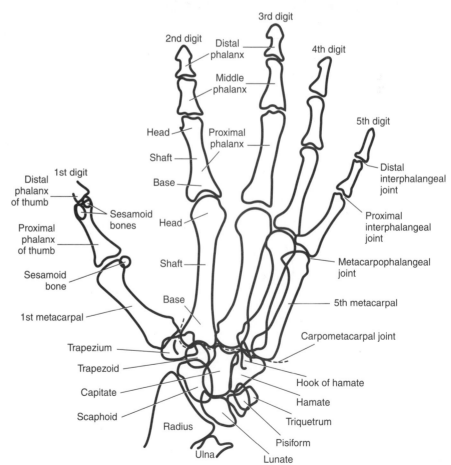

Figure 17-14 Tracing of oblique radiograph of the hand.

Routine Radiologic Evaluation of the Hand

Lateral

This view demonstrates the *hand* and *wrist* from a lateral perspective. The thumb, however, is seen in a true PA projection. Various *sesamoid bones* may be demonstrated on this view.

Radiologic Observations

The important observations are:

1. The ulnar side of the patient's hand and wrist is positioned on the image receptor. As a result, the thumb is farthest from the receptor and thus is magnified.
2. The phalanges and metacarpals are superimposed directly over each other, as are most of the carpals as well as the distal radius and ulna.
3. The normal metacarpal neck-to-shaft angle is 15 degrees.
4. Despite the superimposition of most of the bones of the hand and wrist, *displacement of a fracture fragment* is easily detected on this projection. Note that displacement will be described as being in a *dorsal* or *volar* direction.
5. The longitudinal axes of the radius, lunate, and capitate normally align within 10 degrees of each other (*a* in Fig. 17-15). Significant variations may indicate fracture, dislocation, or ligamentous injury.
6. The longitudinal axes of the radius and the lunate, if not in alignment, should at least be parallel. The angle between them is known as the *radiolunate angle* (*b* in Fig. 17-15). If the lunate is palmarly rotated more than 15 degrees, volar intercalated segmental instability (VISI) is suggested (*c* in Fig. 17-15). If the lunate is extended more than 10 degrees, dorsal intercalated segmental instability (DISI) is suggested (*d* in Fig. 17-15). This relationship is also evaluated on the lateral view of the wrist.

Basic Projections

- PA
- **Lateral**
- Oblique

Setting up the Radiograph

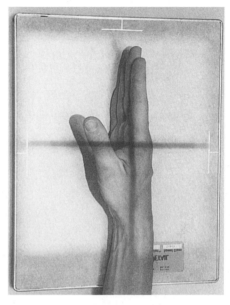

Figure 17-16 Patient position for lateral view of the hand.

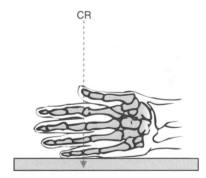

Figure 17-17 The central ray passes through the second metacarpophalangeal joint.

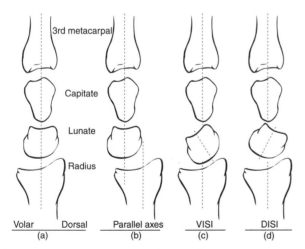

Figure 17-15 Radius–lunate–capitate alignment variations.

What Can You See?

Look at the radiograph (Fig. 17-18) and try to identify the radiographic anatomy. Trace the outlines of the structures using a marker and transparency sheet. Compare results with the book tracing (Fig. 17-19). Can you see the following:

- Bones of the thumb (identify the first metacarpal, proximal phalanx, and distal phalanx)
- Phalanges that are visible (identify the proximal, middle, and distal segments)

- Metacarpals that are visible (identify the proximal, middle, and distal segments)
- Metacarpal neck angle (measure the neck-to-shaft angle)
- Joints of the hand. Identify the distal and proximal interphalangeal joints, the metacarpophalangeal joints, and the carpometacarpophalangeal joints.

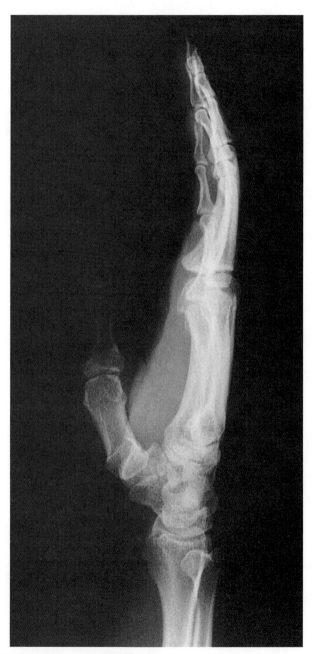

Figure 17-18 Lateral radiograph of the hand.

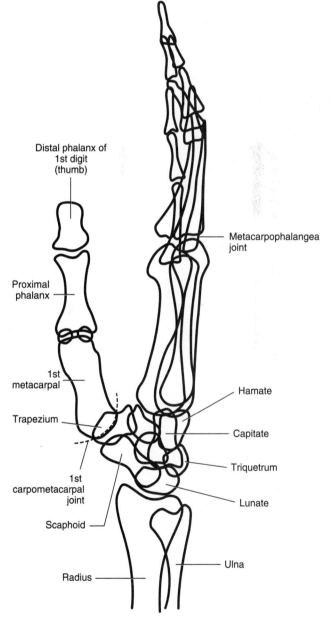

Figure 17-19 Tracing of lateral radiograph of the hand.

Routine Radiologic Evaluation of the Wrist

Posteroanterior

This view demonstrates the middle and proximal portions of the *metacarpals*, the *carpals*, the *distal radius* and *ulna*, and all related *joints*.

Radiologic Observations

The important observations are:

1. The patient's hand is placed palm down on the image receptor and the fingers are then slightly flexed to promote close contact between the wrist and the image receptor.
2. Three arcuate lines can normally be drawn along the articular surfaces of the carpals, outlining the proximal and distal rows (Fig. 17-20):
   - Arc I outlines the proximal convex surfaces of the scaphoid, lunate, and triquetrum.
   - Arc II outlines the distal concave surfaces of the scaphoid, lunate, and triquetrum.
   - Arc III outlines the proximal convex margins of the capitate and hamate. Distortions in these anatomic relationships may be diagnostic of carpal subluxations or dislocations.
3. Note the carpals, which are demonstrated relatively free of superimposition: the scaphoid, lunate, capitate, and hamate. Note the oval image on the hamate, representing the hook of the hamate.
4. Note which carpals are superimposed on this projection: the trapezium and trapezoid, and the triquetrum and pisiform.
5. The relationship of the length of the ulna to the radius is termed *ulnar variance* (Fig. 17-21). Usually the articular surfaces of the ulna and radius are on the same level at the site of articulation with the lunate. This is referred to as *neutral ulnar variance*. In some individuals the ulna is shorter than the radius, and the term *negative ulnar variance* is applied. If the ulna is longer than the radius, the term *positive ulnar variance* is applied. The difference in length is measured in millimeters. This information has practical importance for the orthopedist in assessing fracture displacement, choosing open or closed reduction treatment, and assisting in follow-up evaluation.
6. The *radial articular angle* is another measurement that has significance for the orthopedist (Fig. 17-22). Also referred to as the *ulnar slant of the articular surface of the radius* or the *radial inclination angle*, this angle is formed by the intersection of two lines: a line perpendicular to the long axis of the radius at the level of the radioulnar articular surface (*a* in Fig. 17-22) and a line drawn across the radial articular surface (*b* in Fig. 17-22). Normal values range from 15 to 25 degrees.

Basic Projections

- **PA**
- Lateral
- Oblique

Fundamentals of Orthopedic Radiology

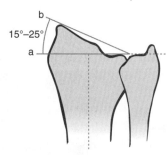

Figure 17-22 The radial angle, or ulnar slant of the articular surface of the radius, is measured as the angle formed by the intersection of the line perpendicular to the long axis (*a*) and the line drawn across the radial articular surface (*b*).

Setting up the Radiograph

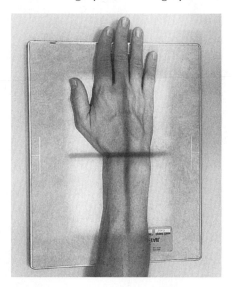

Figure 17-23 Patient position for posteroanterior view of the wrist.

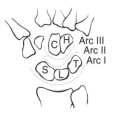

Figure 17-20 Three arcuate lines drawn along the articular surfaces of the carpals designate normal anatomic relationships.

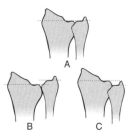

Figure 17-21 (A) Neutral ulnar variance, **(B)** positive ulnar variance, **(C)** negative ulnar variance.

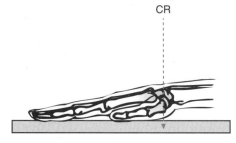

Figure 17-24 The central ray passes through the midcarpal joint.

What Can You See?

Look at the radiograph (Fig. 17-25) and try to identify the radiographic anatomy. Trace the outlines of the structures using a marker and transparency sheet. Compare results with the book tracing (Fig. 17-26). Can you see the following:

- Metacarpals (trace and number each one)
- Carpals (trace and identify each carpal)

- Three arcuate lines formed by the carpals (trace each as described in Fig. 17-20)
- Distal radius and ulna
- Ulnar variance (assess as described in Fig. 17-21)
- Radial articular angle (measure as described in Fig. 17-22)

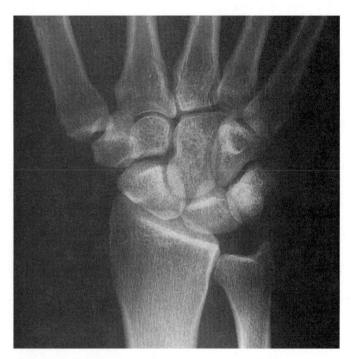

Figure 17-25 PA radiograph of the wrist.

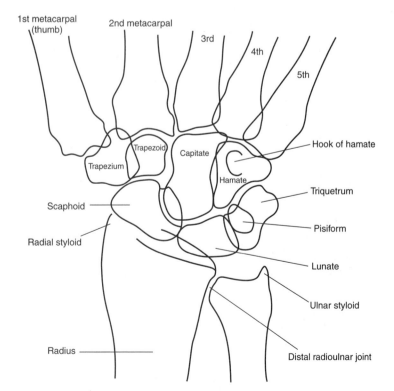

Figure 17-26 Tracing of PA radiograph of the wrist.

Routine Radiologic Evaluation of the Wrist

Oblique

This view demonstrates the middle and proximal *metacarpals,* the *carpals,* and the *distal radius* and *ulna* in an oblique view. Structures best shown are the *trapezium,* the *scaphoid,* and the *first carpometacarpal joint* of the thumb.

Radiologic Observations

The important observations are:

1. The patient's hand and wrist are placed palm-down on the image receptor, and then the thumb side of the hand is lifted, rotating the hand and wrist 45 degrees from the PA position.
2. The first and second metacarpals are viewed with little superimposition.
3. The proximal portions of the third, fourth, and fifth metacarpals overlap.
4. Certain aspects of the carpals are well demonstrated in this projection. Note the following:

   - *Hamate:* The body of the hamate is visualized. The hook of the hamate is not superimposed, as seen in the PA view.
   - *Triquetrum:* The dorsal aspect of this bone is visualized.
   - *Trapezium:* The trapezium itself and its articulations to the trapezoid, scaphoid, and first metacarpal are well visualized (Fig. 17-27).

5. Note that the distal radius and ulna are slightly superimposed. The styloids of each, however, are well visualized.

Basic Projections

- PA
- Lateral
- **Oblique**

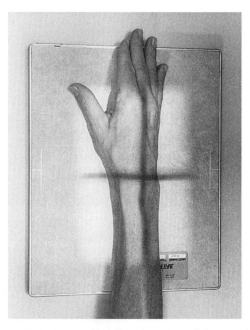

Setting up the Radiograph

Figure 17-28 Patient position for oblique view of the wrist (using thumb to prop hand).

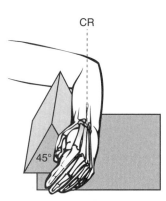

Figure 17-29 The central ray passes through the midcarpal joint. Here a wedge is used to prop the hand.

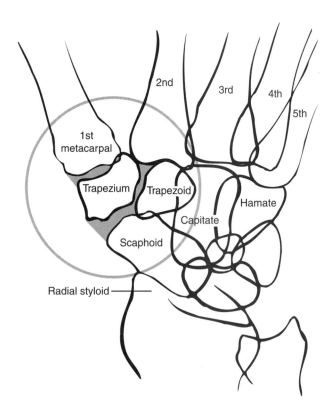

Figure 17-27 The trapezium, and its articulations to the trapezoid, scaphoid, and first metacarpal are well visualized on the oblique view.

What Can You See?

Look at the radiograph (Fig. 17-30) and try to identify the radiographic anatomy. Trace the outlines of the structures using a marker and transparency sheet. Compare results with the book tracing (Fig. 17-31). Can you see the following:

- Metacarpals
- Trapezium, trapezoid, and scaphoid
- Triquetrum and hamate
- Distal radius and ulna

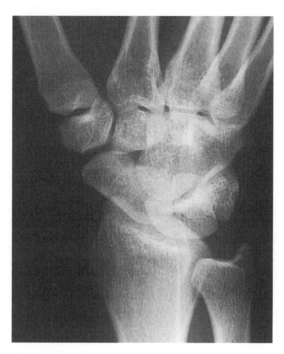

Figure 17-30 Oblique radiograph of the wrist.

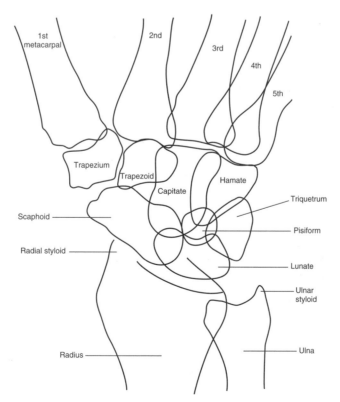

Figure 17-31 Tracing of oblique radiograph of the wrist.

Routine Radiologic Evaluation of the Wrist

Lateral

This view demonstrates superimposed *proximal metacarpals, carpals, distal radius,* and *ulna* as seen from a lateral perspective.

Radiologic Observations

The important observations are:

1. The ulnar side of the hand and wrist is positioned on the image receptor. The metacarpal of the thumb is farthest from the receptor and is somewhat magnified.
2. Despite the superimposition of the wrist and forearm, *displacement of a fracture fragment* is easily detected on this view. Displacement is described as being in a *dorsal or volar* direction.
3. The *volar tilt* of the radial articular surface normally ranges from 16 to 25 degrees (Fig. 17-32). Also known as the *palmar inclination* or *palmar tilt of the radius*, this angle is determined by the intersection of (a) a line perpendicular to the midshaft of the radius and (b) a line drawn across the distal aspects of the radial articular surface. Like the anatomic relationships measured on the PA projection, this angle has practical importance to the orthopedist in assessing fracture displacement, choosing treatment, and assessing follow-up evaluations.
4. The *scapholunate angle* is the intersection of lines drawn along the long axes of the scaphoid and the lunate (Fig. 17-33). The angle of intersection averages 47 degrees, varying between 32 and 62 degrees (an easier way to remember this is 47 ± 15 degrees). If the angle is greater than 80 degrees and the lunate is also dorsiflexed, dorsal intercalated segmental instability (DISI) is suggested.
5. The *capitolunate angle* is the intersection of lines drawn along the long axes of the capitate and the lunate (Fig. 17-34). The angle of intersection should be less than 20 degrees. Carpal instability is suggested if the angle exceeds 20 degrees.
6. Another significant anatomic relationship seen on the lateral views of the wrist or hand is the *alignment of the longitudinal axes* of the *radius, lunate, capitate,* and *third metacarpal bones* (see Fig. 17-15). Variations of up to 10 degrees are considered normal, but major distortions may be diagnostic of fracture or dislocation.

Basic Projections

- PA
- **Lateral**
- Oblique

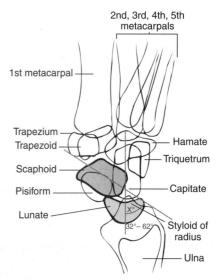

Figure 17-33 The scapholunate angle. The intersection of lines drawn through the long axes of the scaphoid and the lunate forms an angle (*X*) that normally ranges from 32 to 62 degrees.

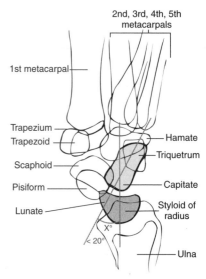

Figure 17-34 The capitolunate angle. The intersection of lines drawn through the long axes of the capitate and the lunate should normally form an angle (*X*) of less than 20 degrees.

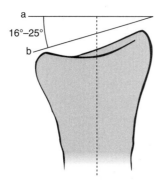

Figure 17-32 The *volar tilt*, or *palmar inclination*, is measured as the angle determined by the intersection of line (*a*), perpendicular to the midshaft of the radius, and (*b*), a line drawn across the distal radial articular surface.

7. Note that the stacked arrangement of the normal radius–lunate–capitate relationship remains true in any degree of wrist flexion or extension. That is, the radial articular surface will always contain the lunate, and the lunate will always cup the capitate in normal conditions.

Setting up the Radiograph

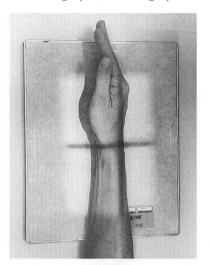

Figure 17-35 Patient position for lateral view of the wrist.

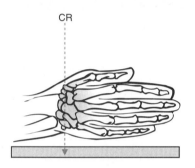

Figure 17-36 The central ray passes through the midcarpal joint.

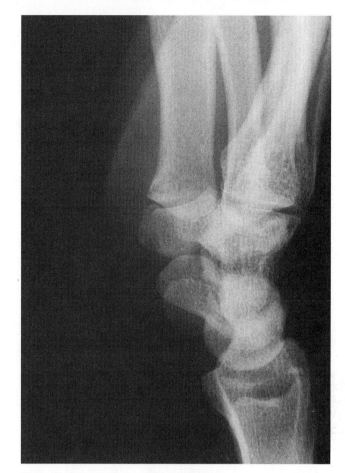

Figure 17-37 Lateral radiograph of the wrist.

What Can You See?

Look at the radiograph (Fig. 17-37) and try to identify the radiographic anatomy. Trace the outlines of the structures using a marker and transparency sheet. Compare results with the book tracing (Fig. 17-38). Can you see the following:

- First metacarpal and trapezium
- Distal radius and ulna
- Volar tilt of the radius (measure as described in Fig. 17-32)
- Scapholunate angle (measure as described in Fig. 17-33)
- Capitolunate angle (measure as described in Fig. 13-34)
- Stacked arrangement of the radius–lunate–capitate relationship

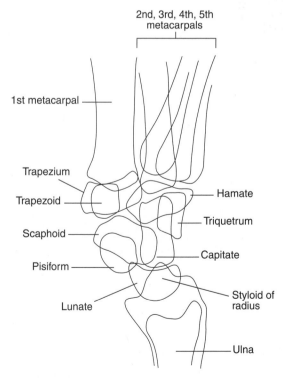

Figure 17-38 Tracing of lateral radiograph of the wrist.

Optional Wrist Views

Ulnar Deviation PA View

This PA view of the wrist is made with the hand positioned in *ulnar deviation* to view the scaphoid and adjacent opened radial intercarpal spaces. Look at the radiograph (Fig. 17-40) and the tracing (Fig. 17-41). The scaphoid normally appears elongated in this projection because of rotation of its distal pole toward the ulna. This elongated appearance verifies normal articulation to the adjacent carpals and excludes scapholunate dislocation.

Setting up the Radiograph

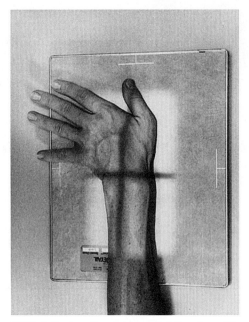

Figure 17-39 Patient position for ulnar deviation view of the wrist.

Optional Projections

- **Ulnar deviation PA view**
- Carpal tunnel view
- Radial deviation PA view

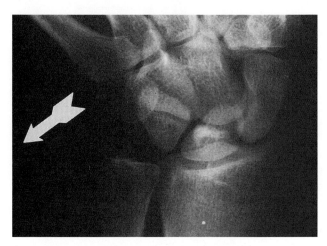

Figure 17-40 Ulnar deviation radiograph of the wrist.

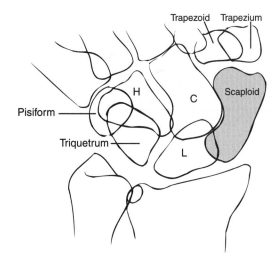

Figure 17-41 Tracing of ulnar deviation radiograph of the wrist.

Optional Wrist Views

Radial Deviation PA View

This PA view of the wrist is made with the hand positioned in *radial deviation* to view the ulnar side carpals and adjacent opened ulnar intercarpal spaces. The lunate, triquetrum, hamate, and pisiform are best shown. Look at the radiograph (Fig. 17-43) and the tracing (Fig. 17-44). Note the foreshortened appearance of the scaphoid. The distal pole of the scaphoid has rotated toward the palm to clear the radial styloid and now is seen end-on.

Setting up the Radiograph

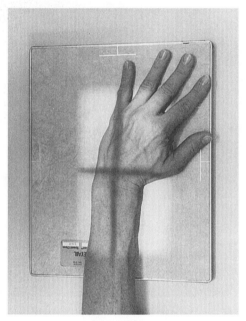

Figure 17-42 Patient position for radial deviation view of the wrist.

Optional Projections

- Ulnar deviation PA view
- Carpal tunnel view
- **Radial deviation PA view**

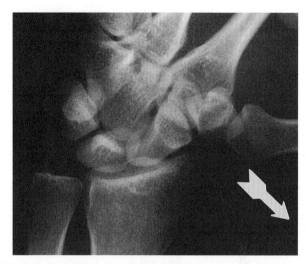

Figure 17-43 Radial deviation radiograph of the wrist.

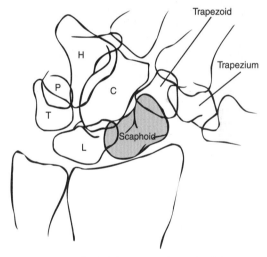

Figure 17-44 Tracing of radial deviation radiograph of the wrist.

Optional Wrist Views

Carpal Tunnel View

This tangential inferosuperior view of the wrist allows visualization of the carpal sulcus. The carpals are demonstrated in a tunnel-like, arched arrangement. This view is usually done to identify abnormalites of the bones or soft tissues that may be compressing the median nerve and flexor tendons that pass through the carpal tunnel. Additionally, fractures involving the hook of the hamate are usually better seen with this projection. Look at the radiograph (Fig. 17-46) and the tracing (Fig. 17-47).

Optional Projections

- Ulnar deviation PA view
- **Carpal tunnel view**
- Radial deviation PA view

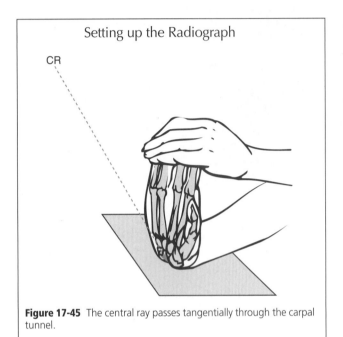

Setting up the Radiograph

Figure 17-45 The central ray passes tangentially through the carpal tunnel.

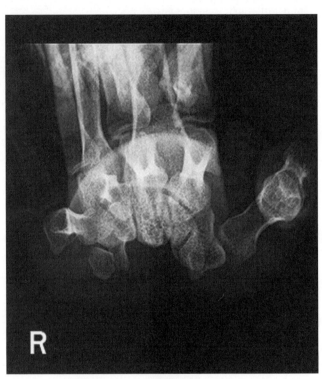

Figure 17-46 Carpal tunnel radiograph of the wrist.

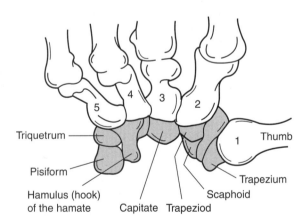

Figure 17-47 Schematic representation of a carpal tunnel radiograph of the wrist. The metacarpals are numbered 1 through 5.

Magnetic Resonance Imaging of the Wrist

Magnetic resonance imaging (MRI) is often recommended as the most appropriate *next study* for the assessment of chronic wrist pain following normal or nondiagnostic radiography. Presented here are coronal, axial, and sagittal MR images of the wrist. On these T1-weighted images, the marrow of bone and fat exhibit high signal intensity (bright), cortical bone and tendons have low signal intensity (dark), and cartilage and muscle have intermediate signal intensity (gray).

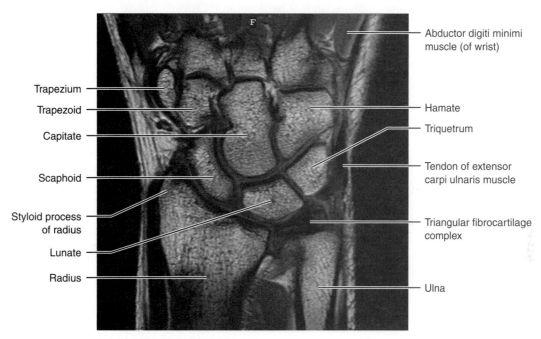

Figure 17-48 Coronal T1-weighted MRI of the wrist.

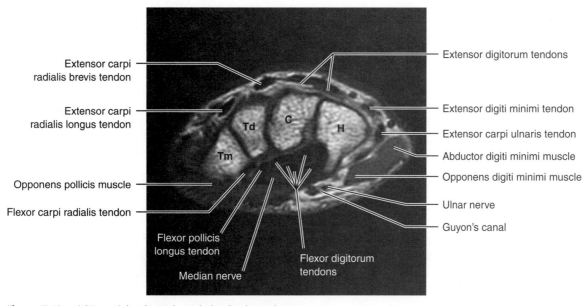

Figure 17-49 Axial T1-weighted MRI through the distal carpal row.

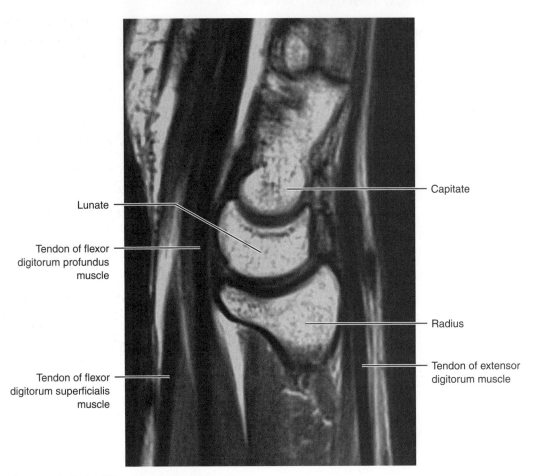

Figure 17-50 Sagittal T1-weighted MRI at mid-wrist.

Lunate

Tendon of flexor digitorum profundus muscle

Tendon of flexor digitorum superficialis muscle

Capitate

Radius

Tendon of extensor digitorum muscle

Fractures of the Hand

The phalanges and metacarpals exhibit fracture patterns like those seen in any long bone. To review, possible fracture lines are transverse, spiral, and oblique. Stable fractures are undisplaced; unstable fractures are displaced and may exhibit rotational or angular deformities. Special features are avulsion and comminution.

A standard of care exists for suspected fractures of the radius or scaphoid. If radiographs are normal, recommendations are to cast and repeat radiographs in 10 to 14 days. At that time, radiographs will confirm or exclude the diagnosis of fracture. However, if immediate confirmation or exclusion of a radial or scaphoid fracture is required, MRI is recommended. Computed tomography (CT) is used if MRI cannot be performed.

If a fracture of the hook of the hamate or a metacarpal is suspected and radiographs are normal, CT is recommended as the next study.

General Treatment Principles

General treatment goals for fractures of the hand are preservation of joint motion and function with protection of underlying soft tissues. Basic principles include:

- *Reduction* as close to anatomic alignment as possible
- *Elevation* of the extremity to limit edema
- *Immobilization* in the *intrinsic* or *protected* position with metacarpophalangeal joints at an angle greater than 70 degrees.
  - Immobilize for 3 to 4 weeks for stable fractures, 4 to 6 weeks for unstable fractures, and 6 to 8 weeks for avulsive fractures, based on radiologic evidence of healing.
  - Complete osseous healing generally takes about 2 weeks longer than the period of recommended immobilization.
- *Mobilization* of the injured finger as soon as possible after cast removal is advised in order to minimize joint stiffness.

Methods of Immobilization

Stable fractures can be treated by "buddy taping" one finger to the other or by splinting. Initially unstable fractures that can be reduced to a stable position are immobilized with a cast or rigid gutter splint or anteroposterior splint. Percutaneous pinning may be used to prevent displacement and permit earlier mobilization (Fig. 17-51).

Unstable fractures that cannot be satisfactorily reduced to near anatomic alignment are treated with open reduction and internal fixation. Methods of fixation include intraosseous wire fixation, tension band techniques, interfragmentary screws, and plate-and-screw combinations.

Clinical Considerations and Pitfalls

Other factors that may influence the type of treatment chosen for an individual patient include the patient's age, hand dominance, occupation, associated soft tissue injury, patient motivation and reliability, and comorbid conditions.

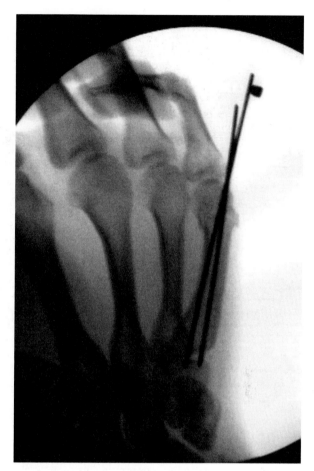

Figure 17-51 Fluoroscopic image after percutaneous pinning of a fracture of the fifth metacarpal neck.

Pitfalls in adequate diagnosis and treatment of hand fractures are noted in the literature: 27% of finger fractures are treated inappropriately in the emergency department; inaccurate reduction and unsatisfactory splinting are the most common errors.[13]

Phalangeal Fractures

Distal phalanges are most often injured by a crushing mechanism that results in comminution of the distal tuft (Fig. 17-52). Significant displacement does not occur owing to the presence of fibrous tissue septa radiating from the bone into the soft tissues. Associated injuries of the nailbed are common and sometimes require repair. Healing is by fibrous rather than bony union. Radiographic evidence of complete bony union may not be evident for several months. Patients may experience pain for this length of time because of bleeding into the fibrous septa.

Fractures of the middle and proximal phalangeal shafts may be classified as *stable, unstable,* or *intra-articular* (Fig. 17-53). Fractures of the proximal phalanx angulate palmarly owing to action of the interosseous muscles, which flex the proximal fragment and extend the distal fragment (Fig. 17-54). Intra-articular fractures may be avulsion-type

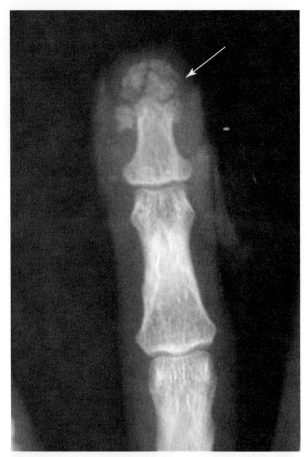

Figure 17-52 Crush injury to the distal phalanx. The arrow points to comminution of the distal tuft.

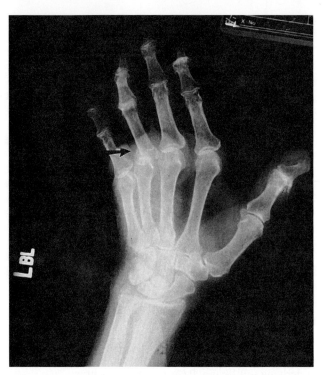

Figure 17-54 Unstable fracture of the proximal phalanx (arrow). On this PA radiograph, a displaced fracture at the base of the fourth proximal phalanx is seen. The distal fragment is angulated ulnarly. Note the soft tissue swelling in the palm and along the extent of the fourth digit. Additionally, osteoarthritic changes are evident at all of the interphalangeal joints, including joint narrowing, subchondral sclerosis, and osteophyte formation. At the distal IP joints the degenrative deformity is known as Herbeden's nodes; at the proximal IP joints it is known as Bouchard's nodes.

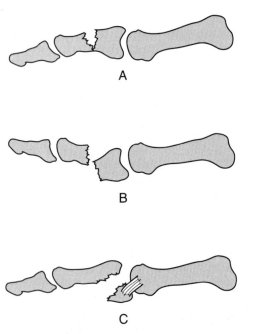

Figure 17-53 Fractures of the middle phalanx: **(A)** stable (nondisplaced), **(B)** unstable (displaced), **(C)** intra-articular.

fractures, with the dorsal aspect of bone disrupted at the attachment of the extensor tendon, or the lateral or volar aspect may be disrupted at the attachment of the collateral ligament. Intra-articular fractures may also involve one or both condyles or exhibit comminution (Fig. 17-55). Most large fragment and comminuted intra-articular fractures require internal fixation to maintain anatomic reduction.

Metacarpal Fractures

Metacarpal fractures are classified by location as fractures of the *head, neck, shaft,* or *base.*

Fractures of the metacarpal *neck* are common. The fifth metacarpal neck is most often involved and is known by the eponym *boxer's fracture.* Characteristic of metacarpal neck fractures is a tendency to impact, shorten, and angulate at the apex dorsally. The consequence of insufficiently corrected angulation is a painful grip due to the protrusion of the head into the palm. Index and middle finger metacarpal neck fractures with angulation greater than 10 degrees are poorly tolerated and often require internal fixation to restore alignment. Remember that the typical metacarpal neck angle, as seen on the lateral radiograph, is 15 degrees. So a measurement of 40 degrees of apex dorsal angulation represents a true angulation of 25 degrees.

Fractures of the metacarpal *shafts* can also cause angular deformities (Fig. 17-56). However, the increased mobility at the carpometacarpal joints of the fourth and fifth digits permits greater tolerance of angulation without the serious functional consequences seen with the metacarpal neck fractures. Up to 30 degrees of angulation is acceptable in fractures of the shaft of the fifth digit and up to 20 degrees in the fourth digit. The second and third metacarpals are less mobile; as a result, only 10 degrees of angulation can be tolerated.

Rotational deformities can be more disabling than angulation because of the tendency for digits to overlap. Rotation is difficult to judge on conventional radiographs and is best judged clinically. Every degree of malrotation in a metacarpal results in 5 degrees of malrotation at a fingertip.

Fractures of the metacarpal *bases* are often associated with carpometacarpal dislocations. These combination injury patterns often require internal fixation to restore alignment and preserve function.

Thumb Metacarpal Fractures

As the thumb is a biomechanically unique digit, fractures of the first metacarpal are distinctly different from fractures at the other metacarpals. The majority of thumb metacarpal fractures occur at or near the *base* and are divided into intra-articular and extra-articular types. Extra-articular types heal well with immobilization in a thumb spica cast. The intra-articular types, commonly known by the eponyms *Bennett fracture* or *Rolando fracture,* are more complicated due to joint disruption.

The Bennett fracture is actually a fracture–dislocation resulting from an axial blow to the partially flexed metacarpal (Fig. 17-57). The base of the metacarpal dislocates and an avulsion fracture occurs at the anterior lip of the base, where strong ligamentous attachment to the trapezium is located. The Rolando fracture is a comminuted version of the Bennett fracture. Treatment methods depend on the size of the fragments. Pin fixation is attempted if the fragments are large enough. In cases of

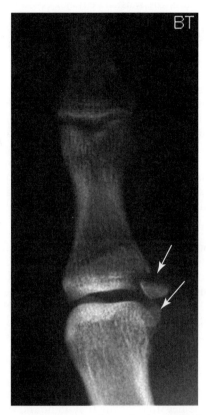

Figure 17-55 Coned-down PA radiograph of a single digit. An intra-articular fracture with comminution and avulsed fragments is seen at the arrows. This is likely to represent avulsion of the collateral ligament due to trauma.

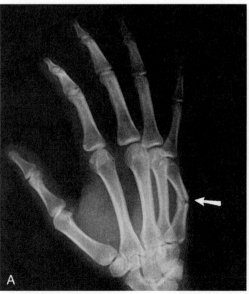
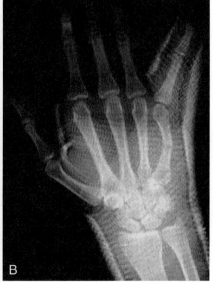

Figure 17-56 Fracture of the fifth metacarpal shaft. **(A)** Oblique view of the hand demonstrates a midshaft fracture of the fifth metacarpal (arrow). The fracture line is complete, transverse, with dorsal angulation of both fracture fragments. **(B)** After closed reduction and casting. Note the configuration of the cast; it has placed the fifth finger in extension in order to prevent finger flexion, which would act to distract the fracture fragments and prevent union.

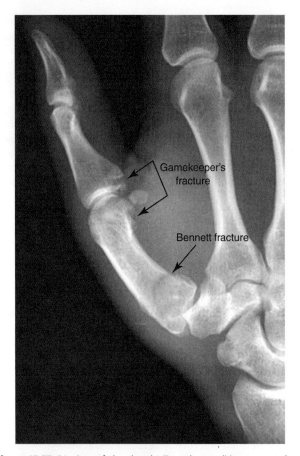

Figure 17-57 PA view of the thumb. Two abnormalities are noted: an acute fracture–dislocation of the base of the first metacarpal, known as a Bennett fracture, and an old avulsion fracture at the site of attachment of the MCP joint ulnar collateral ligament, known as a Gamekeeper's fracture.

compressive forces from the capitate and the thumb axis, and (3) serves as a link between the carpal rows, pushing or pulling the proximal row into position during wrist motions.

Scaphoid fractures occur at three levels: the *distal pole*, the midportion or *waist*, and the *proximal pole* (Fig. 17-58). The majority occur at the waist. The major blood supply of the scaphoid enters through the distal pole. Thus healing of fractures located at the waist or at the proximal pole is rendered less certain and avascular necrosis of the proximal pole is a common complication.

Clinical Considerations The mechanism of injury is a fall on the outstretched hand that imposes a force of dorsiflexion, ulnar deviation, and intercarpal supination. Clinical provocation tests include reproduction of pain to palpation of the space between the extensor pollicis tendons on the dorsal radial aspect of the wrist, known as the anatomic snuffbox: there is pain with dorsal–volar shifting *(scaphoid shift test)* and with passive movement of the wrist from ulnar to radial deviation as the tuberosity undergoes compression *(Watson test)*.

Imaging Routine radiographs plus the ulnar deviation radiograph (scaphoid view) are the first studies recommended. If the radiographs are negative but the clinical exam suggests fracture, protocol is to immobilize and re-radiograph in 10 to 14 days. At that time, if radiographs do not find evidence of fracture but the clinical exam is still significant for fracture, advanced imaging is warranted to reveal occult fractures.

The ACR recommends MRI next, and CT if MRI is not available (Fig. 17-59). Bone scans are recommended only if MRI and CT cannot be performed. Acutely, bone scans may be negative for the first 48 hours, while MRI is positive.

severe comminution, traction and external fixation or brief immobilization with early range-of-motion exercise may remold the articular surface sufficiently to permit functional mobility.

Another eponym, *Gamekeeper's thumb*, describes a common injury at the thumb metacarpophalangeal joint. It is caused by a valgus force that produces a disruption of the ulnar collateral ligament and may also avulse the base of the proximal phalanx (see Fig. 17-57). Originally named for Scottish gamekeepers who sacrificed wounded small game by breaking their necks between the ground and their thumbs and index fingers, a more common mechanism seen today is from the fall of a skier against a planted ski pole.

Fractures of the Wrist

Carpal Fractures

Scaphoid Fractures

Fractures of the scaphoid account for more than 60% of all carpal injuries. The scaphoid's susceptibility to fracture is due in part to its location, where it (1) acts as the principal block to excessive wrist dorsiflexion, (2) accepts

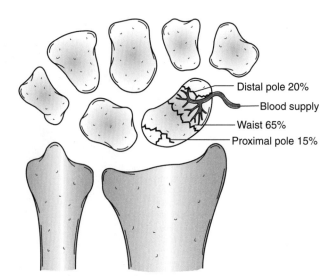

Figure 17-58 The scaphoid is fractured at three levels, the *waist* most frequently. As the major blood supply enters through the distal pole, the proximal pole is often rendered avascular as a complication of fracture across the waist.

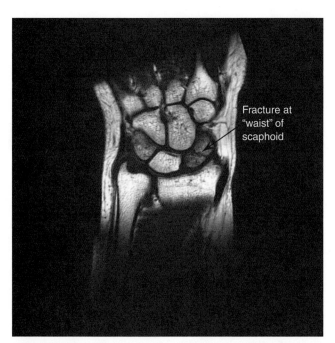

Figure 17-59 T1-weighted coronal MRI of the wrist. A fracture is evident as the low-intensity signal line across the waist of the scaphoid.

Treatment Rates of healing, lengths of treatment immobilization, and complications vary between the fracture locations because of the differentiated vascularity of the scaphoid. Emergency treatment should consist of a thumb spica splint or cast immobilization. Long-arm casting remains controversial, although some studies demonstrate decreased healing time and decreased incidence of nonunion with use of long-arm casts.

Stable nondisplaced fractures are immobilized 6 to 8 weeks in a long-arm thumb spica cast, followed by a short-arm thumb spica cast for an additional 6 to 12 weeks based on radiographic evidence of healing.

Unstable displaced fractures generally require open reduction and internal fixation (ORIF) with wires, pins, or compression screws with or without the use of bone grafts (see Fig. 3-31).

Lunate Fractures

The lunate is a common carpal fracture, second only to the scaphoid.

Clinical Considerations The mechanism of injury is a fall on a hyperextended wrist or a forceful push of the hand with the wrist in hyperextension. Fractures of the lunate often go unrecognized until the bone becomes avascular, at which time Kienbock's disease is diagnosed (see Fig. 3-34).

Imaging MRI is recommended if initial radiographs are nondiagnostic (Fig. 17-60). If radiographs are diagnostic for Kienbock's, CT is recommended only if needed to assess the degree of collapse and associated fractures. The radiographic stages of Kienbock's disease are presented in Figure 17-61.

Treatment Stable nondisplaced lunate fractures are treated with short-arm casting with radiographic follow-up at frequent intervals to evaluate progression of healing. Unstable displaced fractures require ORIF to approximate fragments sufficiently for vascular anastomoses.

Triquetrum Fractures

Clinical Considerations The triquetrum is fractured by either a direct trauma to the ulnar side of the wrist or an avulsion associated with ligament damage. Clinical findings are point tenderness dorsally, 2 cm distal to the ulnar styloid, and reproducible pain with resisted wrist extension.

Imaging Transverse fractures across the body are evident on PA views. Dorsal avulsion fractures may not be evident on the PA view because of superimposition of the lunate; the oblique view is usually diagnostic.

Treatment Nondisplaced fractures are immobilized 6 weeks in a short-arm cast or ulnar gutter splint. Displaced fractures are amenable to open reduction and internal fixation.

Pisiform Fractures

Clinical Considerations Fractures of the pisiform are uncommon and usually undisplaced. The mechanism of injury is a direct blow to the hypothenar eminence. Clinical findings are point tenderness and reproducible pain with

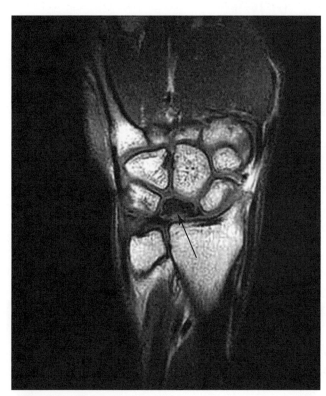

Figure 17-60 Avascular necrosis of the lunate, known as *Kienbock's disease*, seen on a coronal T1-weighted MRI as low intensity signal of the entire lunate with collapse of norml bone architecture. *(Image courtesy of John C. Hunter, MD, University of California, Davis School of Medicine.)*

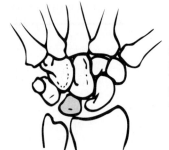

Stage I
Routine radiographs normal. Tomography positive for linear fracture. MRI confirms vascular changes.

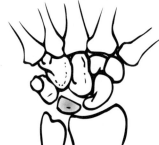

Stage II
Radiographs show sclerosis, fracture line, and cystic changes. No collapse deformity.

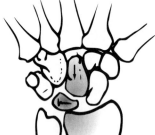

Stage III
Radiographs show advanced bone density changes with fragmentation, cystic resorption, and collapse of lunate, and subluxation of adjacent carpals.

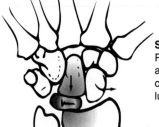

Stage IV
Radiographs show perilunate arthritic changes, complete collapse and fragmentation of lunate.

Figure 17-61 Radiographic staging of avascular necrosis of the lunate, also known as *Kienbock's disease.*

passive extension. This maneuver places the flexor carpi ulnaris (in which the pisiform is embedded) under tension.

Imaging Pisiform fractures are not well demonstrated on routine views. A carpal tunnel view may assist diagnosis.

Treatment Nondisplaced fractures are immobilized in a short-arm cast or ulnar gutter splint 4 to 6 weeks. Displaced fractures often require excision, either early, or late, secondary to nonunion.

Trapezium Fractures

Clinical Considerations Trapezium fractures account for less than 5% of all carpal fractures. They are significant because missed fractures here cause thumb weakness, limited range of motion, and chronic pain. The mechanism of injury is either a direct blow forcing an axial load on an adducted thumb, causing a vertical fracture through the body, or a fall on an extended wrist, causing an avulsion of the trapezial ridge. Clinical findings are reproducible pain on active thumb motion or passive axial compression of the thumb.

Imaging PA views can demonstrate vertical fracture lines. A true AP is often better for diagnosis because of its improved detail. The carpal tunnel view is necessary to visualize trapezial ridge fractures.

Treatment Nondisplaced fractures are immobilized 6 weeks in a thumb spica short-arm cast. Displaced fractures require open reduction and pin or bone graft fixation.

Trapezoid Fractures

Clinical Considerations Isolated trapezoid fractures are rare. The mechanism of injury, an axial force through the second metacarpal, often results in a dislocation of the metacarpal base of the trapezoid. Clinical findings include painful and limited motion of the second metacarpal and a variable dorsal prominence if the trapezoid is dislocated dorsally.

Imaging Routine PA views usually demonstrate this fracture. CT can assist diagnosis if the trapezoid is obscured by overlapping densities.

Treatment Nondisplaced fractures are immobilized 4 to 6 weeks in a short-arm cast. Displaced fractures require open reduction and internal wire fixation to restore carpometacarpal joint congruency.

Capitate Fractures

Clinical Considerations Capitate fractures represent 1% to 2% of all carpal fractures. As with the scaphoid, the proximal pole of the capitate has a tenuous blood supply, which makes it vulnerable to nonunion. The protected position of the capitate makes isolated fractures rare; a fracture of the capitate is more often associated with scaphoid fracture and lunate dislocation. The mechanism of injury is a high-energy blow or crush. Clinical findings are reproducible pain with wrist dorsiflexion.

Imaging Routine views usually demonstrate carpal fractures. CT scans may assist in defining displacement.

Treatment Nondisplaced fractures are immobilized 6 to 8 weeks with interval radiographic evaluation to assess healing. Displaced fractures or combination injuries require ORIF.

Hamate Fractures

Clinical Considerations The hamate may fracture through its distal articular surface from a force transmitted through the fifth metacarpal, as in a fist strike, and the fracture may be accompanied by a dislocation of the fifth metacarpal base.

The hamate may also fracture through its body from direct blow or crush injury. Additionally, the hamate can fracture through its hamulus, or hook. This injury is a frequent athletic injury; the exposed hook is vulnerable to direct blows from bats, hockey sticks, golf clubs, and racquets. The base of the hook is most often involved, although the tip can avulse. The proximity of the ulnar nerve is a concern; injury to the nerve results in paresthesias in the fifth finger and the ulnar aspect of the fourth finger as well as weakness of the intrinsic muscles.

Treatment Nondisplaced fractures are immobilized for 4 to 6 weeks. Displaced fractures may require ORIF with Kirschner wires or screw fixation. Fractures of the hook of the hamate may require excision of the fragment if displaced or in cases of symptomatic nonunion.

Imaging The PA radiograph may demonstrate the fracture, although the radial deviation view and carpal tunnel view remove overlapping superimposition of adjacent structures. If radiography is nondiagnostic, CT is recommended next (Fig. 17-62).

Fractures of the Distal Radius

Incidence

Postmenopausal women incur 60% to 70% of all distal radial fractures as a result of a fall on an outstretched hand. Another 10% to 15% occur in younger adults as a result of violent injuries, as in fistfights, that drive the lunate or scaphoid into the radius, breaking the cortex of the radius like sheet metal being stamped; hence an eponym for these injuries is *die-punch* fractures.

In children, distal radial fractures are the most common of all fractures and heal without difficulty in most cases. The distal third of the radius, or metaphysis, is involved most of the time owing to the decreased bone density at this region of newly formed bone. (Figs. 17-63 and 16-41). The physeal growth plate is involved up to 14% of the time and is the most commonly injured physis in children.

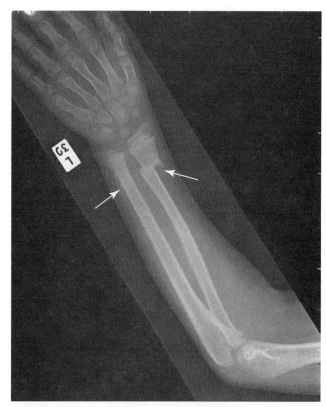

Figure 17-63 Radiograph of the most common fracture in children: fracture of the distal third of the radius due to a fall on an outstretched hand (long arrow). Note also the subtle *torus* or *buckle* fracture at the ulna (short arrow), identifiable by the irregular cortical margin. *(Source of image: http://www.xray2000.co.uk.)*

Eponyms for Distal Radial Fractures

Colles' fracture is an eponym synonomous with distal radial fracture, as 90% of distal radial fractures occur in the pattern described by Abraham Colles almost 200 years ago. The classic Colles' fracture is generally accepted to be an extra-articular fracture located about 1½ inches proximal to the end of the radius, with a volar apex and dorsal angulation or displacement of the distal fragment and with or without an associated ulnar styloid fracture. The attachment of the triangular fibrocartilage complex to the medial side of the radius and to the distal ulna is responsible for the ulnar styloid fractures that frequently accompany distal radial fractures (Figs. 17-64 and 17-65).

The *Smith fracture* (also called a reverse Colles' fracture) is a *dorsal* apex and *volar* angulation of the distal fragment. A *Barton fracture* is a fracture–dislocation injury in which the volar or, more commonly, dorsal radial rim is fractured and displaces with the hand and carpus.

These eponyms are in common use among clinicians but are avoided in radiologic description because of their inexactness and subsequent potential to direct inappropriate treatment.

Clinical Considerations

Complications are involved in approximately 30% of distal radial fractures. The majority of complications are related to

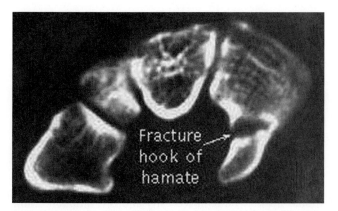

Figure 17-62 Axial CT scan through the distal carpal row demonstrates a fracture of the hook of the hamate. *(Source of image: http://www.xray2000.co.uk.)*

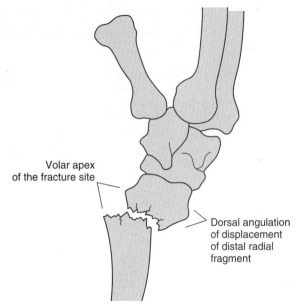

Volar apex
of the fracture site

Dorsal angulation
of displacement
of distal radial
fragment

Figure 17-64 The typical Colles' fracture occurs 1½ inches proximal to the distal end of the radius.

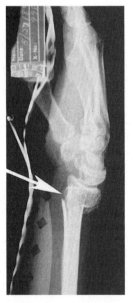

Figure 17-65 Distal radial fracture (Colles' fracture). This lateral view of the wrist demonstrates a volar apex of the fracture site (arrow) with dorsal angulation of the distal fragment. A longitudinal fracture line is also seen extending along the volar aspect of the radial shaft.

malunion deformities that alter the articular relationships at the wrist.

Complications of Malunion

Radial shortening, with loss of the radial angle to less than 15 degrees, is the most disabling deformity after distal radial fracture (Fig. 17-66). Under normal loading of the wrist, the ulnocarpal joint bears 20% and the radiocarpal joint bears 80% of the load. Radial shortening results in a transfer of the majority of loading to the ulnocarpal joint; this results in ulnocarpal impingement, pain, decreased range of motion, and pathology at the triangular fibrocartilage complex. Surgical salvage procedures remove the ulnar head or fuse the distal radioulnar joint.

Loss of the volar tilt of the radius is the most difficult deformity to correct. This malunion results in extrinsic midcarpal instability, increased ulnar loading, and distal radioulnar joint (DRUJ) dysfunction with invariable loss of flexion.

Any articular incongruity after fracture is a malunion that can eventually lead to the development of posttraumatic arthritis. Other complications include median nerve dysfunction, reflex sympathetic dystrophy, rupture of the extensor pollicis longus, and midcarpal instability.

Ligamentous Injuries

Carpal ligament disruption occurs with both extra- and intra-articular fractures of the distal radius. The incidence of scapholunate tears is approximately 30%, and that of lunotriquetral tears is approximately 15%. A clear correlation between specific radial fracture patterns and the extent or location of carpal ligament tears has not as yet been shown.

It is recognized that many partial tears heal uneventfully during the peroid of immobilization necessary for the fracture to unite. Complete tears diagnosed after fracture healing are difficult to treat; options range from conservative measures to ligament reconstruction or carpal fusion.

Imaging

Radiographic examination on the lateral view identifies the amount of fracture fragment angulation relative to the normal volar tilt of the distal radial articular surface. The "dinner fork" deformity sometimes resulting from this fracture is apparent on the lateral films. The volar tilt of the radius is assessed. Restoration of normal volar tilt will help ensure a preserved radiocarpal articular relationship.

The PA view assesses radial shortening caused by overlap of the fracture fragments. Postreduction films should verify that the dorsal displacement of the distal fragment and radial shortening have been corrected. Assessment of ulnar variance helps to confirm this.

Ligamentous lesions are identified with MRI, arthrography, or arthroscopy.

Treatment

Stable, minimally displaced fractures are treated with reduction and immobilization for 6 to 8 weeks. The ideal casting position, duration of immobilization, and use of a long-arm cast remains controversial. When a long-arm cast is used, it is converted to a short-arm cast midway through the immobilization period.

Unstable or displaced fractures may require fixation after reduction. Percutaneous pinning is primarily used for extra-articular fractures and two-part intra-articular fractures. External fixation frames or casting is combined with pin fixation. Pins may be removed early and cast immobilization continued until radiographic evidence of successful healing is demonstrated.

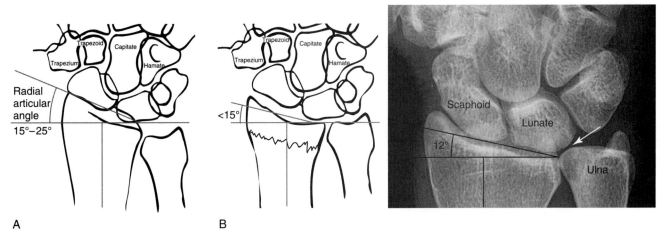

Figure 17-66 (A and B) A complication of fracture of the distal radius is radial shortening, with subsequent loss of the radial articular angle to less than 15 degrees, which results in abnormal ulnocarpal joint loading.

Wrist Instability[36-39,49-66]

The majority of diagnoses of wrist instability are made on the basis of the history and clinical examination. Imaging plays a significant role, however, in the identification of the extent of the pathology, exclusion of differential pathologies, facilitation of a precise diagnosis to direct appropriate treatment, and provision of an informed prognosis for the patient.

In addition, close interaction between the radiologist and the clinician is essential for the correct diagnosis of subtle abnormalities of carpal kinematics. Although general guidelines exist, there are no specific algorithms to diagnose radiologically what is suspected clinically (Fig. 17-67). The complexity of pathology at the wrist demands that each situation be assessed individually. Evaluation of subtle wrist instability requires professional collaboration.

Imaging Techniques to Diagnose Instability

The kinematic concepts of the wrist are complex and remain somewhat controversial. Consequently, the choice of imaging study for a given situation in *chronic* wrist pain is also controversial, and disparity exists between the radiologic and orthopedic literature. Most physicians agree, however, that imaging for the diagnosis of wrist instability begins with routine radiographs and the special views of functional radiographs.

Cineradiography, CT , and bone scans may be appropriate in selected cases. Associated ligamentous lesions can be diagnosed via arthrography, MRI, MR arthrography, CT arthrography, or arthroscopy. The role of these studies in the assessment of instability follows.

Routine Radiographs

The patterns of instability, or *dyskinematic syndromes,* are currently classified by radiologic appearance:

- *Predynamic instability* is a clinical diagnosis without alterations evident on routine radiographs.

- *Dynamic instability* is present if the dyskinematics can be seen only with special techniques such as functional radiographs or motion studies.
- *Static instability* is present if the dyskinematic syndrome is evident on routine radiographs.

It is important to recognize that the value of routine and functional radiographs in the assessment of carpal kinematics depends greatly on accurate patient positioning and true central ray projection to avoid spatial distortion and meaningless measurements.

On routine radiographs, stability is assessed by examining the morphological characteristics of the carpals as well as the radiographic measurements.

Morphological Evaluation

Morphological evaluation on the PA view includes the following:

- Intact, continuous, contours of the three arcuate lines drawn across the proximal and distal surfaces of scaphoid, lunate, and triquetrum and the proximal surfaces of capitate and hamate
- *Parallelism* of the articular surfaces of articulating bones; a lack of parallelism between the scaphoid and the lunate is a subtle sign of disassociation; a prominent sign is a gap greater than 3 mm wide between these bones
- Normal shape of each carpal, particularly of the scaphoid and lunate; the shape of the lunate is trapezoidal in the neutral wrist but alters if the lunate is flexed or extended; if the scaphoid is flexed, it will foreshorten and a cortical ring outline will appear.

Morphological evaluation of the lateral view includes the following:

- Alignment of the radius, lunate, capitate, and third metacarpal; these bones should be collinear although only 11% of wrists show this exact alignment; most wrists exhibit variance within 10 degrees.

Other abnormalites are evaluated on the routine views, including soft tissue swelling, obliteration or bowing of fat spaces, fracture lines, degenerative changes, or inflammatory articular lesions.

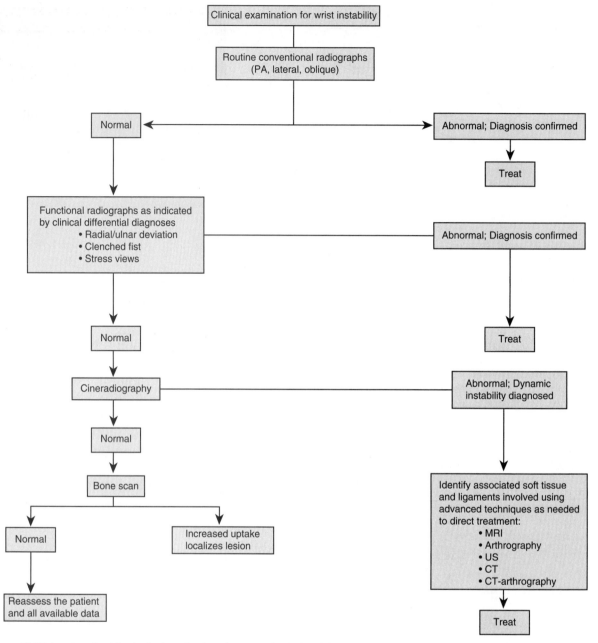

Figure 17-67 Imaging algorithm in the investigation of suspected wrist instability.

Evaluation of Radiographic Measurement

Many parameters exist to help identify carpal instability and assess the potential benefits of various surgical procedures. Databases of normal measurements are helpful if the standard deviation is small. However, wrist morphology shows significant individual variability, which can preclude the detection of subtle instabilities.

It would seem logical to use a patient's healthy wrist as a reference for normal measurement. Interestingly, however, some morphological differences are known to vary significantly between the left and right wrists of the same individual. Radial angle inclination, volar tilt, and ulnar variance can vary significantly in the same individual. Comparison with a database in the general population is suggested for these measurements. Otherwise, carpal height and carpal angle measurements are usually similar bilaterally.

Table 17-1 provides the mean values, standard deviations, and normal limits of common wrist measurement, given for both the PA and lateral views.

Functional Radiographs

Functional radiographs are also called *dynamic views* and *stress views*. The purpose of these views is to study the kinematic behavior of the carpals and detect abnormalities under the influence of tissue tension. These views can be taken of both wrists to compare carpal motion in the healthy wrist with carpal motion in the painful wrist. Functional radiographs include the following:

- PA views in radial deviation, ulnar deviation, and neutral.
- *Clenched-fist PA view:* The patient forcibly clenches the fist as tightly as possible. This results in axial compression,

TABLE 17-1 ● *Measurements of the Wrist, Mean Values, Standard Deviations, and Normal Limits*

Measurement	Definition	Mean	Standard Deviation	Limits of Normal Value
Posteroanterior view				
Inclination angle of the distal radius (degrees)	Angle between a line tangential to the distal articular surface of the radius and a line perpendicular to the shaft of the radius	23.8	2.6	18.8–29.3
Ulnar variance (mm)	Difference between average radius of radial scaphoid lunate fossa and distance between the center of this circle and the cortical rim of the ulnar dome	−0.9	1.5	−4.2 to +2.3
Carpal height (mm)	Distance between the base of the third metacarpal and the point of intersection of the third metacarpal axis with the radiocarpal joint line	33.8	6.1	27.4–40.0
Carpal ulnar distance (mm)	Perpendicular distance between theoretical center of rotation for radial/ulnar deviation of the wrist and longitudinal axis of the ulna projected distally	17.1	3.3	11.4–25.4
Carpal radial distance (mm)	Perpendicular distance between theoretical center of rotation for radial/ulnar deviation of the wrist and a line from the radial styloid that extends distally and parallel to the axis of the distal end of the radius	19.0	1.7	15.9–22.4
Length of the third metacarpal (mm)	Main longitudinal axis	63.2	4.5	55.3–73.2
Length of the capitate (mm)	Main longitudinal axis	21.7	2.1	17.9–25.5
Carpal height ratio	Carpal height/length of the third metacarpal	0.53	0.1	0.46–0.61
Carpal ulnar ratio	Carpal ulnar distance/length of the third metacarpal	0.27	0.03	0.18–0.41
Carpal radial ratio	Carpal radial distance/length of the third metacarpal	0.30	0.02	0.24–0.34
Modified carpal height ratio	Carpal height/length of the capitate	1.56	0.05	
Lateral view				
Palmar tilt of the distal radius (degrees)	Angle between distal articular surface of the radius and perpendicular to the long axis of the shaft of the radius	10.2	2.7	0–20
Carpal height (mm)	See above	35.9	3.2	
Radiolunate angle (degrees)	The lunate axis is defined as the perpendicular to a line joining the palmar and dorsal horns of the bone. Positive with palmar flexion of the lunate	7	6.8	−20 to +10
Scapholunate angle (degrees)	The axis of the scaphoid is defined as tangent to the palmar proximal and distal convexity margins	47.1	6.9	30–70
Capitolunate angle (degrees)	The dorsal margin of the third metacarpal is used as substitute axis for the capitate	10.9	3.5	−20 to +10

Reprinted with permission from Büchler,[21] p. 63.

which pushes the head of the capitate toward the scapholunate interval. If instability is present, the scapholunate space will open, revealing a diastasis (gap) that was not present at rest (Fig. 17-68). Lateral views may also be obtained.

● *Stress views:* These PA or lateral views are made while the examiner passively moves the joint into physiological positions or nonphysiological positions, such as volar or dorsal translation (drawer tests) or ulnar or radial translation or traction. These views may detect a diastasis not apparent on static radiographs.

Cineradiography Motion Studies

Some authors consider cineradiography the imaging method par excellence for diagnosing dynamic carpal instability, particularly at the proximal carpal row level (Fig. 17-69).

Dynamic wrist instability is characterized by rapid abnormal shifts between the carpals, appearing under certain kinematic conditions in response to joint position, joint motion, and loading patterns. Routine and functional radiographs, taken in static positions, are not likely to reveal dynamic imaging instability. If these initial studies are negative in a case of clinically suspected instability, further assessment should include cineradiography.

Cineradiography is the only imaging method that consistently diagnoses dynamic instability.

Components

Cineradiography, also called *cinefluoroscopy*, is a radiographic motion study. The components of this imaging modality include a fluoroscopic unit, a cine camera (similar to a movie camera) and a recording medium. Images may be recorded on 16- or 35-mm film, on videotape, or in digital cinefluoroscopy systems. Studies are evaluated on repeated slow-motion replays.

Examination

The examination is not complex. The patient rests the wrist on the surface of the image intensifier in a PA position. The patient moves the wrist back and forth between radial and ulnar deviation. Next, the patient places the wrist in the lateral view position and moves it back and forth between flexion and extension. If there are complaints of clicking or snapping, the patient is asked to try to reproduce it during these maneuvers.

Normal Cineradiographic Anatomy

The kinematics of the wrist can be explained using the concept of three "rows." The two outer rows are relatively rigid,

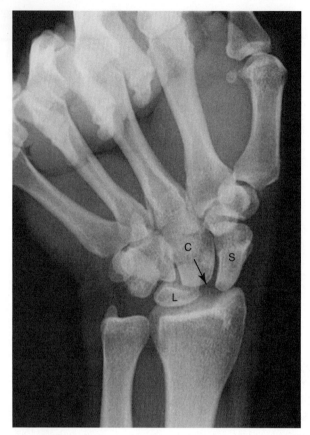

Figure 17-68 Clenched-fist view demonstrates the *dynamic* instability of the scapholunate articulation. A forceful grip produces an axial compression, which pushes the capitate proximally toward the scapholunate interval; this will gap if the scapholunate ligament is insufficient.

while the interposed row is adaptive to the borders of the two outer rows:

- The distal "rigid" row consists of the conjoined trapezium, trapezoid, capitate, and hamate.
- The proximal "rigid" row consists of the radius, triangular fibrocartilage complex, and ulna.
- The interposed row is the adaptive condylar segment and consists of scaphoid, lunate, triquetrum, and pisiform. It is this row (the proximal row of carpals) that makes the most adjustments to allow free movement of the wrist; thus it is also at this row that the dyskinematics of instability are found.

Normally, upon ulnar deviation, the following occurs as seen on the PA view:

- The scaphoid appears long and extended and disengages from the trapezium–trapezoid joint.
- The hamate–triquetral joint approximates and moves lower, adapting to the reduced height of the ulna.
- Extension of the lunate decreases radiocapitate distance and allows the capitate to migrate proximally.

Normally, upon radial deviation, the entire interposed proximal carpal row flexes and the following occurs as seen on the PA view:

- The scaphoid rotates and flexes, allowing approximation of the distal row to the radius.
- The hamate–triquetral joint distracts and moves into a higher position.
- The lunate flexes, permitting adaptive extension of the capitate.

Diagnosis of Dynamic Instability

Diagnosis requires viewing the cineradiographic movie repeatedly, first analyzing the movements of the proximal and distal carpal rows as units and then analyzing the movements of each carpal bone. Diagnosis is made by recognizing momentary abnormalities; these may be diastases, subluxations, or abnormal carpal movement.

For example, isolated sprains or tears of the scapholunate interosseous ligament are demonstrated on the PA view by a momentary gap at the scapholunate articulation and abnormal tilting of the scaphoid. A lateral view demonstrates an abrupt momentary shift of the proximal carpal row.

Advanced Imaging Techniques

Arthrography

If routine and functional radiographs fail to identify a cause for persistant pain, arthrography may be indicated. "Three-phase arthrography" evaluates the radiocarpal, radioulnar, and midcarpal joints by separate injections (Figs. 17-70 and 17-71). Leakage from the radiocarpal joint into the distal radioulnar joint indicates a tear of the triangular fibrocartilage complex. Injections to the remaining joints are spaced by 2 or 3 hours to allow the contrast to clear. Alternatively, digital subtraction techniques can be used for immediate sequential injections. Limitations to arthrography are that it is a two-dimensional investigation of a three-dimensional problem and, significantly, that it is difficult to determine whether a leak is a pathological tear or a degenerative perforation. Leaks of contrast have been shown to be present in the contralateral, asymptomatic wrist and unrelated to trauma.

Bone Scans

As a screening investigation, bone scans can localize the problem but not the pathology. Bone scan is highly sensitive to early joint arthrosis, nonunion, and avascularity.

Ultrasound

Ultrasound has value in the identification of inter- and intraosseous ganglia and synovial cysts of the dorsal wrist and can exclude them as a cause of persistent pain.

CT and CT Arthrography

CT has value in identifying surface irregularities of the joints, identification of exact anatomic location of contrast media leaks, and subtle characteristis of fractures and malunions.

MRI and MR Arthrography

MRI and MR arthrography continue to evolve in value in the specific diagnoses of interosseous ligament tears, intraarticular fractures, vascularity changes, and tears of the triangular fibrocartilage complex.

Instability of the Distal Radioulnar Joint

Wrist instability can be grossly divided into (1) instability at the distal radioulnar joint (DRUJ) and (2) instability between the intercarpal joints. Although these joints are related, they are presented separately here for learning purposes.

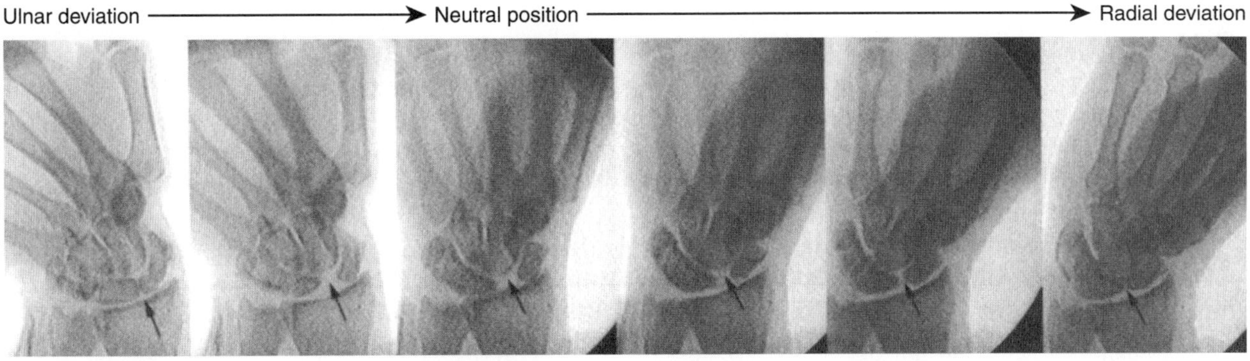

Ulnar deviation ——————————→ Neutral position ————————————————→ Radial deviation

Figure 17-69 Cineradiographic study of a left wrist. Look at the frames from left to right. The arrow points to the scapholunate interval on all frames. As the patient moves the hand from ulnar deviation to neutral, a gap of more than 3 mm appears between the scaphoid and lunate. As the patient continues to move from neutral to radial deviation, this gap closes. All cases of dynamic instability are not the same; in some patients gaps may close in neutral position and widen with either radial or ulnar deviation. *(Reprinted with permission from Buchler,[21] p. 72.)*

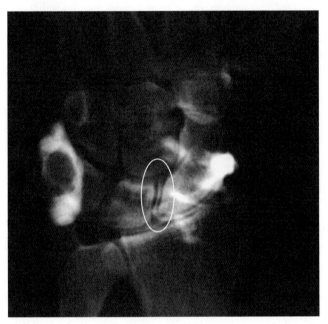

Figure 17-70 Arthrogram of the midcarpal joint. Leakage of contrast into the space between the scaphoid and the lunate indicates a tear of the scapholunate ligament (circled).

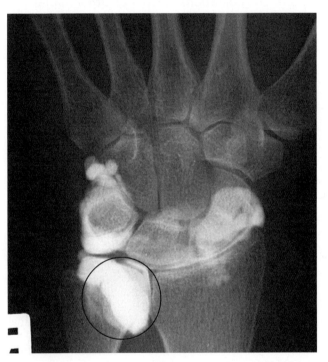

Figure 17-71 Arthrogram of the radiocarpal joint. Leakage of contrast from the radiocarpal joint into the distal radioulnar joint (circled) indicates a tear of the triangular fibrocartilage complex.

In the strict anatomic sense, the distal forearm joint is composed solely of the DRUJ. Functionally, however, the distal forearm joint is composed of the DRUJ, the triangular fibrocartilage complex (TFCC), the ulnocarpal ligaments, and the interosseous membrane. These structures are interlinked, and all contribute to the stability or, after insult, instability of the DRUJ.

Clinical Presentation

DRUJ instability or degenerative arthritis presents with the primary feature of painful forearm rotation. Pain with ulnar deviation suggests TFCC pathology or ulnar impaction. Snapping or popping sensations may represent subluxing or dislocating tendons, carpal instabilities, or TFCC tears.

Chronic instability of the DRUJ can be either dorsal, volar, or global. Dorsal instability causes pain and dislocation in pronation. Volar instability causes pain and dislocation in supination. Global instability causes pain and dislocation in both maneuvers. DRUJ stability must be compared between both of an individual's wrists, because there is considerable variation in "normal" stability among individuals. Because of this, CT imaging studies for instability are done with both wrists simultaneously in neutral, pronation, and supination.

Stability testing is performed in full supination, neutral rotation, and full pronation in both wrists. The volar ligaments are the more important stabilizer in pronation, and the dorsal ligaments are more important in supination. The "piano key" sign is elicited by placing the patient's palm and forearm flat on the table, then having them force the pisiform against the table using the entire upper extremity. The distal ulna will migrate toward the table, the degree determined by the laxity or volar displacement of the radiocarpal unit in the resting position.

Clinical Considerations Related to Distal Radial Fracture

As many as 30% of patients with distal radius fractures have lasting complaints of pain in the DRUJ region. Distal radius fractures may disrupt the DRUJ directly or as a consequence of malunion deformities (radial shortening, angulation) or articular injury. The anatomy of the DRUJ normally accommodates a degree of proximal/distal motion with movement, but dorsal angulation after distal radius fracture can be problematic. More than 20 degrees of dorsal angulation will cause serious restriction of motion and DRUJ degeneration. Orthopedic hand specialists do not like to see any dorsal angulation following a distal radius fracture. They attempt to reduce the angulation to at least a neutral position if the normal volar angulation cannot be restored.

Clinical Considerations Related to Other Injuries

Galeazzi Fracture–Dislocation

The eponym *Galeazzi fracture* refers to a fracture at the junction of the middle and distal thirds of the radius with an associated DRUJ dislocation (Fig. 17-72). Treatment includes radial fixation and reduction of the DRUJ. If the reduction is stable, cast immobilization in supination will suffice. If there is instability but reduction is easily obtained, the DRUJ is reduced and pinned in neutral rotation for 6 weeks. Marked instability or inability to reduce satisfactorily requires open reduction and internal fixation, TFCC and capsule repair, followed by pinning or external fixation to maintain the reduction.

Fractures of the Radial Head

The eponym *Essex–Lopresti fracture–dislocation* refers to fracture of the radial head with dislocation of the DRUJ. This injury involves disruption of the interosseous membrane. After fixation, repair, or replacement of the radial head, the DRUJ must be reduced and pinned until healing can occur, usually in supination. In some cases the interosseous membrane fails to heal; if the radial head is resected, proximal migration of the radius may occur for at least 2 years. This condition disrupts the DRUJ, causing instability and abutment of the ulna to the proximal carpal row.

Fractures of the Ulna

Ulnar styloid fractures occur in more than 50% of fractures of the distal radius. About 25% of ulnar styloid fractures result in nonunion. Instability at the DRUJ results from associated tears of the TFCC. TFCC tears are suspected if there is radial displacement of the styloid or if the fracture is located at the base of the styloid. For these reasons, fractures involving the base of the styloid are fixated to stabilize the TFCC.

Fractures of the distal ulnar shaft may also destabilize the DRUJ. DRUJ incongruency and restricted motion usually become symptomatic with 20 degrees or more of dorsal angulation of the ulnar shaft.

Treatment of DRUJ Instability

Conservative treatment with strengthening of the ulnar wrist motors is rarely successful. A forearm splint molded to support the DRUJ in a reduced position may be of benefit. In more pronounced instability that fails conservative

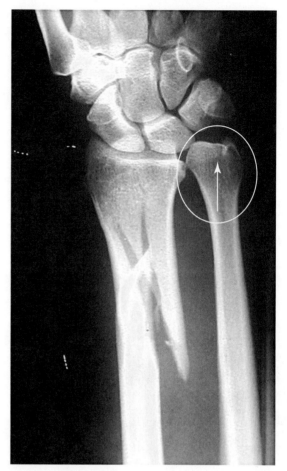

Figure 17-72 Galeazzi fracture. PA view of the wrist demonstrates a spiral, comminuted fracture at the distal third of the radius with dislocation of the distal radioulnar joint (circle) and distal translation (arrow) of the ulna resulting in carpal abutment.

measures, surgery must be considered. Options can include TFCC and distal radioulnar ligament repairs, tethering procedures, or a combination of the two. If the DRUJ is degenerative, some form of resection may be needed. If there is an ulnar positive variance, ulnar shortening will be needed. If there is a distal radial malunion, correction of radial alignment should be performed first and is often all that is needed.

If no degeneration is present, TFCC repair may suffice, but if this is tenuous or no tear is identified, a tethering procedure may be chosen. This may include palmaris longus grafting or using a distal strip of flexor carpi ulnaris or extensor carpi ulnaris, passing these structures though drill holes in the distal ulna and looping the tendon ends back on to themselves, forming a sling.

Classification of Carpal Instabilities

Instability of the wrist is a condition of altered joint kinematics in which one or more carpal bones are permitted abnormal mobility as a result of joint laxity, ligamentous lesions, or bony abnormalities. Several classifications of carpal instability exist. See Table 17-2 for the Mayo Clinic, Taleisnik, and Lichtman classification systems.

TABLE 17-2 ● *Existing Classification Systems for Carpal Instability*

Carpal Instability Dissociative (CID)	Carpal Instability Nondissociative (CIND)	Combined CID/CIND Instability
The Mayo Clinic Classification		
Proximal row CID: • Unstable scaphoid fracture (DISI) • Scapholunate dissociation (DISI) • Lunotriquetral dissociation (VISI) Distal row CID: • Axial–radial (AR) dissociation (radial trans, PM) • Axial–ulnar (AU) dissociation (ulnar trans, PM) • Combined AR–AU dissociation Combined proximal–distal CID Key: DISI: distal intercalated segmental instability VISI: volar intercalated segmental instability Trans: translocation PM: proximal migration	Radiocarpal CIND: • Malunion of the distal radius (DISI, dorsal trans) • Radiocarpal ligament rupture (ulnar trans) • Madelung's deformity (ulnar trans, PM) Midcarpal CIND: • Triquetrum–hamate–capitate ligament rupture (VISI) • Scapho–trapezium–trapezoid ligament rupture (VISI) • Combination Combined radiocarpal–midcarpal instability: • Capitate–lunate instability pattern (CLIP)	Perilunate instability (DISI, ulnar trans)
The Lichtman Classification		

I. Lesser-arc injuries
  • Scapholunate instability, dynamic, partial, static, or complete (DISI)
  • Triquetrolunate instability, dynamic or static (VISI)
  • Perilunate dislocation
II. Greater-arc injuries
  • Scaphoid fractures (stable, unstable)
  • Scaphocapitate injury
  • Variations/combinations
III. Inflammatory disorders
  • Scapholunate instability, static or dynamic
  • Triquetrolunate instability, static or dynamic
IV. Proximal instability
  • Ulnar translocation of the carpus, rheumatoid or post-traumatic
  • Dorsal Barton fracture (intra-articular radial rim fracture)
  • Palmar Barton fracture
V. Miscellaneous		

The Taleisnik Classsification		
Lateral instability: • Scapholunate • Scaphocapitate • Scaphotrapezial	Medial instability: • Triquetrolunate • Triquetrohamate	Proximal instability: • Radiocarpal • Midcarpal

The following text uses the descriptive categories of the Mayo Clinic system. In this system, instabilities are grouped into the following:

- *Carpal instability dissociative (CID)* involves pathology in the intrinsic carpal ligaments and occurs between bones in the same carpal row. (*Dissociative* means that two individual carpals are dissociated from each other.)
- *Carpal instability nondissociative (CIND)* involves pathology of the extrinsic ligaments that leads to abnormal motions of the entire proximal carpal row at both the radiocarpal and the midcarpal joints. (*Nondissociative* means that the pathology is *not* between individual carpals but involves the entire row.)
- *Carpal instability combined (CIC)* involves pathology of both intrinsic and extrinsic ligaments in the wrist.

Carpal Instability Dissociative (CID)

Unstable Scaphoid Fracture

To understand the importance of the scaphoid in wrist stability, recall the three-row concept of the wrist. Now think of the three rows as links in a chain. Like a chain, this construct is stable in tension but unstable in compression. It requires a stabilizing bar to support compression. The scaphoid provides this stability by its connection distally to the capitate and proximally to the lunate. Disruption of the scaphoid renders the carpus unstable and subject to collapse. The radius, lunate, and capitate are then no longer collinear.

Most frequently, the lunate tilts dorsally with the attached proximal pole of the fractured scaphoid. Loading of the distal fragment by the trapezium and trapezoid favors axial compression, causing the distal fragment to flex while the proximal fragment extends, thus creating a volarflexed "humpback" position of the scaphoid. This instability of this fracture contributes to delayed healing because it maintains malalignment across the scaphoid waist.

Scapholunate Dissociation

Scapholunate dissociation is a specific type of instability characterized by malalignment between the scaphoid and lunate. The terms *dorsal intercalated segment instability (DISI)* and *volar intercalated segment instability (VISI)* are used to designate the position of the lunate on the lateral radiograph. Refer back to Figure 17-15 for a schematic that defines these terms.

A uniform pathology is not responsible for scapholunate dissociation; a wide variety of lesions can result in this instability. Commonly, scapholunate dissociation results after injury to the strong scapholunate or lunotriquetral ligaments. The mechanism of injury usually involves a fall on the dorsiflexed, ulnar-deviated wrist. With greater imposed force, this injury can progress to tearing of the scapholunate interosseus ligament, the volar radiocarpal ligaments, and, finally, the dorsal radiocarpal ligaments. Rotary subluxation of the scaphoid, in which the scaphoid rotates toward the palm, occurs with complete disruption of ligamentous stability between the lunate and scaphoid.

The stages of progression of scapholunate instability are described as follows:

- *Predynamic instability* presents with clinical signs, including dorsal wrist pain, but with normal radiographic findings.
- *Dynamic instability* presents with the carpals in normal alignment at rest but collapsed under load. Localized tenderness, provoked by gripping and direct compression over the joint, are frequent complaints. Scapholunate ballottement or shear provokes symptoms. Routine radiographs reveal no dissociation. The lax ligaments are evident only when the wrist is stressed. The diagnosis is confirmed with cineradiographs and ulnar deviation, radial deviation, and clenched-fist radiographs by the following signs: increase in the scapholunate gap (normally less than 2 mm) and a foreshortened appearance of the scaphoid with a "cortical ring" sign. The cortical ring sign is due to overlapping of the cortical waist with volarflexed distal pole of the scaphoid. The widened

scapholunate gap is popularly called the "Terry Thomas sign" after the British actor with a wide gap between his front teeth. Refer to Figure 17-68.

- *Static instability* presents with more advanced clinical findings and is evident on routine PA radiographs as a widening of the scapholunate gap greater than 3 mm (Fig. 17-73A). The lunate, no longer attached to the scaphoid, extends through its attachment to the triquetrum so that its distal surface tilts dorsally. The scaphoid is pulled into flexion (distal pole tilts volarly) through its intact ligamentous attachment with the trapezium and trapezoid. The lateral view will demonstrate DISI and a scapholunate angle greater than 70 degrees.

Scapholunate Advanced Collapse The natural history of a static scapholunate dissociation with a DISI deformity is not entirely delineated; however, it appears that longstanding DISI deformities result in degenerative arthritis. This arthritis first involves the radioscaphoid articulation, particularly at the tip of the radial styloid, and later advances to include capitolunate arthritic changes. Further progression results in degenerative arthritis throughout the carpus, called scapholunate advanced collapse (SLAC) wrist (Fig. 17-73B).

Treatment Patients with scapholunate dissociation are good candidates for surgical repair, with relatively reliable results if treated acutely (within 6 weeks). Nonoperative restoration of scaphoid and lunate alignment is virtually impossible. In chronic cases the ability to repair the scapholunate interosseous ligament directly is lost secondary to atrophy of the ligament remnants.

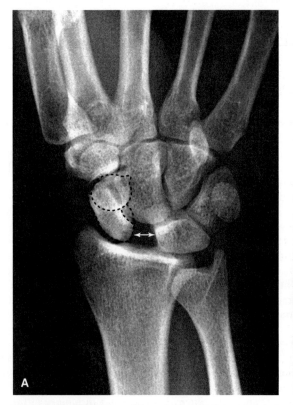
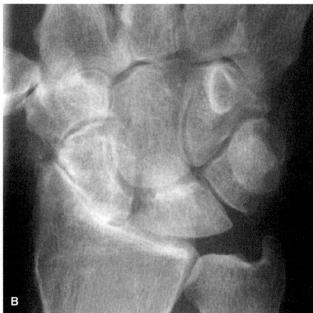

Figure 17-73 **(A)** PA view of the wrist demonstrates a scapholunate dissociation with two classic signs: the *Terry Thomas sign* is an obvious gap in the carpal row and the *signet ring sign* (tracing) is the rotation of the scaphoid, which can occur only with ligamentous instability. **(B)** PA view of chronic scapholunate dissociation resulting in *SLAC,* identified by decreased joint spaces, periarticular sclerosis, scaphoid rotation, and carpal collapse.

Surgical options include: scapholunate ligament repair, dorsal capsulodesis (Blatt procedure), or varieties of intercarpal arthrodesis. Examples of intercarpal arthrodeses are the triscaphe fusion or STT fusion (scaphoid–trapezium–trapezoid), scaphocapitate fusion, or scapholunate fusion. Carpal fusions are durable once union has occurred, but the disadvantages include a high rate of nonunion, decreased motion, and altered carpal mechanics. Salvage procedures include proximal-row carpectomy and wrist arthrodesis.

Intercarpal fusion results in a 50% loss of wrist motion, with the greatest loss in radial deviation. STT fusions have a relatively high rate of nonunion. Proximal-row carpectomy results in weakness of grip, with strength averaging between 50 and 80% of the opposite side. These patients ultimately have a flexion/extension arc of 80 degrees, generally have minimal symptoms, but in some cases may develop secondary degenerative arthritis on the head of the capitate, which necessitates a subsequent fusion.

Patients with total wrist fusion generally have mild persistent pain, decreased grip strength, and minor functional limitations due to lack of movement in the wrist.

Lunotriquetral Dissociation

Lunotriquetral dissociation is a specific type of instability characterized by malalignment between the lunate and triquetrum.

This type of instability can occur secondary to an injury to the ulnar side of the wrist that ruptures the lunotriqetral and triquetrocapitate ligaments. It is also a sequela of rheumatoid arthritis and may develop insidiously in about 20% of the elderly population, possibly as a result of degenerative joint disease.

The VISI deformity is seen in half of the cases of lunotriquetral dissociation. The distal surface of the lunate tilts volarly, and thus the angle between the lunate and scaphoid decreases. On the lateral view, an angle of less then 30 degrees indicates VISI.

Clinically, patients complain of pain on the ulnar aspect of the wrist, which is exacerbated by gripping and ulnar deviation. Dorsal tenderness over the lunotriquetral (LT) ligament may be present. Provocation tests include shearing the triquetrum on a fixed lunate, thereby stressing the LT ligament.

Treatment Most often, lunotriquetral tears do not lead to degenerative joint disease. Nonoperative treatment for acute injuries consists of immobilization for 6 weeks to allow healing of ruptured ligaments. Pinning may be necessary to obtain correct alignment. Failure of nonoperative methods requires surgical ligamentous repair and arthrodesis. Salvage procedures include a four-corner fusion (capitate, lunate, hamate, and triquetrum) and total wrist fusion.

Carpal Instability Nondissociative (CIND)

Carpal instability nondissociative (CIND) includes a complex group of carpal instabilities, which have been labeled midcarpal instability, ulnar translation of the carpus, capitolunate instability, ulnar carpal instability, and triquetral hamate instability. Carpal instability involving the entire proximal carpal row usually occurs in individuals between 20 and 50 years of age. Few patients have wrist-specific ligamentous laxity; most often these patients have generalized ligamentous laxity exhibited by hyperextensibility. Mechanism of injury ranges from minor trauma, to fall on dorsiflexed, rotated hand, to no history of trauma but years of asymptomatic wrist "clunking."

Triquetrum–Hamate–Capitate Ligament Rupture

Most patients with midcarpal CIND have a normal radiographic appearance, but some may exhibit an abnormal VISI resting posture. The classic clinical sign is pain and clicking or clunking sounds when moving the wrist in a circle or when moving from radial to ulnar deviation. This represents dynamic subluxation and a sudden shifting in the position of the proximal carpal row. This painful audible sensation can be eliminated by mechanically positioning the triquetrum dorsally back onto the appropriate facet of the hamate (by pushing the pisiform dorsally) when the wrist is moved in a circular or deviated fashion. The most useful imaging study to diagnose this instability is cineradiography.

Treatment Many patients respond well to nonoperative treatment. Therapeutic measures include strengthening of the hypothenar and extensor carpi ulnaris muscles. The patient can be taught to stabilize the wrist with these muscles prior to ulnar deviation and thus avoid the "clunk." Nonsteroidal anti-inflammatory medications or steroid injections are used to address the synovitis or arthritic components of the symptoms. Splinting is applied in such a way as to stabilize the wrist while providing a pisiform boost.

Surgical treatment for this group of patients is complex and the results are not consistently good. Some procedures in use include triquetral hamate capsular imbrication or triquetral hamate fusion. More recently, soft tissue reconstruction from both a volar and a dorsal approach is recommended. The repair is protected with K-wires for 8 weeks with immobilization in a short-arm cast, followed by 4 more weeks in a splint. The goal is to promote some wrist stiffness in order to control the unstable proximal carpal row.

In symptomatic CIND patients with negative ulnar variance, ulnar lengthening procedures help the carpus return to normal smooth movement.

Carpal Instability Combined (CIC)

Carpal instability combined (CIC) is also referred to as combined CID/CIND. Either term refers to injury patterns involving both the intrinsic carpal ligaments and the extrinsic ligamentous complex.

Perilunate Dislocation

Perilunate dislocation is the complete dislocation of the head of the capitate from the distal surface of the lunate. This is not a common injury; it results from high-energy trauma involving mechanisms of wrist hyperextension or hyperflexion, compression, and intercarpal rotation. A spectrum of progressive ligamentous and osseous lesions is seen, which explains the wide variation in pathology (Fig. 17-74). For this particular injury to occur, the intrinsic ligaments, including the scapholunate and lunotriquetral ligaments as well as the volar radiocarpal ligaments, must be disrupted.

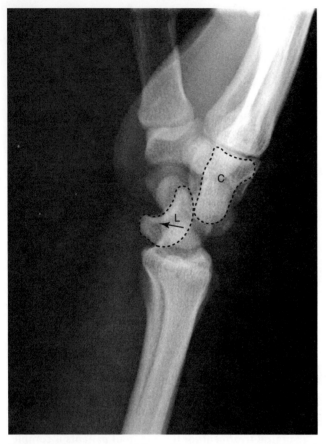

Figure 17-74 Lateral view of the wrist demonstrates a stage II dorsal dislocation of the lunate.

Perilunate dislocation is evident on routine PA and lateral radiographs. On the PA view, the three arcuate lines of the carpal rows are disrupted. On the lateral view, the direction of dislocation and staging are demonstrated as follows (Fig. 17-75):

- *Dorsal, stage I:* Capitate displaces dorsally; lunate remains aligned with radius.
- *Dorsal stage II:* Capitate displaces dorsally; lunate displaces volarly.
- *Volar stage I:* Capitate displaces volarly; lunate remains aligned with radius.
- *Volar stage II:* Capitate displaces volarly; lunate displaces dorsally.

Treatment Treatment of acute perilunate dislocation includes anatomic reduction, which may be obtained by manipulation often necessitating significant traction, followed by percutaneous K-wire fixation to hold this reduction and 8 weeks of thumb spica cast immobilization.

If anatomic reduction cannot be obtained by closed means, open reduction with internal wire or screw fixation is necessary. Dorsal and volar ligaments are also repaired, followed by cast immobilization for 6 to 8 weeks. The expected outcome of adequately reduced and immobilized dislocation is a functional wrist with no or minimal pain, minimal degenerative changes, but significant loss of motion of 40% to 50%.

Treatment for a chronic perilunate dislocation (present for more than 6 weeks) is very different. With chronic dislocation, reduction is no longer an option, and a proximal-row carpectomy or total wrist fusion becomes the treatment of choice. Expected outcomes for chronic perilunate dislocations are similar to those of proximal row carpectomies or total wrist fusions.

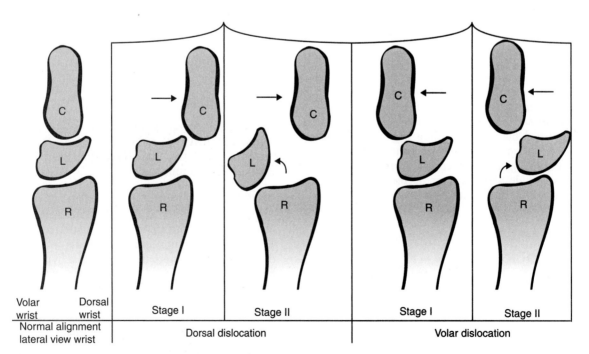

Figure 17-75 Radiographic stages of perilunate dislocation, assessed on the lateral view of the wrist.

Soft Tissue Disorders[13,43–66]

Pathology of the Triangular Fibrocartilage Complex

The triangular fibrocartilage complex (TFCC) serves as an important stabilizer of the distal radioulnar joint, controlling the rotational and sliding movements between the radius and ulna (Fig. 17-76). Additionally, the TFCC absorbs 20% of loading forces through the wrist, whereas the radiocarpal joint transmits approximately 80% of the force.

A lesion of the TFCC is seen as the following:

- An associated injury with distal radial fractures.
- A sequela to malunion of distal radial fractures. Malunions can shift loading to the ulnar carpus; when loads exceed physiological limits, the TFCC fails.
- A sequela to excessive ulnar motion. Ulnar variance changes dynamically with forearm motion, with a shift toward a positive direction with forearm pronation and gripping and toward a negative direction with supination and unfisted hand.
- A result of excessive loading through the ulnar side of the wrist (as when falling on the hand or repetitive loading in athletics—e.g., on the pommel horse in men's gymnastics). Acute trauma usually produces peripheral tears occurring 1 to 2 mm ulnar to the articular disk's attachment to the radius.
- A result of degenerative changes that produce central defects but generally do not contribute to DRUJ instability. The central 80% to 85% of the articular disk is avascular, which often renders this region incapable of healing. The radial aspect of the articular disk does have a vascular plexus and is considered by many to be surgically repairable.

Classification Systems

Several classification systems of TFCC injuries exist, such as the Palmer classification and Mayo Clinic classification. The Palmer system describes two broad types of tears: traumatic and degenerative. The Mayo Clinic classification supplements Palmer's original system in identifying location and directing treatment (see Table 17-3).

Clinical Presentation

Pain is worse with ulnar deviation and most profound when gripping, when ulnarly deviating, and while the forearm is in pronation. Clicking can accompany the pain and tenderness, which is noted within the ulnar snuffbox, on either side of the ulnar styloid, or dorsally just distal to the ulnar head. Once instability of the distal radioulnar joint is ruled out, a number of provocative tests and maneuvers can be attempted to identify tears of the disk. One such test is the articular disk shear test, also known as the ulnomeniscotriquetral dorsal glide. This test involves a dorsal glide of the pisotriquetral complex on the distal ulnar head, thereby shearing the articular disk. Another test is the GRIT (gripping rotatory impaction test). This test involves gripping using a grip dynamometer with the forearm positioned in pronation, neutral, and then supination, maximizing and then minimizing the potential for ulnar impaction.

As these symptoms are also common with DRUJ injuries, high-resolution MRI with a high-field-strength magnet and a dedicated wrist coil is often needed to confirm a diagnosis.

Imaging

Either routine MRI or MR arthrography is recommended to assess the TFCC (Fig. 17-77).

The following describes some basic MRI findings (remember, low signal = darker image, high signal = brighter image):

- The TFCC is a biconcave fibrocartilage band that normally appears dark on all imaging sequences and is surrounded by brighter, higher-signal synovial fluid or hyaline cartilage.

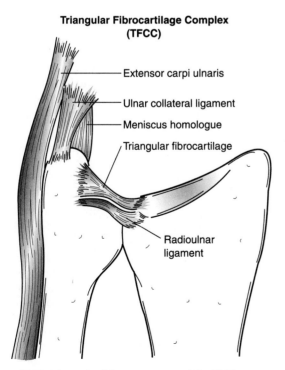

Triangular Fibrocartilage Complex (TFCC)

— Extensor carpi ulnaris

— Ulnar collateral ligament

— Meniscus homologue

— Triangular fibrocartilage

— Radioulnar ligament

Figure 17-76 Schematic of the components of the *TFCC*.

TABLE 17-3 ● Mayo Clinic Classification of Tears of the Triangular Fibrocartilage Complex	
Traumatic Tear (Types)	**Treatment**
I. Radial rim (detachment)	Surgical repair
II. Central	Excision
III. Ulnar (equivalent ulnar styloid fracture)	Surgical repair
IV. Palmar	Surgical repair
Degenerative Tear (Types)	**Treatment**
I. Central tear	Excision
II. Central tear, ulnocarpal impingement	Excision, ulnar recession
III. Central tear, impingement, lunotriquetral ligament tear	Excision, lunotriquetral reconstruction, ulnar recession
IV. Central tear, impingement, lunotriquetral arthritis	Ulnar excision versus ulnar recession

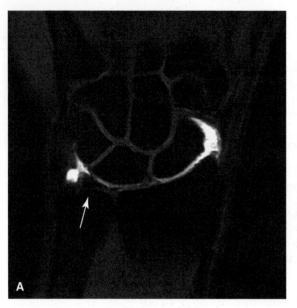
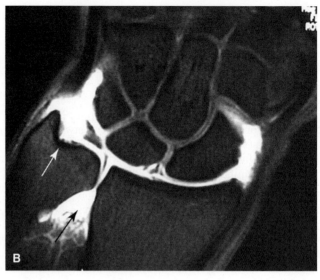

Figure 17-77 MR arthrography studies of the TFCC, which is seen as a triangular structure (arrow), dark on all sequences. **(A)** Normal TFCC. The contrast is confined to the radiocarpal joint, indicating the TFCC is intact. **(B)** Tear of the TFCC. Coronal T2-weighted MR image of a patient with tear in the midportion of the TFCC, as indicated by high-signal fluid leaking into the distal radioulnar joint (black arrow). There also appears to be a tear at the expected site of the attachment to the ulnar fovea (white arrow). Both tears are characteristically posttraumatic.

- The meniscal homolog at the ulnar edge of the TFCC is made up of fibrofatty tissue that appears as high-signal on T1 and proton density images, in contrast to the low-signal TFCC. The meniscal homolog should never appear similar to fluid on T2 images.
- The TFCC is best demonstrated on coronal images, especially in thin-section three-dimensional gradient echo sequences.
- Traumatic tears tend to be perpendicular to the long axis of the TFCC and are associated with fluid in the DRUJ and, to a lesser degree, with excessive fluid in the radiocarpal joint.
- TFCC tears can be partial- or full-thickness injuries. The traumatic TFCC tears are most easily missed on MRI. High signal intensity in this region on T2-weighted sequences is the most reliable finding. Any fluid at the periphery of the TFCC on T2-weighted images that is not in the prestyloid recess or extensor carpi ulnaris (ECU) tendon sheath should be described as a peripheral tear.
- Although the TFCC is usually low in signal on all pulse sequences, increased internal signal may sometimes be seen on T1-weighted images. This represents degeneration of the TFCC and not a true tear. This degenerative signal is globular, is hypointense to cartilage, and does not extend to both sides of the TFCC.
- Another diagnostic pitfall is the line of high-signal hyaline cartilage seen at the insertion of the TFCC into the radius, which can be mistaken for a tear.
- True radial side tears are rare. They are usually caused by acute trauma and consist of a radial avulsion of the TFCC, with increased signal intensity on T2-weighted images. Tears should be seen on at least two pulse sequences.

Treatment

Table 17-3 identifies which TFCC lesions are treated with reconstruction, ulnar recession, or repair.

Carpal Tunnel Syndrome

Carpal tunnel syndrome is a compressive neuropathy of the median nerve at the wrist. It is the most common neuropathy of the upper extremity.

Because the carpal tunnel is an inelastic structure, any condition that increases the volume of the structures in the carpal tunnel will lead to median nerve compression. Some of the possible causes of increased intratunnel pressure include the following:

- Anatomic compression (with fracture–dislocations at the wrist)
- Inflammatory conditions such as diabetes, alcoholism, or thyroid disorder
- Mechanical forces such as joint position, tendon load, or vibration
- Fluid shifts, as in pregnancy and menopause

The ulnar border of the carpal tunnel includes the hook of the hamate, the triquetrum, and the pisiform. The radial border includes the trapezium, scaphoid, and flexor carpi radialis fascia. The roof of the tunnel is made up of the deep forearm fascia, the transverse carpal ligament, and the distal aponeurosis of the thenar and hypothenar muscles. The contents of the tunnel consist of the median nerve and nine flexor tendons: the flexor pollicis longus tendon, four flexor digitorum profundus tendons, and four flexor digitorum superficialis tendons.

Clinical Presentation

The classic clinical presentation of a patient with carpal tunnel syndrome is pain and paresthesias in the median nerve distribution of the hand. Often these symptoms are worse at night or with repetitive hand motions, especially gripping. Patients frequently report clumsiness and weakness of the affected hand.

Clinically, symptoms of paresthesias are limited to the palmar aspect and tips of the thumb, second digit, and half of the third digit. Patients will have a positive *Tinel sign* (tingling produced in the fingers with tapping over the median nerve at the wrist) and a positive *Phalen sign* (symptoms reproduced with wrist flexion test). In cases of chronic median nerve compression, patients may have wasting of the thenar muscles.

Diagnostic Modalities

Although Semmes–Weinstein monofilament testing, which assesses light touch sensibility, is highly sensitive, electrodiagnostic testing is the definitive modality for confirmating carpal tunnel syndrome. Electromyography, which reveals positive waves or fibrillations in the thenar musculature, indicates the severity and chronicity of nerve injury, as does delayed nerve conduction on nerve conduction velocity testing.

Conventional radiographs are useful in ruling out osseous abnormalities or fracture–dislocations at the wrist. MRI currently has a limited role in the evaluation of carpal tunnel syndrome. It may be used occasionally if the symptoms derive from a soft tissue mass or an infection within the carpal tunnel. Indications for wrist MRI include atypical symptoms, a lack of electromyographic findings, high clinical suspicion for a mass, young patient age (possible congenital anomalies), and recurrent symptoms in postoperative patients.

Treatment

Conservative management in mild cases includes splinting, nonsteroidal anti-inflammatory drugs, corticosteroid injection, ultrasound, iontophoresis, and activity modification. Conservative management of moderate to severe carpal tunnel syndrome is not usually an option, especially in patients with muscle atrophy or significant sensory impairment.

An acute increase in carpal tunnel pressure can threaten median nerve viability; prompt open carpal tunnel release is then indicated. General indications for surgical release are clinical or electrodiagnostic evidence of denervation of the median nerve-innervated muscles. Surgical procedures include open carpal tunnel release and endoscopic open carpal tunnel release. There is controversy in the literature regarding outcomes and complication rates of open release versus endoscopic release.

Arthritides[12,13,18,30,34]

Degenerative Joint Disease

Degenerative joint disease (DJD) or *osteoarthritis* is commonly seen in the small joints of the adult hand after the fifth decade. The proximal and distal interphalangeal joints of the fingers and the carpometacarpal joint of the thumb are particularly affected.

Radiologic Characteristics

Radiographic evidence of DJD in the hand, as in other larger joints, is hallmarked by the following:

1. Decrease in the radiographic joint space
2. Sclerosis of subchondral bone
3. Osteophyte formation at joint margins (Fig. 17-78)
4. Joint deformities

When present in the distal interphalangeal joints, the joint deformities are known as *Heberden's nodes*. Similar deformities in the proximal interphalangeal joints are known as *Bouchard's nodes*. Synovial debris engulfed by the joints results in obvious enlargement and pebble-like deformities on the dorsal aspects of the joints (e.g., see Fig. 17-54).

Basal Joint Arthritis

Degenerative joint disease occurring in the first carpometacarpal joint and other adjacent joints at the base of the thumb is sometimes referred to as basal joint arthritis (Fig. 17-79). It occurs most commonly in adults with no prior history of major trauma but is also seen as a sequel to fracture or injury in this area or in patients with rheumatoid arthritis. Arthritic involvement of the thumb base is a painful condition that can seriously impair hand function. The degree of joint damage has been graded radiographically and clinically as follows:

- *Stage 1:* Ligamentous laxity of the thumb carpometacarpal joint is demonstrated on stress views, whereby the metacarpal base subluxes dorsally and laterally as the tips of the thumbs are pressed together.
- *Stage 2:* Chronic subluxation is present at the thumb carpometacarpal joint, and definite radiographic evidence of osteoarthritis is present at this joint.
- *Stage 3:* Osteoarthritis is evident radiographically in adjacent joints, not only the trapezium–first metacarpal joint but also the trapezium–second metacarpal, trapezium–trapezoid, and trapezium–scaphoid articulations.
- *Stage 4:* Osteoarthritis of the thumb metacarpophalangeal joint is present.

Treatment

Treatment of DJD in the hand and thumb is dependent on the degree of involvement present. Rehabilitation plays a significant role. Early stages are often treated with pain management, splinting to prevent or reduce deformity,

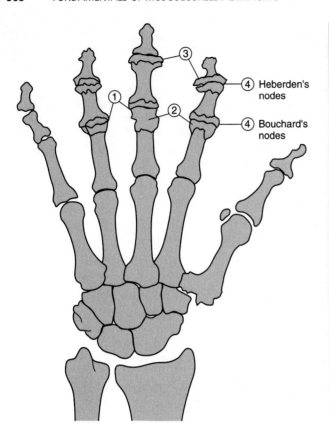

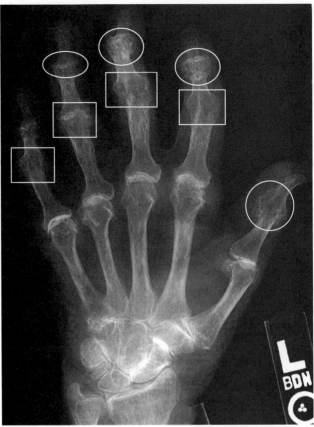

Figure 17-78 DJD present in all the small joints of the hand and wrist. Deformities at the distal interphalangeal joints are known as Heberden's nodes (circled). Deformities at the proximal interphalangeal joints are known as Bouchard's nodes (rectangles). Loss of joint space and periarticular sclerosis is also present at the metacarpophalangeal, carpometacarpal, intercarpal, and radiocarpal joints.

therapeutic exercise to maintain motion, and joint protection education. Later stages may require joint fusion or joint replacement to preserve a pain-free, functional hand.

Rheumatoid Arthritis

Rheumatoid arthritis is characteristically seen in the small joints of the wrist, the metacarpophalangeal joints, and the proximal interphalangeal joints.

Radiologic Characteristics

Radiographic evidence of rheumatoid arthritis in the hand is covered in Chapter 2. Please refer to Figures 2-10, 2-33, 2-34, and 2-37 for corresponding images.

Treatment

Treatment, similar to that of DJD, depends on the degree of involvement and ranges from conservative measures to joint arthroplasties (Fig. 17-80A,B). Rehabilitation is an integral part of management to preserve function.

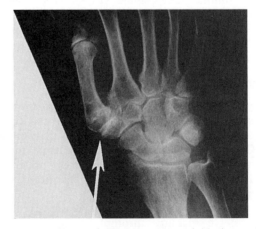

Figure 17-79 Basal joint arthritis. Severe osteoarthritic changes including joint space narrowing, sclerosis, and osteophyte formation, noted at the first carpometacarpal joint and adjacent joints. Degenerative changes involve the trapezium and its surrounding articulations, including the first metacarpal, second metacarpal, trapezoid, and scaphoid articulations.

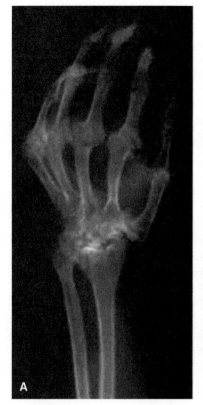
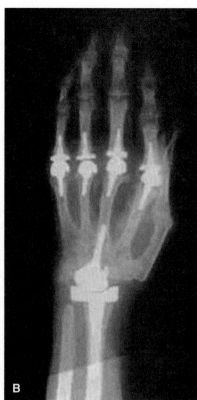

Figure 17-80 Advanced rheumatoid arthritis. **(A)** Pre-operative radiograph demonstates the complete resorptive destruction of all joints, prohibiting function. **(B)** Postoperative radiograph shows total joint replacements at the metacarpal and radiocarpal joints, which will permit basic hinge movements for prehensile function. *(Source of image: http://www.njortho.com.)*

Summary of Key Points

Routine Radiologic Evaluation

1. The routine radiographic evaluation of the hand includes three projections:
   - ➤ *PA*—demonstrates the phalanges, metacarpals, carpals, and joint spaces of the hand
   - ➤ *Lateral*—the long axes of the radius, lunate, capitate, and third metacarpal normally align within 10 degrees of each other
   - ➤ *Oblique*—demonstrates the lateral aspects of the shafts of the long bones of the hand without the superimposition seen in a true lateral view

2. The routine radiographic evaluation of the wrist includes three projections:
   - ➤ *PA*—demonstrates the arcuate lines of the carpal rows, ulnar variance, and the radial articular angle
   - ➤ *Lateral*—demonstrates the volar tilt of the radius, scapholunate angle, and capitolunate angle
   - ➤ *Oblique*—the radial-side carpals and the hamate are well visualized

Optional and Functional Views

3. Three common optional projections of the wrist are the following:
   - ➤ *Ulnar deviation view*—demonstrates the scaphoid and adjacent opened intercarpal spaces

   - ➤ *Radial deviation view*—demonstrates the ulnar-side carpals and intercarpal spaces
   - ➤ *Carpal tunnel view*—demonstrates the arched arrangement of the carpals on the palmar aspect of the wrist
   - ➤ *Clenched-fist view*—gripping produces axial compression that will force the capitate proximally, causing scapholunate dissociation if articulating ligaments are ruptured
   - ➤ *Stress views*—passive motion imposed on the wrist is used to reveal instabilities.

Fractures of the Hand

4. Fractures of the hand are probably the most common fractures of adults. The distal phalanges most often sustain crush-type fractures. Fractures of the remaining phalanges and metacarpals are described by their location at the head, neck, shaft, base, or intra-articular region, including avulsive-type fractures at the attachment sites of tendons and ligaments.

5. Fractures of the metacarpals of the hand occur most frequently at the neck of the shaft.

6. Fractures of the metacarpals of the thumbs occur most frequently at or near the base of the shaft and are divided into intra- and extra-articular types.

Fractures of the Wrist

7. The scaphoid bone is the most frequently fractured carpal bone. The entrance of the blood supply through the distal pole puts fractures occurring at the waist or proximal pole at risk for avascular necrosis.

8. The distal radius is the most frequently fractured bone of the wrist. The eponym *Colles' fracture* generally refers to an extra-articular fracture located about 1½ inches proximal to the distal end of the radius, with dorsal angulation of the distal fragment. Associated fractures of the ulnar styloid are often present.

Wrist Instability

9. Instabilities are generally classified as *predynamic, dynamic,* and *static.*

10. Predynamic instabilities show no radiologic abnormalities; dynamic instabilities are evident only on functional radiographs, stress views, or cineradiography; static instabilities are evident on conventional radiographs.

11. *Cineradiography* is a radiographic motion study. At the wrist it is used to assess the possibility of dynamic instability.

12. Carpal instabilities are classified as carpal instability dissociative (CID), carpal instability nondissociative (CIND), and carpal instability combined (CIC).

Soft Tissue Disorders

13. The *triangular fibrocartilage complex (TFCC)* is an important stabilizer of the distal radioulnar joint. It can be torn in isolation or in association with other injuries. MRI and MR arthrography identify these lesions.

14. *Carpal tunnel syndrome* is the compressive neuropathy of the median nerve as it passes through the wrist. Electrodiagnostic studies are currently the definitive diagnostic modality; however, advanced imaging is being explored as an assessment tool for the characteristics of this syndrome.

Arthritides

15. *Degenerative joint disease (DJD)* is common in the small joints of the hand after the fifth decade of life. Radiologic hallmarks are decreased joint spaces, sclerosis, and osteophytosis.

16. *Heberden's nodes* are DJD deformities in the distal interphalangeal joints; *Bouchard's nodes* are DJD deformities in the proximal interphalangeal joints. *Basal joint arthritis* is DJD at the first carpometacapal joint.

17. *Rheumatoid arthritis* characteristically manifests in the small joints of the wrist, metacarpophalangeal joints, and proximal interphalangeal joints.

18. The radiologic hallmarks of rheumatoid arthritis include uniform joint space narrowing, periarticular rarefaction, articular erosions, synovial cysts, and joint deformities such as *swan-neck deformity* and *boutonnière deformity.*

 Please refer to the text's enclosed CD-ROM for the American College of Radiology's current Musculoskeletal Appropriateness Criteria for the following topics: *Acute Hand and Wrist Trauma, Chronic Wrist Pain.*

CASE STUDIES

CASE STUDY 1

Proximal Phalangeal Fracture With Complications

The patient is a 45-year-old woman referred to physical therapy by an orthopedic surgeon for rehabilitation following fixation of the proximal phalangeal fracture of her third digit.

History of Trauma

The patient was injured by falling on an outstretched left hand when she tripped over a power cord in her garage. She felt immediate pain in the finger and noticed significant swelling in the area. Her husband drove her to the local emergency room.

Initial Imaging

The emergency room physician ordered conventional radiographs of the left hand, including an anteroposterior (AP) of the hand and a lateral of the third digit. A comminuted fracture of the proximal phalanx was diagnosed, and orthopedics was consulted.

Intervention

The patient's finger was immobilized in a splint for 1 week to allow the edema to resolve. The orthopedic surgeon then performed open reduction with internal fixation (ORIF) using two pins (Fig. 17-81).

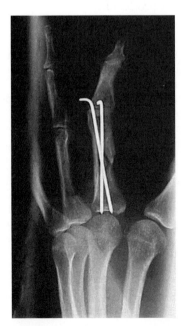

Figure 17-81 Oblique view of comminuted fracture of the proximal phalanx with pin fixation.

Physical Therapy Examination

Patient Complaint

Approximately 4 weeks after surgical fixation, the two pins were removed and the patient started physical therapy. At the initial appointment, the patient reported pain, stiffness, and decreased ability to use her left hand for many activities of daily living. She said she was still not working at her job at a day care center because she is left-hand–dominant and could not complete many of the tasks required of her in caring for the children.

Physical Examination

The patient continued to wear a finger splint for protection and presented with significantly decreased active and passive flexion at the proximal and distal interphalangeal (PIP and DIP) joints of the left middle finger. Extension at these joints was nearly within normal limits. Metacarpophalangeal (MCP) joint flexion and extension were slightly limited. Range of motion in all other joints of the left hand was within normal limits.

Physical Therapy Intervention

Over the next 10 days, the patient started on a treatment regimen to decrease edema in the involved digit and increase passive range of motion in the MCP, PIP, and DIP joints. The therapist also initiated gentle active range-of-motion activities. On the 10th day after beginning physical therapy, the patient reported increased pain and edema in the left middle finger after she accidentally hit her left hand on a wall at home while trying to avoid bumping into her husband in the hallway. She said she was not wearing her protective splint at the time.

Additional Imaging

The therapist examined the hand and noted increased edema in the involved digit, decreased active range of motion, and aberrant movement within the phalanx at the original fracture site. The therapist immediately contacted the orthopedic surgeon and recommended that radiographs be obtained to confirm suspicions of reinjury. The surgeon agreed. Posteroanterior (PA) and lateral radiographs confirmed displacement at the fracture site.

Outcome

The patient underwent ORIF with plate and screws (Fig. 17-82).

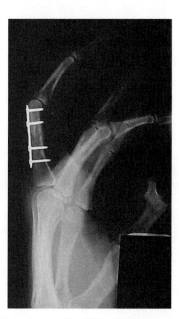

Figure 17-82 Lateral view, after ORIF with plate-and-screw fixation.

Discussion

This case exemplifies the need for caution on the part of a therapist whenever a patient reports some incident that may have affected the involved area. Many times these incidents have little significance and do not critically affect the patient's overall management. Sometimes, however, incidents that appear trivial may change the clinical picture.

This case is summarized in Figure 17-83.

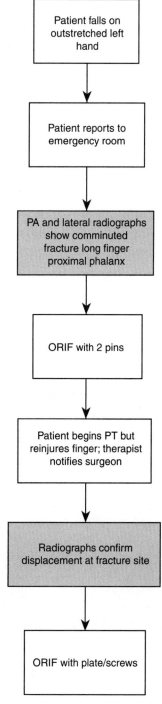

Figure 17-83 Pathway of case study events. Imaging is highlighted.

CRITICAL THINKING POINT

The patient received timely care for the reinjury and therefore may have avoided further complications associated with insufficient immobilization at a fracture site. The key in this incident was the observation of aberrant movement in the proximal phalanx. Unstable fracture sites may be palpated or, as in this case, even observed. Detection of movement at a previous fracture site or increased acute point tenderness at the site requires re-examination by radiography.

CASE STUDY 2

Fracture–Dislocation of the Wrist

The patient is a 31-year-old man referred to physical therapy by an orthopedic surgeon for rehabilitation following ORIF of a fracture–dislocation injury involving the left carpus.

History of Trauma

The patient is a physical laborer who was injured at work when a slab of concrete fell on him, striking his left wrist and hand. He was immediately taken to a local hospital emergency room for evaluation.

Initial Imaging

In the emergency room, conventional radiographs were taken of the left wrist and hand. PA (Fig. 17-84), lateral (Fig. 17-85), and oblique films showed a displaced fracture of the radial styloid process and volar dislocation of the carpus. There was also an intra-articular fracture of the thumb's proximal phalanx.

Intervention

An orthopedic surgeon reduced the wrist dislocation and stabilized the radial styloid fracture with screw fixation. Both the wrist and thumb were splinted for 4 weeks before initiation of physical therapy.

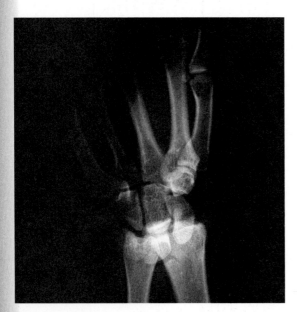

Figure 17-84 PA view of the hand. Displaced fracture of radial styloid, intra-articular fracture of the thumb proximal phalanx, and disruption of carpal arcuate lines.

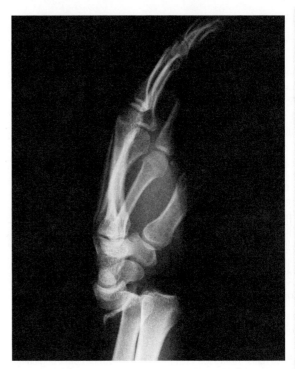

Figure 17-85 Lateral view of the hand demonstrates volar dislocation of the carpus.

Physical Therapy Examination

Patient Complaint

At the patient's first physical therapy appointment, he complained of continued moderate pain and stiffness of the left wrist and hand. He had returned to light duty at work, completing tasks as possible using only his dominant right arm.

Physical Examination

The patient continued to wear splints on the wrist and thumb. He was reluctant to move the hand during the physical exam and demonstrated guarding of the entire left upper extremity. He presented with moderate wrist edema and significant tenderness to palpation about the wrist as well as severe limitations in all wrist and thumb ranges of motion.

Physical Therapy Intervention

The therapist integrated examination findings along with the postoperative radiographic images, which the patient brought to the first visit.

Initially addressed was the patient's fear of moving his hand. Using the radiographs, the therapist was able to explain the injury in greater detail to the patient, point out successful healing of the fracture sites, account for areas of tenderness as related to sites of healing, and answer all his questions related to the injury and surgical repair.

The therapist also noticed the increased scapholunate gap evident on the PA but did not discuss this with the patient at this time.

Therapeutic measures were initiated and progressed as tolerated. These included retrograde massage, joint mobilization, strengthening, splint modifications, and joint protection skills, not only for the recovering acute condition but for the anticipated possibility of carpal instability.

Outcome

At discharge from physical therapy 4 months following the injury, the patient estimated his recovery at 80%. Wrist range of motion and grip strength were within normal limits. He returned to full-time work with some lifting limitations. He did continue to experience pain in the wrist with some movements, especially end-range flexion and extension and with heavy grasping activities.

The therapist discussed concerns with the surgeon regarding scapholunate instability as a source of residual pain; functional radiographs or cineradiography could have confirmed this suspicion. However, because operative treatment is the only course of action for scapholunate instability, the patient declined further imaging that would be done for the purpose of preoperative studies. He was satisfied to return to work and was aware of joint protection strategies to protect the wrist from undue stresses.

Discussion

The therapist used radiographs for two major purposes: treatment planning and patient education.

Visualizing the injury and the surgical repair clarified the extensive nature of structural damage for the therapist, and extrapolations were possible regarding ligamentous damage.

Allowing the patient to view the radiograph, be informed, and have his questions answered was instrumental in giving him the peace of mind that would allow him to participate fully in therapy without undue fears. The patient was better able to understand his injury and the length of time it would take to heal as well as the need for rehabilitation.

This case is summarized in Figure 17-86.

CRITICAL THINKING POINTS

This case demonstrates the following points:

1. In addition to reading a radiologist's report, a therapist should view the images whenever possible to help complete the clinical picture, relating radiologic information with the clinical presentation.

2. Physical therapists are often interested in aspects of imaging that might not be mentioned in a radiologist's report. In this case, the report's information was directed to the surgical repair and state of fracture healing. The therapist was interested in an additional finding—the scapholunate distance.

3. The scapholunate instability was not explored. This was *not* an oversight; it was an *informed choice* made by the patient. The reality of other factors—including job security, insurance issues, or simply the desire to get back to a normal life after a long rehabilitation—may have factored into his decision. The information provided to him regarding his intermittent wrist pain allowed him to make an educated decision and gave him the tools to make modifications in his life that would permit him to live with this pain.

Case studies adapted by J. Bradley Barr, PT, DPT, OCS.

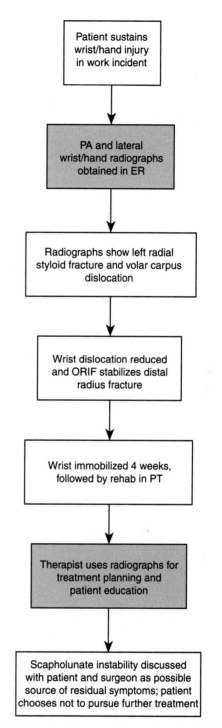

Figure 17-86 Pathway of case study events. Imaging is highlighted.

References

Normal Anatomy

1. Netter, FH: Atlas of Human Anatomy, ed. 4. Saunders, Philadelphia, 2006.
2. Nordin, M, and Frankel, VH: Basic Biomechanics of the Musculoskeletal System, ed. 3. Lippincott Williams & Wilkins, Philadelphia, 2001.
3. Whiting, W, and Zernicke, R: Biomechanics of Musculoskeletal Injury, ed. 2. Human Kinetics, Champaign, IL, 2008.
4. Norkin, CC, and Levangie, PK: Joint Structure and Function: A Comprehensive Analysis, ed. 2. FA Davis, Philadelphia, 1992.
5. Meschan, I: An Atlas of Radiographic Anatomy. WB Saunders, Philadelphia, 1960.
6. Greulich, WW, and Pyle, SI: Radiographic Atlas of Skeletal Development of the Hand and Wrist, ed. 2. Stanford University Press, Stanford, CA, 1999.
7. Gilsanz, V, and Ratib, O: Hand Bone Age: A Digital Atlas of Skeletal Maturity. Springer, New York, 2004.
8. Weber, EC, Vilensky, JA, and Carmichael, SW: Netter's Concise Radiologic Anatomy. WB Saunders, Philadelphia, 2008.
9. Kelley, LL, and Peterson, CM: Sectional Anatomy for Imaging Professional, 2nd ed. Mosby, St. Louis, MO, 2007.
10. Lazo, DL: Fundamentals of Sectional Anatomy: An Imaging Approach. Thomson Delmar Learning, Clifton Park, NY, 2005.

Routine Exam

11. American College of Radiology (ACR): Practice Guideline for the Performance of Radiography of the Extremities. Amended 2006. Accessed October 19, 2008 at http://www.acr.org.
12. Weissman, B, and Sledge, C: Orthopedic Radiology. WB Saunders, Philadelphia, 1986.
13. Greenspan, A: Orthopedic Radiology: A Practical Approach, ed. 4. Lippincott Williams & Wilkins, Philadelphia, 2004.
14. Bontrager, KL: Textbook of Radiographic Positioning and Related Anatomy, ed. 6. Mosby, St. Louis, Mo, 2005.
15. Fischer, HW: Radiographic Anatomy: A Working Atlas. McGraw-Hill, New York, 1988.
16. Wicke, L: Atlas of Radiographic Anatomy, ed. 5. Lea & Febiger, Malvern, PA, 1994.
17. Frank, E, Smith, B, and Long, B: Merrill's Atlas of Radiographic Positions and Radiologic Procedures, ed. 11. Elsevier Health Sciences, Philadelphia, 2007.
18. Squires, LF, and Novelline, RA: Fundamentals of Radiology, ed. 4. Harvard University Press, Cambridge, MA, 1988.
19. Chew, FS: Skeletal Radiology: The Bare Bones, ed. 2. Williams and Wilkins, Baltimore, 1997.
20. Weir, J, and Abrahams, P: An Atlas of Radiological Anatomy. Yearbook Medical, Chicago, 1978.
21. Krell, L (ed): Clark's Positioning in Radiology, vol. 1, ed. 10. Yearbook Medical, Chicago, 1989.

Trauma/Abnormal Conditions

22. ACR: Appropriateness Criteria for Chronic Wrist Pain. Reviewed 2005. Available at http://www.acr.org/SecondaryMainMenuCategories/quality_safety/app_criteria/pdf/ExpertPanelonMusculoskeletalImaging/ChronicWristPainDoc10.aspx.
23. ACR: Appropriateness Criteria for Acute Hand and Wrist Trauma. Reviewed 2008. Available at http://www.acr.org/SecondaryMainMenuCategories/quality_safety/app_criteria/pdf/ExpertPanelonMusculoskeletalImaging/AcuteHandandWristTraumaDoc1.aspx.
24. Bucholz, RW, Heckman, J, and Court-Brown, C (eds): Rockwood and Green's Fractures in Adults, ed. 6. Lippincott Williams & Wilkins, Philadelphia, 2005.
25. Rockwood, CA, and Green, DP (eds): Fractures in Adults, ed. 5. Lippincott Williams & Wilkins, Philadelphia, 2002.
26. Beaty, J, and Kasar, J (eds): Rockwood and Wilkins' Fractures in Children, ed. 6. Lippincott Williams & Wilkins, Philadelphia, 2005.
27. Koval, KJ, and Zuckerman, JD: Handbook of Fractures, ed. 2. Lippincott Williams & Wilkins, Philadelphia, 2002.
28. Eiff, M, et al: Fracture Management for Primary Care. WB Saunders, Philadelphia, 2003.
29. Yochum, TR, and Rowe, LJ: Essentials of Skeletal Radiology, ed. 3. Williams & Wilkins, Baltimore, 2004.
30. Marchiori, DM: Clinical Imaging with Skeletal, Chest, and Abdomen Pattern Differentials. Mosby, St. Louis, MO, 1999.
31. Ip, D: Orthopedic Traumatology: A Resident's guide. Springer, New York, 2006.
32. McConnell, J, Eyres, R, and Nightingale, J: Interpreting Trauma Radiographs. Blackwell, Malden, MA, 2005.
33. Hodler, J, von Schulthess, GK, and Zollikofer, CL: Musculoskeletal Disease: Diagnostic Imaging and Interventional Technology. Springer, Italy, 2005.

34. Daffner, RH: Clinical Radiology: The Essentials, ed. 3. Williams & Wilkins, Baltimore, 2007.
35. Bernstein, J, ed: Musculoskeletal Medicine. American Academy of Orthopedic Surgeons, Rosemont, IL, 2003.
36. Büchler, U: Wrist Instability. Mosby, St. Louis, MO, 1996.
37. Hunter, JM, et al (eds): Rehabilitation of the Hand: Surgery and Therapy, ed. 5, Mosby, St. Louis, MO, 2002.
38. Taleisnik, J: The Wrist, Churchill Livingstone, New York, 1985.
39. Cailliet, R: Hand Pain and Impairment, ed. 4. FA Davis, Philadelphia, 1994.

Fractures

40. Firoozabadi, R, et al: Qualitative and quantitative assessment of bone fragility and fracture healing using conventional radiography and advanced imaging technologies—Focus on wrist fracture. J Orthop Trauma 22(8 Suppl):S83, 2008.
41. Kawamura, K, Chung, KC: Treatment of scaphoid fractures and nonunions. J Hand Surg [Am] 33(6):988, 2008.
42. Cheow, HK, et al: The role of bone scan in the diagnosis of carpal fracture in children. J Pediatr Orthop B 17(4):165, 2008.
43. Kazakos, KJ, et al: Diagnostic value of conventional arthrography in investigating post-traumatic ulnar wrist pain: Are MRI and MR arthrography always necessary? Med Sci Monit 14(4):CS37, 2008.
44. Welling, RD, et al: MDCT and radiography of wrist fractures: Radiographic sensitivity and fracture patterns. AJR Am J Roentgenol 190(1):10, 2008.
45. Morisawa, Y, et al: Dorsoradial avulsion of the triangular fibrocartilage complex with an avulsion fracture of the sigmoid notch of the radius. J Hand Surg Eur 32(6):705, 2007.
46. Karantanas, A, et al: The role of MR imaging in scaphoid disorders. Eur Radiol 17(11):2860, 2007.
47. Cruickshank, J, et al: Early computerized tomography accurately determines the presence or absence of scaphoid and other fractures. Emerg Med Australas 19(3):223, 2007. Erratum in: Emerg Med Australas 19(4):387, 2007.
48. La Hei, N, et al: Scaphoid bone bruising—Probably not the precursor of asymptomatic non-union of the scaphoid. J Hand Surg Eur 32(3):337, 2007.

Wrist Instability/Soft Tissue Disorders

49. Moser, T, et al: Wrist ligament tears: Evaluation of MRI and combined MDCT and MR arthrography. AJR Am J Roentgenol 188(5):1278, 2007.
50. Maizlin, ZV, et al: MR arthrography of the wrist: Controversies and concepts. Hand (NY) 4(1):66, 2009.
51. Moritomo, H, et al: Relationship between the fracture location and the kinematic pattern in scaphoid nonunion. J Hand Surg [Am], 33(9):1459, 2008.
52. Henry, MH: Management of acute triangular fibrocartilage complex injury of the wrist. J Am Acad Orthop Surg 16(6):320, 2008.
53. Lacelli, F: High-resolution ultrasound anatomy of extrinsic carpal ligaments. Radiol Med 113(4):504, 2008.
54. Dodds, SD, et al: Essex-Lopresti injuries. Hand Clin 24(1):125, 2008.
55. Arimitsu, S, et al: Analysis of radiocarpal and midcarpal motion in stable and unstable rheumatoid wrists using 3-dimensional computed tomography. J Hand Surg [Am] 33(2):189, 2008.
56. Chang, W, et al: Arcuate ligament of the wrist: Normal MR appearance and its relationship to palmar midcarpal instability: A cadaveric study. Skel Radiol, 36(7):641, 2007.
57. Giannoulis, FS, and Sotereanos, DG: Galeazzi fractures and dislocations. Hand Clin 23(2):153, 2007.
58. Henry, M: Collapsed scaphoid non-union with dorsal intercalated segment instability and avascular necrosis treated by vascularised wedge-shaped bone graft and fixation. J Hand Surg Eur 32(2):148, 2007.
59. Weiss, S, Schwartz, DA, and Anderson, SC: Radiography: A review for the rehabilitation professional. J Hand Ther 20(2):152, 2007.
60. Young, D, Papp, S, and Giachino, A: Physical examination of the wrist. Orthop Clin North Am 38(2):149, 2007.
61. Ekelund, L, et al: Imaging of four-corner fusion (SLAC arthrodesis) of the wrist with 64-slice computed tomography. Acta Radiol 48(1):76, 2007.
62. Goldfarb, CA: Traumatic wrist instability: What's in and what's out. Instr Course Lect 56:65, 2007.
63. Bencardino, JT, and Rosenberg, ZS: Sports-related injuries of the wrist: An approach to MRI interpretation. Clin Sports Med 25(3):409, 2006.
64. Lubiatowski, P, et al: Instability of the distal radioulnar joint (DRUJ): A description of the problem and own experience. Ortop Traumatol Rehabil 8(3):251, 2006.
65. Dzianach, M, et al: Diagnostic imaging of wrist instability. Ortop Traumatol Rehabil 8(2):150, 2006.
66. Theumann, NH, et al: Association between extrinsic and intrinsic carpal ligament injuries at MR arthrography and carpal instability at radiography: Initial observations. Radiology 238(3):950, 2006.

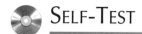 SELF-TEST

Radiograph A

1. Identify the *projection.*

2. A surgical procedure has been done to alleviate the pain and limitation of *osteoarthritis at the first carpometacarpal joint.* Which *carpal* has been resected?

3. The *palmaris longus* has been coiled into the resected area in order to preserve joint space. How is this soft tissue secured in place?

Radiograph B

4. Identify the *projection.*

5. The bony findings are normal. The location and expanse of the *soft tissue swelling* (arrows) suggest that what structures are involved?

6. If the patient's history and clinical findings narrowed the possibilities to trauma caused by *repetitive mechanical stresses,* what is a likely diagnosis?

Radiograph C

7. Identify the *projection.*

8. What radiographic findings suggest that a *disease* state exists?

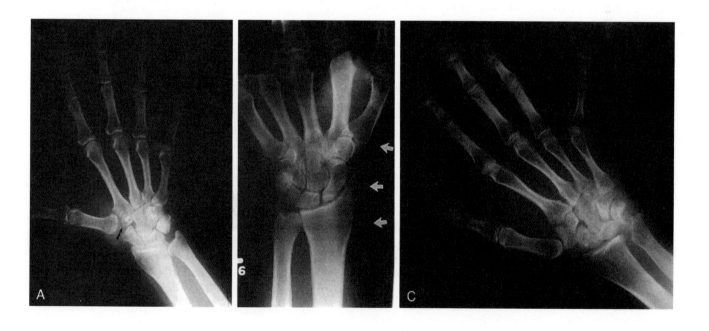

Chapter 18

INTEGRATION OF IMAGING INTO PHYSICAL THERAPY PRACTICE

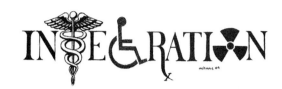

J. Bradley Barr, PT, DPT, OCS

Changing Perspectives on Diagnostic Imaging in Physical Therapy Education

The Traditional Model

Physical therapy has gradually evolved into a profession with specialized areas of practice, including primary care, which requires considerable expertise in musculoskeletal evaluation. In response, the professional education of physical therapists in the United States has undergone many changes in recent decades.

Until recently, most physical therapy education programs contained very little if any curricular content related to diagnostic imaging. In the past, the exclusion of diagnostic imaging education was perhaps based on an assumption that because physical therapists do not make medical diagnoses, the study of diagnostic imaging added little to the expertise of physical therapists as rehabilitation specialists. The prevailing perception was that diagnostic imaging was not useful in daily physical therapy practice. The value of integrating diagnostic

imaging information into the physical therapy evaluation was not recognized or explored. Rather, the absence of diagnostic imaging instruction from physical therapy curricula appeared to reflect the traditional model of medicine as well as the physical therapist's restricted scope of practice.

An Evolving Model

In recent decades the response of the physical therapy profession to modern patient needs has resulted in an expanded professional identity and higher professional standards. These developments have been and continue to be the catalyst for legislative changes relating to state practice acts. Laws permitting clients *direct access* to physical therapy have been enacted in 44 states in the United States (Table 18-1).[1] This political shift has altered the way many physical therapists practice. Physical therapists, now more than ever, may be the first health-care professionals patients encounter. The potential for the physical therapist to be a *primary care* provider is one significant factor that has changed the profession's perception of the importance of

TABLE 18-1 ● States Allowing Physical Therapists Direct Access to Patients, as of July 2007			
Under Provisions	**By Omission**	**Evaluation Only**	**No Direct Access**
Arkansas	Alaska	Hawaii	Alabama
California	Arizona	Michigan	Indiana
Connecticut	Colorado	Missouri	
Delaware	Idaho	Oklahoma	
District of Columbia	Maryland		
Florida	Massachusetts		
Georgia	Nebraska		
Illinois	Nevada		
Iowa	North Dakota		
Kansas	South Dakota		
Kentucky	Utah		
Louisiana	Vermont		
Maine			
Minnesota			
Mississippi			
Montana			
New Hampshire			
New Jersey			
New Mexico			
New York			
North Carolina			
Ohio			
Oregon			
Pennsylvania			
Rhode Island			
South Carolina			
Tennessee			
Texas			
Virginia			
Washington			
West Virginia			
Wisconsin			
Wyoming			

Source: American Physical Therapy Association.[1]

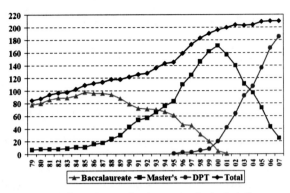

Number of Accredited PT Programs by Degree Offered 1979 – 2007

Figure 18-1 Number of accredited entry-level physical therapy programs by degree offered, 1979–2007. (*Adapted from American Physical Therapy Association,*[2] *p. 2.*)

TABLE 18-2 ● APTA Vision Statement 2020
Physical therapy, by 2020, will be provided by physical therapists who are doctors of physical therapy and who may be board-certified specialists. Consumers will have direct access to physical therapists in all environments for patient/client management, prevention, and wellness services. Physical therapists will be practitioners of choice in clients' health networks and will hold all privileges of autonomous practice. Physical therapists may be assisted by physical therapist assistants who are educated and licensed to provide physical therapist-directed and supervised components of interventions.
Guided by integrity, life-long learning, and a commitment to comprehensive and accessible health programs for all people, physical therapists and physical therapist assistants will render evidence-based service throughout the continuum of care and improve quality of life for society. They will provide culturally sensitive care distinguished by trust, respect, and an appreciation for individual differences.
While fully availing themselves of new technologies, as well as basic and clinical research, physical therapists will continue to provide direct care. They will maintain active responsibility for the growth of the physical therapy profession and the health of the people it serves.

Source: American Physical Therapy Association.[3]

diagnostic imaging in the education of physical therapists. As a result, diagnostic imaging is now an integral component of many physical therapy education programs.

The current physical therapy model of practice is defined by documents put forth by the principal professional and educational accreditation organization of physical therapists, the American Physical Therapy Association (APTA). Integration of diagnostic imaging into physical therapy practice is supported by the following documents: "Vision Statement 2020," the "Guide to Physical Therapist Practice, A Normative Model of Physical Therapist Professional Education," and the "Orthopaedic Physical Therapy Description of Specialty Practice." These documents are described in the following sections.

Vision Statement 2020

The most obvious change in the identity of the physical therapy profession is seen in the degrees awarded by educational institutions. The number of entry-level and transitional doctor of physical therapy (DPT) education programs has grown rapidly from 1990 through 2010 (Fig. 18-1).[2] Doctoral-level physical therapy education is formally supported by "Vision Statement 2020" (Table 18-2), which sets forth the goal that all physical therapists will be "doctors of physical therapy."[3] The statement also urges physical

therapists to "avail themselves of new technologies . . . to provide direct care."[3] These evolutionary changes in our profession have necessitated increased knowledge in the area of medical imaging on the part of both students and practicing clinicians. The depth to which the profession needs to explore diagnostic imaging, however, is not yet defined. What is implied is that physical therapists must seek enough understanding to allow them to provide a comprehensive level of professional care.

Evidence Supporting Increased Imaging Education

The central practice document for the profession, the "Guide to Physical Therapist Practice," defines the elements of patient–client management.[4] As part of these elements, the guide describes how physical therapists integrate data from comprehensive screening in their examination with the evaluative process to "identify possible problems that require consultation with or referral to another provider."[4] This language supports referral to experts in other areas and referral for tests or measures physical therapists do not directly provide. To fulfill the guide's expectations for patient management, physical therapists must become educated users of diagnostic imaging capable of making appropriate referrals to the experts in imaging: radiologists.

"A Normative Model of Physical Therapist Professional Education: Version 2004" serves as a guide for accreditation of physical therapist education programs.[5] This document provides many examples of how physical therapy students should be prepared to make decisions regarding patient referral for diagnostic imaging. For instance, one of the patient–client management expectations regarding the evaluation process states: "The graduate identifies additional diagnostic tests (imaging, laboratory tests, electrophysiological tests, EMG, etc.) needed to develop an accurate diagnosis and refers for testing as indicated".[5]

The normative model also emphasizes the physical therapist's ability to incorporate the imaging information contained in the radiologist's written report into the decision-making process. Sample behavioral objectives from the document include, "the student will be able to use results of various imaging procedures for connective tissue in patient/client management" and "the student will be able to compare physical examination results with MRI results in the patient/client diagnosed with HNP."[5]

The "Orthopaedic Physical Therapy Description of Specialty Practice" describes expert orthopedic physical therapy practice, dimensions, professional responsibilities, knowledge areas, and procedures.[6] It was created by the Specialty Council on Orthopaedic Physical Therapy and subject matter experts and approved by the American Board of Physical Therapy Specialties. The purpose of this description of specialty practice is to help facilitate the process of specialist certification in orthopedic physical therapy. The document specifically lists imaging studies as a knowledge area expected of orthopedic clinical specialists.[6] Case examples in the document outline the physical therapist's use of diagnostic imaging as a part of the clinical decision-making process.[6]

A New Perception Emerges

The foregoing examples support the integration of diagnostic imaging content into the education of a physical therapist. In concept, this knowledge should support the ability of the physical therapist to do the following:

1. Recognize when diagnostic imaging is needed to complete a comprehensive examination
2. Integrate information from the radiologist's written report into the physical therapy treatment plan
3. Understand the diagnostic image visually to obtain information that may not be stated on the radiologist's report but may be useful to the physical therapist
4. Recognize when diagnostic imaging is needed *and when it is not needed* to promote an optimal patient outcome
5. Communicate effectively regarding diagnostic imaging with the referring physician, the radiologist, and others involved in the care of the patient

The Physical Therapist as a Primary Care Provider in the United States

As defined in the "Guide to Physical Therapist Practice," primary care is "the provision of integrated, accessible health-care services by clinicians who are accountable for addressing a large majority of personal health-care needs, developing a sustained partnership with patients, and practicing within the context of family and community."[4] The role of the physical therapist as a primary care provider is most obvious in direct-access settings but may also include other situations, such as industrial settings or home health settings, where physical therapists coordinate and integrate a number of services.[4]

The Physical Therapist as the Referral Source

For health-care professionals involved in primary management of musculoskeletal disorders, diagnostic imaging is an essential tool for differential diagnosis and medical screening purposes. Traditionally, only the physician bore the responsibility for referrals for diagnostic testing. Today, many routine orders may be generated by other health-care professionals. For example, physician assistants, nurse practitioners, and physical therapists in select settings may triage patients for musculoskeletal problems. The responsibility of recognizing when diagnostic imaging is needed begins with this initial screening of the patient (Fig. 18-2).

These professionals have the authority to order diagnostic imaging either to confirm a diagnosis or to rule out diagnoses that would change the course of treatment. This access to imaging is crucial for medical screening in primary care practice, because *diagnostic imaging sometimes provides diagnostic information not available through the interview and physical examination.* For example, in the case of a typical ankle inversion injury, a radiograph may be diagnostic for an avulsion fracture, which necessitates referral to a physician for management, or it may rule out a fracture, confirming that the soft tissue injury can be managed by the physical therapist. Furthermore, in the case of a more serious ankle sprain with instability, the physical therapist may conclude that the radiograph is not useful in evaluating ligaments and may suggest that magnetic resonance imaging (MRI) be performed to define which tissues are involved.

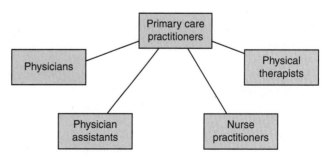

Figure 18-2 Primary care practitioners.

The Physical Therapist as an Educated User of Diagnostic Imaging

As part of any interdisciplinary health-care team, physical therapists must be able to confer with physicians about diagnostic imaging, suggest appropriate diagnostic imaging to the patient's primary care physician, and refer directly to the radiologist if needed. To do these things effectively, physical therapists must be educated about the many parameters associated with diagnostic imaging, such as cost, availability, radiation exposure, and contraindications for some diagnostic studies that may apply to individual patients.

Additionally, physical therapists, like any other providers who make decisions regarding the need for diagnostic imaging, must know what information may potentially be provided by the selected diagnostic study. Extensive research exists on the diagnostic utility of the various imaging modalities. Although the radiologist possesses the greatest expertise in all of these factors, it is not practical or logistically possible to consult a radiologist for every patient. Physical therapists must have an awareness of the most appropriate diagnostic imaging studies for the musculoskeletal conditions they treat.

The U.S. Military Health System

In the U.S. Department of Defense Military Health System, physical therapists have been providing primary care to patients with musculoskeletal conditions since the early 1970s.[7–10] In response to a growing need for primary care providers, physical therapists in the army were granted expanded privileges, including the authority to refer patients for radiography and other imaging tests.[8] This army model is now used in some form by all of the other uniformed services, including the U.S. Navy, U.S. Air Force, and U.S. Public Health Service.[8]

Today these expanded privileges for physical therapists are considered necessary to perform neuromusculoskeletal evaluations safely as nonphysician health-care providers.[9] Military therapists may now refer patients to radiology for conventional radiographs, bone scans, and magnetic resonance (MR) images, depending upon local policy, which varies according to the needs of the particular facility.[9] The policy does not vary according to state practice act, because the federal laws governing the military override state regulations.[8]

The military experience has shown that giving ordering privileges to physical therapists may be effective in reducing the number of extraneous images ordered, presumably due to the physical therapist's expertise in the initial screening process. James and Stuart[10] first studied the use of physical therapists as primary screeners in 1973. The physical therapists were able to reduce the number of radiological examinations by more than 50% in a population of 2,117 patients with low back pain.[10] Military therapists' expertise as primary musculoskeletal examiners is also evidenced by a recent retrospective study of 560 patients referred for magnetic resonance imaging (MRI). The study found that physical therapists' clinical diagnostic accuracy, as compared with MRI findings, was similar to that of orthopedic surgeons and significantly greater than that of nonorthopedic providers.[11]

Military physical therapists participate in additional specialized training in order to practice as *physician extenders*—clinicians who are responsible for some duties normally performed by the physician. In the army, the preferred training method is a 2-week neuromusculoskeletal course at the U.S. Army–Baylor University Program in Physical Therapy.[8] As a part of this course, the therapist receives specialized instruction in radiology. After the course, physical therapists practice and study under supervision for a 4- to 6-month period prior to beginning independent practice.[8]

Other Practice Environments in the United States

Recently, physical therapists in some health maintenance organizations and the Veterans Administration Health System have been working in roles similar to those of the U.S. military model. With the public currently being allowed direct access to physical therapists by 44 states' practice acts,[1] many civilian physical therapists currently function in the role of primary care practitioners. It is not currently prevalent in any nonmilitary setting, however, for physical therapists to order diagnostic imaging studies. Physical therapist access to diagnostic imaging is accomplished in other ways, almost always via physicians in the same health-care system.

Access to Imaging and Relationships With Physicians

Currently, physical therapists' ability to obtain diagnostic imaging is dependent upon the clinical practice environment. Outside of the military, physical therapists must look for points of access other than direct referral to radiology.

Most commonly, physical therapists rely on their relationships with referring physicians to request diagnostic imaging studies. A number of factors determine the ease of access of this method, including pre-established working relationships with physicians and a physical therapist's level of experience and knowledge about appropriate imaging studies. Figure 18-3 illustrates various points of access physical therapists may have to diagnostic imaging.

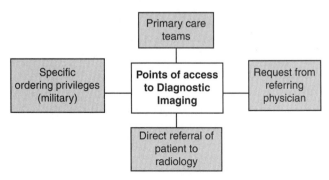

Figure 18-3 Possible points of access to diagnostic imaging for physical therapists.

Primary Care "Teams"

Some physical therapists' practices streamline the process of obtaining diagnostic imaging by pairing physical therapists with other primary care practitioners in primary care clinics or "teams." Through a brief screening or triage process, patients who are likely to have a primary musculoskeletal complaint are seen by a physical therapist for an initial appointment. The physical therapist completes a musculoskeletal examination that includes thorough screening for medical disease that may mimic musculoskeletal conditions. If the physical therapist recognizes a need for radiologic evaluation to define a musculoskeletal problem, the therapist need only request the study and have a physician in the same primary care clinic "sign off" on the request. If a serious pathology is suspected, the patient is referred to the physician for diagnostic decisions. Once trusting relationships between the physical therapists and physicians working in these clinics are developed, this model can work efficiently.

Private Practice

For physical therapists in private practice and other settings more remote from larger health-care systems, access to diagnostic imaging is more problematic. In these environments, physicians must be contacted in order to obtain imaging. Clear communication among physical therapists, referring physicians, and radiologists can help facilitate the process of obtaining appropriate diagnostic imaging.

Referral to a Radiologist

Another potential point of access to diagnostic imaging for the physical therapist is direct referral of a patient from a physical therapist to a radiologist or radiology clinic. Currently, this mode of access is not commonly employed by physical therapists. With direct access to physical therapists (and reimbursement for such access) becoming more commonplace in practice, however, direct referral to a radiologist for diagnostic imaging may be efficient and cost-saving in some settings.

The "Guide to Physical Therapist Practice," "A Normative Model of Physical Therapist Professional Education," and the "Orthopaedic Physical Therapy Description of Specialty Practice" all provide supportive language and examples for this type of referral. Physical therapists are expected to refer patients to other physician specialists when necessary (such as orthopedic surgeons, internal medicine specialists, and neurologists); radiologists would not seem to be an exception. An example of direct referral to a radiologist already exists in practice: patients with chronic pain who fail to improve with conservative treatment may be referred to radiology clinics for interventional (pain management) procedures.

Third-party reimbursement presents a potential practical barrier to direct referral of patients from a physical therapist to a radiologist. Radiology is unique among medical specialties in that patients are almost always referred for services from another physician. An insurance company's willingness to reimburse a radiologist based upon referral from a physical therapist, instead of a physician, is relatively

untested. Even if this mode of referral were to become accepted by physicians and physical therapists, in practice it would be an unlikely occurrence if patients were forced to pay out of pocket for imaging studies and interpretation.

State Practice Acts

Related to the issue of physical therapists' access to diagnostic imaging is the question of legal scope of practice as defined in each state's practice act (Table 18-3).[12] Twenty-nine states in the United States specifically prohibit the use of roentgen rays and radioactive materials for diagnosis and/or therapeutic purposes by physical therapists within the state practice act. This topic is usually addressed within the definition section, under "physical therapy." Twenty states neither prohibit nor mention use of roentgen rays and radioactive materials, x-rays, plain film materials, or imaging as defined within the scope of practice for physical therapy. One state, New Mexico, did not list its definitions for physical therapy within the general provisions of the practice act and instead uses the word *reserved* within that section.

Ramifications of Older Practice Acts

Most physical therapists are probably unaware that "the use of roentgen rays and radioactive materials for diagnosis and/or therapeutic purposes" is mentioned at all in their state practice acts. Presumably, this language was originally

TABLE 18-3 ● *State Practice Acts Concerning Radiology: Legal Status of Use of X-rays and Radioactive Materials by Physical Therapists*

Prohibited	Neither Prohibited Nor Mentioned
Alabama	Arizona
Alaska	Delaware
Arkansas	Georgia
California	Hawaii
Colorado	Indiana
Connecticut	Iowa
Florida	Massachusetts
Idaho	Michigan
Illinois	Minnesota
Kansas	Montana
Kentucky	New Hampshire
Louisiana	New Jersey
Maine	North Dakota
Maryland	Oregon
Mississippi	Pennsylvania
Missouri	Rhode Island
Nebraska	South Dakota
Nevada	Tennessee
New York	Texas
North Carolina	Vermont
Ohio	
Oklahoma	
South Carolina	
Utah	
Virginia	
Washington	
West Virginia	
Wisconsin	
Wyoming	

Adapted from American Physical Therapy Association.[12]

intended to define a territory between chiropractors, physicians, and physical therapists. The designers of older practice acts may also have been attempting to protect patients, especially in an era when the dangers of radiation exposure were not fully understood. The history behind such language in older practice acts is difficult to decipher, as are the ramifications for modern day clinical practice.

Current Updating of Practice Acts

The Federation of State Boards of Physical Therapy has created a Model Practice Act to serve as a guide for states considering or in the process of updating their practice acts. The language it contains is considered by the Federation to be ideal in legally defining the physical therapist's scope of practice. The Model Practice Act does not have any references to radiology or diagnostic imaging in physical therapy practice, nor does it specifically address referral to other practitioners.[13]

Undefined Issues

From a legal standpoint, some ambiguity exists regarding the role of diagnostic imaging in physical therapy practice. It is clear that physical therapists in many states are specifically prohibited from physically creating patient images using radiology equipment. No current state practice act includes language specifically authorizing a physical therapist to make x-ray images or other diagnostic images, and neither does the Model Practice Act. Often left open to interpretation, however, are issues such as direct referral to radiologists and physical therapists' interpretation of imaging studies.

As the profession of physical therapy continues to evolve, the following issues will require closer scrutiny and eventually demand clarification:

- Can nonmilitary physical therapists legally (according to each state's practice act) refer patients directly to a radiologist to obtain diagnostic imaging and receive a written report? The question is fairly new to the profession and has yet to be fully explored.
- Can radiologists legally receive referrals from and generate written reports for nonphysicians, such as physical therapists, according to their state practice acts?
- Will insurance companies reimburse radiologists for technical and professional fees generated through direct referral from a physical therapist to a radiologist?
- What is the physical therapist's legal scope of practice regarding the use of diagnostic imaging information, including both visual information and information from the written radiologist's report?

Physiotherapists and Diagnostic Imaging Outside the United States

Outside of the United States, many physiotherapists practice as primary care providers. As such, they often incorporate referral for diagnostic imaging into their clinical decision making. Physiotherapists working in Australia, New Zealand, and the United Kingdom, for example, all possess some ability to refer patients for imaging studies.[14–17]

In Australia, physiotherapists provide first contact, primary care services to patients in both the public and private sectors.[14,15] They are able to order a number of imaging studies as part of the diagnostic process, although there are differences in the reimbursement schedules for some physiotherapist-ordered studies as compared with physician-ordered studies.[15] A survey of Australian physiotherapists in private practice was conducted in 2004 by the Australian Physiotherapy Association (APA). The study found that 74% of physiotherapists do refer patients for radiographs at an overall annual rate of 8.3 referrals per physiotherapist.[15]

Physiotherapists in New Zealand were recognized by the Accident Compensation Commission (ACC) in 1999 as providers able to refer patients for both conventional radiographs and ultrasound imaging.[17] A study published in 2006 reported on the imaging referral habits of New Zealand physiotherapists.[14] Of the clinical decision rules identified (Ottawa Ankle Rules, Ottawa Knee Rules, and the ACC New Zealand acute low back pain guidelines), only the Ottawa Ankle Rules were used regularly in practice. The authors concluded that there was a widespread desire for more education among New Zealand physiotherapists on the use of clinical decision rules to guide radiology referral.[14]

Perhaps the most clearly defined role for physiotherapists in regards to imaging comes from the United Kingdom. There, physiotherapists who are registered as extended scope practitioners (ESPs) explicitly possess the ability to refer patients for diagnostic imaging.[16] ESP physiotherapists are categorized with practitioners like nurses and radiographers as non–medically qualified professionals who may legally request any clinical imaging procedure (including both ionizing and nonionizing modalities) as part of their role as primary care providers.[18] The specific set of eligibility criteria ESP physiotherapists must meet to request diagnostic imaging are (among others) as follows[18]:

- They must be currently registered with the Health Professions Council and Chartered Society of Physiotherapy (CSP).
- They must have completed Ionising Radiation (Medical Exposure) Regulations (IR[ME]R) training and any local clinical imaging training. They must also undertake continuing education related to IR(ME)R guidelines.
- They must understand their professional accountability arising from the current CSP Rules of Professional Conduct, Core Standards of Physiotherapy Practice and medico-legal issues arising from their extended role.
- They must have knowledge to request the appropriate investigations for their patients, understand findings of radiologic investigations and reports, and have the ability to act on them.
- They must be fully familiar with current, local clinical imaging protocols.
- They must undertake evaluation of their clinical imaging referrals regularly.

Although these criteria define the privileges and responsibilities of ESP physiotherapists in the United Kingdom, the regulations stop short of using the term *interpret* as part of the therapists' role. It would appear that interpreting radiographic images remains outside the scope of physiotherapists' practice in the United Kingdom.

The Role of Imaging in the Diagnostic Process

When to Recommend Imaging

The most important aspect of using diagnostic imaging effectively in primary care practice is *making an appropriate judgment about whether diagnostic imaging is needed*. The critical question clinicians must ask themselves when making a decision about diagnostic imaging is, "Will the results of this study change the course of treatment or alter the outcome of the problem?" Imaging modalities are often essential in the investigation of differential diagnoses. On the other hand, imaging is certainly not necessary in all cases. Many times the patient interview and physical examination are sufficient to lead a clinician to the correct diagnosis and appropriate intervention.

In all cases, diagnostic imaging should be recommended only if it is likely that the findings will have an impact on the patient's management.[19] Imaging studies are expensive compared to the physical examination and are reported to be overutilized.[20,21] Reasons include the execution of a facility's standard routine, fulfillment of patient expectations, or use of imaging studies as a protective measure against lawsuits.[22] As primary care clinicians, physical therapists must take on the same responsibility as other primary care practitioners for weighing the relative value of a diagnostic procedure and considering the cost to the health-care system.

Value of the Information

Physical therapists should consider a number of factors when determining the relative weight to place on information obtained through diagnostic imaging. First of all, was the imaging study appropriate, considering the working hypotheses? Each type of study has relative strengths and weaknesses in providing information about different tissues. For example, conventional radiography is most valuable for imaging bone, whereas MRI is superior for imaging soft tissues. Thus, when an injury to a tendon or ligament is suspected, the information provided by conventional radiography may be of little value except to rule out associated fractures. A physical therapist must be aware of these diagnostic strengths and weaknesses when recommending studies and when considering the information coming from studies that were ordered by other practitioners.

Sensitivity and Specificity

The physical therapist must be aware of the sensitivity and specificity of different imaging techniques. A diagnostic test's sensitivity may be defined as the "test's ability to obtain a positive test when the target condition is really present, or a true positive."[23] Specificity may be defined as the "test's ability to obtain a negative test when the condition is really absent, or a true negative"[23]—in other words, how discriminating is the imaging technique in identifying the suspected pathology? A diagnostic imaging modality's sensitivity and specificity values will vary according to the individual pathology or lesion. For example, a bone scan may be the most sensitive modality for determining that a skeletal lesion does indeed exist, but it has poor specificity in determining the characteristics of that lesion.

An imaging procedure's sensitivity and specificity values for a particular diagnosis are determined by clinical research comparing how accurate the diagnostic modality has been at identifying that lesion over a large number of cases. However, sensitivity and specificity for a particular imaging modality's ability to identify a lesion is not fixed. Imaging techniques continue to improve as technology improves. Subsequently, the best test for confirming a particular diagnosis may change over time. Because of the rapid progress in imaging technology, primary care practitioners should rely on the radiologist's expertise in determining the best current test for identifying a particular lesion.

Factors Affecting the Value of an Imaging Study

A variety of factors may influence the value of information from a particular diagnostic imaging study. Some imaging studies, such as ultrasonography, are operator-dependent, and the image is directly related to the operator's skill level. Other imaging studies, such as computed tomography (CT) or MRI, are dependent upon correctly chosen scanning planes. Although basic scanning planes are usually sufficient, imaging in areas of complex or small anatomy, such as the temporomandibular joint (TMJ), can be challenging. MRI involves further complexity in the choice of technical parameters in a given imaging sequence. Some diagnostic imaging studies may not be sensitive to a pathology at a certain phase of its development. Finally, the interpretive skill of the professional who reads and reports on the resulting images is critical to the value of any diagnostic study.

Therefore it is critically important that the clinician be able to link diagnostic imaging information with clinical presentation. Any imaging study is worthless if the clinician cannot apply clinical judgment to the individual patient, giving due consideration to the imaging results within the context of the overall clinical picture.[19]

Inconsistencies Between Imaging Results and Clinical Examination

When the results of an imaging study or series of studies do not correlate well with the overall clinical picture, how should a clinician proceed? The answer depends on the nature of the inconsistency. The possibilities include the following:

1. Imaging was negative for pathology that was strongly suspected clinically.
2. Imaging was positive for an abnormality that was not suspected.

In either case, the clinician's hypothesis was not confirmed by imaging. The pretest likelihood and the test result were not consistent with each other. When these circumstances arise, *clinicians should place no more or less weight on the imaging than on other aspects of the diagnostic process.*

Clinicians may choose to follow one of several possible actions depending upon the situation. As an example of the first type of inconsistency, a strong pretest likelihood or clinical suspicion of a carpal fracture and a negative radiograph result may require re-examination with a special projection or another imaging modality with better sensitivity for the suspected pathology. However, in terms of cost, it may be more prudent simply to treat the wrist with immobilization and obtain radiographs again in 1 to 2 weeks, when fracture healing would be evident.

For the second type of inconsistency, an unexpected abnormality may simply be an incidental anomaly that requires no further action. This scenario is a more common occurrence than incidental findings of a serious nature, such as the discovery of a neoplasm. Such findings necessitate immediate involvement of other professionals and minimize the physical therapist's role in patient management.

A common example for a physical therapist would be a report including findings like degenerative changes or bulging intervertebral disks. Pre-existing conditions, as well as findings that may or may not be responsible for the present complaint, are relatively common in the general population. The clinician must use sound clinical judgment to decide how relevant these findings are in the context of the patient's signs and symptoms.

Clinical Decision Making and Clinical Practice Guidelines

Hypothetico–Deductive Reasoning

Both novice and expert orthopedic physical therapists utilize the hypothetico–deductive reasoning process in patient management.[24] This process involves the initial generation of multiple hypotheses based on both patient- and therapist-generated information. The therapist tests these hypotheses in a structured way, employing interview and physical examination data. Other forms of data, such as diagnostic imaging, can play a critical role in the reasoning process of the therapist engaged in primary musculoskeletal screening. (Case Study 1, below, provides an example of the use of diagnostic imaging in physical therapy decision making.) Once interventions have been chosen, the therapist assesses the patient's response to the chosen interventions and modifies the hypothesis and interventions, if necessary. Diagnostic imaging can also play an important role in this process, providing information about issues such as the stage of tissue healing and anatomic alignment. Case Study 2 is an example of using diagnostic imaging in a patient's intervention planning.

Clinical Decision Rules and Appropriateness Guidelines

Physical therapists should be familiar with decision-making guides published in the literature. Some of these guides have undergone a rigorous development and testing process; these are usually referred to as clinical decision rules (CDRs). In radiology, a number of CDRs have been developed to help first-contact clinicians decide whether imaging is necessary in cases of trauma. Other sets of evidence-based guidelines, often referred to as appropriateness guidelines or criteria, have been developed and approved by a group of experts to assist clinicians in choosing imaging modalities for both acute and chronic conditions. This type of guideline is usually approved by a professional body based on expert consensus.

In general, a CDR exists to assist clinicians in making diagnostic and prognostic assessments.[25] A CDR is established by compiling existing clinical assessments that have been found to have predictive power, are validated for accuracy, and analyzed for clinical impact in terms of patient outcomes and costs.[25] Prior to widespread adoption of a CDR, the rule should be tested in formal implementation studies. The Ottawa Knee Rules, Ottawa Ankle Rules, and Canadian C-Spine Rule are all examples of formal CDRs that have successfully met standards of derivation, validation, and implementation.[26–33]

Guides for Knee Trauma

Two sets of CDRs have been developed to guide clinicians following acute knee injuries. Development of these guides was prompted by the frequent use of radiographs following trauma to the knee. It was found that radiographs were being ordered for 85% of patients, when only 6 to 12% of those patients were found to have a fracture.[34] The Ottawa Knee Rules and the Pittsburgh Decision Rules were created to help clinicians use radiography more appropriately to identify fractures and to minimize the unnecessary use of radiographs.[35] Both of these guides provide the clinician with criteria to assist in deciding whether to order conventional radiographs to screen for fractures about the knee joint.

Pittsburgh Decision Rules[34–36] The Pittsburgh decision rules (Table 18-4) are quite simple,[34–36] calling for conventional radiographs when a patient has had "blunt trauma or a fall as a mechanism of injury plus either or both of the following:

- Age younger than 12 years or older than 50 years
- Inability to walk four weight-bearing steps in the emergency department

This guide has shown excellent sensitivity (99%) and specificity (60%) for identifying knee fractures.[34,35] In terms of predictive value, a fracture was actually found 24.1% of the time when the rules indicated fracture (positive predictive value). When the rules indicated no fracture, there was none 99.8% of the time (negative predictive value).[34,35] Given this performance, Seaberg concludes that the Pittsburgh decision rules could decrease the use of radiographs in this patient population by 52%.[34]

Ottawa Knee Rules[34,35,37] Unlike the Pittsburgh Decision Rules, which are applicable to patients of all ages, the Ottawa Knee Rules (Table 18-5) were originally intended to apply only to patients under the age of 18. The Ottawa rules call for

TABLE 18-4 • Pittsburgh Decision Rules for Knee Trauma
Conventional radiographs should be ordered for patients with the following characteristics: Blunt trauma or fall mechanism of injury AND . . . • Age under 12 or over 50 **AND/OR**. . . • Inability to walk four weight-bearing steps in the emergency department
Sources: Seaberg et al;[34] Tandeter et al;[35] and Bauer et al.[36]

TABLE 18-5 ● *Ottawa Knee Rules*
Conventional radiographs should be ordered after trauma to the knee for patients with any of the following characteristics[a]: • Age greater than 55 years • Tenderness at fibular head • Isolated tenderness of patella • Inability to flex knee to 90° • Inability to walk four weight-bearing steps immediately after injury and in the emergency department
[a]Rules should not be applied to patients younger than 18 years. *Sources:* Seaberg et al;[34] Tandeter et al;[35] and Stiell et al.[37]

TABLE 18-6 ● *Ottawa Ankle Rules for Ankle/Foot Trauma*	
Conventional radiographs should be ordered after trauma to the ankle/foot for patients with any of the following characteristics:	
Ankle	**Foot**
Pain in the malleolar zone (about the medial or lateral malleolus) AND… • Tenderness at the posterior aspect or tip of the lateral malleolus, **OR…** • Tenderness at the posterior aspect or tip of the medial malleolus, **OR…** • Inablility to bear weight both immediately and in the emergency department	Pain in the midfoot zone (about the midfoot) AND… • Tenderness at the fifth metatarsal base, **OR…** • Tenderness at the navicular bone, **OR…** • Inability to bear weight both immediately and in the emergency department
Source: Stiell et al.[38,39]	

conventional radiographs following knee trauma in any of the following cases[34,35,37]:

● Patient older than 55 years
● Tenderness at the head of the fibula
● Isolated tenderness of the patella
● Inability to flex the knee to 90 degrees
● Inability to walk four weight-bearing steps immediately after the injury *and* in the emergency department

The Ottawa rules have shown a measure of sensitivity of 97% and specificity of 27%.[34,35] Given its performance, Seaberg concludes that this tool could reduce the use of radiographs in patients following knee trauma by 23%.[34] Since development, the rules have been validated in one study for use with children aged 2 to 16.[28]

Ottawa Rules for Trauma to the Ankle and Foot[38,39]

The Ottawa Ankle Rules (Table 18-6) were developed to help clinicians to decide whether to order conventional radiographs following trauma to the ankle. There is a set of rules for the ankle and a separate set for the foot (midfoot specifically), depending on which region is affected.

Following trauma to the ankle, the rules state that conventional radiographs should be ordered only if there is pain in the "malleolar zone" (surrounding one or both of the malleoli) *and* one or more of the following[38,39]:

● Tenderness at the posterior aspect or tip of the lateral malleolus
● Tenderness at the posterior aspect or tip of the medial malleolus
● Inability to bear weight, both immediately and in the emergency department

Following trauma to the foot, the rules state that conventional radiographs should be ordered only if there is pain in the "midfoot zone" (about the midfoot) *and* one or more of the following[38,39]:

● Tenderness at the fifth metatarsal base
● Tenderness at the navicular bone
● Inability to bear weight both immediately and in the emergency department

Sensitivity and specificity values have been reported for the Ottawa Ankle Rules, which include the ankle and foot guides applied together: The sensitivity and specificity were found to be 100% and 40%, respectively.[38] Based upon this clinical tool's performance, Stiell concludes that implementation of the Ottawa Ankle Rules could reduce the use of conventional radiography following ankle trauma by 30%.[38] Owing to the

relatively low specificity of the Ottawa Ankle Rules, resulting in many false positives, a few studies have suggested that the use of additional clinical examination techniques may further reduce the unnecessary use of radiographs. The methods have included application of vibration with a tuning fork or indirect stress to the ankle with force applied proximal to the site of injury.[40–41]

The Canadian C-Spine Rule[42] and NEXUS Criteria[43]

The Canadian C-Spine Rule[42] and the National Emergency X-Radiography Utilization (NEXUS) Study[43] provide clinicians guidelines to aid decision making following suspected trauma to the cervical spine.

The Canadian C-Spine Rule (CCR) applies to patients who are *alert and medically stable*. The tool is designed to help clinicians decide whether conventional radiography of the cervical spine is necessary for patients who have sustained a traumatic injury involving the head or neck. The guide is specifically meant to identify patients at risk for "clinically important cervical spine injury, defined as any fracture, dislocation, or ligamentous instability demonstrated by diagnostic imaging."[42]

The decision whether to order conventional radiographs is based on answers to three questions[42]:

1. Are there any high-risk factors that mandate radiography? Examples include age greater than or equal to 65 years, a dangerous mechanism of injury, or paresthesias in the extremities. If the answer is yes, then radiographs should be obtained.
2. Are there any low-risk factors that allow safe assessment of range of motion? Examples include a simple rear-end motor vehicle accident, a normal sitting position, a patient being ambulatory at any time, delayed onset of neck pain, or absence of midline cervical spine tenderness. If the answer is no, then radiographs should be obtained. If the answer is yes, then the clinician can move to question 3.
3. Is the patient able to rotate the neck actively at least 45 degrees to the right and left? If the patient is unable, then radiographs should be obtained. If the patient is able, then no radiographs are necessary.

Based on the prospective study by Stiell, the CCR had a sensitivity of 100% and a specificity of 43%.[42] The authors estimated that, using the decision rule, the radiography ordering rate would have been 58% for the patients in their study, compared to the actual rate of almost 70%.[42]

The NEXUS low-risk criteria were developed to help identify patients following trauma who *do not need* diagnostic imaging for the cervical spine based on their clinical presentation. This guideline states that radiography is indicated following trauma unless a patient meets all five criteria[43]:

1. No posterior midline cervical tenderness
2. No evidence of intoxication
3. Normal level of alertness and consciousness
4. No focal neurological deficit
5. No painful distracting injuries (e.g., an injury in an area other than the cervical spine that may distract the patient from neck pain)

A validity study by the NEXUS researchers reported a sensitivity of 99.6% and a specificity of 12.9% when applying the criteria to a population of 34,069 patients.[43]

Appropriateness Criteria

The American College of Radiology (ACR), the primary professional society for radiologists, has produced clinical guidelines for over 160 topics.[44] These *appropriateness criteria* are designed to help providers choose the best imaging study for a given clinical situation, based upon evidence and expert concensus. In the musculoskeletal realm, the ACR makes criteria available to providers on topics ranging from acute hand and wrist trauma to chronic hip pain to suspected spine trauma.[45] Table 18-7 summarizes some recommendations from the ACR Appropriateness Criteria for suspected spine trauma, which utilizes risk criteria from the Canadian C-Spine Rule (CCR) and the National Emergency X-Radiography Utilization Study (NEXUS) criteria,[45] both described in the previous section. The supplementary information in the table compares the NEXUS and CCR high and low risk criteria. Table 18-8 provides a partial summary of the ACR appropriateness criteria for patients with chronic elbow pain.[45]

Diagnostic Imaging Guidelines for Acute Low Back Pain

With many musculoskeletal conditions, including low back pain, a level of uncertainty concerning diagnosis can persist throughout the patient's episode. This uncertainty *may or may not* have a negative impact on the clinician's ability to formulate an effective set of interventions. Because low back pain often resolves without a definitive diagnosis, the utility of diagnostic imaging in cases of acute low back pain has been questioned. In this area, in particular, conventional radiographs are overutilized by primary care providers.[46] In most cases of acute low back pain, a patient's symptoms will resolve within 4 weeks with proper conservative management, without the need for any diagnostic imaging.[47] In these patients whose symptoms are expected to resolve relatively quickly, ordering imaging studies is unnecessary and not consistent with recommendations found in the literature.[46–48]

Practice guidelines from the Agency for Health Care Policy and Research (AHCPR) published in 1994 address the imaging of patients with acute low back pain.[48] Although these guidelines are found within a larger set of clinical guidelines for the management of low back pain that is no longer considered current, the specific imaging recommendations are still useful. The AHCPR guidelines recommend no imaging in the first month of onset of low back pain, in the absence of certain "red flag" items at initial clinical examination: cauda equina syndrome, fracture, tumor, infection, and nonspinal sources of low back pain, such as abdominal or pelvic pathology.[48]

An extensive search of the literature by Jarvik and Deyo,[49] spanning the period 1966 to 2001, reviewed evidence for the diagnostic accuracy of clinical information and imaging for patients with acute low back pain in primary care settings. These authors' conclusions, published in 2002, suggest a diagnostic strategy similar to that of the 1994 AHCPR guidelines[49]:

1. For adults younger than 50 years of age with no signs or symptoms of systemic disease, symptomatic therapy without imaging is appropriate.
2. For patients 50 years and older or those whose findings suggest systemic disease, conventional radiography and simple laboratory tests can almost completely rule out underlying systemic disease.
3. Advanced imaging should be reserved for patients who are considering surgery or those in whom systemic disease is strongly suspected.

The Role of Imaging in Physical Therapy Intervention

What Do Physical Therapists Look For?

The radiologist bears the ultimate responsibility for the radiological diagnosis. In brief, the orthopedic radiologist attempts to diagnose an unknown disorder, demonstrate the exact location, identify the distribution of the lesion in the skeleton, gain pertinent information for the surgeon, and monitor the response of the lesion to medical intervention. Once a disorder is identified in this way, the function of diagnostic imaging is complete as far as the physician is concerned.

A physical therapist, however, may use imaging studies for purposes other than diagnosis but related to rehabilitation of the diagnosed pathology. Because the radiology report is written to serve the physician's decision-making needs, information specific to the physical therapist's intervention planning is not usually provided. The ability to comprehend the image itself, then, is valuable for the physical therapist. See Table 18-9 for examples of how physicians and physical therapists might use imaging studies differently.

Incorporating Imaging Into Treatment Planning

How can the physical therapist take the wealth of information contained on an image and incorporate it into treatment planning? A challenge for the physical therapist armed with knowledge of diagnostic imaging is to explore the possibilities offered by the image itself.

TABLE 18-7 ● *Spine Trauma Imaging Recommendations: ACR Appropriateness Criteria and NEXUS vs. CCR Criteria*

Clinical Condition: Suspected Spine Trauma

Radiologic Exam or Procedure	Appropriateness Rating	Comment
Variant 1: Cervical spine imaging not indicated by NEXUS or CCR clinical criteria. Patient meets low-risk criteria.		
X-ray cervical spine	1	
CT cervical spine without contrast	1	With sagittal and coronal reformat
Myelography and post myelography CT cervical spine	1	
CTA head and neck	1	
MRI cervical spine without contrast	1	
MRA neck with contrast	1	
Arteriography cervicocerebral	1	
Variant 2: Suspected acute cervical spine trauma. Imaging indicated by clinical criteria (NEXUS or CCR). Not otherwise specified.		
CT cervical spine without contrast	9	With sagittal and coronal reformat
X-ray cervical spine	6	Lateral view only. Useful in CT reconstructions are not optimal
Myelography and post myelography CT cervical spine	1	
CTA head and neck	1	
MRI cervical spine without contrast	1	
MRA neck with contrast	1	
Arteriography cervicocerebral	1	

Supplementary: High risk vs. low risk according to NEXUS and Canadian C-Spine Rule

High risk criteria (CCR, imaging indicated)

Altered mental status

Multiple fractures

Drowning or diving accident

Significant head or facial injury

Age >65 years

"Dangerous Mechanism"*

Paresthesias in extremities

Rigid spinal disease (ankylosing spondylitis, DISH)

Low risk criteria (no imaging required)

CCR: simple rear end MVC, sitting position in ED, ambulatory at any time, delated onset of neck pain, absence of midline cervical tenderness, able to actively rotate neck 45° left and right

NEXUS: no midline cervical tenderness, no focal neurologic deficits, no intoxication or indication of brain injury, no painful distracting injuries, normal alertness

---

*"Dangerous Mechanism" defined as: Fall from an elevation of 3 ft. or 5 stairs, axial load to the head (eg, diving), motor vehicle collision at high speed (>100 km/hr) or with rollover or ejection, collision involving a motorized recreational vehicle or bicycle collision.
Appropriateness criteria scale 123456789
1 = Least appropriate
9 = Most appropriate
Available at www.acr.org. Updated 2009.

Consider this basic scenario. Physical therapists are typically responsible for restoring normal movement to a joint that has been directly or indirectly affected by a disorder. Before choosing specific treatment techniques to address the movement limitations, physical therapists want to know:

1. What barriers to normal movement might exist at the joint? Surgical fixation devices, loose bodies, and excessive callus can all be problematic.
2. Which interventions (passive, active, resistive maneuvers) for restoring movement are safe and appropriate at any given point in a patient's rehabilitation?
3. How much stress applied to healing tissues will promote the return of normal function without compromising optimal healing?
4. Where should the limb be stabilized to avoid movement at a fracture site? Can an adjacent joint be mobilized without endangering the fracture site?
5. How much weight-bearing is safe at this time?

Sometimes viewing available imaging studies can help answer these questions. If not, consultation with the physician regarding the images may answer them. Even a consultation, however, requires that the physical therapist understand an image well enough to discuss it.

TABLE 18-8 ● *American College of Radiology Appropriateness Criteria*

Clinical Condition: Chronic Elbow Pain

Radiologic Exam or Procedure	Appropriateness Rating	Comment
Variant 1: Initial evaluation for chronic elbow pain. First test.		
X-ray elbow	9	
MRI elbow without contrast	1	
MR arthrography elbow	1	
CT elbow without contrast	1	
CT arthrography elbow	1	
US elbow	1	
Tc-99m bone scan elbow	1	
Variant 3: Suspect occult injury; e.g., osteochondral injury; radiographs nondiagnostic.		
MRI elbow without contrast	9	
CT elbow without contrast	2	
MR arthrography elbow	2	
CT arthrography elbow	2	
Tc-99m bone scan elbow	2	
US elbow	1	
Variant 9: Suspect nerve abnormality; radiographs nondiagnostic.		
MRI elbow without contrast	9	
US elbow	8	An alternative to MRI if expertise is available. Dynamic US is ideal for assessing ulnar nerve dislocation and snapping triceps syndrome
MR arthrography elbow	1	
CT elbow without contrast	1	
CT arthrography elbow	1	
Tc-99m bone scan elbow	1	

Appropriateness criteria scale 123456789
1 = Least appropriate
9 = Most appropriate
Available at www.acr.org. Updated 2009.

TABLE 18-9 ● *Examples of How Physicians and Physical Therapists May Use Musculoskeletal Imaging Studies*

Physicians, Including Radiologists (Medical Diagnosis)
- Screen for serious pathology, such as bony or soft-tissue neoplasms.
- Identify and classify fractures.
- Identify dislocations.
- Identify ligament, tendon, and cartilage lesions.
- Assess nerve tissue.
- Identify disease processes affecting bone.
- Identify and characterize degenerative processes.
- Identify soft-tissue swelling.
- Characterize fracture healing.

Physical Therapists (Intervention Planning)
Consider all of the above, plus any of the following that may affect normal movement:
- Assess bony alignment.
- Identify bony blocks to movement.
- Visualize exact location of fractures to plan interventions.
- Identify exact position of fixation devices.
- Assess bone healing to make decisions about movement and weight-bearing.

What Does the Future Hold?

Interaction between the fields of rehabilitation and diagnostic imaging is relatively new territory for most physical therapy education programs and for most practicing clinicians. The vision outlined for the future of the physical therapy profession clearly incorporates basic knowledge of diagnostic imaging. The undefined challenges of this vision include how to integrate diagnostic imaging information significantly into physical therapy intervention, the possibility of professional collaboration between the two fields, and the research potential afforded by this collaboration.

Summary of Key Points

1. The growth of direct access, with physical therapists assuming primary care roles, and the transition to the doctor of physical therapy degree are among the changes related to practice and education in the physical therapy profession that have increased physical therapists' need to be knowledgeable about diagnostic imaging.

2. The APTA documents "Vision Statement 2020," "Guide to Physical Therapist Practice," "A Normative Model of Physical Therapist Professional Education," and "Orthopaedic Physical Therapy Description of Specialty Practice" all contain language supportive of physical therapists' use of diagnostic imaging information in clinical practice.

3. A physical therapist who is an educated user of diagnostic imaging should be able to recognize when imaging is appropriate, integrate information from the radiologist's report into treatment planning, understand diagnostic images visually, and communicate effectively with other providers about a patient's imaging studies.

4. In the United States, physical therapists practicing in the military, in private practice, in health maintenance organizations, in the Veterans Administration, and in other settings may all assume primary care roles, thus necessitating knowledge of and access to diagnostic imaging.

5. Physical therapists in the United States most commonly gain access to diagnostic imaging via their relationships with physicians. Direct access to radiology services for physical therapists is a complicated issue involving state practice acts, reimbursement considerations, and physician relationships.

6. Physiotherapists in Australia, New Zealand, and the United Kingdom all have the ability to directly obtain diagnostic imaging for patients within their roles as primary care providers.

7. Diagnostic imaging is a critical piece of the diagnostic process that assists clinicians in screening for serious pathology and in defining musculoskeletal conditions.

8. Decisions to recommend diagnostic imaging should always be based on clinical evidence, as gathered through the clinical examination.

9. Clinical practice guidelines, such as clinical decision rules and appropriateness criteria, exist to aid clinicians in making choices about diagnostic imaging. These guidelines include the Pittsburgh Decision Rules, the Ottawa Knee Rules, the Ottawa Ankle Rules, the Canadian C-Spine Rule, ACR Appropriateness Criteria, and guidelines for acute low back pain imaging.

10. Physical therapists may incorporate diagnostic imaging information into intervention planning to help them identify barriers to normal movement, to choose safe and appropriate treatment techniques, to decide where to stabilize a limb during movement following a fracture, and to make decisions about weight-bearing.

CASE STUDIES

The two cases presented here illustrate a physical therapist's integration of diagnostic imaging information into the decision-making process. These examples demonstrate how access to imaging can play a critical role in patient management when the therapist has the ability to recommend (or order) an appropriate imaging study.

CASE STUDY 1

Differential Diagnosis: Strain or Stress Fracture?

The patient is a 40-year-old female triathlete treated by a physical therapist via direct access. The patient complains of pain in the lateral aspect of the right lower leg and ankle. She reports that she is training for her first Half Ironman distance triathlon and has been running approximately 25 miles per week the past month, an increase over her usual distance of 15 miles per week. Initially she experienced pain for about an hour after finishing a training run, but she has recently begun to experience pain during her runs, and the pain lasts for 2 hours after finishing.

Physical Examination

The patient is examined after running on a treadmill in the clinic until she begins to experience some lateral leg pain. Her running biomechanics are good without abnormal or compensatory motions observed. In standing, her feet show good longitudinal arches with little movement into pronation with single-limb standing. Screening examination maneuvers for the lumbar spine and knee reveal no abnormalities and do not provoke symptoms. Ankle active range of motion is normal, but overpressure applied to inversion and eversion does provoke her lateral leg pain. Manual muscle testing of the lower leg muscles produces pain with resisted eversion. She is tender to palpation over the middle to distal third of the lateral leg along the fibula.

Working Hypotheses

The physical therapist suspects a stress fracture of the fibula but also considers differential diagnoses of compartment syndrome or fibularis longus strain.

Diagnostic Imaging

To test the hypothesis of stress fracture, the physical therapist contacts the patient's primary care provider to discuss the possibility of obtaining conventional radiographs. The physician agrees, and radiographs of the right leg are obtained (anteroposterior [AP] and lateral). A radiologist reads the films and identifies no fracture or other abnormality.

Intervention

The physical therapist decides to proceed with an intervention plan based on a hypothesis of overuse of the lateral compartment musculature (fibularis muscles). The physical therapist recommends modification of training, including a significant decrease in running mileage and an increased focus on swimming and cycling training. The therapist also recommends another model of running shoes and treatment of symptoms with ice and soft tissue massage. After 4 weeks, the triathlete reports that her lateral leg pain has decreased but not disappeared. She continues to experience symptoms when running. There are no changes in the findings on the physical examination. The therapist contacts the physician again to discuss the situation and suggests a bone scan to rule out a stress fracture.

Additional Imaging

The bone scan shows a "hot spot" of increased tracer uptake in the right lateral leg, suggestive of a stress fracture. Conventional radiographs are taken again at the same time, this time showing some callus formation in the right distal fibula above the malleolus, confirming a stress fracture (Fig. 18-4).

Discussion

The physical therapist in this case suspected a stress fracture of the fibula from the initial examination. The history of gradual onset of pain concurrent with an increase in training load, combined with the physical examination findings of bone tenderness, pointed to this hypothesis. The initial conventional radiographs appeared normal, which is not unusual in cases of stress fracture. Often a stress fracture becomes evident on conventional radiographs only when callus forms at the fracture site. A more sensitive imaging test for stress fracture is a bone scan. There was a strong enough pretest likelihood of stress fracture that a bone scan would have been appropriate at the time of the initial radiographs (see Fig. 18-5 for the actual and alternative decision-making pathways). It is likely that the test would have suggested stress fracture at that time. The test is not specific enough to make a diagnosis of stress fracture by itself; but if it had been combined with the whole clinical picture, the hypothesis could have been confirmed earlier. At that time, complete rest and reduced weight-bearing could have been prescribed, probably resulting in a quicker recovery and eventually a gradual return to the patient's training schedule.

CASE STUDY 2

Physical Therapy Intervention: Postsurgical Shoulder Rehabilitation

The patient is a 25-year-old man referred to physical therapy for rehabilitation 6 weeks after surgical intervention of a proximal humerus fracture–dislocation.

History of Trauma

The patient was mountain biking on an expert path when he hit a large rock and was thrown over the handlebars, falling directly onto his left shoulder. Conventional radiographs of the left shoulder taken in the emergency department showed a comminuted fracture–dislocation involving the proximal humerus and humeral head (Fig. 18-6). The patient underwent open reduction and internal fixation (Fig. 18-7).

Physical Therapy Intervention Considerations

The severity of this patient's injury is better appreciated visually than by reading the radiologist's report. Direct visualization of the original injury and subsequent surgical fixation improves the physical therapist's awareness of the patient's condition. In addition to the structures known to be at risk with this injury, including the axillary nerve and circumflex humeral arteries, the physical therapist must consider the stability and degree of healing of the proximal humerus and humeral head at all stages during rehabilitation. Using the patient's imaging studies, along with regular contact with the patient's orthopedic surgeon, the therapist is able to plan safe interventions that will allow for progress while minimizing the risks of problems such as avascular necrosis and malunion.

Passive and active range-of-motion, joint mobilization, stretching, and strengthening activities for the glenohumeral joint and

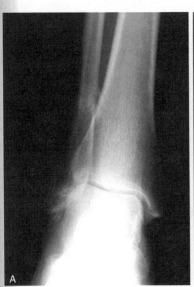
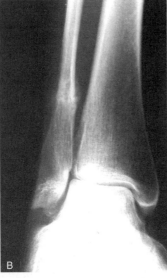

Figure 18-4 Conventional radiographs showing a stress fracture of the right distal fibula for the patient in Case Study 1. **(A)** AP right ankle, **(B)** mortise view right ankle.

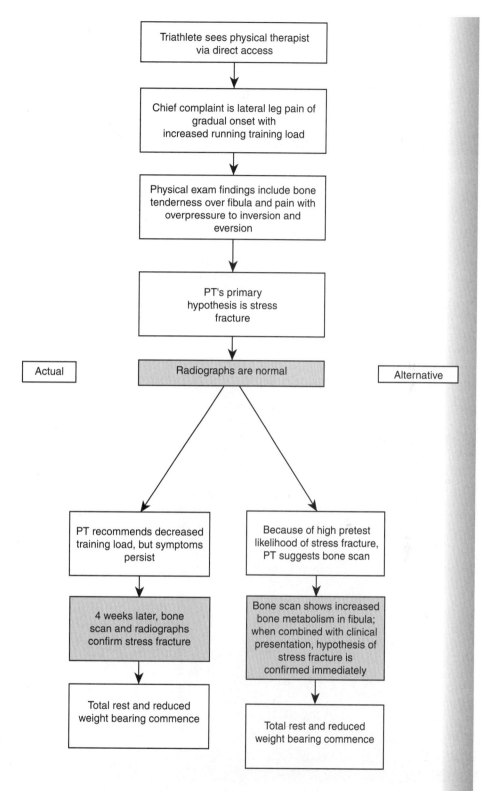

Figure 18-5 Diagnostic imaging decision-making pathway for Case Study 1, including actual and alternative paths.

scapula will all be necessary to achieve an optimal outcome. The physical therapist will be able to make well-informed decisions about when to initiate each of these activities, how far in the range-of-motion exercises they can be taken, where stabilization must be placed, and how much force to use, by examining the patient's radiographs. The therapist can use the images to educate

the patient about the fragile postsurgical condition of his shoulder and why some movements must be avoided.

Discussion

A common challenge to physical therapists designing intervention plans for patients following fractures is to stress the involved

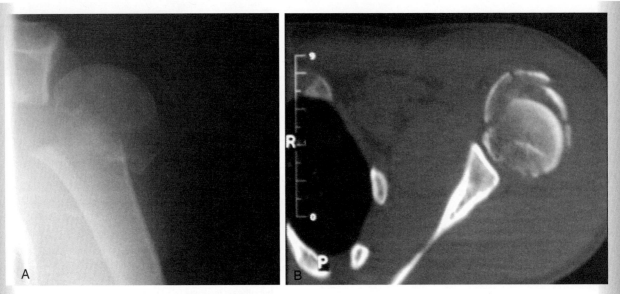

Figure 18-6 **(A)** Conventional radiograph (AP shoulder) and **(B)** axial CT image showing the proximal humerus and humeral head comminuted fracture–dislocation for the patient in Case Study 2.

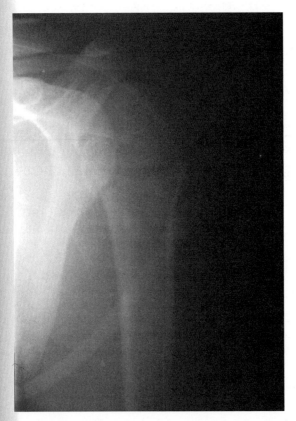

Figure 18-7 AP shoulder radiograph for Case Study 2 showing the patient's injury after open reduction and internal fixation.

tissues enough to promote healing without causing gross movement at the fracture site that will delay healing. As this case exemplifies, therapists can use patients' imaging studies to guide them in deciding where to place their hands when moving a limb or mobilizing a joint. The detrimental effects of prolonged immobilization are well known, and it is known that movement of the soft tissues and joints around the fracture is beneficial. Yet the fracture site also needs to be protected while the movements are performed. Imaging provides a very useful clinical tool to physical therapists so that guesswork can be eliminated by visualization of the severity and exact location of fractures and visualization of the methods of fixation and any possible barriers to movement.

References

1. American Physical Therapy Association (APTA): A summary of direct access language in state physical therapy practice acts. Accessed September 13, 2008 at http://www.apta.org/AM/Template.cfm?Section=Top_Issues2& CONTENTID=43482&TEMPLATE=/CM/ContentDisplay.cfm.
2. APTA: 2007–2008 Fact Sheet, Physical Therapist Education Programs. APTA, Alexandria, VA, May 2008.
3. APTA: APTA Vision Sentence and Vision Statement for Physical Therapy 2020. Accessed September 13, 2008 at http://www.apta.org/AM/Template. cfm?Section=Vision_20201&Template=/TaggedPage/TaggedPageDisplay .cfm&TPLID=285&ContentID=32061.
4. Rothstein, JM (ed): Guide to Physical Therapist Practice, ed. 2. Phys Ther 81:9, 2001.
5. APTA: A Normative Model of Physical Therapist Professional Education: Version 2004. APTA, Alexandria, VA, 2004.
6. American Board of Physical Therapy Specialties Specialty Council on Orthopaedic Physical Therapy: Orthopaedic Physical Therapy Description of Specialty Practice. APTA, Alexandria, VA, 2002.
7. Benson, CJ, et al: The role of Army physical therapists as nonphysician health care providers who prescribe certain medications: Observations and experiences. Phys Ther 75:380, 1995.
8. Dininny, P: More than a uniform: The military model of physical therapy. PT Magazine 3(3):40, 1995.
9. Greathouse, DG, et al: The United States Army physical therapy experience: Evaluation and treatment of patients with neuromusculoskeletal disorders. J Orthop Sports Phys Ther 19:261, 1994.
10. James, JJ, and Stuart, RB: Expanded role for the physical therapist: Screening musculoskeletal disorders. Phys Ther 55:121, 1975.
11. Moore, JH, et al: Clinical diagnostic accuracy and magnetic resonance imaging of patients referred by physical therapists, orthopaedic surgeons, and nonorthopaedic providers. J Orthop Sports Phys Ther 35:67, 2005.
12. APTA: Directory of state practice acts, government affairs. Accessed September 13, 2008 http://www.apta.org/AM/Template.cfm?Section= Professional_Resources&Template=/TaggedPage/TaggedPageDisplay.cfm& TPLID=201&ContentID=40335.
13. Federation of State Boards of Physical Therapy: Model Practice Act for Physical Therapy, ed. 3. Federation of State Boards of Physical Therapy, Alexandria, VA, 2001.
14. Littlejohn, F, Nahna, M, Newland, C, et al: What are the protocols for imaging referral by physiotherapists? N Z J Physiother 34(2):81, 2006.
15. Australian Physiotherapy Association: Physiotherapists Diagnostic Imaging Referral Patterns, Presented to the Department of Health and Aging. Australian Physiotherapy Association, August 2004.
16. The Chartered Society of Physiotherapy: Chartered physiotherapists working as extended scope practitioners. Information paper No. PA29. London, 2002.
17. Scrymgeour, J: Moving on: A history of the New Zealand Society of Physiotherapists, Inc. 1973–1999. Wellington, The New Zealand Society of Physiotherapists Inc., 2000.
18. Royal College of Nursing: Clinical Imaging Requests from Non-medically Qualified Professionals. Royal College of Nursing, London, 2006.
19. Chang, PJ: The rational selection and interpretation of diagnostic tests. In Erkonen, WE, and Smith, WL (eds). Radiology 101: The Basics and Fundamentals of Imaging. Lippincott-Raven, Philadelphia, 1998, pp 57–67.
20. Hall, FM: Overutilization of radiological examinations. Radiology 120:443, 1976.
21. Abrams, HL: The overutilization of x-rays. N Engl J Med 300:1213, 1979.
22. Long, AE: Radiographic decision-making by the emergency physician. Emerg Med Clin North Am 3:437, 1985.
23. Portney, LG, and Watkins, MP: Foundations of Clinical Research: Applications to Practice, ed. 2. Prentice Hall, Upper Saddle River, NJ, 2000.
24. Jones, M, et al: Clinical reasoning in physiotherapy. In Higgs, J, and Jones, M (eds): Clinical Reasoning in the Health Professions. Butterworth-Heinemann, Oxford, UK, 2000, pp 117–127.
25. McGinn, T, et al: Users' guides to the medical literature XXII: How to use articles about clinical decision rules. JAMA 284(1):79, 2000.
26. Stiell, IG, and Bennett, C: Implementation of clinical decision rules in the emergency department. Acad Emerg Med 14(11):955, 2007.
27. Perry, JJ, and Stiell, IG: Impact of clinical decision rules on clinical care of traumatic injuries to the foot and ankle, knee, cervical spine, and head. Injury 37(12):1157, 2006.
28. Bulloch, B, Neto, G, Plint, A, et al: Validation of the Ottawa knee rule in children: A multicenter study. Ann Emerg Med 42(1):48, 2003.
29. Broomhead, A, and Stuart, P: Validation of the Ottawa ankle rules in Australia. Emerg Med (Fremantle) 15(2):126, 2003.
30. Wynn-Thomas, S, Love, T, McLeod, D, et al: The Ottawa ankle rules for the use of diagnostic x-ray in after hours medical centres in New Zealand. N Z Med J 115(1162):U184, 2002.
31. Papacostas, E, Malliaropoulos, N, Papadopouolos, A, and Liouliakis, C: Validation of Ottawa ankle rules protocol in Greek athletes: Study in the emergency departments of a district general hospital and a sports injuries clinic. Br J Sports Med 35(6):445, 2001.
32. Yuen, MC, Sim, SW, Lam, HS, and Tung, WK: Validation of the Ottawa ankle rules in a Hong Kong ED. Am J Emerg Med 19(5):429, 2001.
33. Kerr, D, Bradshaw, L, and Kelly, AM: Implementation of the Canadian C-spine rule reduces cervical spine x-ray rate for alert patients with potential neck injury. J Emerg Med 28(2):127, 2005.
34. Seaberg, DC, et al: Multicenter comparison of two clinical decision rules for the use of radiography in acute, high-risk knee injuries. Ann Emerg Med 32:8, 1998.
35. Tandeter, HB, et al: Acute knee injuries: Use of decision rules for selective radiograph ordering. Am Fam Physician 60:2599, 1999.
36. Bauer, SJ, et al: A clinical decision rule in the evaluation of acute knee injuries. J Emerg Med 13:611, 1995.
37. Stiell, I, et al: Prospective validation of a decision rule for the use of radiography in acute knee injuries. JAMA 275(8):611, 1996.
38. Stiell, I, et al: Decision rules for the use of radiography in acute ankle injuries: refinement and prospective validation. JAMA 269(9):1127–1132, 1993.
39. Stiell, I, et al: Implementation of the Ottawa ankle rules. JAMA 271(11):827, 1994.
40. Dissmann, PD, and Han, KH: The tuning fork test—A useful tool for improving specificity in "Ottawa positive" patients after ankle inversion injury. Emerg Med J 23:788, 2006.
41. Eggli, S, et al: The Bernese ankle rules: A fast, reliable test after low-energy, supination-type malleolar and midfoot trauma. J Trauma 59(5):1268, 2005.
42. Stiell, I, et al: The Canadian C-spine rule for radiography in alert and stable trauma patients. JAMA 286(15):1841, 2001.
43. Hoffman, JR, et al: Validity of a set of clinical criteria to rule out injury to the cervical spine in patients with blunt trauma. National Emergency X-Radiography Utilization Study Group. N Engl J Med 343(2):94, 2000.
44. Demmerle, C, and Glaudermanns, J: Diagnostic Imaging/Spending Trends and the Increasing Use of Appropriateness Criteria and Accreditation. Avalere Health, Washington, DC, July 2008.
45. American College of Radiology: Musculoskeletal Imaging ACR Appropriateness Criteria. Accessed October 23, 2009 at http://www.acr.org/ SecondaryMainMenuCategories/quality_safety/app_criteria/pdf/Expert PanelonMusculoskeletalImaging.aspx.
46. Acute Low Back Problems Guideline Panel: Acute low back problems in adults: Assessment and treatment. Am Fam Physician 51:469, 1995.
47. Staiger, T, et al: Imaging studies for acute low back pain: When and when not to order them. Imaging 105:161, 1999.
48. Bigos, SJ: Acute low back problems in adults. ACHPR publication no. 95–0642. U.S. Department of Health and Human Services, Public Health Service, Agency for Health Care Policy and Research; Clinical Practice Guidelines no. 14. Rockville, MD, 1994.
49. Jarvik, JG, and Deyo, RA: Diagnostic evaluation of low back pain with emphasis on imaging. Ann Intern Med 137:586, 2002.

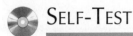 SELF-TEST

1. Why is it important that physical therapists functioning in direct access roles have access to diagnostic imaging?

2. Describe how the information obtained from imaging studies should best be used in the diagnostic process.

3. Name three published decision-making guidelines, sometimes referred to as *clinical decision rules*, that were developed to help clinicians decide when to order radiographic studies.

4. Identify three different pieces of information for which a physical therapist may look for when using a patient's imaging studies to help design an intervention plan.

5. Why should diagnostic imaging modalities never be used in isolation to make a diagnosis?

6. True or false: Conventional radiography is recommended for most patients with acute low back pain (present fewer than 4 weeks).

ANSWERS TO SELF-TEST QUESTIONS

CHAPTER 1

Radiograph A

1. Low contrast is present, as there is little variation between the soft tissue and bone radiographic densities.

2. This is a chest film, as the low contrast makes the soft tissues of the lungs and heart more visible.

3. Yes. The film is positioned correctly for viewing the patient in anatomic position. The shadow of the heart to the patient's left side verifies this.

Radiograph B

4. No. The film is *not* being viewed as if the patient is in anatomic position. The shadow of the heart should appear to the patient's left.

5. The small oval-shaped area of increased density is likely to be of metallic composition, as can be inferred by its solid white radiographic density.

6. No. Without a lateral projection made at right angles to this AP projection, the depth of the location of the foreign object in the body cannot be determined. The object could represent a bullet lodged in a thoracic vertebra, or it could just as well represent a harmless medallion on a necklace resting on the skin.

Radiograph C

7. A barium contrast study of the gastrointestinal tract.

8. The technician forgot to have the patient empty his pockets. Fortunately, the area of interest was not obscured by the metallic key, so a repeat study was not necessary.

Radiograph D

9. A cat.

10. The cat swallowed its owner's pierced earring! The missing jewelry is visualized in the cat's stomach. Note that because of the small part-thickness of this animal, technical adjustments in mAs and kVp are necessary to produce a radiograph that demonstrates bony anatomy as well as the soft tissue anatomy. The heart, liver, stomach, and intestines are easily identifiable.

CHAPTER 2

Radiograph A

1. AP projection of the right femur.

2. The bone density of the distal femoral shaft is abnormally uneven. There is loss of a distinct cortical shell and

no interface between the cortex and the medullary canal. The external architecture of the distal shaft is also uneven and deformed. These gross changes in mineralization are indications of a pathological state.

3. No. The upper half of the femoral shaft and the pelvis do not show the bony changes as listed in answer 2. However, the neck of the femur does exhibit osteopenia and thinned cortical margins. This could be related to disuse atrophy.

4. No. The evidence of previous surgical intervention is revealed by the regularly spaced radiolucent lines representing the removal of sideplate fixation screws.

5. No. The hip joint space is decreased, a radiographic sign of degenerative joint disease.

Radiograph B

6. AP projection of the right distal femur.

7. See answer 2.

8. Neoplasm. The most obvious reason is that the pathology has not crossed the joint space. Tumors may extend to the margin of the joint but do not cross the joint space. Infections and inflammatory processes usually involve the joint space and both articulating surfaces.

CHAPTER 3

1. A lateral projection and an AP projection of the left lower leg.

2. The fracture is located at the midshaft of the tibia.

3. The fracture is complete because the fracture line extends through all of the cortex of the shaft.

4. The distal fragment is displaced laterally and anteriorly. There is minimal angulation, and some overriding of the fragments is present.

5. The fracture line is transverse with comminution.

CHAPTER 4

Image A

1. The structures marked are (1) psoas major, (2) iliacus, (3) gluteus medius, and (4) multifidus.

2. The joint marked (5) is the L5/S1 facet joint. The "joint" marked (6) is a fracture through the pars interarticularis; this 19-year-old male has bilateral spondylolysis at L5. This phenomenon, so well displayed with CT, is referred to as the "double facet" sign.

3. The upper image is more caudal by the following: (1) The psoas major muscle is further from the vertebral body. (2) The vertebral body has a triangular shape, making it the S1 body. (3) The iliacus and gluteus medius muscles are thicker, while the multifidus is smaller.

Image B

4. The numbered structures are (1) coracobrachialis, (2) anterior deltoid, (3) lesser tuberosity, (4) bicipital groove, (5) greater tuberosity, (6) posterior deltoid, (7) glenoid, and (8) subscapularis.

5. The anterior part of the head of the humerus is relatively radiolucent. There is a distinct border between the healthy and the diseased part of the bone, pointing to a benign process. This 21-year-old male has chondroblastoma, a benign cartilaginous tumor that primarily affects the epiphyses of long bones in young patients.

CHAPTER 5

Image A

1. All intervertebral disks show some degree of abnormality. There is decreased signal intensity and horizontal bands of fibrous tissue ("nuclear clefts") extending through the nucleus. The disk height at L5/S1 is decreased and there is no nuclear signal within the disk. At that level, there is a large, extruded herniation (3) that occupies two-thirds of the spinal canal.

2. All vertebral end plates show some abnormality. At the T12–L1, L1–L2, and L2–L3 spaces there are intervertebral herniations through both the inferior and superior endplates. Not the irregularity of the superior endplate at L5–S1.

3. This is a fluid-filled lesion. Note that it is only bright on T2, which rules out hemangioma, which normally shows slightly increased signal intensity on T1 as well.

4. This represents type II degenerative vertebral body marrow changes (Modic, MT, and Ross, JS: Lumbar degenerative disk disease. Radiology 245:43, 2007). These changes, associated with disk disruption, manifest as increased signal intensity both on T1 and T2, since they both have increased fluid and lipid content.

Image B

5. The structures are (1) subcutaneous fat, (2) quadriceps tendon, (3) fat folds in the superior recess (previously visualized on ultrasound, which could not distinguish the nature of this abnormality), (4) biceps femoris muscle, (5) cartilage of lateral femoral condyle, (6) cortex, (7) infrapatellar fat pad, (8) posterior horn of lateral meniscus, (9) tibia, and (10) superior tibio-fibular joint.

6. The signal characteristics are (1), (3), and (7) fat is bright on T1 and dark on T2; (2) tendons are dark on all sequences; (4) muscles are light gray on T1 and dark gray on T2; (5) and (10) cartilage is light gray on T1 and dark gray on T2; (6) the bony cortex is dark on all sequences; (8) healthy menisci are dark on all sequences; (9) cancellous bone is bright on T1 and dark on T2.

CHAPTER 6

Image A

1. The structures are (1) skin, (2) subcutaneous fat, (3) Achilles tendon, (4) soleus muscle, (5) flexor hallucis longus muscle, (6) fascia, (7) cortex of tiba, and (8) posterior malleolus of tibia.

2. Keep in mind the acoustic properties of various tissues, as well as how these properties are affected by reflection at the interfaces of different tissues. (1) Skin is relatively hyperechoic; (2) fat is hypoechoic; (3) tendons are best identified by hyperechoic superficial and deep margins and a distinct parallel fiber pattern; (4) and (5) muscles are hyperechoic relative to fat with parallel hyperechoic bands (not as regular as that of tendons); (6) fasciae (intramuscular or intermuscular) is hyperechoic relative to muscle; (7) cortex forms a regular hyperechoic line; and (8) bone, deep to the cortex, is hypoechoic or anechoic.

Image B

3. The middle image shows effusion in the suprapatellar recess (*a*) and a partial tear of the articular surface of the quadriceps tendon (*b*). The transverse sonogram on the right shows echogenic exostoses (*c*), probably resulting from inflammatory enthesopathy. Note how these rise above the cortical outline of the patella (2) and cast an acoustic shadow.

CHAPTER 7

Radiograph A

1. Lateral view of the cervical spine.

2. Grossly normal vertebral structures with irregularites of the anterior borders of C5 and C6; note anterior and posterior osteophytes at the vertebral endplates.

3. C5–C6 and C6–C7 disk spaces show diminished height.

4. Decreased disk space height with sclerosis and osteophytes (spondylosis) at the vertebral endplates.

Radiograph B

5. Oblique view of the cervical spine.

6. The intervertebral foramina.

Radiograph C

7. Lateral view of the cervical spine.

8. Disk space narrowing and spondylosis is evident at all cervical segments.

Radiograph D

9. Oblique view of the cervical spine.

10. C4–C5 foramen appears the most constricted; thus the C5 nerve root is vulnerable to compression.

Comparing both patients

11. Patient C/D has greater degrees of degenerative changes at more levels, and this would seem to implicate patient C/D as having greater loss of range of motion. However, remember that the degree of joint degeneration seen radiographically does not always correlate with clinical findings. Other factors, such as soft tissue or mechanical

joint dysfunction, can restrict or alter joint motion either acutely or chronically. Patient A/B may just as well have greater restricted range of motion. The correct answer is that it is not possible to determine based on radiographic evidence alone.

CHAPTER 8

Image A

1. (a) external auditory meatus, (b) condyle mandibular fossa, (c) articular eminence, (d) mandibular fossa, (e) petrous line.

2. Figure 1 shows an abnormally placed condyle; the condyle is situated high in the fossa and against the posterior wall of the fossa. Figure 2 shows a hypermobile condyle, that has translated past the slope of the eminence.

Image B

3. The atlas is rotated to the left, as evidenced by the wider radiolucent space on the left between atlas and dens.

4. The axis is rotated to the right, as seen by the fact that its spinous process is to the left of a midline drawn through the dens.

5. The atlas is side-bent to the right. You can either compare the inferior borders of the lateral masses of the atlas, or draw horizontal lines through the transverse processes.

CHAPTER 9

Radiograph A

1. This is an AP projection of the posterior left ribs, below the diaphragm.

2. The symmetrical position of the spinous processes between the equally spaced pedicles of the thoracic vertebrae tells you that this is not a lateral or oblique view. The image of the pairs of ribs attaching to the vertebrae shows that they are posterior ribs, and, because they must be closest to the image receptor to be so well visualized, this must be an AP projection. (If this were a PA projection, the costocartilaginous portions of the anterior rib cage closest to the film plate would image much differently.) The left-side ribs of the patient are being evaluated, which is obvious by the area exposed by the central ray. That they are below the diaphragm is known because you can see the lumbar spine (possessing no rib attachments) and can then identify the lower thoracic vertebrae and ribs by number. Ribs 8 through 12 are well demonstrated.

Radiograph B

3. AP projection of the thoracic spine.

4. All thoracic vertebrae, T1–T12, are visible. The attachment of the first ribs is also visible at T1. L1 and L2 of the lumbar spine are visible. They are identified by their lack of rib attachments. (Note, however, that this is not always foolproof. T12 may lack ribs, or L1 may have ribs.)

5. A right major thoracic curve is present, seen in the long right-side convexity extending from T1 to T12 or L1.

6. Without viewing the entire lumbar spine, it cannot be said whether a secondary or minor compensatory curve exists in the lumbar spine. (Likewise, identifying a compensatory curve above the thoracic curve requires cervical spine films.)

7. Erect AP lateral flexion projections of the entire spinal column, taken at the end ranges of side-bending right and side-bending left, would reveal the amount of flexibility present.

CHAPTER 10

Image A

1. PA.

2. An implanted defibrillator or pacemaker with a lead into the heart is seen in the left upper chest. Two electrodes are seen in the upper outer borders of the chest.

3. The width of the heart far exceeds the normal "50% the width of the chest" cardiothoracic ratio estimate.

4. Cardiomegaly.

5. Pleural effusion.

6. Congestive heart failure.

Image B

7. PA.

8. The heart width is far less than 50% the width of the chest.

9. The mediastinum appears narrowed, and the vessels appear pulled downward.

10. The lung fields appear abnormally dark, or hyperinflated.

11. The diaphragm is depressed and the domes are flattened as well as scalloped on the left.

12. There is airspace between the heart and the diaphragm, because the diaphragm is depressed due to increased volume in the lungs.

13. A chronic obstructive pulmonary disease has all of the above characteristics.

CHAPTER 11

Radiograph A

1. This is a lateral projection of the lumbar spine.

2. The L4–L5 and L5–S1 disk spaces are narrowed.

3. L5. If you trace lines along the anterior and posterior vertebral bodies, you will find that L5 disrupts the continuity of these two curving parallel lines with a sharp step-off.

4. There appears to be a retrolisthesis of L5.

5. Osteophyte or spur formation is present along the margins of the anterior vertebral bodies. Spondylosis deformans describes the condition whereby anterior protrusion of the intervertebral disk nucleus elevates the anterior longitudinal ligament and leads to spur formation. *Traction spurs* is the term used to denote spur formation caused by tension at the sites of attachment of the anterior longitudinal ligament on the vertebral bodies. Note the different configurations of the spurs. At T12–L1, the clawlike spurs have bridged together. At L3, a clawlike spur is present on the inferior margin, and a sharp spur is present on the

superior margin. Some authors believe that the claw-type spurs are related to disk degeneration, whereas the sharp-type spurs are related to traction.

Radiograph B

6. This is a lateral projection of the lumbosacral junction, or an L5–S1 spot film.

7. An abnormal fusion is present between the bodies of L4 and L5, noted by the lack of an intervertebral disk space and by the malformation of the diameter of the bodies. This congenital anomaly is known as a block vertebra. Because of lack of motion at this segment, compensatory excessive motion may be present at adjacent segments, possibly accelerating degenerative joint changes. Another consequence of this anomaly is that the bodies may have developed asymmetrically and contributed to a scoliosis. Additional films are necessary to visualize the anomaly fully.

Chapter 12

Radiograph A

1. This is an AP projection of the pelvis.

2. The heart-shaped pelvic inlet is generally attributed to men; however, the wide flared expanse of the greater pelvis is generally attributed to women. The angle of the pubic arch is not visible, nor is the soft tissue outline of the genitalia. Therefore, because of individual variations, it is not possible to determine the sex of the patient by this film.

Radiograph B

3. The bilateral hip joint spaces exhibit severe concentric narrowing. Some regions appear to be bone on bone.

4. The femoral heads have migrated superiorly and medially into the acetabulum. This can also be described as axial migration.

5. *Acetabular protrusion* (or *protrusio acetabuli*) is the term that denotes the outpouching of the medial wall of the acetabulum in response to axial migration of the femoral head.

6. Both processes are evident. Signs present that are characteristics of rheumatoid arthritis include the bilateral, symmetrical involvement of the joints, the concentric joint space narrowing, and the acetabular protrusion. Signs present that are characteristics of degenerative joint disease include sclerotic repair and spur formation. Both processes can exist simultaneously; degenerative processes can proceed while the joints are in a remission from rheumatoid arthritis.

Chapter 13

Radiographs A, B, and C

1. A, intercondylar notch or tunnel view of the knee; B, lateral view of the knee; C, tangential view of the patellofemoral joint.

2. The object lies within the joint capsule. The location of the object cannot be determined by the AP view alone.

From the lateral view it is obvious the object is not anterior or posterior to the joint; it is thus being obscured within the joint.

3. One possibility is an osteochondral fragment.

4. The medial compartment and the patellofemoral compartment show mild degenerative changes.

5. Degenerative changes present include subchondral sclerosis and joint space narrowing.

Chapter 14

Radiograph A

1. This is an AP or dorsoplanar projection of the foot.

2. Hallux valgus. This term describes a condition whereby the first metatarsal is deviated medially and the first phalanx is deviated laterally.

3. A bony exostosis, or bunion, is present on the medial aspect of the metatarsal head.

4. The great toe and second toe are crossed over each other.

Radiograph B

5. This is an AP projection of the bilateral ankles.

6. There appears to be gross inversion and pronation of the ankles and feet, although complete collapse of normal bony architecture would also describe this deformity. Bilaterally, the joints of the ankle, hindfoot, and midfoot appear to be fused. This severe condition represents the burned-out stage of rheumatoid arthritis.

Chapter 15

Radiograph A

1. This is an AP projection of the left shoulder.

2. Abnormal findings include the following: the humeral head has been completely resorbed and the surgical neck has migrated superiorly into the joint space; no lytic lesions are present in the humerus but demineralization is evident; the minimal soft tissue shadows indicate gross muscle wasting.

Radiograph B

3. This is an AP projection of the right shoulder.

4. The acromioclavicular joint is stabilized via internal fixation.

Radiograph C

5. This is an AP projection of the left shoulder.

6. A severely comminuted fracture pattern is present.

7. A gunshot wound or any other high-velocity trauma that would leave the telltale metal shards, as seen on this film.

Chapter 16

Radiographs A, B, and C

1. All three are AP projections of the left elbow.

2. A, 10-year-old; B, 30-year-old; C, 5-year-old.

3. The presence of open epiphyseal plates tells you that patients A and C are the children. The younger child is determined by noting the smaller size and thus earlier stage of development of the epiphyses, especially the epiphyses for the radial head and medial epicondyle, which have just begun ossification.

CHAPTER 17

Radiograph A

1. This is a PA or dorsoplanar projection of the hand.

2. The trapezium has been resected.

3. A metallic device is visible at the trapezoid. This Mytex suture anchor secures the soft tissue to bone. (This procedure has been dubbed the *anchovy* procedure, because the palmaris longus is coiled into the resected space like anchovies packed in a can.)

Radiograph B

4. This is a PA or dorsoplanar projection of the wrist.

5. The soft tissues present at this location are the tendons and muscles of the extensor pollicis brevis and the abductor pollicis longus.

6. Tenosynovitis of the first dorsal compartment of the wrist, also known as DeQuervain's disease.

Radiograph C

7. This is a PA or dorsoplanar projection of the hand.

8. Abnormal findings include resorption or malformation of the distal radius, distal ulna, and distal phalanges of all the digits. Additionally there are irregularities in the density of all the bones. The shafts of the phalanges are sclerotic while the proximal ends of each phalanx are demineralized. There also is rarefaction of the metacarpal heads. The trabeculae of the carpals appear sparse and distinct. This young adult had been diagnosed years earlier with osteogenesis imperfecta.

CHAPTER 18

1. Diagnostic imaging generates information the patient interview and physical examination cannot. Access to imaging is critical for primary care practitioners to screen for serious pathology and confirm diagnoses such as fractures and ligament tears.

2. Diagnostic imaging should always be used to test hypotheses generated through the patient interview and physical examination. Imaging should be ordered only when the results will have an impact on patient management.

3. Pittsburgh decision rules (knee), Ottawa knee rules, Ottawa ankle rules (including ankle and foot), Canadian C-spine rule (cervical trauma).

4. Examples include assessment of bony alignment, identification of bony blocks to movement, visualizing the exact location of fractures, identifying the exact location of orthopedic fixation devices, and assessing bone healing to make decisions about movement and weight bearing.

5. Although diagnostic imaging modalities are excellent for visualizing a patient's tissues, pathology can be missed due to inadequate sensitivity of the test or errors in reading the images. Also, findings from diagnostic imaging may not correlate with the patient's overall clinical picture.

6. False. According to guidelines from the Agency for Health Care Policy and Research, most patients with acute low back pain will experience symptom resolution with conservative management within 4 weeks. So, in the absence of red flags for serious pathology, imaging is not necessary.

INDEX

G